Creating a Lifestyle Medicine (

Jeffrey I. Mechanick • Robert F. Kushner

Editors

Creating a Lifestyle Medicine Center

From Concept to Clinical Practice

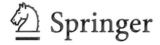 Springer

Editors
Jeffrey I. Mechanick
The Marie-Josée and Henry R. Kravis Center for
Cardiovascular Health at Mount Sinai Heart, and
the Division of Endocrinology, Diabetes and Bone
Disease
Icahn School of Medicine at Mount Sinai
New York, NY
USA

Robert F. Kushner
Departments of Medicine and Medical Education
Northwestern University
Chicago, IL
USA

ISBN 978-3-030-48090-5   ISBN 978-3-030-48088-2   (eBook)
https://doi.org/10.1007/978-3-030-48088-2

This Springer imprint is published by the registered company Springer Nature Switzerland AG
The registered company address is: Gewerbestrasse 11, 6330 Cham, Switzerland

We wish to thank our friends and colleagues at the Kravis Center for Cardiovascular Health at Mount Sinai Heart and Northwestern Medicine Center for Lifestyle Medicine who share our passion and commitment to providing exceptional care, our patients who teach us how to be better doctors, and our families who keep us grounded.

– JM and RK

Foreword

Cardiovascular disease is the number one cause of mortality worldwide and impels the coordinated quest for scientifically valid strategies, along with safe and effective actions. Unfortunately, humans have had to bear witness to the many false starts, misdirections, and premature conclusions to what have been regarded as best laid plans. Where are the failings? What are we doing wrong inasmuch as epidemiological evidence continues to demonstrate worsening of cardiovascular disease and prevalence rates of modifiable risk factors in certain populations?

My lifelong aspiration is to better understand not only the nature of human disease, but more importantly the nature of human health. It is the purpose of our healthcare system to optimize human health for all people, taking into account pathophysiology and diversity. The framework I have structured and formally detailed [1] focuses on prevention. In a nutshell, rather than the conventional way of waiting for disease to take root and cause harm before any meaningful intervention is performed, a diligent process of screening, case finding, and intervention to abrogate or mitigate the disease process, in a manner that improves health, is implemented. At first, this may be on a small scale, but the ultimate goal is far-reaching, grounded in science, with demonstrable wellness for individuals and populations.

There are six dimensions to this plan. First, we focus on the eight behavioral aspects of cardiometabolic prevention: healthy eating, healthy weight and body composition, healthy glucose levels, healthy blood pressure, healthy cholesterol levels, plenty of physical activity, avoidance of tobacco products, and psychological health. Second, the term "health" is classified as poor, intermediate, and ideal for the purposes of study and messaging. Third, there must be a global scope that involves people of all ethnicities, cultures, and ways of living. Fourth, mitigation strategies are included for other chronic diseases, such as cancer and degenerative disease prevention. Fifth, there are important roles of technology, economics, education, quality of life, and behavior that must be considered and leveraged for best outcomes. And sixth, prevention programs must be implemented early and in a sustainable fashion; this means targeting our children and creating an infrastructure that works over a relatively long timeframe.

It is this last dimension that has proven to be the most challenging, yet most intriguing and rewarding when one devotes energy and thoughtfulness to the problem. The FAMILIA Trial, published last year, was a cluster-randomized controlled study of 562 children aged 3–5 years, demonstrating that a multidimensional school-based educational intervention strategy (a form of primordial prevention) can improve healthy behaviors in a diverse, socioeconomically disadvantaged community [2]. No doubt, this model will need to be scaled up and validated in different settings—but here is the rub. How do we actually build physical structures with successful operations and management to truly realize superior outcomes on a scale that durably transforms healthcare? This is the practice gap that has been so elusive over the years and must be closed in the lifestyle medicine space so that scientifically sound strategies can result in a pervasive elevation of health.

This book by my colleagues, Drs. Jeffrey Mechanick and Robert Kushner, succeeds in providing the blueprint for closing this practice gap. This book builds on the concepts, theory, and science of lifestyle medicine in their first book, and now provides not only the broad strokes on what a Lifestyle Medicine Center is, but also the details for how to imagine, build, and operate this enterprise in a host of settings. Challenges, examples, and technical factors are all discussed in a way that captures interest and spurs on action. My dream is to improve health for all people at all points in the lifecycle. A book on implementation fills the gap to enable me, and you, to realize this shared dream.

References

1. Turco J, Inal-Veith A, Fuster V. Cardiovascular health promotion. J Am Coll Cardiol. 2018;72:908–13.
2. Fernandez-Jimenez R, Jaslow R, Bansilal S, et al. Child health promotion in underserved communities: the FAMILIA Trial. J Am Coll Cardiol. 2019;73:2011–21.

Valentin Fuster
Physician-in-Chief, The Mount Sinai Hospital
Director, Mount Sinai Heart
New York, NY, USA

Preface

Lifestyle medicine is a discipline that is growing in popularity for three reasons. First, there are more scientific studies supporting the role of structured lifestyle change, benefits of healthy behaviors, and positive impact of individual lifestyle components on nearly every chronic disease state examined. Second, lifestyle medicine can be clinically delivered in the outpatient setting to produce these benefits for the patient. Third, educational programs have promulgated the message of lifestyle medicine to healthcare professionals, other stakeholders, and the general public. The net effect of these three drivers is the transformation of how we think about and deliver healthcare. This is a much-needed event, given the confused medical economic climate, growing nature of healthcare inequities in society, and unfortunate disenchantment of many workers in the medical profession.

Yet, a gap exists between the enthusiasm for lifestyle medicine and its implementation. Despite all the accumulated scientific evidence in the lifestyle medicine literature, the increasing expertise and experience acquired by students of lifestyle medicine, and the overt successes resulting from the instances where lifestyle medicine is practiced, there is still a lack of large-scale, pervasive use of this new discipline. The clinical demand to deliver lifestyle medicine programs is overwhelming based on the rarity of good health practices among Americans and the very small percentage of patients (<5%) who are completely free of modifiable chronic disease risks. The benefits of providing lifestyle medicine lie in prevention, abrogation, or mitigation of the risks for or progression of chronic disease. As a result, it is anticipated that healthcare expenditures would be reduced, quality of life improved, and end-of-life morbidity compressed.

In 2016, we co-edited *Lifestyle Medicine: A Manual for Clinical Practice* to provide a corpus of information about the burgeoning lifestyle medicine field. In this book, pertinent elements of lifestyle medicine were discussed within a comprehensive framework. This was intended to empower the reader to embark on a journey that included lifestyle medicine in his or her own clinical practice. A couple of years later, we realized that in order to successfully realize the larger-scale practice of lifestyle medicine, a follow-up book was needed to provide the pragmatic tools to actually build a Lifestyle Medicine Center.

Our companion book, *Creating a Lifestyle Medicine Center: From Concept to Clinical Practice*, is divided into three sections, with introductory chapters establishing the rationale, middle chapters expounding on the details, and end chapters providing real-world examples. Each of the chapters is based on scientific evidence and written by experts in the field by their own right. Editing by us was focused on delivering a particular message that fit squarely within the implementation tactic: planning, building, and managing a successful and sustainable Lifestyle Medicine Center.

Once again, we thank our colleagues at Springer, namely Kristopher Spring, Megan Ruzomberka, and Michael Griffin, for making this process streamlined and rewarding. Our families have endured yet again with another book and we thank them for their support and encouragement. We also thank you, our readers, for the wonderful feedback, and our colleagues and contributors, from whom we learn far more than we could ever teach.

New York, NY, USA   Jeffrey I. Mechanick
Chicago, IL, USA   Robert F. Kushner

Contents

Contributors

Prajakta Adsul, MBBS, MPH, MPH Department of Internal Medicine, University of New Mexico, Albuquerque, NM, USA

Mohamed Al-Kazaz, MD, FACC Icahn School of Medicine at Mount Sinai, Department of Cardiology, New York, NY, USA

Patricia P. Araujo, RD Northwestern Medicine, Center for Lifestyle Medicine, Chicago, IL, USA

Marc Braman, MD, MPH Lifestyle Medicine Pro, LLC, Salem, OR, USA

David A. Chambers, DPhil Division of Cancer Control and Population Sciences, National Cancer Institute, Rockville, MD, USA

Zorina Costello, DMin, MS Center for Spirituality and Health, Mount Sinai Health System, Icahn School of Medicine, New York, NY, USA

Robert L. Crocker, MD Director, Strategic Clinical Planning and Implementation, Andrew Weil Center for Integrative Medicine, Clinical Assistant Professor of Medicine, College of Medicine, University of Arizona, Tucson, AZ, USA

Catherine L. Davis, PhD Georgia Prevention Institute, Department of Medicine, Medical College of Georgia at Augusta University, Augusta, GA, USA

Bethany Doerfler, MS, RDN Northwestern Medicine, Digestive Health Center, Chicago, IL, USA

Zach Seth Dovey, BSc, MRCP, FRCS (Urol) Department of Urology, Icahn School of Medicine at Mount Sinai, New York, NY, USA

Altaf Engineer, PhD, March, BArch University of Arizona CAPLA, School of Architecture and UA Institute on Place, Wellbeing, and Performance, Tucson, AZ, USA

Anne Findeis, MS, RN (Retired), Patient Education Department, Northwestern Memorial Hospital, Chicago, IL, USA

Yoni Freedhoff, MD Department of Family Medicine, University of Ottawa, Bariatric Medical Institute, Ottawa, ON, Canada

Juan P. González-Rivas, MD International Clinical Research Center, St Anne's University Hospital, Brno, Czech Republic

Harvard TH Chan School of Public Health, Harvard University, Boston, MA, USA

Foundation for Clinical, Public Health, and Epidemiological Research of Venezuela (FISPEVEN), Caracas, Venezuela

Sherri Sheinfeld Gorin, PhD, FSBM The University of Michigan, Department of Family Medicine, Ann Arbor, MI, USA

Henry, MPH Mount Sinai Hospital, Population Health Science & Policy, New
York, NY, USA

Holly R. Herrington, MS, RD, CDE Northwestern Memorial Hospital, Center for Lifestyle
Medicine, Chicago, IL, USA

Janet H. Johnson, DNP, APRN-BC, CDE, FAANP The Mount Sinai Hospital, Marie-Josée
and Henry R. Kravis Center for Cardiovascular Health at Mount Sinai, New York, NY, USA

Scott Kahan, MD, MPH National Center for Weight and Wellness; Faculty, Department of
Health Policy & Administration, Johns Hopkins Bloomberg School of Public Health,
Washington, DC, USA

Robert F. Kushner, MD, MS Departments of Medicine and Medical Education, Northwestern
University, Chicago, IL, USA

Simin Liu, MD, ScD Center for Global Cardiometabolic Health, Brown University,
Epidemiology, Medicine and Surgery, Providence, RI, USA

Kenneth Lo, PhD Center for Global Cardiometabolic Health, Brown University,
Epidemiology, Medicine and Surgery, Providence, RI, USA

Deborah B. Marin, MD Center for Spirituality and Health, Icahn School of Medicine at
Mount Sinai, New York, NY, USA

Mark P. Mattson, PhD Department of Neuroscience, Johns Hopkins University School of
Medicine, Baltimore, MD, USA

Edwin McDonald, IV, MD University of Chicago Medicine, Section of Gastroenterology,
Hepatology, and Nutrition, Chicago, IL, USA

Mary Ann McLaughlin, MD, MPH, FACC Icahn School of Medicine at Mount Sinai,
New York, NY, USA

Marie-Josee and Henry R. Kravis Center for Cardiovascular Health at Mount Sinai Heart,
New York, NY, USA

Jeffrey I. Mechanick, MD The Marie-Josée and Henry R. Kravis Center for Cardiovascular
Health at Mount Sinai Heart, and the Division of Endocrinology, Diabetes and Bone Disease,
Icahn School of Medicine at Mount Sinai, New York, NY, USA

David Meltzer, MD, PhD University of Chicago Medicine, Department of Medicine, Section
of Hospital Medicine, Chicago, IL, USA

Karl Nadolsky, DO Michigan State University College of Human Medicine, Spectrum
Health Medical Group, Department of Diabetes & Endocrinology, Grand Rapids, MI, USA

Spencer Nadolsky, DO, BA UCSD, Preventive Medicine, Family Medicine, San Diego, CA,
USA

Ramfis Nieto-Martínez, MD, MSc LifeDoc Health, Memphis, TN, USA

Harvard TH Chan School of Public Health, Harvard University, Boston, MA, USA

Foundation for Clinical, Public Health, and Epidemiological Research of Venezuela
(FISPEVEN), Caracas, Venezuela

April Oh, PhD, MPH Division of Cancer Control and Population Sciences, National Cancer
Institute, Rockville, MD, USA

Norma A. Padrón, MA, MPH, PhD American Hospital Association, Center for Health
Innovation, Chicago, IL, USA

Magdalyn Patyk, MS, RN, BC Patient Education Department, Northwestern Memorial Hospital, Chicago, IL, USA

Lilian G. Perez, PhD, MPH Behavioral and Policy Sciences Department, RAND Corporation, Santa Monica, CA, USA

Emily Perish, MPP University of Chicago Medicine, Department of Medicine, Section of Hospital Medicine, Chicago, IL, USA

Joe Raphael, DrPH, MBA, MA, LMFT, CHES Lifestyle Medicine Pro, LLC, Salem, OR, USA

James M. Rippe, MD Rippe Lifestyle Institute, Shrewsbury, MA, USA

Vanshdeep Sharma, MD Center for Spirituality and Health, Mount Sinai Hospital, Department of Psychiatry, New York, NY, USA

Ash K. Tewari, MD Department of Urology, Icahn School of Medicine at Mount Sinai, New York, NY, USA

Frank Vera, MS Marie-Josee and Henry R. Kravis Center for Cardiovascular Health at Mount Sinai Heart, New York, NY, USA

John B. Wetmore, BA Icahn School of Medicine at Mount Sinai, Population Health and Health Policy, New York, NY, USA

Shan Zhao, MD, PhD Department of Anesthesiology, Icahn School of Medicine at Mount Sinai, New York, NY, USA

Daniel K. Zismer, PhD Professor Emeritus and Chair, Division of Health Policy and Management, School of Public Health, University of Minnesota, Minneapolis, MN, USA

Co-Chair and Chief Executive Officer, Associated Eye Care Partners, LLC, Stillwater, MN, USA

Statement of Purpose

Jeffrey I. Mechanick and Robert F. Kushner

Introduction

In 2016, *Lifestyle Medicine: A Manual for Clinical Practice* was published [1], ushering in another scientifically based perspective of nonpharmacological and nonsurgical/nonprocedural strategies to manage chronic disease. The rapid expansion of interest in this new medical specialty parallels the increased burden of chronic disease in the USA and globally. Lifestyle medicine comprises direct and indirect multiscale effects on health and well-being. If sufficiently pervasive and durable, the ramifications of a new healthcare culture that embraces lifestyle medicine could relieve enormous economic burdens by interrupting the natural progression of disease much earlier on a population scale and by averting high costs of tertiary prevention. Fortunately, the role of a lifestyle medicine approach is becoming more prominent even in the midst of the remarkable progress in and attractiveness of biomedical technology. Indeed, within the context of a preventive care paradigm, every patient encounter should, and ideally must, include some aspect of preventing pathophysiological events that lead to disease progression with the mainstay of intervention being lifestyle change. The components of this argument for the transformative role of lifestyle medicine to create a new culture of healthcare are illustrated in Fig. 1.1.

What are the challenges to lifestyle medicine garnering further traction? First and foremost is to perform high-quality scientific research to substantiate the use of lifestyle medicine. The second challenge is to incorporate lifestyle medicine evidence, not only in written clinical practice guidelines but also in actual clinical practice to achieve optimal health status for individuals and populations, as well as manifest clear benefits for wider recognition. A favorable by-product of increased lifestyle medicine research and practice is the generation of data in electronic health records, registries, and other formats amenable to data mining. The third challenge lies in education and real-life experiential training. Though budding lifestyle medicine programs exist, they are not yet routinely and formally part of our medical education curriculum. Once lifestyle medicine research, clinical practice, and education are operational, they can be leveraged in a dedicated entity or facility – the Lifestyle Medicine Center – to effect change on a larger scale.

Potential strategies for the application of lifestyle medicine have a very far reach, extending from more obvious and high-impact chronic diseases, such as cardiovascular disease and cancer, to those less obvious, such as neurodegenerative, infectious, and inflammatory diseases. Moreover, primordial and primary prevention strategies in those without apparent disease and generally considered as "well" are also part of lifestyle medicine. However, there is a striking gap between theory/strategy and practice/tactics in the lifestyle medicine space, particularly in the extant published literature. It is this vulnerability in the successful evolution of lifestyle medicine that becomes a viable target for improvement. In fact, it is the creation of a *bona fide* Lifestyle Medicine Center or Clinical Service Line that acts as a force multiplier to close this gap and create a new healthcare culture.

J. I. Mechanick (✉)
The Marie-Josée and Henry R. Kravis Center for Cardiovascular Health at Mount Sinai Heart, and the Division of Endocrinology, Diabetes and Bone Disease, Icahn School of Medicine at Mount Sinai, New York, NY, USA
e-mail: jeffrey.mechanick@mountsinai.org

R. F. Kushner
Departments of Medicine and Medical Education, Northwestern University, Chicago, IL, USA
e-mail: rkushner@northwestern.edu

The Strategic Target: Chronic Disease

Lifestyle medicine strategies are discussed and organized by basic principles, tools, and chronic diseases in *Lifestyle Medicine: A Manual for Clinical Practice* (Table 1.1) [1]. The focus in this first book was to provide a scientific basis

© Springer Nature Switzerland AG 2020
J. I. Mechanick, R. F. Kushner (eds.), *Creating a Lifestyle Medicine Center*, https://doi.org/10.1007/978-3-030-48088-2_1

Fig. 1.1 The Lifestyle Medicine Center as a Force Multiplier for Healthcare Change*. (*Force multipliers are tools that can amplify the effects of effort to achieve greater results)

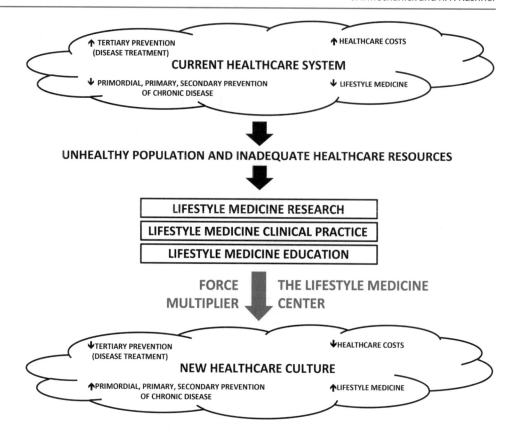

for preventive and therapeutic strategic planning, establishing the foundation for lifestyle medicine actions by the health care professional (HCP). The main components of any lifestyle medicine strategy are as follows:

- Detecting, diagnosing, and then targeting a particular chronic disease problem
- Classifying interventions in terms of preventive care modalities, which can overlap as needed: primordial, primary, secondary, and/or tertiary, with ongoing quaternary prevention that reduces over-medicalization
- Generating a list of evidence-based interventions and then prioritizing in terms of anticipated benefits, risks, and costs
- Taking inventory of accessible resources, timeframes, and metrics prior to actual implementation

As more scientific evidence becomes available with an increasing number of high-quality preclinical studies and clinical trials, strategies, particularly in the form of clinical practice guidelines and algorithms, will become more detailed and amenable to personalization. More specifically, lifestyle medicine interventions will better align with a growing genetic/epigenetic, environmental, and behavioral knowledge base. The question now is how do HCPs translate this knowledge and planning into successful action.

The Tactical Plan: A Lifestyle Medicine Center

Whereas strategy deals with longer-term plans of action and why certain actions should be considered, tactics deal more with implementation, generally over a shorter time frame, and how these actions are applied. Reviewing the evidence and debating the relative risks and benefits can yield a plan, but building an infrastructure to execute many small and concurrent actions – in a safe and effective manner, within resource and cost constraints, and adapting to unexpected obstacles – is a major challenge to lifestyle medicine and the deliverable of improved individual patient- and population-based outcomes. In reality, this challenge primarily focuses on the adverse economics resulting from low reimbursement structures and high expenses [2]. Lifestyle medicine tactics should be explored in terms of research, clinical practice, and education to arrive at a better understanding of the problem, before actually embarking on the technical aspects of building a Center to be discussed in subsequent chapters.

Research

Research publications in the field of lifestyle medicine continue to increase with clear expansion of original clinical trials during the 2010–2014 period, extending to the present period (Table 1.2). This is an illuminating finding as academic

Table 1.1 Summary of topics in *Lifestyle Medicine: A Manual for Clinical Practice*[a]

Section topics	Chapter topics
Basic principles	Why lifestyle medicine
	Healthy living and defining lifestyle medicine
	Communication and behavioral change
	Paradigms of care
	Behavioral factors with weight loss treatment
	Chronic care model and primary care
Tools	Composite risk scores
	Anthropometrics and body composition
	Physical activity measures
	Metabolic profiles
	Healthy eating
	Weight loss programs
	Physical activity programs
	Cognitive-behavioral therapy
	Tobacco cessation programs
	Alcohol use
	Sleep management
	Integrative medicine
	Transcultural applications
	Community engagement
	Lifestyle medicine checklist
Chronic diseases	Obesity
	Diabetes
	Cardiometabolic risk
	Cancer
	Depression
	Chronic pain
	Age-related brain disorders
	Chronic kidney disease
	Non-alcoholic fatty liver disease and steatohepatitis
	Gastrointestinal disease
	Chronic pulmonary disease
	Human immunodeficiency virus infected patients

[a]The first book focused on scientific substantiation in lifestyle medicine and clinical strategies [1]. In contrast, this second book focuses on implementation and building a Lifestyle Medicine Center

Table 1.2 Expanding literature on "lifestyle medicine" in PubMed[a]

	Total citations	Total citation		
Years	(N [%] Clinical Trials)	Growth (%)	Interpretation	
1995–1999	2228 (142 [6.4])	n/a	Initial figures	
2000–2004	4162 (205 [4.9])	86.8	Significant increase in the number of total citations but same percent of clinical trials	
2005–2009	6983 (408 [5.8])	67.8	Mild decrease in the number of total citations but same percent of clinical trials	
2010–2014	10,076 (**1042 [10.3]**)	44.3	Continuous deceleration in the number of total citations and a clear increase in the number and percent of clinical trials	
2015–2019	17,136 (**1843 [10.8]**)	70.1	A **recovered increase in the number of total citations** with consistent percent of clinical trials	

[a]This PubMed search was conducted on December 29, 2019, using the keywords "lifestyle medicine," with inclusive dates as given in column 1, and for humans only. Total citation growth is expressed as percentage increase from one 5-year period to the next. The percent of total citations and number of clinical trials are each presented to differentiate original information from less rigorous clinical studies and reviews. Interpretation of data finds a clear increase (**in bold**) in clinical trials in lifestyle medicine beginning in the 2010–2014 time period

interest has evolved from just writing about lifestyle medicine, outlining problems and need for improvements, to conducting clinical trials and publishing results that can drive an evidence-based clinical practice. There are also many clinical studies in lifestyle medicine that are retrospective, observational, single-arm prospective cohort trials with an intervention, or comparison studies, but with significant methodological flaws. Hence, stronger studies are needed, such as prospective, randomized controlled studies, which are adequately powered, with appropriate comparator groups, representing current standards of care for a true state of clinical equipoise. Studies should determine optimal intensity, duration, and mode of delivery for lifestyle interventions [3]. Ideally, these studies should concentrate on lifestyle medicine care pathways and relevant long-term clinical outcomes, instead of single interventions and surrogate markers.

Lifestyle Medicine Centers play a role in the translation of academic knowledge to clinical practice. This is accomplished on two fronts. First, through a deliberate and diligent process of analyzing and curating research findings, new information can guide adaptations in policies and protocols within a center's operations. For instance, as new data become available demonstrating the efficacy of certain types of strength training in patients of South Asian ancestry to reduce cardiometabolic risk, a Center's medical fitness program can collaborate with HCPs and incorporate these exercises in the comprehensive care plan, as well as develop wearable technologies with apps that provide animation or avatar-based exercise (event) nudges and demonstrations. Second, as a Center matures and has built a registry of clinical data, additional programs can be developed and implemented based on needs. One of these may be a dedicated research program for the Center, where data mining can be performed with the Center's own registry (or the registry could be part of the sponsoring healthcare system). Relevant research questions can be formulated based on the needs of the Center or general needs of the healthcare system. Ultimately, the generation of new information will be used to improve clinical practice.

Clinical Practice

The formal practice of lifestyle medicine has been relatively marginalized from the traditional Western biomedical model of medicine, which emphasizes biological factors to the exclusion of behavioral, social, and environmental factors. With the continued rise in chronic disease prevalence and adverse impact of morbidities, disabilities, and costs, there is a need to transform healthcare and place lifestyle medicine squarely in routine clinical practice [4, 5]. Factors that currently drive interest and action with respect to lifestyle medicine include:

1. New scientific data - these prompt the synthesis of new care pathways and chronic care models that require implementation in order to exert real benefit.
2. Urban infrastructure - this now mandates a healthier population, which can only occur with much earlier intervention to avert chronic diseases and their sequelae.
3. Healthcare - this is much more fragmented and inpatient/outpatient care needs to be better integrated using comprehensive approaches and innovative care models to apply team approaches and tackle a multiplicity of risk factors, not just one risk factor at a time when they present or become symptomatic.
4. Behavioral factors - these are recognized as important drivers of motivation, adherence, and sustainability for successful chronic disease care.

There are also certain unique aspects to practicing lifestyle medicine that have not historically been part of medical education and postgraduate training. These include not only the broad disciplines of nutrition, medical fitness, and behavior but also lesser-known principles about physician personal behaviors, immersive therapeutic environments, and high-touch patient care. In a review by Bodai et al. [5], there is a core need to focus on patient adherence with recommendations to improve healthy eating (77% not adherent), active living (60% not adherent), healthy weight (60% not adherent), and emotional resilience (50% not adherent). There are many new techniques that are based on evidence to assist with messaging healthy lifestyle information and recommendations, such as storytelling to promote self-management [6, 7] or cultural adaptions for different ethnicities [8]. For instance, spontaneous and stimulated laughter, in the setting of professionalism, can improve hemodynamics, pain thresholds, mood, and stress hormones [9].

Although traditional practice models in lifestyle medicine have succeeded (e.g., private practice and free-standing Centers, multispecialty practice, and clinical service lines in sponsoring healthcare systems), innovations in care are also needed (e.g., group visits [10], micropractice community partnerships [11], concierge medicine models [12], and bun-dled services [13]), especially when confronted with inadequate reimbursement structures. The other variables at play are a changing landscape for third-party payers and whether alternative models of payments (e.g., actuarial- or value-based) are beneficial to those practicing lifestyle medicine [14, 15]. Lastly, performance metrics reflect clinical, biochemical, and other biological and behavioral variables, as well as wearable technology outputs, questionnaire responses about how patients are faring long term, and survey data related to the Center (physical attributes and human resources).

Education

Research studies and clinical practice generate new information, both academic and pragmatic, which needs to be taught to contemporary HCPs, as well as next-generation HCPs, to ensure the viability of the lifestyle medicine specialty. There are different formats available for lifestyle education, though many have not been fully developed since this is a young medical specialty. Various professional medical organizations have developed their own programs and resources, which can be accessed through each Society's website. Notably, according to the American College of Preventive Medicine, in partnership with the American College of Lifestyle Medicine, the Lifestyle Medicine Core Competencies program was developed based on five domains:

1. Leadership
2. Knowledge
3. Assessment Skills
4. Management Skills
5. Use of Office and Community Support [16]

In general, medical students receive inadequate training in lifestyle medicine, including healthy eating, physical activity, motivational interviewing, tobacco cessation, and sleep [17, 18]. In 2017, the American Medical Association House of Delegates passed resolution 959, which supports processes that incorporate lifestyle medicine and social determinants of health education in undergraduate, graduate, and continuing medical education [19]. The Lifestyle Medicine Education Collaborative provides undergraduate curricula, faculty and student champion support, influence on policy, and assessments [20, 21]. At Stanford University School of Medicine, a lifestyle medicine course is available to any Stanford university student [22]. A reasonable starting point for medical school deans to transform curricula is the incorporation of evidence-based nutrition [23]. Time constraints are considerable challenges to medical school curricula for the development of comprehensive and complete courses.

One solution would be implementation of active learning resources, or pedagogies, on advanced lifestyle medicine skills that require only a 90-minute block of time [24].

Within postgraduate residency programs, there are efforts to integrate lifestyle medicine into existing curricula (e.g., primary care, family medicine, cardiology, and endocrinology), as well as create dedicated programs for lifestyle medicine (e.g., community-engaged general preventive medicine/public health training with a focus on building health equity [25, 26]). There is even a call-for-action to create a clinical lifestyle medicine specialty fellowship to train physicians in both acute medical care and public health promotion settings to address problems related to chronic disease [27, 28].

In order for lifestyle medicine messaging to be effective, there needs to be consistency with respect to knowledge and experience among HCPs. To this end, lifestyle medicine should be a core curricular component for advanced practice providers, such as physician assistants [29] and nurse practitioners. In another paradigm, undergraduate, medical, and allied health students engage community middle and high school students in interactive lifestyle medicine workshops [30]. As a sign of the times, NextGenU.org, through partnerships with universities and professional organizations, offers free online training in lifestyle medicine (https://nextgenu.org/course/view.php?id=205 [accessed on December 30, 2019]) [31]. A semester-long, web-based lifestyle medicine curriculum was also developed by the Harvard Extension School, though how this activity affects population health remains to be seen [32]. Lastly, there are processes for board certification in the field of lifestyle medicine as with other medical specialties [33].

The Deliverable: A how-to Medical Textbook on Lifestyle Medicine

The purpose of this book is to present information in such a way that the reader can build a Lifestyle Medicine Center. Specifically, the information takes the form of theory, scientific evidence, and experience proffered to support decision-making by individuals, informal groups, or formal committees tasked with building a Lifestyle Medicine Center. Since the definition of lifestyle medicine is inexact, and since the goals of lifestyle medicine HCPs may differ depending on their own backgrounds, target patients, and perceptions of the specialty, the structure and function of one Lifestyle Medicine Center may be vastly different from another. Consequently, the information in this book will combine principles that are common to virtually all Lifestyle Medicine Centers, while also providing principles that may be applicable to one sort or another.

This book is organized into three parts: introductory, conceptual modeling, and case studies. The idea here is to bring all readers up to speed in the first part, which reviews the basic principles of lifestyle medicine and sets the stage for translating knowledge into action. The second part presents in-depth topics that may be new to most readers on specific pragmatic aspects of justifying, building, organizing, and operating a Lifestyle Medicine Center. The third part is critical as it formally presents examples of a broad range of successful Lifestyle Medicine Centers, with the forethought that each reader has their own interpretation of lifestyle medicine, for their own unique setting.

It is clear that there are different models of clinical practice, reflecting the histories and biases of the HCPs, administrators, and support staff that build the facilities. The nature of lifestyle medicine is neither uniform nor static – it is fluid and adaptable to changes in the environment that affect human behavior, healthcare management, and the expression of chronic disease. The deliverable of this second book is not only to provide knowledge but also to systematically and explicitly provide guidance on how to effectively translate that knowledge into real action and undeniable success.

References

1. Mechanick JI, Kushner RF. Lifestyle medicine – a manual for clinical practice. New York: Springer; 2016.
2. Braman M, Edison M. How to create a successful lifestyle medicine practice. Am J Lifestyle Med. 2017;11:404–7.
3. Doughty KN, Del Pilar NX, Audette A, et al. Lifestyle medicine and the management of cardiovascular disease. Curr Cardiol Rep. 2017;19:116. https://doi.org/10.1007/s11886-017-0925-z.
4. Williams MA, Kaminsky LA. Healthy lifestyle medicine in the traditional healthcare environment – primary care and cardiac rehabilitation. Prog Cardiovasc Dis. 2017;59:448–54.
5. Bodai BI, Nakata TE, Wong WT, et al. Lifestyle medicine: a brief review of its dramatic impact on health and survival. Perm J. 2018;22:17–25.
6. Gucciardi E, Jean-Pierre N, Karam G, et al. Designing and delivering facilitated storytelling interventions for chronic disease self-management: a scoping review. BMC Health Serv Res. 2016;16:249. https://doi.org/10.1186/s12913-016-1474-7.
7. Kim YC, Moran MB, Wilkin HA, et al. Integrated connection to neighborhood storytelling network, education, and chronic disease knowledge among African Americans and Latinos in Los Angeles. J Health Commun. 2011;16:393–415.
8. Mechanick JI, Davidson JA, Fergus IV, Galindo RJ, KcKinney KH, Petak SM, Sadhu AR, Samson SL, Vedanthan R, Umpierrez GE. Transcultural diabetes care in the United States – a position statement by the American Association of Clinical Endocrinologists. Endocr Pract. 2019; https://doi.org/10.4158/PS-2019-0080.
9. Louie D, Brook K, Frates E. The laughter prescription: a tool for lifestyle medicine. Am J Lifestyle Med. 2016;10:262–7.
10. Pegg Frates E, Morris EC, Sannidhi D, et al. The art and science of group visits in lifestyle medicine. Am J Lifestyle Med. 2017;11:408–13.
11. Graff K. Micropractice/community partnership model for lifestyle medicine. Am J Lifestyle Med. 2018;12:124–7.
12. Serna DC. Lifestyle medicine in a concierge practice: my journey. Am J Lifestyle Med. 2019;13:367–70.

13. Raphael J. Applying the business of lifestyle medicine. Am J Lifestyle Med. 2017;11:227–9.

14. Cupples ME, Byrne MC, Smith SM, et al. Secondary prevention of cardiovascular disease in different primary healthcare systems with and without pay-for-performance. Heart. 2008;94:1594–600.

15. Beckman K. New approach for lifestyle medicine payment. Am J Lifestyle Med. 2019;13:36–9.

16. Pere D. Building physician competency in lifestyle medicine: a model for health improvement. Am J Prev Med. 2017;52:260–1.

17. Sayburn A. Lifestyle medicine: a new medical specialty? BMJ. 2018;363:k4442. https://doi.org/10.1136/bmj.k4442.

18. Radenkovic D, Aswani R, Ahmad I, et al. Lifestyle medicine and physical activity knowledge of final year UK medical students. BMJ Open Sp Ex Med. 2019;5:e000518. https://doi.org/10.1136/bmjsem-2019-000518.

19. Trilk J, Nelson L, Briggs A, et al. Including lifestyle medicine in medical education: rationale for American College of Preventive Medicine/American Medical Association resolution 959. Am J Prev Med. 2019;56:e169–75.

20. Trilk JL, Muscato D, Polak R. Advancing lifestyle medicine education in undergraduate medical school curricular through the lifestyle medicine education collaborative (LMEd). Am J Lifestyle Med. 2018;12:412–8.

21. Muscato D, Phillips EM, Trilk JL. Lifestyle medicine education collaborative (LMEd): "champions of change" medical school leaders workshop. Am J Lifestyle Med. 2018;12:382–6.

22. Zhou J, Bortz W, Fredericson M. Moving toward a better balance: Stanford School of Medicine's lifestyle medicine course is spearheading the promotion of health and wellness in medicine. Am J Lifestyle Med. 2017;11:36–8.

23. Reddy KR, Freeman AM, Esselstyn CB. An urgent need to incorporate evidence-based nutrition and lifestyle medicine into medical training. Am J Lifestyle Med. 2019;13:40–1.

24. Pasarica M, Kay D, Cameron R. Using active pedagogies to advance learning for lifestyle medicine: an approach for medical students. Adv Physiol Educ. 2019;43:191–5.

25. Krishnaswani J, Jaini PA, Howard R, et al. Community-engaged lifestyle medicine: building health equity through preventive medicine residency training. Am J Prev Med. 2018;55:412–21.

26. Malatskey L, Zeev YB, Tzuk O, et al. Lifestyle medicine course for family medicine residents: preliminary assessment of the impact on knowledge, attitudes, self-efficacy and personal health. Postgrad Med. 2017;93:549–54.

27. Kelly J, Shull J. A comprehensive clinical lifestyle medicine specialty fellowship program: what intensive lifestyle treatment can do. Am J Lifestyle Med. 2017;11:414–8.

28. Shull JA. Navigating the uncharted waters of a lifestyle medicine fellowship. Am J Lifestyle Med. 2017;11:318–20.

29. Keyes S, Gardner A. Should lifestyle medicine be a core curricular component for physician assistant students? J Phys Assist Educ. 2017;28:125–6.

30. Wolferz R Jr, Arjani S, Bolze A, et al. Students teaching students: bringing lifestyle medicine education to middle and high schools through student-led community outreach programs. Am J Lifestyle Med. 2019;13:371–3.

31. Rossa-Roccor V, Malatskey L, Frank E. NextGenU.org's free, globally available online training in lifestyle medicine. Am J Lifestyle Med. 2017;11:132–3.

32. Pegg Frates E, Xiao RC, Sannidhi D, et al. A web-based lifestyle medicine curriculum: facilitating education about lifestyle medicine, behavioral change, and health care outcomes. JMIR Med Educ. 2017;3:e14. https://doi.org/10.2196/mededu.7587:10.2196/mededu.7587.

33. Herzog S, Dysinger W. The American Board of Lifestyle Medicine. Am J Lifestyle Med. 2017;11:230–1.

The Burden of Chronic Disease and the Role of Lifestyle Medicine

2

Robert F. Kushner and Jeffrey I. Mechanick

Abbreviations

CVD   cardiovascular disease
DALYs   disability-adjusted life years
EHR   electronic health record
FDA   Food and Drug Administration
NCD   non-communicable diseases
SDOH   social determinants of health

Introduction

The purpose of writing this companion textbook to our earlier book, *Lifestyle Medicine: A Manual for Clinical Practice* [1], is to present existing and emerging information on the current state of lifestyle medicine and the foundational knowledge needed to build a successful Lifestyle Medicine Center. Interest in lifestyle medicine has grown considerably over the past 5 years as demonstrated by continued development of educational training programs [2–4], growth of professional societies [5], and increased focus on healthcare professionals [6–9]. Underpinning this interest is the increasing number of publications of evidence-based, basic science, and clinical outcome data that support the role of health-promoting habits on the prevention and treatment of non-communicable diseases (NCDs). Here, we revisit the determinants and burden of NCDs in greater detail and the components and impact of lifestyle habits on NCDs.

R. F. Kushner
Departments of Medicine and Medical Education,
Northwestern University, Chicago, IL, USA
e-mail: rkushner@northwestern.edu

J. I. Mechanick (✉)
The Marie-Josée and Henry R. Kravis Center for Cardiovascular
Health at Mount Sinai Heart, and the Division of Endocrinology,
Diabetes and Bone Disease, Icahn School of Medicine at Mount
Sinai, New York, NY, USA
e-mail: jeffrey.mechanick@mountsinai.org

The Epidemiology and Contributions of Non-communicable Diseases

Non-communicable diseases include a broad range of conditions such as cardiovascular diseases (CVDs), cancers, diabetes, chronic respiratory diseases, and mental and neurological illnesses [10, 11]. This group of diseases accounts for 70 percent of global mortality [12] and a large proportion of years lived with disability [13]. The regional differences in morbidity and mortality patterns among high-, middle-, and low-income countries reflect multiple determinants, including economics, governmental policies, health system delivery, social and cultural factors, racial and ethnic biological differences, and personal lifestyle behaviors. Thus, it is becoming clear that public health and lifestyle medicine are interwoven.

In the USA, the five leading causes of death are [1] ischemic heart disease, [2] tracheal, bronchial, and lung cancers, [3] chronic obstructive pulmonary disease, [4] Alzheimer's disease and other dementias, and [5] colon and rectum cancers [14]. Diet, tobacco use, and high systolic blood pressure were the leading risks causing deaths, while tobacco use, high body mass index [obesity], and diet were the leading risk factors for disability-adjusted life years (DALYs) [14]. The same study found that 45% of total DALYs were attributable to risk factors, of which behavioral risk factors accounted for the largest percentage attributable fraction (43.5%) [14]. In contrast, low back pain and major depressive disorder were the leading causes of years lived with disability [14].

Among the many causative factors for NCD are the social determinants of health (SDOH) – the conditions in which people are born, grow, live, work, and age [15]. They include socioeconomic status, education, neighborhood and physical environment, employment, and social support networks, as well as access to healthcare (Fig. 2.1). These factors, in turn, influence the decisions people make in their personal lives. The causal relationship between SDOH and health behavior is demonstrated in a recent dataset from the USA [16].

© Springer Nature Switzerland AG 2020
J. I. Mechanick, R. F. Kushner (eds.), *Creating a Lifestyle Medicine Center*, https://doi.org/10.1007/978-3-030-48088-2_2

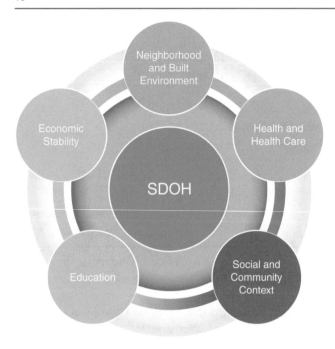

Fig. 2.1 Social determinants of health*. (*See Healthy People 2020 [15])

Chetty et al. [16] found that the most significant predictive variables of life expectancy in the USA relate to socioeconomic and race/ethnicity factors, such that life expectancy increased continuously with income. At the extremes, men in the top 1% of the income distribution lived 14.6 years longer than those in the bottom 1% [16]. The corresponding disparity for women between the two income brackets was 10.1 years. In turn, differences in life expectancy were highly correlated with health rates of smoking ($r = -0.69$; $p < 0.001$) and obesity ($r = -0.47$; $p < 0.001$), and positively correlated with exercise rates ($r = 0.32$; $p = 0.004$) among individuals in the bottom income quartile [16]. In a cohort study among older adults in the USA and England, low wealth was shown to be associated with increased death and disability [17]. The authors conjectured that those with lowest wealth are least likely to mobilize financial resources to successfully adapt to disabilities through interventions, such as hiring private help or accessing an assisted living facility.

In the Atherosclerosis Risk in Communities study of over 15,000 participants, educational attainment was inversely associated with the lifetime risk of CVD [18] such that men and women with the lowest educational level had lifetime CVD risks of approximately 60% and 50%, respectively, while those at the highest educational level had approximately 40% and 30% lifetime CVD risk. Although the mechanisms of this association were not explored in the study, other studies [19] have shown that behavioral risk factors partially mediate the effect of education on CVD, particularly smoking and obesity. In another cross-sectional study by Sasson et al. [20] in 2000 and 2017, adult life expectancy

increased among college-educated persons, but declined among persons without a 4-year college degree. The authors speculated that much of the increasing educational differences in years of life lost might be related to deaths attributed to drug use.

These studies highlight the importance of building Lifestyle Medicine Centers that are comprehensive and consider multiple contributors to population and individual health regardless of the center's focus. The complex interplay between individual factors with the SDOH can be captured by obtaining a thorough social history. Benforouz et al. [21] suggest the inclusion of six new categories beyond the common topics of marital status, occupation, tobacco, alcohol use, etc. – individual characteristics, life circumstances, emotional health, perception of healthcare, health-related behaviors, and access and utilization of healthcare. Canter and Thorpe [22] proposed five categories by collating data from three different sources: those generally collected by electronic health records (EHRs), safety issues, financial issues, behavioral health, and other demographic characteristics. Despite a 2014 report of the National Academies of Medicine [23] that SDOH should be integrated into EHRs, little progress has been made due to lack of policy standards around which data should be captured [24]. Until then, Lifestyle Medicine Centers will need to develop their own systems to acquire this information.

Creating a New Paradigm for and Redefining Lifestyle Medicine

Lifestyle medicine entails more than just focusing on health behaviors. It must incorporate socioeconomic and environmental factors that influence individual habits. Borrowing from the concept of the twentieth-century germ theory, Egger [25] proposed the term *anthropogens* as a unifying terminology to describe the man-made environments, their byproducts, and/or lifestyles encouraged by these to describe the emergence of NDC. Similarly, Ziegelstein [26, 27] has extended the concept of precision medicine from genomics, proteomics, pharmacogenomics, metabolomics, and epigenomics to include *personomics*, a new term used to refer to an individual's unique life circumstances that influence disease susceptibility, phenotype, and response to treatment. The term incorporates the psychological, social, cultural, behavioral, and economic factors of each person [26].

At the same time as the concept of lifestyle medicine has been broadened, there has been further emphasis on merging precision medicine with healthy living. In 2011, the National Research Council defined precision medicine as "an emerging approach for disease treatment and prevention that takes into account individual variability in genes, environment, and lifestyle for each person" [28]. A recent theme issue with

15 articles on merging precision medicine and healthy living was published in 2019 [29] and included a myriad of topics ranging from nutritional phenotypes [30] to cardiorespiratory fitness [31], the built environment [32], heart health [33], and weight loss [34]. This work is based on the idea that one size does not fit all for individuals when it comes to lifestyle interventions [35]. According to Ma et al. [35], precision lifestyle medicine is the blueprint for the next generation of lifestyle interventions that will be adaptive to variations in individual biology, life course behavior, and environment at baseline and over time. However, despite the promise of precision medicine, more research needs to be done to identify the individual characteristics that can more accurately predict one's response to a particular lifestyle intervention.

Update on Recommendations for Lifestyle Medicine

The benefit and importance of incorporating healthy living practices into medical care are supported by numerous evidence-based guidelines and recommendations that address the prevention and treatment of multiple diseases. Table 2.1 lists the current guidelines and consensus statements that include recommendations that relate to elements of lifestyle medicine [36–45]. Two of the guidelines address the importance of a healthy dietary pattern [36] and physical activity [37] for all Americans. The mechanisms linking various dietary components to CVD [46] and the association of leisure time physical activity with total mortality [47] and cancer [48] were recently reviewed. The other guidelines and recommendations target the prevention and treatment of CVD, hyperlipidemia, hypertension, diabetes, obesity, and the metabolic syndrome.

The guidelines particularly emphasize the four tenets of healthy living medicine that recognize the importance of moving more and sitting less, consuming a healthy diet at the appropriate calorie load, maintaining a healthy body weight, and not smoking [49]. From a practical and clinical point, it is apparent that the majority of recommendations apply to all of the NCDs, thus making counseling generalizable to the majority of patients and communities. Furthermore, many of the behaviors do not occur alone, but rather, cluster together; that is, individuals who are physically active are more likely to follow a healthy diet [50]. For example, data from the 2003–2006 National Health and Examination Survey cycles showed that after controlling for age, sex, body mass index, poverty-to-income ratio, cotinine level, and comorbidities, participants were 32% more likely to consume a healthy diet if they met physical activity guidelines [50]. The interconnection or bundling of multiple health behaviors into habit change formation can be leveraged in the delivery of care in Lifestyle Medicine Centers [51].

Although smoking is not listed as a recommendation in many of the guidelines since they are primarily focused on diet, physical activity, and healthy body weight, tobacco use ranks as the leading risk factor for US morbidity and mortality combined, represented by DALYs [14]. It increases the risk of multiple chronic diseases including heart disease and stroke, diabetes, and cancer [52]. We also know that smoking cessation reduces the subsequent risk of CVD. Among heavy smokers ($\geq$20 pack-years) in the Framingham Heart Study, CVD was significantly lower within 5 years of smoking cessation relative to current smokers (hazard ratio = 0.6) but remained significantly elevated for at least 5–10 years and possibly 25 years after cessation relative to never-smokers [53]. Recommendations for smoking cessation by behavioral counseling and pharmacotherapy interventions have been promoted by the US Preventative Services Task Force [54].

Among all of the health behavior recommendations listed in Table 2.1, only two have shown significant progress due to the aid of enforced policy regulation: *trans* fats and tobacco. The Food and Drug Administration (FDA) ruled in 2015 that artificial *trans* fats were unsafe to eat and gave food-makers 3 years to eliminate them from the food supply, with a deadline of June 18, 2018. However, to allow for an orderly transition in the marketplace, FDA allowed more time for products produced prior to June 18, 2018, to work their way through distribution. FDA extended the compliance date for these foods to January 1, 2020. The second "winnable battle" to reach target rates is tobacco use. Strengthened by the collaboration between the public health policies of taxation and clean indoor laws along with changes in social norms, the prevalence of adults who smoke cigarettes has declined from 43% in 1964 to just 15% in 2016 [55].

The impact of lifestyle medicine on other chronic diseases not addressed by the guidelines and consensus statements listed in Table 2.1 has also appeared over the past 5 years. Notable examples include non-alcoholic fatty liver disease [56, 57], chronic obstructive pulmonary disease [58], chronic kidney disease [59, 60], and HIV [61], among others.

Sleep and Stress

There are two additional components of lifestyle medicine that are not included in national guidelines and have emerged as important determinants of health: sleep and stress. Data from a cumulative total of 5,172,710 participants collected from 53 studies showed that compared with normal sleep, short sleep duration [<6 hours of sleep] is associated with a significant increase in mortality due to all causes at a relative risk of 1.12 [62]. There was an absolute increase of 37% for diabetes, 17% for hypertension, 16% for CVD, and 38% for obesity. Shortened sleep is also associated with depres-

Table 2.1 The Commonality of Lifestyle Medicine Themes in Guidelines and Consensus Statements[a]

Topic	Dietary guidelines	Physical activity	Lifestyle and diabetes	Nutrition and physical activity in cancer	Primary prevention in cardiovascular disease	Hypertension	Overweight and obesity	Cancer	Lipids	Metabolic syndrome
Organization	USDA	DHHS	ADA	ACS	AHA/ACC	ACC/AHA/ABC/ACPM/AGS/APhA/ASH/ASPC/NMA/PCNA	AHA/ACC/TOS	AICR/WCRF	AHA/ACC/AACVPR/AAPA/ABC/ACPM/ADA/AGS/APhA/ASPC/NLA/PCNA	International panel
Date (year)	2015–2020	2018	2019	2012	2019	2017	2013	2018	2019	2017
Reference number	36	37	38	39	40	41	42	43	44	45
Healthy body weight	✓	✓	✓	✓	✓	✓	✓	✓	✓	✓
Engage in physical activity	✓	✓	✓	✓	✓	✓	✓	✓	✓	✓
Increase fruits and vegetables	✓		✓	✓	✓				✓	
Choose whole grains (high-fiber foods)	✓		✓	✓	✓				✓	
Limit salt	✓		✓		✓	✓				✓
Limit saturated fat, *trans* fat, and cholesterol	✓		✓		✓				✓	✓
Limit consumption of alcoholic beverages	✓		✓	✓		✓		✓		✓
Minimize intake of added sugars	✓		✓		✓			✓	✓	✓
Limit consumption of processed meat and meat products	✓			✓	✓			✓	✓	✓
Limit consumption of refined grains	✓		✓		✓					
Smoking cessation					✓					✓

[a]This is a representative sample and not a complete listing of guidelines and position papers. Abbreviations: *AACVPR* American Association of Cardiovascular and Pulmonary Rehabilitation, *AAPA* American Academy of Physician Assistants, *ABC* Association of Black Cardiologists, *ACC* American College of Cardiology, *ACPM* American College of Preventive Medicine, *ACS* American Cancer Society, *ADA* American Diabetes Association, *AGS* American Geriatrics Society, *AHA* American Heart Association; *AICR* American Institute for Cancer Research, *APhA* American Pharmacists Association, *ASH* American Society of Hypertension, *ASPC* American Society of Preventive Cardiology, *DHHS* Department of Health and Human Services, *NMA* National Medical Association, *PCNA* Preventive Cardiovascular Nurses Association, *TOS* The Obesity Society, *USDA* United States Department of Agriculture, *WCRF* World Cancer Research Fund International

sion and other psychiatric disorders, neurodegenerative diseases, and Alzheimer's disease [62]. Although the mechanisms are uncertain, sleep restriction is associated with metabolic alterations in appetite regulation, sympathetic nervous system activity, insulin sensitivity, and changes in circadian rhythm [63]. Based on these data, "sleep health" (or sleep hygiene) has emerged as a new concept that contains multiple domains of sleep characteristics, including regularity, alertness, timing, efficiency, and satisfaction [64]. This new concept harmonizes with the 2018 Sleep in America® poll that found that sleep was ranked fourth among the top five items that were most important to responders [65]. The first three were fitness/nutrition, work, and hobbies/interests. Sleep health conforms to the socio-ecological model construct that posits multiple factors that contribute to sleep and, thus, multiple targets of intervention exist. Examples include individual behavioral factors (e.g., regular bedtimes and wake times, limiting caffeine and alcohol, creating a cool, dark, and quite bedroom, and restricting digital media in the hour before bedtime), interpersonal factors (e.g., supportive relationships), and community factors (e.g., physical conditions such as buildings, roads, and traffic patterns, and ambient environment such as noise, temperature, and light pollution) [64].

Stress (or stress reduction) is the second component of lifestyle medicine that is not routinely included in prevention guidelines. Two recent surveys highlight the common experience of stress among Americans. In the Gallup 2019 Global Emotions Report, the majority of Americans (55%) said they had experienced stress during a lot of the day, and nearly half (45%) said they felt worried a lot [66]. In the 2019 Stress in America® survey [67], around six in ten adults identified work (64%) and money (60%) as significant sources of stress, making them the most commonly mentioned personal stressors.

The impact of stress on physical and mental health has been defined by the terms allostasis, allostatic state, and allostatic load [68]. *Allostasis* refers to the physiological process of achieving stability through change in response to our environment. The primary drivers are the hormones of the hypothalamic-pituitary-adrenal (HPA) axis, catecholamines, and cytokines. *Allostatic state* refers to the altered and sustained activity levels of these primary mediators. *Allostatic load* is the wear and tear on the body and brain resulting from chronic overactivity or inactivity of physiological systems that are normally involved in adaptation to environmental change. This, in turn, leads to glucocorticoid dysregulation and dysfunction of the network of mediators involving the automatic, endocrine, metabolic, and inflammatory systems [69]. The definition of allostatic load reflects the cumulative effects of experiences of daily life and the resulting health-damaging behaviors, including poor sleep, social isolation, lack of exercise, and unhealthy diet [70].

Table 2.2 Allostatic load battery[a]

Primary mediators
Salivary cortisol
Interleukin-6
C-reactive protein
Fibrinogen
Heart rate variability
24-hour urinary norepinephrine and epinephrine
Secondary mediators
Blood pressure
Glycosylated hemoglobin
Glucose
Insulin
Lipid profile
Waist circumference

[a]See reference [71]

Clinical measurement of allostatic load varies among studies based upon the available dataset of parameters obtained. However, a suggested allostatic load battery has been proposed by McEwen [71] that reflects primary and secondary mediators (Table 2.2). In a Scottish population health study of 6300 adults, allostatic load was associated with a 46% increased risk of dying from all-causes at 10 years follow-up [72]. However, after adjusting for age, allostatic load was attenuated to an 8% increased risk of death at 10 years. The authors interpreted the association between increasing age and allostatic load as a marker of cumulative physiological burden.

A plethora of studies have been published that have assessed the utility of employing a variety of stress-reducing techniques on multiple disease states, including depression [73], anxiety [74], cancer [75], CVD [76], diabetes [77], hypertension [78], and osteoarthritis [79]. Collectively termed mind-body therapies, they encompass modalities such as yoga, meditation, mindfulness, guided imagery, tai chi, and mindfulness-based stress reduction. Despite the limitations among the studies regarding study design, sample size, duration of treatment, and primary outcomes, these techniques have generally shown promise in reducing stress and improving disease burden.

Conclusion

Lifestyle medicine continues to evolve in theory and practice grounded by an expanding scientific and clinical evidence-based medical literature. The importance of incorporating SDOH and the principles of population health into the tenets of lifestyle medicine is becoming more apparent. At the same time, the evolution of precision medicine and the new concept of personomics will make its way into the assessment and delivery of lifestyle medicine over the coming years. It is important for Lifestyle Medicine Centers to stay abreast of and assimilate the continuing advancements in the field.

References

1. Mechanick JI, Kushner RF. Lifestyle medicine – a manual for clinical practice. New York: Springer; 2016.
2. Hivert MF, McNeil A, Lavie CJ, et al. Training health professionals to deliver healthy living medicine. Prog Cardiovasc Dis. 2017;59:471–8.
3. Wylie A, Leedam-Green K. Health promotion in medical education: lessons form a major undergraduate curriculum implementation. Ed Primary Care. 2017;28:325–33.
4. Trilik JL, Muscato D. Progress of lifestyle medicine education. Curr Inventory in Context. 2019;6:1–7.
5. American College of Lifestyle Medicine. https://www.lifestyle-medicine.org/. Accessed 22 Jan 2020.
6. Grabovac I, Smith L, Stefanic S, et al. Health care providers' advice on lifestyle modification in the US population: results from the NHANES 2011-2016. Am J Med. 2019;132:489–97.
7. Rippe JM. Are we ready to practice lifestyle medicine? Am J Med. 2019;132:6–8.
8. Rognmo O, Wisloff U. Exercise is medicine. Prog Cardiovasc Dis. 2019;62:85. https://doi.org/10.1016/j.pcad.2019.03.001.
9. Rippe JM. Lifestyle medicine: The health promoting power of daily habits and practices. Am J Lifestyle Med. 2018;12:499–512.
10. Hunter DJ, Reddy KS. Noncommunicable diseases. N Engl J Med. 2013;369:1336–43.
11. Ali MK, Jaacks LM, Kewalski AL, et al. Noncommunicable diseases: three decades of global data show a mixture of increases and decreases in mortality rates. Health Aff. 2015;34:1444–55.
12. Global Burden of Disease Study 2013 Collaborators. Global, regional, and national incidence, prevalence, and years lived with disability for 301 acute and chronic diseases and injuries in 188 countries, 1990–2013: a systematic analysis for the Global Burden of Disease Study 2013. Lancet. 2015;386:743–800.
13. Murray CJ, Vos T, Lozano R, et al. Disability-adjusted life years (DALYs) for 291 diseases and injuries in 21 regions, 1990-2010: a systematic analysis for the global burden of disease study 2010. Lancet. 2012;380:2197–223.
14. The US. Burden of diseases collaborators. Mokdad AH, Ballestros K, Echko M· et al. The state of the US health, 1990-2016. Burden of diseases, injuries, and risk factors among US states. JAMA. 2018;319:1444–72.
15. Office of Disease Prevention and Health Promotion. Healthy People 2020. https://www.healthypeople.gov/. Accessed 19 Jan 2020.
16. Chetty R, Stepner M, Abraham S, et al. The association between income and life expectancy in the United States, 2001-2014. JAMA. 2016;315:1750–66.
17. Makaroun LK, Brown RT, Dia-Ramirez LG, et al. Wealth-associated disparities in death and disability in the United States and England. JAMA Intern Med. 2017;177:1745–53.
18. Kubota Y, Heiss G, MacLehose R, et al. Association of educational attainment with lifetime risk of cardiovascular disease. The atherosclerosis risk in communities study. JAMA Intern Med. 2017;177:1165–72.
19. Nordahl H, Rod NH, Frederiksen BL, et al. Education and risk of coronary heart disease: assessment of mediation by behavioral risk factors using the additive hazards model. Eur J Epidemiol. 2013;28:149–57.
20. Sassin I, Hayward MD. Association between educational attainment and causes of death among white and black US adults, 2010-2017. JAMA. 2019;322:756–63.
21. Behforouz HL, Drain PK, Rhatigan JJ. Rethinking the social history. N Engl J Med. 2014;371:1277–9.
22. Cantor MN, Thorpe L. Integrating data on social determinants of health into electronic health records. Health Aff. 2018;37:585–90.
23. Committee on the Recommended Social and Behavioral Domains and Measures for Electronic Health Records, Board on Population Health and Public Health Practice, Institute of Medicine. Capturing Social and Behavioral Domains and Measures in Electronic Health Records: Phase 2. Washington DC: National Academies Press (US); 2015.
24. Freij M, Dullabh P, Lewis S, et al. Incorporating social determinants of health in electronic health records: qualitative study of current practices among top vendors. JMIR Med Informatics. 2019;7:e13849. https://doi.org/10.2196/13849.
25. Egger G. In search of a germ theory equivalent for chronic disease. Prev Chronic Dise. 2012;9:E95. https://doi.org/10.5888/pcd9.110301.
26. Ziegelstein RC. Personomics. JAMA Intern Med. 2015;175:888–9.
27. Ziegelstein RC. Personomics: the missing link in the evolution from precision medicine to personalized medicine. J Pers Med. 2017;7:11, 10.3390.
28. National Research Council. Toward Precision Medicine. Building a knowledge network for biomedical research and a new taxonomy of disease. Washington, DC: The National Academies Press; 2011.
29. Arena R, Laddu D. Merging precision and healthy living medicine: individualizing the path to a healthier lifestyle. Prog Cardiovasc Dis. 2019;62:1–2.
30. Laddu D, Hauser M. Addressing the nutritional phenotype through personalized nutrition for chronic disease prevention and management. Prog Cardiovasc Dis. 2019;62:6–14.
31. Ozemek C, Arena R. Precision in promoting physical activity and exercise with the overarching goal of moving more. Prog Cardiovasc Dis. 2019;62:3–8.
32. Hills AP, Farpour-Lambert NJ, Byrne NM. Precision medicine and healthy living: The importance of the built environment. Prog Cardiovasc Dis. 2019;62:33–8.
33. Kaminsky LA, Myers J, Arena R. Determining cardiorespiratory fitness with precision: compendium of findings from the FRIEND registry. Prog Cardiovasc Dis. 2019;62:76–82.
34. Severin R, Sabbahi A, Mahmoud AM, et al. Precision medicine in weight loss and healthy living. Prog Cardiovasc Dis. 2019;62:15–20.
35. Ma J, Rosas LG, Lv N. Precision lifestyle medicine. A new frontier in the science of behavior change and population health. Am J Prev Med. 2016;50:395–7.
36. U.S. Department of Health and Human Services and U.S. Department of Agriculture. 2015–2020 Dietary Guidelines for Americans. 8th ed; 2015. Available at http://health.gov/dietaryguidelines/2015/guidelines/. Accessed 19 Jan 2020.
37. U.S. Department of Health and Human Services. Physical Activity Guidelines for Americans. 2nd ed. Washington, DC: U.S. Department of Health and Human Services; 2018. https://health.gov/paguidelines/. Accessed 19 Jan 2020.
38. American Diabetes Association. Lifestyle management: standards of medical care in diabetes – 2019. Diabetes Care. 2019;42(Supplement 1):S46–60.
39. Kushi LH, Doyle C, McCullough M, et al. American Cancer Society guidelines on nutrition and physical activity for cancer prevention. CA Cancer J for Clinicians. 2012;62:30–67.
40. Arnett DK, Khera A, Blumenthal RS. 2019 ACC/AHA guideline on the primary prevention of cardiovascular disease: part 1, lifestyle and behavioral factors. JAMA Cardiol. 2019;4:1043–4.
41. Whelton PK, Carey RM, Aronow WS, et al. 2017 ACC/AHA/AAPA/ABC/ACPM/AGS/APhA/ASH/ASPC/NMA/PCNA guideline for the prevention, detection, evaluation, and Management of High Blood Pressure in adults: a report of the American College

of Cardiology/American Heart Association task force on clinical practice guidelines. Circulation. 2018;138:e484–594.

42. Jensen MD, Ryan DH, Apovian CM, et al. 2013 AHA/ACC/TOS guideline for the management of overweight and obesity in adults: a report of the American College of Cardiology/American Heart Association task force on practice guidelines and The Obesity Society. Curculation. 2014;129(25 Suppl 2):S102–38.

43. World Cancer Research Fund/American Institute for Cancer Research. Diet, Nutrition, Physical Activity, and Cancer. A global perspective. Continuous update project expert report 2018. https://www.wcrf.org/dietandcancer/about. Accessed 19 Jan 2020.

44. Grundy SM, Stone NJ, Bailey AL, et al. 2018 AHA/ACC/AACVPR/AAPA/ABC/ACPM/ADA/AGS/APhA/ASPC/NLA/PCNA guideline on the Management of Blood Cholesterol: a report of the American College of Cardiology/American Heart Association task force on clinical practice guidelines. Circulation. 2019;139:e1082–143.

45. Pérez-Martínez P, Mikhailidis DP, Athyros VG, et al. Lifestyle recommendations for the prevention and management of metabolic syndrome: an international panel recommendation. Nutr Rev. 2017;75:307–26.

46. Stanhope KL, Goran MI, Bosy-Westphal A, et al. Pathways and mechanism linking dietary components to cardiovascular disease: thinking beyond calories. Obes Rev. 2018;19:1205–35.

47. Arem H, Moore SC, Patel A, et al. Leisure time physical activity and mortality. A detailed pooled analysis of the dose-response relationship. JAMA Intern Med. 2015;175:959–67.

48. Moore SC, Lee IM, Weiderpass E, et al. Association of leisure-time physical activity with risk of 26 types of cancer in 1.44 million adults. JAMA Intern Med. 2016;176:816–25.

49. Arena R, Ozemek C, Laddu D, et al. Applying precision medicine to healthy living for the prevention and treatment of cardiovascular disease. Curr Probl Cardiol. 2018;43:448–83.

50. Loprinzi PD, Smit E, Mahoney S. Physical activity and dietary behavior in US adults and their combined influence on health. Mayo Clin Proc. 2014;89:190–8.

51. Spring B, Moller AC, Coons MJ. Multiple health behaviours: overview and implications. J Public Health. 2012;34(Suppl 1):i3–i10.

52. U. S. Department of Health and Human Services. The Health Consequences of Smoking: 50 Years of Progress. A report of the Surgeon General. Altlanta, GA: U. S. Department of Health and Human Services, Center for Disease Control and Prevention, National Center for Chronic Disease Prevention and Health Promotion, Office on Smoking and Health; 2014.

53. Duncan MS, Freiberg MS, Greevy RA, et al. Association of smoking cessation with subsequent risk of cardiovascular disease. JAMA. 2019;322:642–50.

54. Patnode CD, Henderson JT, Thompson JH, et al. Behavioral counseling and pharmacotherapy interventions for tobacco cessation in adults, including pregnant women. A review for the US services preventive task force. Ann Intern Med. 2015;163:608–21.

55. Koh HK, Parekh AK. Toward a United States of Health: implications of understanding the US burden of disease. JAMA. 2018;319:1438–40.

56. Saeed N, Nadeau B, Shannon C, et al. Evaluation of dietary approaches for the treatment of non-alcoholic fatty liver disease: a systematic review. Nutrients. 2019;11:3064. https://doi.org/10.3390/nu11123044.

57. Romero-Gomez M, Zelber-Sagi S, Trenell M. Treatment of NAFLD with diet, physical activity and exercise. J Hepatol. 2017;67:829–46.

58. Lewthwaite H, Effing TW, Olds T, et al. Physical activity, sedentary behavior and sleep in COPD guidelines: a systematic review. Chronic Resp Dis. 2017;14:231–44.

59. Evangelidis N, Craig J, Bauman A, et al. Lifestyle behavior change for prevention the progression of chronic kidney disease: a systematic review. BMJ Open. 2019;9:e031625. https://doi.org/10.1136/bmjopen-2019031625.

60. Bach KE, Kelly JT, Palmer SC, et al. Healthy dietary patterns and incidence of CKD. A meta-analysis of cohort studies. CJASN. 2019;14:1441–9.

61. Fitch KV. Contemporary lifestyle modification interventions to improve metabolic comorbidities in HIV. Curr HIV/AIDS Reports. 2019;16:482–91.

62. Itani O, Jike M, Watanabe N, et al. Short sleep duration and health outcome: a systematic review, meta-analysis, and meta-regression. Sleep Med. 2017;32:246–56.

63. Reutrakul S, Van Cauter E. Sleep influences on obesity, insulin resistance, and risk of type 2 diabetes. Metabolism. 2018;84:56–66.

64. Hale L, Troxel W, Buysse DJ. Sleep health: an opportunity for public health to address health equity. Ann Rev Public Health. 2020;41:81–99. https://doi.org/10.1146/annurev-publhealth-040119-094412.

65. National Sleep Foundation. 2018 Sleep in America Poll. https://www.sleepfoundation.org/press-release/national-sleep-foundations-2018-sleep-americar-poll-shows-americans-failing. Accessed 19 Jan 2020.

66. Gallup. Gallup 2019 Global Emotions Report. https://www.gallup.com/analytics/248909/gallup-2019-global-emotions-report-pdf.aspx. Accessed on 26 Jan 2020.

67. American Psychological Association. Stress in American: Stress and Current Events. Stress in America™ Survey; 2019.

68. McEwen BS, Wingfield JC. The concept of allostasis in biology and biomedicine. Horm Behav. 2003;43:2–15.

69. Fava G, McEwen BS, Guidi J, et al. Clinical characterization of allostatic overload. Psychoneuroendocrinology. 2019;108:94–101.

70. Suvarna B, Suvarna A, Phillips R, et al. Health risk behaviours and allostatic load: a systematic review. Neurosci Biobehav Rev. 2020;108:694–711.

71. McEwen BS. Biomarkers for assessing population and individual health and disease related to stress and adaptation. Metabolism. 2015;64(3 Suppl 1):S2–S10.

72. Robertson T, Beveridge G, Bromley C. Allostatic load as a predictor of all-cause and cause-specific mortality in the general population: evidence from the Scottish Health Survey. Plos One. 2017;12:e0183297. 10.1371.

73. Streeter CC, Gerbarg PL, Whitfield TH, et al. Treatment of major depressive disorder with Iyengar yoga and coherent breathing: a randomized controlled dosing study. Altern Complement Ther. 2017;23:236–43.

74. Sharma M, Haider T. Tai chi as an alternative and complimentary therapy for anxiety: a systematic review. J Evid Based Complement Altern Med. 2015;20:143–53.

75. Rush SE, Sharma M. Mindfulness-based stress reduction as a stress management intervention for cancer: a systematic review. J Evidence Based Complement Altern Med. 2017;22:347–59.

76. Levine GN, Lange RA, Bairey-Merz CN, et al. Meditation and cardiovascular risk reduction. A scientific statement from the American Heart Association. J Am Heart Assoc 2017; 6: pii: e002218, https://doi.org/10.1161/JAHA.117.002218.

77. Medina WL, Wilson D, de Salvo V, et al. Effects of mindfulness on diabetes mellitus: rationale and overview. Curr Diabetes Rev. 2017;13:141–7.

78. Shi L, Zhang D, Wang L, et al. Meditation and blood pressure: a meta-analysis of randomized clinical trials. J Hypertens. 2017;35:696–706.

79. Lee AC, Harvey WF, Price LL, et al. Mindfulness is associated with treatment response from nonpharmacologic exercise interventions in knee osteoarthritis. Arch Phys Med Rehabil. 2017;98:2265–73.

Translating Knowledge and Implementing a Successful Lifestyle Medicine Center

3

Jeffrey I. Mechanick and Robert F. Kushner

Abbreviations

APP   Advanced practice provider
HCP   Healthcare professional
RDN   Registered dietitian nutritionist
T2D   Type 2 diabetes

Introduction

The goal of lifestyle medicine is to reduce the risk and impact of chronic disease by using nonpharmacological and nonsurgical/nonprocedural interventions. Once a scientifically based clinical practice guidelines and/or algorithm is established to guide actions, resources need to be identified, organized, and leveraged to implement these plans. Implementation consists of translation of ideas into action, materialization of a physical space (consisting of conceptualization and operationalization of the physical space), and then optimization of the process. The net result is the creation of a Lifestyle Medicine Center (Fig. 3.1).

Knowing what lifestyle medicine is, how the supporting evidence can be translated and applied, and which guidelines one must adhere to requires a categorically different skillset than actually performing the service in the real world with demonstrable benefits. Practically speaking, this requires the build-out of a physical setting that can enable implementation. Materialization applies to transforming an idea or body of

J. I. Mechanick (✉)
The Marie-Josée and Henry R. Kravis Center for Cardiovascular Health at Mount Sinai Heart, and the Division of Endocrinology, Diabetes and Bone Disease, Icahn School of Medicine at Mount Sinai, New York, NY, USA
e-mail: jeffrey.mechanick@mountsinai.org

R. F. Kushner
Departments of Medicine and Medical Education, Northwestern University, Chicago, IL, USA
e-mail: rkushner@northwestern.edu

knowledge into something real, something with perceptible existence. This materialization process consists of multiple actions that are goal oriented, generally over the short term, and can be codified in terms of clinical research, clinical practice, and education. The success of this materialization process depends on the status of certain variables: environment, chronic disease pathophysiology, chronic care models within the prevailing healthcare system, and logistical ease or operations.

For those who are unclear about the need for an emphasis on implementation, consider the following exemplar.

> Patient LC is referred by their cardiologist having had a myocardial infarction and coronary artery bypass grafting in the setting of uncontrolled type 2 diabetes, hypertension, and class II obesity. A detailed history and focused physical examination is performed, followed by phlebotomy for laboratory testing concentrated on biomarkers related to cardiometabolic risk and goals for secondary prevention. In addition to medication changes, recommendations are provided for the patient to see a registered dietitian nutritionist (RDN), participate in a formal cardiac rehabilitation program, purchase an activity wearable device, and participate in a lifestyle medicine educational program at the nearby community center.

This case study is not unusual and includes generally accepted, evidence-based recommendations. The problem is that many patients will find it challenging to adhere with each of these recommendations, particularly on a long-term basis commensurate with the nature of chronic disease. Thus, it is not surprising that despite all the available evidence, knowledge, and even experience with the type of clinical encounter described above, there are still high prevalence rates of chronic disease. Now, consider the alternate exemplar below with changes underlined.

> Patient LC is referred by their cardiologist having had a myocardial infarction and coronary artery bypass grafting in the setting of uncontrolled type 2 diabetes, hypertension, and class II obesity. A detailed history and focused physical examination is performed, followed by phlebotomy for laboratory testing concentrated on biomarkers related to cardiometabolic risk and goals for secondary prevention. In addition to medication changes, the patient is introduced to the RDN with a warm

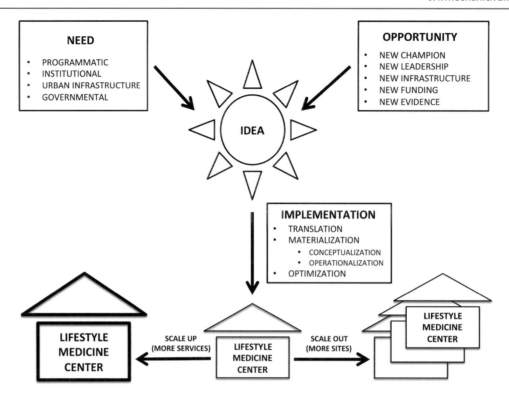

Fig. 3.1 Materialization of a Lifestyle Medicine Center*. (*The process of building a Lifestyle Medicine Center begins with an idea that is spawned by a convergence of need and opportunity. The implementation process begins with knowledge (e.g., scientific evidence enriched with expert experience), translation into action (programs, clinical service lines, and other organizational entities), materialization or physical construction into a suitable space (consisting of conceptualization of care models and operationalization by planning, building, and managing), and then a long-term process for clinical and financial optimization for sustainability. Overtime, with various successes, and through collaborative leadership among HCPs and administrators, the Lifestyle Medicine Center can be scaled up by adding more services and scaled out over a larger geographic area.)

handoff from the physician. Another warm handoff and introduction to the exercise physiologist is conducted and then the patient is navigated in the Lifestyle Medicine Center to the advanced practice provider (APP; nurse practitioner and clinical director) who reviews the comprehensive care plan, including placement of the glucose sensor, provision of the center's App for the patient's smartphone, provision and instructions for a wearable accelerometer, and scheduling for free educational classes in the center on aspects of lifestyle medicine.

It should be obvious that this sequence of events should be more successful as a result of convenience, but it is also the immersive and positive experience that contributes to desirable clinical outcomes. The challenges should also be obvious: critical evidence demonstrating superior outcomes, durability/sustainability of a therapeutic/preventive effect, and having the wherewithal to actually build a Lifestyle Medicine Center capable of these activities. The third challenge about building a Lifestyle Medicine Center is the prime focus of this book, but a derivative feature will be the first and second challenges – the realization of sustainable benefits as more and more Lifestyle Medicine Centers are activated, optimized based on new data, and part of a new culture of population health. Many of the

concepts described in this introductory chapter are presented in greater detail in subsequent chapters.

Implementation Modalities

Research

Lifestyle Medicine Centers are conceived and constructed based on empirical evidence gleaned from a larger body of relevant scientific studies. Using nutritional research as an example, Satija et al. [1] argue that the best scientific approach is to improve study design, reduce measurement errors, and leverage new technologies. The weight of evidence needs to include multiple study designs and methods [1], and then be curated in terms of validity, scientific substantiation, relevance, topic, and miscellaneous interest for translation into policy, protocols, practice, and physical infrastructure.

Research findings are used to guide decision-making for the design of physical components, human resources, and policies/protocols that constitute a Lifestyle Medicine

Center. One example of this process is the translation of research on maternal obesity, excessive gestational weight gain, and the global obesity problem, into a policy of comprehensive lifestyle interventions for target populations in the community [2]. Another aspect highlighting the need for specialized research relates to the problem of implementation. Since cost factors, third-party reimbursements, staff turnover, institutional commitment, self-efficacy, and highly diverse target populations represent significant obstacles to success, high-quality research studies need to be designed and carried out to determine how Lifestyle Medicine Centers can succeed and endure [3]. For instance, there are care models that can be replicated in different settings that successfully transition from research-funded resources to institution-funded resources [3]. There are also different lifestyle surveillance systems that are optimized for implementation of chronic disease prevention activities [4].

How can a research program be integrated into the physical Lifestyle Medicine Center space? Clinical trials and epidemiological studies will require administrative resources, recruitment and support of scientists, space that is scaled for on-site patient care and data collection, technology and informatics for data analysis, and the flexibility to adapt to different protocols over time. If biochemical and molecular studies are involved, then there needs to be adequate space allocated, such as phlebotomy and/or tissue sampling and specimen processing areas and, if unavailable, provisions for referrals to another facility.

Clinical Practice

Lifestyle medicine is directed at the prevention of chronic diseases, e.g., cardiometabolic-based chronic disease (including cardiovascular disease [CVD], dyslipidemia, hypertension [HTN], obesity [or adiposity-based chronic disease {5}], and type 2 diabetes [T2D, or dysglycemia-based chronic disease {6}]; [7, 8]), cancer, chronic obstructive pulmonary disease, chronic kidney disease, neurodegenerative diseases, and depression. It is important to note that the dimension of this problem is larger in lower-income, urban populations where multiple chronic conditions (>2) are more prevalent than the national average [9]. In various chronic care models, the emphasis is on interceding as early as possible to abrogate, or at least mitigate, the natural progression of disease in a sustainable manner [5–8].

In a clinical model, health status can be viewed as health, disease, or suboptimal (an intermediate state) [10]. Healthy lifestyles and mitigation of risk factors are associated with regression of suboptimal health status to the healthy state [11]. These actions are informed by research findings in basic science on pathophysiology and clinical trials on the efficacy of various lifestyle interventions, e.g., healthy eating patterns, physical activity, tobacco cessation, behavior change, and sleep hygiene. For instance, among 20,721 men, of age 45–79 years, without cancer, CVD, diabetes, HTN, or high cholesterol, adherence with regular physical activity (walking/bicycling ≥40 minutes/day and exercising ≥1 hour/week), healthy eating (plant-based food, low-fat food, fish, and minimally processed food), moderate alcohol use (~1 drink/day), no smoking, and achieving normal abdominal adiposity (waist circumference <95 cm) was associated with a 79% lower risk for myocardial infarction [12]. However, the problem is that exhibiting all these healthy attributes was only found in 1% of the sample population, further extolling the need for effective lifestyle medicine implementation tactics [13].

For the most part, strategies to actualize lifestyle medicine have been anchored in the development of clinical practice guidelines and belief that their promulgation and general acceptance were tantamount to successful implementation [14]. Many lifestyle medicine programs are based on these guidelines and purport to be evidence-based and *de facto* implementation solutions. Much attention has been paid to behavioral medicine within these strategic approaches to promote patient adherence and improve clinical outcomes, but actually changing patient behaviors has proven to be very difficult.

There are different behavioral methods within patient-centered care. Thomas et al. [15] presented a substantive theory of being healthy in a primary care setting, composed of conditions, management, and interactions. Using interview data, four patient trajectories were revealed: resigned (passive role without internal or external resources to be healthy), receivers (passive role without internal resources to be healthy, but with external sources that can prompt healthy change), coworkers (active role due to internal responsibility and collaboration with healthcare professional [HCPs] to achieve their own health), and leaders (active role due to internal responsibility and are primary stakeholders in achieving their own health) [15]. Ideally, care plans and HCP-patient interactions can be optimized with successful screening tools to accurately detect these patient trajectory potentials [15]. Interestingly, nurse-led communication of risk was associated with improved patient perceptions and satisfaction [16]. Shared or group medical appointments (e.g., with the physician, health coach, culinary instructor, exercise physiologist, RDN, or mind-body therapist) can improve results while also satisfying budgetary constraints [17]. The incorporation of spirituality, or interior life, is a feature of behavioral medicine and an intriguing aspect of effective lifestyle medicine, representing a unique challenge to healthcare systems in general and budding Lifestyle Medicine Centers in particular [18]. Unfortunately, the implementation of guidelines on lifestyle medicine, which provides the content and impetus for communication, has been historically disappointing, despite efforts to optimize methodologies, create electronic versions and educational resources, focus on patient adherence, develop public campaigns, and forge community-based collaborations [19, 20]. These disappointments can be traced, first to the relative de-emphasis on behavioral medicine and second to the relative lack of coordinated physical space to harness all aspects of lifestyle medicine and promote positive attitudes.

What has become apparent is that successful implementation of lifestyle medicine requires a physical enterprise, or "Center," that translates strategy into effective action. This point was emphasized during a recent expert panel discussion on lifestyle medicine implementation that concentrated on the physical Center as a common denominator for success [21]. The Centers ranged from an Ornish program in a Cardiac Rehabilitation Center in Morristown, New Jersey, to a Lifestyle Medicine Institute in Loma Linda, California, to the Complete Health Improvement Program at Lee Health in Florida, to the Cummins LiveWell Center for employees of Cummins, Inc., in Columbus, Ohio, to Community Integrated Health at Young Men's Christian Associations (YMCAs) across the country [21].

It is apparent that physical Centers in lifestyle medicine can take the form of academic programs, divisions, or departments; qualified clinical service lines within a sponsoring organization; or free-standing organizations as a clinic or institute, each with their own clinical and business parameters and strategic geographic settings. As an example, in a study of Hispanic pregnant women with overweight/obesity, group sessions for lifestyle interventions were best conducted in a Center in or near the patient's community, with text messages and social media as reinforcements [22]. In fact, the mission of a Lifestyle Medicine Center to reduce chronic disease risk factors can be enhanced through collaborations with community health promotion programs under stable leadership [23].

Once a physical Lifestyle Medicine Center is planned, attention needs to be given to creating the proper culture. Carlfjord et al. [24] found that a single, shared culture is best when transferring new knowledge into healthcare practice, as opposed to multiple subcultures, which can create mixed messaging and confusion for the patient, as well as different experiences for personnel. Furthermore, during the initialization phase, leadership should be prepared to "re-invent" aspects of lifestyle medicine taking into account the context [25], competing natures of different programs, as well as the imperatives of implementation versus sustainability [26].

It is unclear how to create a proper culture, but several examples can provide guideposts. Various studies have shown that configuring a nurse in a central role for coordination of care can improve lifestyle counseling implementation [16, 27]. Wierenga et al. [28] found that for

non-research worksite health promotion programs, evidence-based interventions are not as important for implementation as logistical ease, low cost, and minimal effort. Healthy nutrition is a cornerstone of lifestyle medicine and has been a considerable barrier for many patients. This is particularly true for those with polycystic ovary syndrome, a condition with high prevalence rates of abnormal adiposity and dysglycemia, and a paucity of knowledge about lifestyle medicine implementation [29, 30]. In terms of physical activity, particularly for the elderly, implementation obstacles can be overcome with on-site screening, recruitment strategies, education, social interactions, and follow-up with inclusion of family members and/or friends [31]. For patients with T2D, translation of implementation strategies (risk assessment, motivational interviewing, increasing patient adherence, community engagement, and education [32]) can be facilitated by the Lifestyle Medicine Center.

Another active ingredient for a nurturing culture in a Lifestyle Medicine Center is personalized coaching activity, which facilitates care and can be delivered by the physician, APP, RDN, and even medical student [33, 34]. By having a physical place with resources at the ready, each patient can be provided with the following:

- Healthy foods and menus along with commercial sites and smartphone apps for ordering and delivery
- Aerobic and strength-training exercises with equipment demonstrations and then sites where the patient can be assisted with ordering items (e.g., dumbbells, stationary bicycle, and elliptical trainer) for delivery to home or even office
- Demonstrations of different smartphone apps providing behavioral modification and then assistance with ordering and downloading
- Presentations of wearable technologies that target specific symptoms and personal preferences, and assistance with ordering and delivery

Education

Once a Lifestyle Medicine Center is operational, educational activities must be expanded, to teach not only theory and rationale but also the logistics and technical aspects of building infrastructure. The target audience for these pragmatic educational programs includes personnel inside the Center to continue further development (e.g., physicians, other HCPs, and staff), and also other interested stakeholders outside the Center to increase influence within a geographic region. Through this extension, others are encouraged to build additional centers and can be provided with the details to replicate successes and avoid common pitfalls.

Educational events can be organized on-site or in venues locally, regionally, nationally, and internationally in, for example, private spaces, academic centers, and professional society conferences. If on-site education is part of the Center's design, then space needs to be allocated as a lecture, multipurpose, or laboratory demonstration room, with adequate audiovisual and demonstration (e.g., gym and culinary arts) equipment. If the Center is a clinical service line and part of a larger organization, then more advanced technology may be needed for distribution of material in real time, or as enduring cloud-based content, or both. Full-fledged educational programs in lifestyle medicine can be developed at essentially all levels, from elementary school to middle/high school, to college and undergraduate medical education, residency, and fellowship training, to continuing medical education. At a systems level, the net effect of ongoing educational initiatives to develop a pragmatic lifestyle medicine discipline is a transformative event for the healthcare culture.

Materialization: Conceptualization Variables

Once scientific and experiential knowledge are translated into ideas about actions, a framework, or model, is conceptualized in the context of real-life variables that have a direct impact on success. This is a critical step in the cognitive process of lifestyle medicine implementation and emphasizes the interactive dynamics of environment and chronic disease.

Environment

Primary drivers of chronic disease are genetic, environmental, and behavioral, each acting independently and also in combination [7, 8]. Secondary drivers are physiological, such as dysglycemia, abnormal adiposity, inflammation, and degenerative [7, 8]. There are several environment factors that are associated with increased risk for chronic disease, e.g., crime and discrimination, pollution, urban residence, lower neighborhood walkability, and decreased green space [35]. By leveraging systems science, a local health department can predict the effects of certain population health metrics (e.g., 1% decrease in A1C leads to reduction of 20-year prevalence of end-stage renal disease from 1.7 to 0.9%) and then derive a business model on this larger scale [36]. Unhealthy systems, or cultures, are found in high-risk locales, especially where there is structural violence (e.g., individual and institutional racism, and inequitable social policy/practice) [37, 38]. One way to address this geographic heterogeneity in lifestyle is by scaling out prevention programs nationally, such as the collaboration between the UnitedHealth Group and YMCA [39]. Another way is to integrate cultural adaptations in lifestyle medicine programs [37], such as in cardiac rehabilitation programs [40]. In addition, the use of the patient-centered medical home promises to improve clinical outcomes with reduced cost, though further study is required [41]. Lastly, faith-based lifestyle programming can improve health metrics. In a study by Rhodes et al. [42], an 18-session, church-based Fit Body and Soul program led to healthy weight loss and decreased waist circumference.

Chronic Disease Care Models

The chronic care model was developed in the 1990s by Wagner et al. [43] and consists of community linkages, clinical information sharing, delivery system design, self-management, and clinical support. However, in a structured review by Sendall et al. [44], few published studies actually utilize all of these components. Furthermore, anywhere from 20% [45] to over 60% [9] of patients have multiple chronic disease morbidities with a level of complexity that breeds overmedicalization. This has prompted development of new care models that prioritize what is termed "minimally disruptive medicine," which is a form of quaternary prevention [46]. Reducing the burden of treatment offers advantages in cost, adherence, and clinical outcomes. Healthcare systems tend to be more fragmented in terms of services provided; this can be addressed with comprehensive, patient-centered coordinated care, informed by patient-reported measures, and practiced on a large scale [47–49]. In other words, physical build-outs of ambulatory care centers that practice lifestyle medicine and efficiently incorporate practical resources (e.g., assistance with finances and transportation) [46], as well as coordinate seamless care between outpatient and inpatient settings, can defragment healthcare in society [50]. Another aspect of chronic disease in many patients involves the management of demoralization – an existential conflict with loss of purpose and meaning of life – seen for example in heart transplant patients [51]. Using the comprehensive task-model approach, patients can focus on adaptation and then reconstruct their personal existence [52]. Taken together, the translation of knowledge into physical Centers will need to significantly focus on behavioral medicine.

Cardiovascular Disease

Comprehensive primary and secondary prevention models for CVD have been successfully implemented. In one example, Gordon et al. [53] chronicle program development, beginning with non-physician HCPs working with physician HCPs, incorporation of behavioral change models (e.g., social learning theory, stages of change, and single concept learning theory), and then physical presence in hospitals, physician practices, cardiac rehabilitation programs, work sites, shopping malls, and health clubs, with call centers and web-based engagement. Cardiovascular disease is the leading cause of mortality worldwide, and not surprisingly, among women in the USA. There are several key reasons for this: awareness (27% believe breast cancer is their greatest health threat), more chronic comorbidities (likely due to the older age at presentation), and disparities in implementation (e.g., screening programs, prevention strategies, and lifesaving measures) [54]. The *Healthy People 2010®* is an evidence-based, comprehensive heart care program for women that improves CVD knowledge and awareness, as well as clinical and biochemical metrics of health [54].

Part and parcel of CVD prevention programs is attention to component cardiometabolic risks (e.g., dysglycemia, abnormal adiposity, hypertension, dyslipidemia, tobacco use, physical inactivity, and unhealthy eating patterns). The metabolic syndrome is a clustering of drivers and features that lead to CVD. Any successful intervention would need to have durable effects, beyond simple short-term benefits. One example is the Obesity-Related Behavioral Intervention Trials model that achieved 53.8% remission after a median of 2.5 years [55]. In general, translating evidence-based recommendations from numerous professional medical societies into formal programs that emphasize primary and secondary preventions (in addition to usual tertiary prevention approaches), and then into physical Centers that incorporate structured lifestyle medicine, face several challenges. Barriers to implementation are centered on personalization, such as adherence with appropriate exercise programs, meal planning that addresses behaviors, social variables, and tastes; manageable technologies to monitor glycemic status; as well as other markers of health [56]. Adherence is addressed with behavioral modification. For instance, in a study by Abbasi et al. [57], implementation of a "credit system" for adopting various health behaviors was associated with improved diabetes and CVD outcomes.

Cancer

In patients with cancer, healthy lifestyle modifications are generally regarded as elements of tertiary prevention: to manage symptoms and complications of the underlying malignancy as well as the effects of cancer therapy. The value of a Lifestyle Medicine Center in the routine management of patients with cancer, of all types and at all stages, is more apparent when considering new approaches for primary and secondary preventions to minimize the number of chronic comorbidities. One example of a successful comprehensive lifestyle modification intervention is *Lifestyle 180®* [58]. Of the initial 400 patients studied in 2011, 58 had a diagnosis of past cancer [58]. Of these 58, 47% had hyperlipidemia, 57% hypertension, 22% diabetes, 50% prediabetes, 45% obese, 24% overweight, and 16% depression [58].

Twelve months after the completion of the 6-month program with 64 hours of intensive nutrition, culinary medicine, physical activity, and stress relief, there were significant improvements in body mass index, waist circumference, high-density lipoprotein, triglycerides, C-reactive protein, fasting insulin, homeostatic model assessment – insulin resistance, perceived stress, and quality of life [58]. However, there were no detectable differences in depressive symptoms or blood pressure [58].

Cognitive Health

Cognitive health encompasses chronic neurodegenerative disease and is approached not only with pharmacology and procedures but also with structured lifestyle medicine interventions, including certain eating patterns, physical activity, and behavioral approaches (e.g., positive psychology) [59–61]. Implementation of this wide range of interventions has been proposed as part of a comprehensive, cognitive wellness clinical service line [59]. Primary and secondary prevention strategies are important in patients with mental illness and require a trusting and empathetic environment [62]. In addition, chronic pain conditions can be managed with healthy eating patterns, representing another opportunity for programmatic collaboration [63].

Materialization: Operationalization Variables

The implementation process includes translation, materialization (consisting of conceptualization and operationalization), and optimization. The materialization process begins with conceptualization (modeling the translated concepts of lifestyle medicine, such as how interactions between environment and the chronic care model can be addressed in a physical setting) and continues with operationalization (defining variables in terms of measurable factors in the real world: planning, building, and managing). The Lifestyle Medicine Center is the instrument by which health variables can be measured – before, during, and after strategic interventions – and improved.

Planning

Sound business models are important for the success of a Lifestyle Medicine Center. Cost containment needs to be a priority, especially during the early developmental stages [64]. On the other hand, payment models can take several forms: cash, direct primary care, fee-for-service with third-party (insurance) reimbursement, and concierge [64]. In another format, where startup finances may be limiting, a micropractice can be partnered with community resources (e.g., health systems and culinary centers). In this format, physical space is limited to just what is needed for clinical encounters, with minimal human resources and a dependence on web-based coordination and messaging [65].

Building

The center's décor can influence healing potential, particularly through the use of paint, revealing positive imagery, such as happy faces and moods [66]. Survey data indicate that patients prefer transparent waiting areas with views of nature, daylight, perceived warmth, non-institutional furniture arrangements, visual orientation, and the use of natural materials for interior design [67]. The design of physical environments in healthcare should also reflect cultural preferences, allow for social interactions, and be sustainable [68]. For the elderly, daylighting is important, along with high contrast handrails, slip-free flooring, sound/noise mitigation, biophilic spaces (e.g., photos with natural landscapes), and exposure to wearable technologies and the Internet of Medical Things [69]. Height-adjustable workstations reduce work-sitting times for personnel, while also contributing to the immersive health-conscious environment [70]. Medical fitness facilities require specialized equipment, but in contrast to gyms, they are fully integrated into the Lifestyle Medicine Center with the use of protocols and a network of HCPs that have degrees and certifications. When renovating the Lifestyle Medicine Center, it is important to note that any patient experience metrics may be positively biased for a year or more [71].

Managing

The successful practice in a dedicated Lifestyle Medicine Center relies on implementation science, which targets increased incorporation of evidence-based innovations into routine settings to improve the quality and outcomes of services [72, 73]. On one level, this can simply be the electronic implementation of clinical practice guidelines [19]. However, on more pragmatic and ambitious levels, implementation science consists of behavioral changes that close the evidence-practice gap, engage stakeholders in the community (individuals [micro-level], organizations [meso-level], and populations [macro-level]), and exhibit flexibility with nonlinear (e.g., cyclical over time) approaches in real-world scenarios [74]. In a critical review and synthesis, McIsaac et al. [75] found that many implementation science theories were not applicable to macro-level factors, and those that were applicable lacked

Table 3.1 Management of a Lifestyle Medicine Center[a]

Core services	Business
Mission statement	Successful core services
Vision statement	Cost containment
Positive health messaging	Flexible payment models
Evidence-based care	Marketing and branding
Individual clinical outcomes	Balance sheet targets
Population health	Sustainability

[a]Both categories require knowledge and implementation science. Mission and vision statements may include clinical, research, and educational objectives about health. Balance sheet targets can range from profitability, to revenue neutrality, to acceptable losses based on the mission statement and organizational structure (e.g., freestanding medical practice versus clinical service line in a larger sponsoring health system)

sufficient guidance on structural factors, such as social determinants of health. In fact, as lifestyle medicine practices become more and more complex, non-evidence-based policies and protocols will need to be de-implemented [73]. Moreover, failures of effective implementation strategies that recognize the behavioral uniqueness of certain populations can lead to health inequities in the community [76].

The management of ongoing activities in the Lifestyle Medicine Center can be considered in two broad categories: core services and business. The core services of the Center are related to health with deliverables that are related to the mission/vision statements and clinical outcomes; the business of the center is related to fiscal soundness with deliverables that are related to the balance sheet and organizational sustainability (Table 3.1). Marketing can subserve both categories with social marketing improving healthy behaviors (health marketing) [77–81] and traditional commercial marketing improving patient referrals and retention. Research Centers may have different care and business models than clinical Centers, but the deliverables are still the same: accomplishing the mission and sustainability. Informatics, registries, and technology play an increasing role in the success of all types of Lifestyle Medicine Centers, and the relatively high initial and ongoing costs for this infrastructure pose a significant challenge.

Within the context of a clinical service line and available payment models, organizational structure needs to be aligned with a shared focus of attention (operational tactics, personnel roles and relationships, and patient-centered needs and engagement) [82]. With value-based services in an academic setting, organizational structures require recruitments of key physician leaders who can positively engage matrixed models of governance, management, clinical care, education, and research to create streamlined and coordinated workflows that transcend historical department-based silos and cultures [83].

Conclusion

Lifestyle medicine is centered on chronic disease risk management through nonpharmacological and nonprocedural means, on both individual- and population-based scales. However, despite the expanding evidence base and even awareness of how healthy lifestyles promote well-being and decrease chronic disease risk, there is still a significant chronic disease burden in society, particularly multi-morbid disease states. The explanation of this discrepancy is based on implementation, which consists of translating knowledge into action plans, and then materializing and optimizing a Lifestyle Medicine Center. The materialization process consists of conceptualization based on the environment and chronic care model (research, clinical practice, and education) and operationalization based on implementation science (planning, building, and managing).

Optimization is an adaptive process that responds to positive and negative events with a resultant trend toward superior effectiveness. The main dimensions of optimization are clinical and financial. Optimization includes scale-up and scale-out growth and is necessary for sustainability. Though fairly ambitious, as more Lifestyle Medicine Centers are built, providing more and more clinical services, a new culture of health and healthcare can be realized.

References

1. Satija A, Stampfer MJ, Rimm EB, et al. Perspective: are large, simple trials the solution for nutrition research? Adv Nutr. 2018;9:378–87.
2. Hill B, McPhie S, Moran LJ, et al. Lifestyle intervention to prevent obesity during pregnancy: implications and recommendations for research and implementation. Midwifery. 2017;49:13–8.
3. Pagoto S. The current state of lifestyle intervention implementation research: where do we go next? TBM. 2011;1:401–5.
4. Unim B, De Vito C, Massimi A, et al. The need to improve implementation and use of lifestyle surveillance systems for planning prevention activities: an analysis of the Italian regions. Public Health. 2016;130:51–8.
5. Mechanick JI, Hurley DL, Garvey WT. Adiposity-based chronic disease as a new diagnostic term: American Association of Clinical Endocrinologists and the American College of Endocrinology position statement. Endocr Pract. 2017;23:372–8.
6. Mechanick JI, Garber AJ, Grunberger G, Handelsman Y, Garvey WT. Dysglycemia-based chronic disease: an American Association of Clinical Endocrinologists position statement. Endocr Pract. 2018;24:995–1011.
7. Mechanick JI, Farkouh ME, Newman JD, Garvey WT. Cardiometabolic-based chronic disease – adiposity and dysglycemia drivers. J Am Coll Cardiol. 2020; [In Press].
8. Mechanick JI, Farkouh ME, Newman JD, Garvey WT. Cardiometabolic-based chronic disease – addressing knowledge and clinical practice gaps in the preventive care plan. J Am Coll Cardiol. 2020; [In Press].
9. Majumdar UB, Hunt C, Doupe P, et al. Multiple chronic conditions at a major urban health system: a retrospective cross-sectional analysis of frequencies, costs and comorbidity patterns. BMJ Open. 2019;9:e029340. https://doi.org/10.1136/bmjopen-2019-029340.
10. Bi J, Huang Y, Xiao Y, et al. Association of lifestyle factors and suboptimal health status: a cross-sectional study of Chinese students. BMJ Open. 2014;4:e5156.
11. Chen J, Xiang H, Jiang P, et al. The role of healthy lifestyle in the implementation of regressing suboptimal health status among college students in China: a nested case-control study. Int J Environ Res Publ Health. 2017;14:240. https://doi.org/10.3390/ijerph14030240.
12. Åkesson A, Larsson SC, Discacciati A, et al. Low-risk diet and lifestyle habits in the primary prevention of myocardial infarction in men: a population-based prospective cohort study. J Am Coll Cardiol. 2014;64:1299–306.
13. Mozaffarian D. The promise of lifestyle for cardiovascular health. J Am Coll Cardiol. 2014;64:1307–9.
14. Weaver CM, Gordon CM, Janz KF, et al. The National Osteoporosis Foundation's position statement on peak bone mass development and lifestyle factors: a systematic review and implementation recommendations. Osteoporos Int. 2016;27:1281–386.
15. Thomas K, Bendtsen P, Krevers B. Implementation of healthy lifestyle promotion in primary care: patients as coproducers. Patient Educ Couns. 2014;97:283–90.
16. Koelewijn-van Loon MS, van der Weijden T, Ronda G, et al. Improving lifestyle and risk perception through patient involvement in nurse-led cardiovascular risk management: a cluster-randomized controlled trial in primary care. Prev Med. 2010;50:35–44.
17. Schneeberger D, Golubic M, Moore HCF, et al. Lifestyle medicine-focused shared medical appointments to improve risk factors for chronic diseases and quality of life in breast cancer survivors. J Altern Complement Med. 2018; https://doi.org/10.1089/acm.2018.0154.
18. Pujol N, Jobin G, Beloucif S. 'Spiritual care is not the hospital's business': a qualitative study on the perspectives of patients about the integration of spirituality in healthcare settings. J Med Ethics. 2016;42:733–7.
19. Mechanick JI, Pessah-Pollack R, Camacho P, et al. American Association of Clinical Endocrinologists and American College of endocrinology protocol for standardized production of clinical practice guidelines, algorithms, and checklists – 2017 update. Endocr Pract. 2017;23:1–16.
20. Fisch MJ, McNeill LH, Basen-Engquist KM. Helping colorectal cancer survivors benefit from changing lifestyle behaviors. JAMA Oncol. 2018;4:777–8.
21. Rippe JM, Campanile G, Diehl H, et al. American College of Lifestyle Medicine expert panel discussion: implementing intensive therapeutic lifestyle change programs. Am J Lifestyle Med. 2017;11:375–86.
22. Torres R, Soltero S, Trak MA, et al. Lifestyle modification intervention for overweight and obese Hispanic pregnant women: development, implementation, lessons learned and future applications. Contemporary Clin Trials Communic. 2016;3:111–6.
23. Dennis S, Hetherington SA, Borodzicz JA, et al. Challenges to establishing successful partnerships in community health promotion programs: local experiences from the national implementation of healthy eating activity and lifestyle (HEAL™) program. Health Promotion J Austr. 2015;26:45–51.
24. Carlfjord S, Andersson A, Lindberg M. Experiences of the implementation of a tool for lifestyle intervention in primary health care: a qualitative study among managers and professional groups. BMC Health Serv Res. 2011;11:195. http://www.biomedcentral.com/1472-6963/11/195.
25. Cabassa LJ, Stefancic A. Context before implementation: a qualitative study of decision makers' views of a peer-led healthy lifestyle intervention for people with serious mental illness in supportive housing. TBM. 2019;9:217–26.

26. Berendsen BAJ, Kremers SPJ, Savelberg HHCM, et al. The implementation and sustainability of a combined lifestyle intervention in primary care: mixed method process evaluation. BMC Fam Pract. 2015;16:37. https://doi.org/10.1186/s12875-015-0254-5.

27. van de Glind IM, Heinen MM, Evers AW, et al. Factors influencing the implementation of a lifestyle counseling program in patients with venous leg ulcers: a multiple case study. Implementation Sci. 2012;7:104. http://www.implementationscience.com/content/7/1/104.

28. Wierenga D, Engbers LH, Empelen PV, et al. The implementation of multiple lifestyle interventions in two organizations. JOEM. 2014;56:1195–206.

29. Jarrett BY, Lin AW, Lujan ME. A commentary on the new evidence–based lifestyle recommendations for patients with polycystic ovary syndrome and potential barriers to their implementation in the United States. J Acad Nutr Dietet. 2019;119:205–10.

30. Blackshaw LCD, Chhour I, Stepto NK, et al. Barriers and facilitators to the implementation of evidence-based lifestyle management in polycystic ovary syndrome: a narrative review. Med Sci. 2019;7:76. https://doi.org/10.3390/medsci7070076.

31. Gibbs JC, McArthur C, Milligan J, et al. Measuring the implementation of lifestyle-integrated functional exercise in primary care for older adults: results of a feasibility study. Can J Aging. 2019; https://doi.org/10.1017/S0714980818000739.

32. Roumen C, Blaak EE, Corpeleijn E. Lifestyle intervention for prevention of diabetes: determinants of success for future implementation. Nutr Rev. 2009;67:132–46.

33. Polak R, Finkelstein A, Axelrod T, et al. Medical students as health coaches: implementation of a student-initiated lifestyle medicine curriculum. Isr J Health Policy Res. 2017;6:42. https://doi.org/10.1186/s13584-017-0167-y.

34. Kaye S, Pathman J, Skelton JA. Development and implementation of a student-led lifestyle medicine curriculum. Am J Lifestyle Med. 2019;13:253–61.

35. Den Braver NR, Lakerveld J, Rutters F, et al. Built environmental characteristics and diabetes: a systematic review and meta-analysis. BMC Med. 2018;16:12. https://doi.org/10.1186/s12916-017-0997-z.

36. Li Y, Padrón NA, Mangla AT, et al. Using systems science to inform population health strategies in local health departments: a case study in San Antonio, Texas. Public Health Rep. 2017;132:549–55.

37. Mechanick JI, Davidson JA, Fergus IV, et al. Transcultural diabetes care in the United States – a position statement by the American Association of Clinical Endocrinologists. Endocr Pract. 2019; https://doi.org/10.4158/PS-2019-0080.

38. Browne AJ, Varcoe C, Lavoie J, et al. Enhancing health care equity with indigenous populations: evidence-based strategies from an ethnographic study. BMC Health Serv Res. 2016;16:544. https://doi.org/10.1186/s12913-016-1707-9.

39. Vojta D, Koehler TB, Longjohn M, et al. A coordinated national model for diabetes prevention. Am J Prev Med. 2013;44:S301–6.

40. Look MA, Kaholokula JK, Carvahlo A, et al. Developing a culturally based cardiac rehabilitation program: the HELA study. Prog Community Health Partnersh. 2012;6:103–10.

41. Philpot LM, Stockbridge EL, Padrón NA, et al. Patient-centered medical home features and health care expenditures of Medicare beneficiaries with chronic disease dyads. Popul Health Manag. 2016;19 https://doi.org/10.1089/pop.2015.0077.

42. Rhodes EC, Chandrasekar EK, Patel SA, et al. Cost-effectiveness of a faith-based lifestyle intervention for diabetes prevention among African Americans: a within-trial analysis. Diab Res Clin Pract. 2018; https://doi.org/10.1016/j.diabres.2018.09.016.

43. Wagner EH, Austin BT, Michael VK. Organizing care for patients with chronic illness. Milbank Q. 1996;7:511–44.

44. Sendall M, McCosker L, Crossley K, et al. A structured review of chronic care model components supporting transition between healthcare service delivery types for older people with multiple chronic diseases. Health Inform Manage J. 2017;46:58–68.

45. Barnett K, Mercer S, Norbury M, et al. Epidemiology of multimorbidity and implications for health care, research, and medical education: a cross-sectional study. Lancet. 2012;380:37–43.

46. Boehmer KR, Abu Dabrh AM, Giofriddo MR, et al. Does the chronic care model meet the emerging needs of people living with multimorbidity? A systematic review and thematic synthesis PLoS ONE. 2018;13:e0190852.

47. Sugavanam T, Fosh B, Close J, et al. Codesigning a measure of person-centred coordinated care to capture the experience of the patient: the development of the P3CEQ. J patient Experience. 2018;5:201–11.

48. Lloyd H, Wheat H, Horrell J, et al. Patient-reported measures for person-centered coordinated care: a comparative domain map and web-based compendium for supporting policy development and implementation. J Med Internet Res. 2018;20:e54. https://doi.org/10.2196/jmir.7789.

49. Lloyd HM, Pearson M, Sheaff R, et al. Collaborative action for person-centred coordinated care (P3C): an approach to support the development of a comprehensive system-wide solution to fragmented care. Health Res Policy Syst. 2017;15:98. https://doi.org/10.1186/s12961-017-0263-z.

50. Meltzer DO, Ruhnke GW. Redesigning care for patients at increased hospitalization risk: the comprehensive care physician model. Health Aff. 2014;33:770–7.

51. Wu YC, Tung HH, Wei J. Quality of life, demoralization syndrome and health-related lifestyle in cardiac transplant recipients – a longitudinal study in Taiwan. Eur J Cardiovasc Nurs. 2018; https://doi.org/10.1177/1474515118800397.

52. Samson A, Siam H. Adapting to major chronic illness: a proposal for a comprehensive task-model approach. Patient Educ Counsel. 2008;70:426–9.

53. Gordon NF, Salmon RD, Mitchell BS, et al. Innovative approaches to comprehensive cardiovascular disease risk reduction in clinical and community-based settings. Curr Atheroscler Rep. 2001;3:498–506.

54. Villablanca AC, Beckett LA, Li Y, et al. Outcomes of comprehensive heart care programs in high-risk women. J Women's Health. 2010;19:1313–25.

55. Powell LH, Appelhans BM, Ventrelle J, et al. Development of a lifestyle intervention for the metabolic syndrome: discovery through proof-of-concept. Health Psychol. 2018;37:929–39.

56. Yacoub TG. Combining clinical judgment with guidelines for the management of type 2 diabetes: overall standards of comprehensive care. Postgrad Med. 2015;126:85–94.

57. Abbasi AA, Grunberger G, Parikh S, et al. Diabetes care credit system: a model for comprehensive and optimal diabetes care. Endocr Pract. 2004;10:187–94.

58. Golubic M, Schneeberger D, Kirkpatrick K, et al. Comprehensive lifestyle modification intervention to improve chronic disease risk factors and quality of life in cancer survivors. J Altern Complement Med. 2018; https://doi.org/10.1089/acm.2018.0193.

59. Pimental PA, O'Hara JB, Jandak JL. Neuropsychologists as primary care providers of cognitive health: a novel comprehensive cognitive wellness service delivery model. Appl Neuropsychol Adult. 2018;25:318–26.

60. Shakersain B, Rizzuto D, Wang HX, et al. An active lifestyle reinforces the effect of a healthy diet on cognitive function: a population-based longitudinal study. Nutrients. 2018;10:1297. https://doi.org/10.3390/nu10091297.

61. Chan AS, Cheung WK, Yeung MK, et al. Sustained effects of memory and lifestyle interventions on memory functioning of older adults: an 18-month follow-up study. Front Aging Neurosci. 2018;10:240. https://doi.org/10.3389/fnagi.2018.00240.

62. Yarborough BJH, Stumbo SP, Cavese JA, et al. Patient perspectives on how living with a mental illness affects making and maintain-

ing healthy lifestyle changes. Patient Educ Couns. 2018; https://doi.org/10.1016/j.pec.2018.08.036.

63. De Gregori M, Belfer I, De Giorgio R, et al. Second edition of SIMPAR's "Fedd Your Destiny" workshop: the role of lifestyle in improving pain management. J Pain Res. 2018;11:1627–36.

64. Braman M, Edison M. How to create a successful lifestyle medicine practice. Am J Lifestyle Med. 2017;11:404–7.

65. Graff K. A micropractice/community partnership model for lifestyle medicine. Am J Lifestyle Med. 2018;12:124–7.

66. Toll E, Melfi BS. The healing power of paint. JAMA. 2017;317:1100–2.

67. Jiang S, Powers M, Allison D, et al. Informing healthcare waiting area design using transparency attributes: a comparative preference study. Health Environ Res Des J. 2017;10:49–63.

68. Anaker A, Heylighen A, Nordin S, et al. Design quality in the context of healthcare environments: a scoping review. Health Environ Res Des J. 2017;10:136–50.

69. Engineer A, Sternberg EM, Najafi B. Designing interiors to mitigate physical and cognitive deficits related to aging and to promote longevity in older adults: a review. Gerontology. 2018; https://doi.org/10.1159/000491488.

70. Li I, Mackey MG, Foley B, et al. Reducing office workers' sitting time at work using sit-stand protocols: results from a pilot randomized controlled trial. JOEM. 2017;59:543–9.

71. Gauthey J, Tieche R, Streit S. Interior renovation of a general practitioner office leads to a perceptual bias on patient experience for over one year. PLoS One. 2018;13:e0193221.

72. Eccles MP, Mittman BS. Welcome to implementation science. Implementa Sci. 2006;1:1–3. https://doi.org/10.1186/1748-5908-1-1.

73. Wolk CB, Beidas RS. The intersection of implementation science and behavioral health: an introduction to the special issue. Behav Ther. 2018;49:477–80.

74. Handley MA, Gorukanti A, Cattamanchi A. Strategies for implementing implementation science: a methodological overview. Emerg Med J. 2016;33:660–4.

75. McIsaac JL, Warner G, Lawrence L, et al. The application of implementation science theories for population health: a critical interpretive synthesis. AIMS Public Health. 2018;5:13–30.

76. Napoles AM, Stewart AL. Transcreation: an implementation science framework for community-engaged behavioral interventions to reduce health disparities. BMC Health Serv Res. 2018; https://doi.org/10.1186/s12913-018-3521-z.

77. Carins JE, Rundle-Thiele SR. Eating for the better: a social marketing review (2000-2012). Public Health Nutr. 2013;17:1628–39.

78. Liu E, Stephenson T, Houlihan J, et al. Marketing strategies to encourage rural residents of high-obesity countries to buy fruits and vegetables in grocery stores. Prev Chronic Dis. 2017;14:170109.

79. Aceves-Martins M, Llaurado E, Tarro L, et al. A school-based, peer-led, social marketing intervention to engage Spanish adolescents in a healthy lifestyle ("We Are Cool" – Som la Pera Study): a parallel-cluster randomized controlled study. Childhood Obes. 2017;13:300–13.

80. Chichirez CM, Purcarea VL, Davila C. Health marketing and behavioral change: a review of the literature. J Med Life. 2018;11:15–9.

81. Chau JY, McGill B, Thomas MM, et al. Is this health campaign really social marketing? A checklist to help you decide. Health Promot J Austral. 2018;29:79–83.

82. Louis CJ, Clark JR, Gray B, et al. Service line structure and decision-maker attention in 3 health systems: implications for patient-centered care. Health Care Management Rev. 2017; https://doi.org/10.1097/HMR.0000000000000172.

83. Phillips RA, Cyr J, Keaney JF, et al. Creating and maintaining a successful service line in an academic medical center at the dawn of value-based care: lessons learned from the heart and vascular service line at UMass memorial health care. Acad Med. 2015;90:1340–6.

Implementation Science Across Lifestyle Medicine Interventions

Prajakta Adsul, Lilian G. Perez, April Oh, and David A. Chambers

Abbreviations

CFIR	Consolidated Framework for Implementation Research
EBI	Evidence-based intervention
HCP	Healthcare professional
LC	Learning collaborative
NIH	National Institutes of Health
PTSD	Posttraumatic stress disorder
TLC	Telephone lifestyle coaching
VA QUERI	Veterans Affairs Quality Enhancement Research Initiative
WATI	Web-assisted tobacco interventions

The Research-to-Practice Gap

In the USA and across the globe, the primary risk factors for disability and premature death in adults are largely related to lifestyle behaviors (e.g., smoking, poor diet, and physical inactivity), which contribute to the rising prevalence of non-communicable diseases such as type 2 diabetes, hypertension, and cancer, among others [1–3]. Lifestyle medicine – defined as "the non-pharmacological and non-surgical management of chronic disease" – provides an approach to address the complexity of non-communicable diseases, including their behavioral root causes, in a clinical setting [4]. The past few decades in health behavior research have produced a growing database of lifestyle interventions including programs, practices, procedures, products, prescriptions, and policies. Such interventions can target individuals, groups, or populations. Interventions that have explicit evidence of improving health outcomes are considered "evidence-based," per the evidence-based medicine movement [5–7]. Although there are a growing number of evidence-based lifestyle interventions for improving health behaviors and related outcomes, such as those listed in the Research Tested Intervention Programs web database [8], the US Preventive Task Force preventive clinical services recommendations [9], and the Community Guide to Preventive Services [10], many challenges remain in implementing such interventions in clinical "real-world" settings.

Traditionally, systematic reviews and clinical and community guidelines [11, 12] have been the primary resources to guide practitioners on what should be implemented in clinical practice. However, relying on this passive way of diffusing information to clinical practitioners has only limited benefit. It is estimated that it takes an average of 17 years for research findings to be incorporated into clinical practice, and even then, only a small fraction of evidence-based interventions (EBI) are incorporated into real-world settings [13, 14]. Such efforts have done little to help individuals adopt and sustain healthy behaviors to improve health outcomes [15].

A key challenge to implementation of EBIs is the lack of understanding of how lifestyle EBIs should be translated into clinical practices and policies. In general, EBIs are implemented in controlled conditions, such as in clinical trials, which do not represent real-world, non-research settings. Differences between research and real-world settings can occur at multiple levels: patient (e.g., education), clinical team or group (e.g., team function/coordination), organizational (e.g., quality assurance and organizational culture), or larger system/environment (e.g., national organizations and payment policies) [16]. Furthermore, there are differences in context (geographic, cultural, etc.) and practical issues (cost, feasibility, acceptability, etc.), which can also influence the implementation of EBIs [17].

P. Adsul (✉)
Department of Internal Medicine, University of New Mexico, Albuquerque, NM, USA
e-mail: padsul@salud.unm.edu

L. G. Perez
Behavioral and Policy Sciences Department, RAND Corporation, Santa Monica, CA, USA
e-mail: lperez@rand.org

A. Oh · D. A. Chambers
Division of Cancer Control and Population Sciences, National Cancer Institute, Rockville, MD, USA
e-mail: April.oh@nih.gov; dchamber@mail.nih.gov

© Springer Nature Switzerland AG 2020
J. I. Mechanick, R. F. Kushner (eds.), *Creating a Lifestyle Medicine Center*, https://doi.org/10.1007/978-3-030-48088-2_4

Implementation science bridges this research-to-practice gap by building a knowledge base about how EBIs are integrated into clinical and community settings for public health and healthcare services. The National Institutes of Health (NIH) defines implementation science as "the study of methods to promote the integration of research findings and evidence into healthcare policy and practice." [18]. More specifically, implementation research in healthcare is the scientific study of strategies that adopt and integrate health-related EBIs into clinical and community settings to improve patient- and population-based clinical outcomes.

While implementation science shares common ancestry with centuries-old activities targeting improvements in medical care, it has become far more systematic in its conceptual models, research designs, and measures over the past 20 years. The US federal agency efforts, including the "Translating Research into Practice" by the Agency for Healthcare Research and Quality ([Accessed: August 29, 2019]), Veteran's Affairs (VA) Quality Enhancement Research Initiative (QUERI) (https://www.queri.research. va.gov/ [Accessed: August 29, 2019]), and NIH Dissemination and Implementation Research funding announcements ([Accessed: August 29, 2019]), aim to expand the quality and quantity of implementation science.

Lifestyle medicine has been at the leading edge of many of these efforts. For example, the National Institute of Mental Health held multiple workshops and conferences in the early 2000s to increase implementation science activities in depression, bipolar illness, and child trauma, among other topics. The Veterans Affairs (VA) Quality Enhancement Research Initiative (QUERI) centers concentrated on mental health, substance abuse, diabetes, and other lifestyle medicine priorities [19]. The National Cancer Institute's "Designing for Dissemination" meetings focused on improving the fit among research, practice, and public health for known cancer risk factors (e.g., diet, physical activity, and tobacco use) [20]. These initiatives have culminated in ongoing funding opportunities that have supported hundreds of implementation studies, an annual meeting bringing together well over 1200 participants, training programs, multiple journals, and even a Society for Implementation Research Collaboration.

Fundamentals of Implementation Science

Theories, Frameworks, and Models

Implementation research typically involves the use of theories and frameworks from a variety of fields of health research. Specifically, up to 159 theories, frameworks, and models are aggregated across multiple individual, organizational, and community levels [21, 22]. These theories can provide overarching guidance for understanding implemen-

tation context, processes, and outcomes. A commonly used framework has been the Consolidated Framework for Implementation Research (CFIR). The CFIR was developed in an attempt to reduce redundancy and integrate previously published theories to provide researchers with a core comprehensive and standardized list of determinants of the implementation process [23]. The authors of the framework propose using CFIR as a roadmap to understand these concepts across multiple interventions and contexts to build a deeper understanding of the complexity of implementation.

Investigators studying the Better Exercise Adherence After Treatment for Cancer (BEAT-Cancer) intervention used the CFIR model to inform the development of an implementation toolkit [24]. BEAT-Cancer is a three-month intervention to improve physical activity among rural women cancer survivors through supervised exercise sessions, counseling, and home exercise programs [25]. Following confirmation of efficacy, the investigators used the toolkit to guide implementation in other community research sites. The toolkit was informed by qualitative interviews with potential program interventionists and other stakeholders (e.g., hospital administrators, healthcare professionals [HCP], and advocacy groups), who identified multiple CFIR constructs relevant to study parameters. Example constructs included implementation process (e.g., engaging, reflecting, and evaluating), intervention characteristics (e.g., design quality, cost, and adaptability), and individual characteristics (e.g., knowledge and beliefs). The interventionists and other stakeholders also identified strategies to target those constructs at multiple levels (individual, organizational, and community) – e.g., physician buy-in, community involvement, evaluation data, and fundraisers – which can help enhance implementation success.

Implementation Outcomes and Strategies

An important advance in the field of implementation science has been the conceptualization of implementation outcomes [26]. These are distinguished from service delivery (e.g., efficiency, equity, and patient-centered care) and health outcomes and include acceptability, appropriateness, adoption, costs, feasibility, fidelity, penetration, and sustainability [26, 27]. When translating EBIs to practice settings, these implementation outcomes can help specify processes and measures for success. Furthermore, contextual factors for success are identified when these outcomes are considered on multiple levels within a socioecologic framework (e.g., individual, HCP, and healthcare organizational frameworks).

The instruments available to measure implementation outcomes have been recently reviewed [27]. In addition to quantitative measures, there are resources that provide guidance and examples for the use of qualitative methods to measure implementation outcomes [28–30]. The selection

Table 4.1 Implementation outcomes[a]

Implementation outcomes	Definitions [26,27]	Measures available (27)	Relevant examples or resources
Acceptability	Satisfaction or agreement with various aspects of the intervention among implementation stakeholders	50 instruments	Evidence-based practice attitude scale for measuring providers attitudes [51]
Adoption	The initial decision, intention, or action to try and use an evidence-based intervention; also referred to as uptake or utilization	19 instruments	Adoption of Information technology Innovation [52]
Appropriateness	Perceived fit, relevance, or compatibility of the intervention with the implementation problem or issue; also referred to as compatibility	7 instruments	Factors influencing the adoption of an innovation [53]
Feasibility	The extent to which an intervention can be successfully implemented in a given practice setting	8 instruments	Feasibility of intervention measure [54]
Fidelity	Degree to which an intervention was implemented as intended by the intervention developers	No instruments	Data collection methods for measuring fidelity [55]
Implementation cost	The financial impact of an implementation effort	8 instruments	Utilization and cost questionnaire [56]
Penetration	Integration of an intervention within a practice setting	4 instruments	Levels of institutionalization scale [57]
Sustainability	The extent to which an intervention is maintained or institutionalized within a practice setting	8 instruments	Program sustainability assessment tool [58]

[a]References provided in brackets

of methods and measures depends on the research question, and several resources, such as web-based repositories and tools, are available to guide their selection [31, 32]. Table 4.1 provides a list of selected implementation outcomes, their definitions, the number of quantitative measures available, and examples of studies assessing each outcome.

The Telephone Lifestyle Coaching (TLC) program is an example of a program that assessed an implementation outcome [33]. This program examined a telephone-based coaching intervention targeting lifestyle behaviors in VA facilities and focused on penetration [33]. Specifically, the program evaluated the extent to which referral processes were integrated into the clinical settings of the participating VA facilities [33]. The direct measure used was the facility referral rate, defined as the number of TLC referrals divided by the monthly average number of veterans enrolled in primary care at each facility in the first 12 months of the program [33]. An evaluation showed successful implementation of the TLC program, with about 13 referrals made per 1000 veterans, of whom 57% enrolled and participated in at least one telephone coaching session.

Besides implementation outcomes, there has been extensive focus on implementation strategies, which are conceptualized as the specific means or methods for adopting and sustaining interventions [34]. Waltz et al. [35] compiled implementation strategies in the Expert Recommendations for Implementing Change study. This study identified 73 distinct strategies and grouped them into 9 categories: engaging consumers, using evaluative and iterative strategies, changing infrastructure, adapting and tailoring to context, developing stakeholder relationships, utilizing financial strategies, supporting clinicians, providing interactive assistance, and training and educating stakeholders [35].

In the TLC program example, investigators used multiple implementation strategies to promote penetration, such as training and educating stakeholders, developing stakeholder relationships (e.g., creating an advisory board and identifying points of contact at each facility), and using financial strategies (e.g., providing the program at no cost to patients) [33]. VA facilities with the most skilled implementation leaders who effectively led the multicomponent implementation strategies showed the greatest penetration, whereas facilities with less support had the lowest [33].

Another example investigated a diabetes care intervention that was implemented within small, autonomous primary care clinics using practice facilitation as an implementation strategy to overcome challenges to providing care according to the Chronic Care Model [36]. A trained facilitator assisted clinicians using multiple tools: group/shared medical appointments, diabetes registry, point-of-care hemoglobin A1c testing, resources/approaches to patient education/activation, and planned diabetes visits with clinical reminders and decision support for clinical staff. The facilitator worked with clinicians and staff to adapt the tools to their patient and clinical context. Evaluation of the practice facilitation implementation strategy showed that it significantly improved delivery of diabetes care consistent with the Chronic Care Model and this was sustained at one-year post-implementation.

Methods and Study Designs

To reduce the time lag between research discovery and clinical uptake, some researchers have also suggested blending effectiveness and implementation study designs, referred to as "hybrid designs" [37]. These hybrid designs typically take on three approaches: [a] testing effectiveness of interventions while gathering information on implementation, [b] simultaneously testing effectiveness and implementation of interventions, and [c] testing implementation while gathering information on effectiveness of interventions.

A hybrid implementation-effectiveness study often evaluates the implementation strategy and the clinical intervention's effects [38]. One such study was the Quality Improvement in Tobacco – Provider Referrals and Internet-Delivered Microsystem Optimization (QUIT-PRIMO) trial, a national study that evaluated the clinical practice innovation (implementation strategy), specifically using an e-portal to refer smokers to Web-Assisted Tobacco Interventions (WATIs), and the effects of the WATI components on smoking cessation (clinical intervention). Practices were randomized to either the paper-referral (comparison condition) or the e-portal referral group (intervention). Those referred to the e-portal received e-mails encouraging them to register to a WATI. For their implementation aims, the researchers measured the number of smokers referred and smokers registering to a WATI. To test the effects of the WATIs, registered smokers were randomized to receive either standard features (e.g., a tailored, interactive smoking cessation website) or enhanced features (either standard features plus automated motivational e-mail messages or standard features plus automated motivational e-mail messages, access to an online support group, and access to a tobacco treatment specialist).

To facilitate the implementation of the referrals, the program identified and trained implementation coordinators (e.g., physicians, nurses, or other staff) at each practice on the referral procedures and to facilitate adoption of the referral system. The implementation coordinators could decide on how to adopt and use the referral system in their practice. This facilitation strategy was based on the Promoting Action on Research Implementation in Health Services (PARIHS) framework [39]. Results of the trial showed that although the mean number of smokers referred to the WATIs did not differ by mode (paper vs. e-portal), the rate of smoker registration in the e-portal referral group was nearly triple that of the paper-referral group [39]. In terms of clinical effectiveness, the smokers randomized to the WATIs with enhanced features were significantly more likely to quit than those in the standard-features WATIs [39].

An additional methodology that is currently gaining traction in its efforts to reduce the research-to-practice gap is the use of learning systems or collaboratives, which typically comprise multiple partners from a system joining forces to create knowledge around change [40]. For example, the VA used a Learning Collaborative (LC) model to facilitate implementation of incorporating integrated care for smoking cessation into routine treatment for veterans with posttraumatic stress disorder (PTSD) [41]. The first step to creating the LC was to establish an expert panel of individuals who were deemed integral to the implementation of integrated care for smoking cessation (veterans, VA administrators, experts in PTSD treatment, etc.). The panel identified a set of overarching goals and key objectives for achieving those goals across three domains – organizational support and capacity, clinical competence, and effective veteran engagement. Then, a separate group of experts was tasked to design and implement the LC across 12 VA PTSD facilities. This group identified three to five staff from each facility considered key to implementing integrated care. One of those staff members was identified as the clinical champion tasked to train other PTSD providers at their facility. In this study, a clinical champion was considered as someone who was key for implementation and could lead the trainings for other clinical staff in the setting.

The expert panels and facility teams held learning sessions focused on different topics, such as clinical skill building and quality improvement tools, to identify and address barriers to implementation. After the learning sessions, the teams focused on several integrated care activities such as educating patients about cessation resources, engaging tobacco users in treatment, delivering integrated care, and addressing implementation barriers, among other activities. Delivery of integrated care was documented in electronic health records to produce cumulative reports, which allowed for assessment of progress toward implementation of integrated care across facilities. Overall, an evaluation of the LC showed that approximately 400 veterans received integrated care for smoking cessation following the first learning session and that additional clinic staff (trained by the clinical champions) began delivering integrated care in that period, pointing to the feasibility of spreading the intervention at some sites.

Specific Recommendations

Engage a Broad Range of Stakeholders to Coproduce Knowledge Regarding Implementation

Successful implementation of evidence-based lifestyle interventions depends on involving a broad range of stakeholders among the HCP team (e.g., physicians, advanced practice providers, nutritionists, counselors, and physician assistants) and non-professional staff. These stakeholders span multiple disciplines in academic communities and can cross boundaries to include community perspectives [42]. Traditional, linear processes may be limited in gathering perspectives from these stakeholders, and using implementation science can help accelerate the uptake of interventions by its inherent ability to encourage partnerships across different disciplines.

Furthermore, understanding diverse stakeholder perspectives early in the design and intervention development phase can reduce the time it takes for an intervention to be adopted into clinical practice.

For example, implementing health information technologies in the healthcare setting has been influenced by technical, social, organizational, and wider social-political factors [43]. Using a systematic approach to information technology interventions with careful planning can be helpful in achieving rapid large-scale impact. Other approaches may include internal and external advisory boards that consider patient and community roles, human-centered design approaches, knowledge integration pathways, and community-based participatory research activities. Specifically, participatory implementation science has been considered as an important tool to support the increased adoption and implementation of EBI in real-world settings [44]. Additionally, gathering stakeholder perspectives can often result in collaborations and engagements needed for evaluating the effectiveness of lifestyle medicine programs in clinical settings.

Build Capacity to Optimize Delivery of Lifestyle Interventions

Among the many requirements for a Lifestyle Medicine Center are considerations for how best to address the contextual variables that may influence implementation and adaptation of interventions to ensure they are appropriate for the target settings and populations. Several frameworks in implementation science can help systematically assess and address context and increase capacity for delivery, such as the CFIR [45], Exploration, Preparation, Implementation and the Sustainment (EPIS) [46], and the Practical Robust Implementation and Sustainability Model (PRISM) [47]. A recent scoping review that assesses emerging evidence highlighted four widely addressed context dimensions: organizational support, financial resources, social relations and support, and leadership [48]. Although it can be difficult to explore all dimensions of context in which an intervention is implemented, it remains critical to acknowledge and recognize at minimum the most relevant dimensions to lifestyle medicine.

Successful implementation of lifestyle medicine EBIs also requires the consideration of how well they fit within existing healthcare systems (Table 4.2). Implementors need to proactively and iteratively determine any necessary adaptations to an intervention. A recent review identified 13 frameworks that could help guide the process of adaptation in healthcare settings and engagement of a diverse set of stakeholders to gather perspectives [49]. Some researchers have described the idea of an "adaptome," which reflects a data platform that systematically captures information across settings and populations on adaptations in the delivery and/or intervention, and can help provide essential feedback to implementers [50]. The availability of such data can have an important influence on the implementation of EBIs across lifestyle modalities.

Table 4.2 Interventions across the lifestyle modalities[a]

Intervention	Setting studied	Target audience	Barriers and facilitators	Examples of implementation strategies used	Indicators of success
Diabetes prevention program [59, 60]	Veteran affairs clinics across the USA	Staff, coordinators, managers, clinical leaders, primary care personnel	REAIM specific at the organizational level	Champion/ training/ adaptation	Participant's satisfaction, implementation cost, delivery fidelity
Telephone Lifestyle Coaching [33]	24 veteran affairs clinics	VA personnel	Challenges in referring and recruiting target individuals	Changing infrastructure, engaging stakeholders, altering patient fees	Penetration, referral rates,
Team-based diabetes care based on the chronic care model [36]	Primary care	Primary care staff and clinicians	Organization of the staff through redesign and improvement	Practice facilitation	Delivery of team-based care consistent with the chronic care model
Web-assisted tobacco intervention (WATI) [38]	Community-based primary care practices	Clinical practice	Paper referrals in clinical systems do not work	Practice innovation (e-portal to refer smokers to WATI)	Referral rates

[a]References in brackets. Abbreviations: *REAIM* Reach Effectiveness Adoption Implementation Maintenance, *VA* Veterans Affairs

Training and Resources for the Science of Implementation

Training programs in implementation science provide opportunities to realize the full potential of the discipline. For example, the NIH Training Institute for Dissemination and Implementation in Health has been providing short-course trainings for doctoral level investigators (e.g., PhD and MD) each year since 2011 (https://www.scgcorp.com/tidirh2019/index.html [Accessed August 10, 2019]). The NIH Clinical and Translational Science Awards Program also supports implementation research training to faculty and scholars at medical research institutions. An increasing number of graduate and doctoral programs are now available with an emphasis on implementation science such as Master's in Clinical Research, Certificate Programs in Implementation Science, and PhD programs in translational science. Additional training opportunities and resources are provided by the US Department of Veterans Affairs (https://www.queri.research.va.gov/ [Accessed August 29, 2019]).

A mainstay of implementation science is the incorporation of transdisciplinary approaches such as organizational change, business, cost-effectiveness, and behavioral medicine, across the design, planning, and evaluation of implementation studies. Resources and toolkits such as the Implementation Science at a Glance (https://cancercontrol.cancer.gov/IS/docs/NCI-ISaaG-Workbook.pdf [Accessed August 25, 2019]) can help guide practitioners in considering the implementation of EBIs in their settings. Furthermore, there are implementation science funding opportunities to assist researchers and practitioners across health domains, such as cancer, cardiovascular, and aging, that are included in the NIH Funding Opportunity Announcement (https://grants.nih.gov/grants/guide/pa-files/PAR-19-274.html [Accessed August 25, 2019]). Organizations supporting implementation science include US federal agencies, such as the NIH (www.grants.gov [Accessed August 25, 2019]) and VA (https://www.research.va.gov/funding/ [Accessed August 25, 2019]), academic institutions, and the Patient-Centered Outcomes Research Institute (https://www.pcori.org/ [Accessed August 25, 2019]).

Conclusion

Integrating implementation science within lifestyle medicine programs can offer the theoretical and methodological tools to improve clinical practice and achieve health impact. Table 4.3 highlights some core aspects of implementation science studies. The lifestyle medicine community can use these tools to engage stakeholders and build capacity to optimize the delivery of interventions using the existing resources available within the field of implementation science. It is a collective hope that the science of implementation helps accelerate efforts in adopting healthy behaviors, preventing chronic disease, and reducing mortality worldwide.

Table 4.3 Fundamentals of implementation science

Concept	Definition/explanation
Implementation science	The study of methods to promote the integration of research findings and evidence into healthcare policy and practice [18]
Implementation theories, frameworks and models	Over 100 theories, models, and frameworks have been developed to explain the process of integrating research findings into practice. These frameworks help identify key influences on implementation, multiple actors within local and national contexts, and stages of change [21, 22]
Implementation outcomes	These include acceptability, appropriateness, adoption, costs, feasibility, fidelity, penetration, and sustainability [26, 27]
Implementation strategies	These are specific means or methods for adopting and sustaining interventions in community or clinical practice. Examples include engaging consumers, using evaluative and iterative strategies, changing infrastructure, adapting and tailoring to context, developing stakeholder relationships, utilizing financial strategies, supporting clinicians, providing interactive assistance, and training and educating stakeholders [35, 61]
Implementation science methods	Implementation scientists use a range of study designs, including observational, experimental, and quasi-experimental, and include quantitative, qualitative, and mixed methods [62]

References

1. Mokdad AH, Marks JS, Stroup DF, et al. Actual causes of death in the United States, 2000. JAMA. 2004;291:1238–45.
2. Ford ES, Bergmann MM, Boeing H, et al. Healthy lifestyle behaviors and all-cause mortality among adults in the United States. Prev Med. 2012;55:23–7.
3. US Burden of Disease Collaborators, Mokdad AH, Ballestros K, Echko M, et al. The state of US health, 1990-2016: Burden of diseases, injuries, and risk factors among US states. JAMA. 2018;319:1444–72.
4. Kushner RF, Mechanick JI. The importance of healthy living and defining lifestyle medicine. Lifestyle Medicine: Springer; 2016. p. 9–15.
5. Masic I, Miokovic M, Muhamedagic B. Evidence based medicine – new approaches and challenges. Acta Inform Med. 2008;16:219–25.
6. Sackett DL, Rosenberg WMC, Gray JAM, et al. Evidence based medicine: what it is and what it isn't. BMJ. 1996;312:71–2.
7. Rychetnik L, Hawe P, Waters E, et al. A glossary for evidence based public health. J Epidemiol Comm Health. 2004;58:538–45.
8. National Cancer Institute. Research-Tested Intervention Programs (RTIPs). https://rtips.cancer.gov/rtips/index.do. Updated 11/21/19. Accessed 24 Jan 2020.
9. U.S. Preventive Services Task Force. U.S. Preventive Services Task Force Recommendations for Primary Care Practice 2019. https://

www.uspreventiveservicestaskforce.org/Page/Name/recommenda-tions. Accessed 24 Jan 2020.

10. Centers for Disease Control and Prevention. Community Preventive Services Task Force Findings: The Community Guide, 2019. https://www.thecommunityguide.org/task-force-findings. Accessed on 24 Jan 2020.

11. Briss PA, Zaza S, Pappaioanou M, et al. Developing an evidence-based guide to community preventive services--methods. The task force on community preventive services. Am J Prev Med. 2000;18:35–43.

12. Krist AH, Bibbins-Domingo K, Wolff TA, et al. Advancing the methods of the U.S. preventive services task force. Am J Prev Med. 2018;54:S1–3.

13. Balas EA, Boren SA. Managing clinical knowledge for health care improvement. Yearbook of medical informatics 2000: Patient-Centered Systems; 2000.

14. Morris ZS, Wooding S, Grant J. The answer is 17 years, what is the question: understanding time lags in translational research. J Royal Soc Med. 2011;104:510–20.

15. Prochaska JJ, Prochaska JO. A review of multiple health behavior change interventions for primary prevention. Am J Lifestyle Med. 2011;5. https://doi.org/10.1177/1559827610391883.

16. Ferlie EB, Shortell SM. Improving the quality of health care in the United Kingdom and the United States: a framework for change. Milbank Q. 2001;79:281–315.

17. Ockene JK, Edgerton EA, Teutsch SM, et al. Integrating evidence-based clinical and community strategies to improve health. Am J Prev Med. 2007;32:244–52.

18. Department of Health and Human Services. PAR-19-274 Dissemination and Implementation Research in Health 2019. https://grants.nih.gov/grants/guide/pa-files/PAR-19-274.html. Accessed on 24 Jan 2020.

19. Chambers DA, Pintello D, Juliano-Bult D. Capacity-building and training opportunities for implementation science in mental health. Psychiatry Res. 2020;283:112511. https://doi.org/10.1016/j.psychres.2019.112511.

20. Chambers DA, Vinson CA, Norton WE. Advancing the science of implementation across the cancer continuum: Oxford University Press; 2018.

21. Tabak RG, Khoong EC, Chambers DA, et al. Bridging research and practice: models for dissemination and implementation research. Am J Prev Med. 2012;43:337–50.

22. Strifler L, Cardoso R, McGowan J, et al. Scoping review identifies significant number of knowledge translation theories, models, and frameworks with limited use. J Clin Epidemiol. 2018;100:92–102.

23. Damschroder LJ, Aron DC, Keith RE, et al. Fostering implementation of health services research findings into practice: a consolidated framework for advancing implementation science. Implementation Sci. 2009;4:50. https://doi.org/10.1186/1748-5908-4-50.

24. Rogers LQ, Goncalves L, Martin MY, et al. Beyond efficacy: a qualitative organizational perspective on key implementation science constructs important to physical activity intervention translation to rural community cancer care sites. J Cancer Surviv. 2019;13:537–46.

25. Rogers LQ, Courneya KS, Anton PM, et al. Effects of the BEAT Cancer physical activity behavior change intervention on physical activity, aerobic fitness, and quality of life in breast cancer survivors: a multicenter randomized controlled trial. Breast Cancer Res Treat. 2015;149:109–19.

26. Proctor E, Silmere H, Raghavan R, et al. Outcomes for implementation research: conceptual distinctions, measurement challenges, and research agenda. Admin Pol Ment Health. 2011;38:65–76.

27. Lewis CC, Fischer S, Weiner BJ, et al. Outcomes for implementation science: an enhanced systematic review of instruments using evidence-based rating criteria. Implement Sci. 2015;10:155. https://doi.org/10.1186/s13012-015-0342-x.

28. Ayala GX, Elder JP. Qualitative methods to ensure acceptability of behavioral and social interventions to the target population. J Public Health Dentistry. 2011;71(Suppl 1):S69–79.

29. O'Cathain A, Hoddinott P, Lewin S, et al. Maximising the impact of qualitative research in feasibility studies for randomised controlled trials: guidance for researchers. Pilot Feasibility Stud. 2015;1:32. eCollection 2015.

30. Holtrop JS, Rabin BA, Glasgow RE. Qualitative approaches to use of the RE-AIM framework: rationale and methods. BMC Health Serv Res. 2018;18:177. https://doi.org/10.1186/s12913-018-2938-8.

31. Rabin BA, Lewis CC, Norton WE, et al. Measurement resources for dissemination and implementation research in health. Implement Sci. 2016;11:42. https://doi.org/10.1186/s13012-016-0401-y.

32. Ford B, Rabin B, Morrato EH, et al. Online resources for dissemination and implementation science: meeting demand and lessons learned. J Clin Translat Sci. 2018;2:259–66.

33. Damschroder LJ, Reardon CM, Sperber N, et al. Implementation evaluation of the telephone lifestyle coaching (TLC) program: organizational factors associated with successful implementation. Translat Behav Med. 2017;7:233–41.

34. Proctor EK, Powell BJ, McMillen JC. Implementation strategies: recommendations for specifying and reporting. Implement Science. 2013;8:139. https://doi.org/10.1186/1748-5908-8-139.

35. Waltz TJ, Powell BJ, Matthieu MM, et al. Use of concept mapping to characterize relationships among implementation strategies and assess their feasibility and importance: results from the expert recommendations for implementing change (ERIC) study. Implement Sci. 2015;10:109. https://doi.org/10.1186/s13012-015-0295-0.

36. Parchman ML, Noel PH, Culler SD, et al. A randomized trial of practice facilitation to improve the delivery of chronic illness care in primary care: initial and sustained effects. Implement Sci. 2013;8:93. https://doi.org/10.1186/1748-5908-8-93.

37. Curran GM, Bauer M, Mittman B, et al. Effectiveness-implementation hybrid designs: combining elements of clinical effectiveness and implementation research to enhance public health impact. Med Care. 2012;50:217–26.

38. Houston TK, Sadasivam RS, Allison JJ, et al. Evaluating the QUIT-PRIMO clinical practice ePortal to increase smoker engagement with online cessation interventions: a national hybrid type 2 implementation study. Implement Sci. 2015;10:154. https://doi.org/10.1186/s13012-015-0336-8.

39. Rycroft-Malone J. The PARIHS framework—a framework for guiding the implementation of evidence-based practice. J Nurs Care Qual. 2004;19:297–304.

40. Wenger E, McDermott RA, Snyder W. Cultivating communities of practice: a guide to managing knowledge: Harvard business press; 2002.

41. Ebert L, Malte C, Hamlett-Berry K, et al. Use of a learning collaborative to support implementation of integrated care for smoking cessation for veterans with posttraumatic stress disorder. Am J Public Health. 2014;104:1935–42.

42. Colditz GA, Emmons KM, Vishwanath K, et al. Translating science to practice: community and academic perspectives. J Public Health Management Pract. 2008;14:144–9.

43. Cresswell KM, Bates DW, Sheikh A. Ten key considerations for the successful implementation and adoption of large-scale health information technology. J Am Med Informatics Assoc. 2013;20:e9–e13.

44. Ramanadhan S, Davis MM, Armstrong R, et al. Participatory implementation science to increase the impact of evidence-based cancer prevention and control. Cancer Causes Control. 2018;29:363–9.

45. Damschroder LJ, Aron DC, Keith RE, et al. Fostering implementation of health services research findings into practice: a consolidated framework for advancing implementation science. Implement Sci. 2009;4:50. https://doi.org/10.1186/1748-5908-4-50.

46. Aarons GA, Hurlburt M, Horwitz SM. Advancing a conceptual model of evidence-based practice implementation in public service sectors. Adm Policy Ment Health. 2011;38:4–23.

47. Feldstein AC, Glasgow RE. A practical, robust implementation and sustainability model (PRISM) for integrating research findings into practice. Joint Comm J Qual Patient Safety. 2008;34:228–43.

48. Nilsen P, Bernhardsson S. Context matters in implementation science: a scoping review of determinant frameworks that describe contextual determinants for implementation outcomes. BMC Health Serv Res. 2019;19:189. https://doi.org/10.1186/s12913-019-4015-3.

49. Escoffery C, Lebow-Skelley E, Udelson H, et al. A scoping study of frameworks for adapting public health evidence-based interventions. Translat Behav Med. 2018;9:1–10.

50. Chambers DA, Norton WE. The adaptome: advancing the science of intervention adaptation. Am J Prev Med. 2016;51(4 Suppl 2):S124–31.

51. Aarons GA, Cafri G, Lugo L, et al. Expanding the domains of attitudes towards evidence-based practice: the evidence based practice attitude scale-50. Adm Policy Ment Health. 2012;39:331–40.

52. Moore GC, Benbasat I. Development of an instrument to measure the perceptions of adopting an information technology innovation. Inform Syst Res. 1991;2:192–222.

53. Scott SD, Plotnikoff RC, Karunamuni N, et al. Factors influencing the adoption of an innovation: an examination of the uptake of the Canadian heart health kit (HHK). Implement Sci. 2008;3:41. https://doi.org/10.1186/1748-5908-3-41.

54. Weiner BJ, Lewis CC, Stanick C, et al. Psychometric assessment of three newly developed implementation outcome mea-

sures. Implement Sci. 2017;12:108. https://doi.org/10.1186/s13012-017-0635-3.

55. Breitenstein SM, Gross D, Garvey CA, et al. Implementation fidelity in community-based interventions. Res Nurs Health. 2010;33:164–73.

56. Kashner MT, Rush JA, Altshuler KZ. Measuring costs of guideline-driven mental health care: the Texas medication algorithm project. J Mental Health Policy Econ. 1999;2:111–21.

57. Goodman RM, McLeroy KR, Steckler AB, et al. Development of level of institutionalization scales for health promotion programs. Health Educ Quart. 1993;20:161–78.

58. Luke DA, Calhoun A, Robichaux CB, et al. The program sustainability assessment tool: a new instrument for public health programs. Prevent Chronic Dis. 2014;11:130184.

59. Pagoto SL, Kantor L, Bodenlos JS, et al. Translating the diabetes prevention program into a hospital-based weight loss program. Health Psychol. 2008;27:S91–8.

60. Whittemore R, Melkus G, Wagner J, et al. Translating the diabetes prevention program to primary care: a pilot study. Nurs Res. 2009;58:2–12.

61. Powell BJ, Waltz TJ, Chinman MJ, et al. A refined compilation of implementation strategies: results from the expert recommendations for implementing change (ERIC) project. Implement Sci. 2015;10:21. https://doi.org/10.1186/s13012-015-0209-1.

62. Brown CH, Curran G, Palinkas LA, et al. An overview of research and evaluation designs for dissemination and implementation. Ann Rev Public Health. 2017;38:1–22.

Models for Caring for Patients with Complex Lifestyle, Medical, and Social Needs

5

Emily Perish, David Meltzer, and Edwin McDonald

Abbreviations

C4P   Comprehensive Care, Community and Culture Program
CCP   Comprehensive Care Physician
CMMI   Center for Medicare and Medicaid Innovation
NCD   Non-communicable disease
PCP   Primary care physician

Introduction

Overview of Current State of the US Healthcare System

The United States spends far more than other developed countries on healthcare, with ~18% of its gross domestic product attributed to healthcare spending in 2017 [1]. However, despite higher spending, the United States performs worse across a range of population health outcomes [2]. Hospital utilization among a small fraction of the population constitutes a large fraction of this cost. Chronic diseases contribute importantly to these costs. This is not surprising because nearly half of all Americans suffer from at least one chronic condition, and people who are frequently hospitalized are even more likely to have ≥1 chronic condition, such as diabetes, hypertension, heart disease, obesity, and respiratory diseases [3]. Moreover, the prevalence of these conditions is increasing with the aging of the population so that effectively managing chronic conditions is one of the greatest challenges facing patients and healthcare systems.

The management of chronic conditions for patients who are hospitalized is often complicated by fragmentation between inpatient and outpatient care that may increase healthcare spending and adversely impact their health outcomes. This has been especially true as the US healthcare system has become increasingly specialized and hospitalists have increasingly provided hospital care instead of the traditional model in which primary care physicians (PCPs) cared for their own patients in clinic and in the hospital. The traditional model fell into decline as PCPs no longer typically had enough patients in the hospital for it to be economically viable for them to see patients in the hospital.

As high spending and poor outcomes in the United States have increasingly driven efforts toward value-based health, costs related to hospitalization have been targeted by a range of interventions that aim to improve health outcomes and decrease healthcare spending. Many of these interventions involve hiring additional staff and clinical team members, e.g., nurses and social workers, to coordinate care for patients who are deemed "high-risk." These interventions involve additional hiring costs, which make it difficult to reduce the total cost of care because those additional costs must be recouped before net savings can be achieved. Moreover, care still tends to be fragmented, as patients must typically graduate from these care coordination models after a few months because of their high ongoing costs. Thus, there is an important need for patient-centered care coordination programs to meet both the medical and social needs of frequently hospitalized patients while not increasing, and ideally decreasing, the total cost of care.

E. Perish (✉) · D. Meltzer
University of Chicago Medicine, Department of Medicine, Section of Hospital Medicine, Chicago, IL, USA
e-mail: eperish@medicine.bsd.uchicago.edu;
dmeltzer@medicine.bsd.uchicago.edu

E. McDonald
University of Chicago Medicine, Section of Gastroenterology, Hepatology, and Nutrition, Chicago, IL, USA
e-mail: emcdonald1@medicine.bsd.uchicago.edu

© Springer Nature Switzerland AG 2020
J. I. Mechanick, R. F. Kushner (eds.), *Creating a Lifestyle Medicine Center*, https://doi.org/10.1007/978-3-030-48088-2_5

Overview of Lifestyle Factors Impacting Health

The role of an unhealthy lifestyle in the development of chronic non-communicable diseases (NCDs) and premature mortality is well established [4]. In 1996, the Danish Twin Study, an exploration of a cohort of 2872 twin pairs, found that genetics accounted for only 26% of longevity in men and 23% in women, while environmental factors and lifestyle played a larger role in determining the subjects' lifespans [5]. Similarly, a recent analysis of the UK Biobank study, a cohort of more than 500,000 individuals with genetic data, found that genetics and poor lifestyle were independent risk factors for the development of NCDs such as coronary artery disease, stroke, hypertension, atrial fibrillation, and diabetes [6]. Khera et al. [7] evaluated the genetic risk for coronary artery disease in three large prospective cohorts in the United States and found that a healthy lifestyle may offset the genetic risk of coronary disease. The investigators concluded that a healthy lifestyle was associated with a 46% lower relative risk of coronary events among genetically high-risk individuals compared to an unhealthy lifestyle [7].

The rise in NCDs, both globally and nationally, provides another argument for developing interventions to address unhealthy lifestyles. Globally, the decline of infectious disease made NCDs (e.g., ischemic heart disease and stroke) the leading causes of death [8], while increasing urbanization promoted a "nutritional transition" toward adoption of less-healthy "Westernized" dietary patterns and overall lifestyles [9–11].

Similar patterns exist within the United States. The Hawaii, Los-Angeles, Hiroshima study has illustrated how Japanese-Americans adopt Western lifestyles and high fat, simple carbohydrate dietary patterns compared to their native Japanese counterparts and accordingly had higher rates of obesity and diabetes [12]. These findings elucidate how lifestyle behaviors influence the health of Americans, with heart disease, stroke, diabetes, and cancer accounting for the top 10 leading causes of death in the United States [13].

Unhealthy dietary patterns are a major contributor to the burden of NCDs in the United States [14], with an estimated 650,000 deaths annually attributed to dietary factors. Using data from the National Health and Nutrition Examination Surveys, Micha et al. [15] estimated that 318,656 deaths from cardiometabolic conditions (heart disease, stroke, and diabetes) in 2012 were associated with dietary factors (corresponding to 45.4% of all deaths associated with these conditions). The dietary factors with the greatest impact included high intake of sodium (9.5% of cardiometabolic deaths), low intake of nuts/seeds (8.5%), low consumption of vegetables (7.6%), high intake of processed meats (8.2%), low intake of fruits (7.5%), and high consumption of sugar-sweetened beverages (7.4%) [15].

Unhealthy dietary patterns are not the only lifestyle behavior contributing to NCDs and mortality in the United States. An investigation of three large cohorts, including over 120,000 US adult men and women, revealed that smoking, alcohol use, sleep, and television viewing were also independently associated with weight gain [16]. A similar study found an association between decreased all-cause mortality, including cardiovascular mortality, and adopting five low-risk lifestyle factors—abstaining from smoking, maintaining a healthy body weight, having a high-quality (healthy) diet, moderating alcohol consumption, and participating in 30 min of moderate exercise daily [17]. Adopting these healthy behaviors at the age of 50 years was estimated to extend life expectancy by 14 years in women and 12 years in men [17].

Many unhealthy lifestyle behaviors that influence the risk of NCDs also have psychosocial determinants. For example, the types of grocery stores in a neighborhood have implications for health outcomes. In the Atherosclerosis Risk in Communities cohort, living in areas where grocery stores are more prevalent was associated with a lower prevalence of being overweight or obese [18]. Another comparable study showed that food insecurity was associated with reduced dietary quality, including more frequent consumption of high-fat dairy products, salty snacks, sugar-sweetened beverages, and red/processed meats [19]. To be food insecure means that an individual does not have reliable access to affordable, nutritious food due to lack of money or resources [20].

The types of grocery stores in a community and food insecurity are both surrogates for income level, which is also a key social determinant of health. Individuals who fall near or below the poverty line are also more likely to face challenges in managing their healthcare, including affording medications and accessing space to exercise and purchase/prepare healthy food, which can lead to or exacerbate chronic conditions. Using income data from tax records and mortality data from Social Security Administration records, Chetty et al. [21] demonstrated a significant difference in life expectancy between the wealthiest 1% and the poorest 1% of the population: 14.6 years (95% CI, 14.4–14.8 years) for men and 10.1 years (95% CI, 9.9–10.3 years) for women. However, the gap in life expectancy varied across geographic areas and was associated with differences in health behaviors and local characteristics [21]. As such, income is not the only social determinant that influences behavior.

Social isolation is an important and underappreciated psychosocial factor that affects lifestyle behaviors and health outcomes. The definition of social isolation entails an absence of social relationships [22]. Based on data from the National Health and Aging Trends Study, social isolation affects 24% of self-responding adults over age 65 [23]. Risk factors for social isolation include being male, not married, having low education, and a low income [23]. Given the prevalence of social isolation in the United States, social isolation has gained interest as a modifiable risk factor for NCDs and mortality. In one study, researchers demonstrated that loneliness doubled the risk of developing dementia among individuals living in senior facilities in Chicago [24]. An analysis of adults enrolled in the American Cancer Prevention Study II cohort ($n = 580,182$) found that social isolation was associated with all-cause mortality in all the population subgroups studied [25].

The diverse set of lifestyle behaviors and their respective impacts on NCDs suggests that care models are needed to address these relationships, as well as diagnose, treat, and monitor disease progression. Furthermore, care models must address psychosocial factors that drive unhealthy lifestyle behaviors. For example, social isolation and loneliness have been associated with higher risks for general and mental health conditions, including high blood pressure, heart disease, obesity, anxiety, depression, and cognitive decline [26]. Given the complex connections among the social, psychological, and behavioral drivers of chronic health conditions, comprehensive approaches hold great promise for improving health outcomes.

Comprehensive Care Physician Program and Center for Medicare and Medicaid Innovation Study

With the passage of the Affordable Care Act in 2010, the Center for Medicare and Medicaid Innovation (CMMI) was established to find, implement, and fund new models of care to improve health outcomes and decrease costs [27]. Patients at increased risk of hospitalization were a natural target for new models of care due to the concentration of health spending and adverse outcomes observed. The need for new models was reinforced by evidence that care by "hospitalist" physicians produced, at best, only small improvements in costs or outcomes [28]. Such modest results were not surprising. Hospitalists were viewed by many as displacing traditional PCPs from providing inpatient care, shepherding continuity of care, and nurturing enduring doctor-patient relationships. Most notable in this literature on the value of continuity of care is a randomized trial performed by Wasson [29] that randomized participants to receive care from either the same or different PCP each visit. This study showed large decreases in hospital day, length of stay, and emergency department visits [29].

Given this evidence on the value of receiving care from a physician with whom one has a continuing relationship, as well as the known discontinuities of care in the hospitalist model, one can question whether there are opportunities to revamp inpatient care by focusing on clinicians with whom patients have an ongoing relationship. In considering this question, the traditional model was reexamined where PCPs provide care in and out of the hospital without hospitalists. Based on an economic analysis comparing the traditional model of combined inpatient and outpatient care with the newer model of segregated inpatient (hospitalist-based) and outpatient (PCP-based) care, there was insufficient hospital-based income for PCPs to justify blocking out clinic hours for inpatient rounding. This result led to the core idea of the Comprehensive Care Physician (CCP) model. In this model, physicians who focus their practice on patients at increased risk of hospitalization might find it easier to provide care in both the clinic and hospital. Focusing on patients at increased risk of hospitalization is critical in the CCP model because it allows participating physicians to manage a small panel of ambulatory patients. In other words, the physicians can provide their higher-risk patients with the ambulatory care they need, while also limiting clinic time for inpatient rounding on other high-risk patients in their practice. This not only averts a loss of income but also potentially develops an economically successful practice [30].

Having developed the idea behind the CCP model, an application to CMMI was made to fund implementation and evaluation processes at the University of Chicago. Though the core idea behind the CCP model is about reorganizing physicians' work, it is also a team-based model, including CCP physicians, a licensed clinical social worker, registered nurse, medical assistant, and clinic coordinator. The team works together to produce the key elements of the CCP program: an integrated approach to care, trusted doctor-patient relationship, ready access to outpatient care, and a proactive interdisciplinary team tailored to patient needs [31].

In 2012, CMMI funded this project and a 2000-person randomized trial was started comparing the CCP model, in which there is relational continuity with the same physician across settings to standard care, in which patients receive care from different physicians in the hospital and the clinic. Findings to date, based on patient reported outcomes, suggest significant improvements in patient experience and mental health status, with a 15–20% decrease in hospitalization, implying savings of $3000–$4000 per patient per year [32]. Analysis of hospitalization data based on Medicare claims and State of Illinois Hospitalization records is nearing completion. The positive initial findings have already motivated dissemination strategies and work with hospitals and healthcare systems around the United States and internationally.

The Comprehensive Care, Community and Culture Program

Notwithstanding the encouraging findings from the CCP study, there are additional opportunities to improve the health and well-being of patients with complex needs. Notably, these benefits accrued, even though nearly 30% of patients who chose to enroll in the CCP program did not fully engage in it, either never making appointments or not keeping their appointments if they made them. Hypothetically, social determinants prevented these patients from engaging with the program. To address these unmet social needs and increase patient engagement, the Comprehensive Care, Community and Culture Program (C4P) was established and funded in 2016 by the Robert Wood Johnson Foundation. The C4P enhances the CCP model by adding [1] systematic assessment of 17 domains of unmet social needs, [2] access to a community health worker, and [3] access to community-based arts and culture programming (Fig. 5.1).

C4P research coordinators screen study participants every 3 months about their magnitude of need across 17 domains of social needs. These include traditional needs such as housing, food, public benefits, transportation, and less traditionally recognized needs such as healthy eating, physical activities, social engagement, and spiritual needs. The screening tool is meant to identify the broad class of need and initiate more specific conversations with the clinical team. The C4P community health worker is integrated closely within the clinical team and receives ongoing training and mentorship from a licensed clinical social worker. The community health worker and social workers receive automated alerts in real time as patients identify social needs in the quarterly survey

and begin work with patients to address those specific needs. Another method to address unmet social needs of patients is through the Artful Living Program, which is grounded by growing evidence of positive effects of various types of art on adults' physical, mental, and social health [33, 34]. Group activities bring individuals together around a common goal as they share the experience of observing, exploring, and creating together [35].

Figure 5.2 describes the conceptual model underlying C4P. Patients at increased risk of hospitalization have varying levels of healthcare activation. Activation describes a set of beliefs and actions a patient may possess related to their ability to positively impact their health outcomes. The conceptual model posits that patients who are more activated are more likely to engage in CCP and benefit from its care, while those who are less activated are less likely to engage in care. C4P is hypothesized to increase patient activation, resulting in increased engagement in CCP and improved outcomes. This theoretical model predicts that patients who are least activated at baseline may benefit most from C4P if it is able to increase their level of activation.

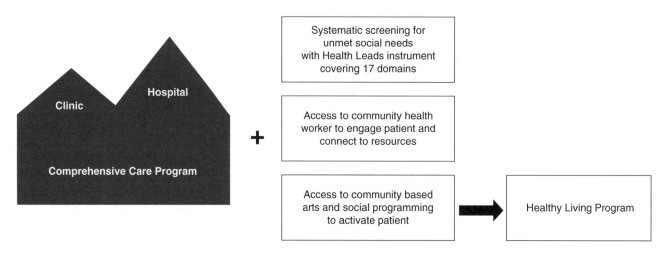

Fig. 5.1 Comprehensive Care, Community and Culture Program (C4P) Model. See Ref. [36] for the HealthLeads instrument

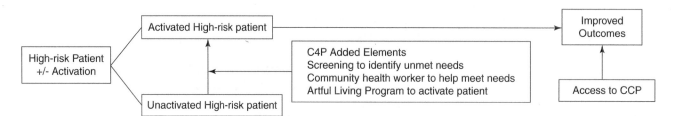

Fig. 5.2 Comprehensive Care, Community and Culture Program (C4P) Conceptual Model. This figure describes the conceptual model underlying Comprehensive Care, Community and Culture Program (C4P). Patients at increased risk of hospitalization have varying levels of healthcare activation. Activation describes a set of beliefs and actions a patient may possess related to their ability to positively impact their health outcomes. The conceptual model posits that patients who are

more activated are more likely to engage in the Comprehensive Care Program (CCP) and benefit from its care, while those who are less activated are less likely to engage in care. C4P is hypothesized to increase patient activation, resulting in increased engagement in CCP and improved outcomes. This theoretical model predicts that patients who are least activated at baseline may benefit most from C4P if it is able to increase their level of activation

Preliminary Findings Concerning Unmet Social Needs

The unmet social need data has been highly informative. The 17 areas of unmet social needs identified at screening are highly concentrated [36]. Specifically, 87% of all unmet needs are concentrated in the 41% of patients who have three or more unmet needs and the patterns of needs among these high-need individuals are highly diverse. Discussions with patients and healthcare professionals highlighted the many challenges faced by individuals with multiple needs. As a result, interventions were designed to address multiple patient needs using a core strategy. To identify the clusters of unmet social needs in the study patient population, a latent class analysis was performed. Five unique clusters of unmet social needs were identified: few needs, many needs (average about five or more), financial and insurance needs, child-related needs and legal needs, and needs for healthy eating, physical activities, and social engagement. With renewed funding, the C4P model evolved and included interventions that focused on these different clusters of unmet social needs.

Design of C4P Healthy Living Program

The C4P Healthy Living Program was developed to address the unmet social needs of the group of patients identified in the latent class analysis. These unmet needs cluster as healthy eating, physical activity, and engaging in social activities elements. The C4P Healthy Living Program incorporates the Artful Living Program, which offers community-based arts and socialization.

Element 1: Healthy Eating Curriculum

The first element of the program is a healthy eating curriculum. For many Americans, both cooking and consumption of food prepared at home have declined since the 1960s [37]. A large number of patients in the program have chronic conditions in which diet is a modifiable risk factor. Furthermore, many of the patients in the program live in areas where unhealthy food options overshadow healthy ones (e.g., "food deserts" and "food swamps") [38]. Evidence suggests that teaching patients with diabetes how to cook in a healthy way can improve blood pressure, hemoglobin A1c, and cholesterol [39]. Accordingly, a healthy eating curriculum was developed that educates patients on healthy food choices when eating out, as well as cooking techniques to promote healthy eating at home. The primary goals of the curriculum are to increase the frequencies of preparing, cooking, and eating healthy foods, including fruits, vegetables, nuts, and whole grains, and limiting unhealthy items, such as sugar-sweetened beverages, added sugars, ultra-processed foods, sodium, and saturated fats.

The curriculum occurs over 12 monthly sessions. Each session lasts at least an hour and a half. At each class, a culinary-trained physician provides a lecture that covers various nutrition topics and demonstrates a recipe corresponding to the information included in the lecture. The sessions occur in a medical center conference room that lacks specialized equipment. The physician/chef brings portable equipment for cooking demonstrations, including cutting boards, prep-bowls, knives, induction burners, toaster ovens, etc. The patients have the opportunity for hands-on participation. Participation includes cutting vegetables, tasting the recipes, and discussing recipes/taste preferences. Tasting the recipes is a critical part of the demonstrations because it allows patients to try new foods and recognize that healthy recipes are also quite palatable. The recipes demonstrated are intentionally inexpensive, easy to prepare, and use ingredients sourced from grocery stores in the neighborhoods surrounding the hospital.

Several sources are used to create a healthy eating curriculum. The Conceptual Model of Healthy Cooking provides a framework for using cooking as a tool to impact chronic disease [40]. The model focuses on increasing cooking frequency, using healthy cooking techniques, decreasing unhealthy items, incorporating various flavorings, and supplementing with healthy additions/replacements [40]. Lecture topics are also based on the 2015–2020 Dietary Guidelines for Americans [41]. These guidelines provide an overview of healthy food patterns. Overall, the curriculum focuses on whole foods, instead of a reductionist, nutrient-oriented approach.

Element 2: Physical Activities

The second element of the C4P Healthy Living Program focuses on physical activity. Patients in C4P often experience several chronic conditions and disabilities, which make it challenging to exercise. Many of these patients are also socially isolated and find it difficult to leave their homes. To address needs for physical activities in this patient population, regularly occurring events are conducted in the program. These activities include monthly walking groups, yoga and mindfulness exercises, dancing classes, and gardening sessions. These physical activities are chosen based on the interests of patients, keeping in mind mobility and health limitations. For example, dance is popular with many patients but difficult to perform, so strategies were developed to adapt popular dances to persons with limited mobility. These events are all staffed by social workers, community health workers, and research coordinators embedded in the program. The continuity of this team across events, and integration with the ongoing clinical care and research activities, builds relationships with patients to improve health outcomes.

Element 3: Community Gardens

The third component to the C4P Healthy Living Program is access to community gardens and gardening events. With grant funding, a small garden – the Learning Garden – was built on a patio space in the medical center. This garden includes several handicap-accessible raised garden beds and pots. Each spring, plantings are organized with patients, family, friends, and staff. Throughout the summer and fall, cooking demonstrations, yoga sessions, and other events in the Learning Garden are hosted. The limited space available in the Learning Garden means that the amount of produce yielded is modest, but the community health worker identifies patients with food insecurity needs and provides them with fresh produce if available. There is also a popular end-of-season harvest event that typically provides enough produce to allow all participating patients to have something to take home.

There are partnerships with three community gardens in neighborhoods on the south side of Chicago near where most of the patients in the program live. These partnerships vary in the level of engagement. In each of the partner community gardens, patients who are interested are welcome to garden in the communal garden beds. This means patients are able to engage with other community members and assist with maintaining the beds and harvesting the produce for themselves or their families. Two of the gardens have also offered to reserve a few individual plots for patients in the program to maintain and harvest independently; these are not shared plots and often are in high demand in urban community gardens. Moreover, the program co-hosts Healthy Living Program events in one of these partner gardens, which includes healthy cooking demonstrations, mindfulness exercises, and dance classes. Instead of bringing in C4P program staff, these events are hosted by facilitators that further engagement with the community. This partnership has been particularly effective because patients are not only engaging in the C4P Healthy Living Program events with one another but are also being integrated in their communities and interacting with individuals across generations and states of wellness. These participating garden programs benefit not only from the modest financial resources provided by the C4P program but also by the new members from their community. There are also benefits to the C4P program in terms of recruiting new study and program participants.

Finally, there are plans to build a new garden in a neighboring vacant lot. Vacant land presents a significant challenge to cities. The presence of vacant space in communities is not only an economic challenge, but it has also been shown to adversely impact the overall well-being, physical health, and mental health of communities as they often attract crime, rodents, and trash [42]. Converting vacant lots into community gardens has been a beneficial approach to making these spaces productive and safe. Community gardens can increase property values, provide safe space for public community gatherings, offer fresh produce in communities that often lack healthy food options, and in some cases create jobs. Successful gardens have the ability to address a myriad of social needs: food insecurity, financial insecurity, healthy eating needs, physical activities, and social engagement.

Another promising venture in development is a job-readiness program targeting young men at increased risk of incarceration. One aspect is engaging the men in work preparing vacant lots for use as gardens. Once opened, this community garden will accommodate community events that promote intergenerational engagement and furnish not just gardening opportunities for patients in the C4P program, and their families and friends, but also opportunities for young men gaining experience engaging older adults. This activity can lead to potential career opportunities serving the needs of older adults.

Community engagement is a critical piece of lifestyle medicine. Each of these garden components, the Learning Garden, partnerships with existing community gardens, and prospect of building and operating a new community garden address a range of social needs and offer a place to engage with community in a meaningful way. Adopting a community-based approach and co-creating these activities and spaces increase the efficacy and sustainability of the C4P program.

Element 4: Social Engagement

Each of the C4P Healthy Living Program elements addresses healthy eating and physical activity needs with opportunities for social engagement. This is done intentionally to address issues of social isolation that are prevalent in the C4P patient population. At each of the C4P Healthy Living Program events, patients can socialize with one another, C4P staff, facilitators, doctors, social workers, and other clinical team members who care for them. The continuity among the staff is critical for this and is purposively leveraged to engage those individuals seen as most vulnerable to becoming less engaged and most likely to benefit from engagement. There are also patients in the program who have become self-appointed ambassadors of the program, proactively engaging new participants who attend an event or members of the C4P patient advisory group. Recognizing the importance of these interactions among C4P members at Healthy Living Program events, techniques were implemented for patients to get to know one another and team members. These include unstructured interactions during events to socialize, using name tags, and having staff facilitate reflective discussion about the event content, whether it is new cooking techniques, gardening, or other topics of interest.

There are ways in which these activities can be brought to patients who are homebound or find it difficult to leave their homes to join. For example, community health workers bring blank canvases and painting supplies to patients in their homes. The patients painted the canvases on their own or with the assistance of family members. These canvases were then collected and gathered in a larger art instillation that was revealed during a Learning Garden opening.

Healthy Living Program Evaluation

The C4P Healthy Living Program and its components are evaluated using several approaches. First, patients are asked to complete a feedback survey at the end of each event. This survey asks patients about whether they enjoyed the event, whether they learned something new, what can be improved for future events, etc. The C4P staff review feedback from these surveys regularly and adjust programming as needed, including timing and content of events. Feedback about the Healthy Living Program events collected to-date has been highly positive. Patients state that they especially enjoy the cooking demonstrations and learning new recipes or tips on healthy substitutes for their favorite meals. Patients have also shared that they prefer attending these events in the late morning or early afternoon. Events late in the day or evening can mean that patients are traveling home in the dark, leading to concerns about personal safety.

In addition, as more specific learning goals are formulated, a pre/post survey is administered to patients who participate in the Healthy Living Program cooking event. This survey is adapted from Cooking Matters [43], an organization that empowers families with skills to cook healthy meals, while also extending their food budgets. Through this survey, the Healthy Living Program is evaluated with respect to its ability to impact participant frequency of consuming healthy foods and beverages, healthy cooking skills, and knowledge of healthy foods and beverages. These surveys include identifiers that link responses of an individual over time.

Lastly, the Healthy Living Program sits within the larger C4P intervention, which also houses systematic screening for unmet social needs, access to community health workers, and additional arts and culture events. The C4P model is being evaluated in a randomized trial, compared to the CCP model, in which patients receive care from the same physician in both the hospital and the clinic but do not receive added social supports or fragmented care from different physicians when hospitalized. With the promising findings already realized, it is hoped that the targeted interventions, including the Healthy Living Program, are aiding the C4P model in better addressing clusters of unmet social needs and community engagement.

Dissemination of the C4P and the Healthy Living Programs

Cost and Scalability Factors

One of the goals when designing and implementing the C4P program is to ensure that its comprehensive care coordination elements are scalable to other settings. In order to do this, the model is initially designed to be very lean from a staffing perspective, limiting the number of clinical team members and program staff to those that are necessary. Because the team is multidisciplinary and co-located, the clinicians often share responsibilities and benefit from the expertise of one another. For instance, the physicians have increased capacity to manage some of the psychosocial issues that arise in clinic appointments because of their close and sometimes overlapping professional relationships. Additionally, the team that supports C4P non-clinical programming is small and includes the program director and two research coordinators who involve clinic team members and students as needed in project implementation, community-based event facilitation, etc. Similarly, the C4P Healthy Living Program is a low-cost program to start and operate. With careful attention to cost-effective purchasing, the budget needed to fund the cooking demonstrations, community garden events, and physical activities is minimal. The C4P program purchases basic refreshments for events, ingredients for cooking demonstrations, and supplies and plants for gardening.

Keeping the programming simple and cost-efficient allows for easier scaling and implementation in other communities and health systems. Future plans are underway to expand the C4P and the Healthy Living Program to reach more patients in new settings, such as expanding relationships with existing community gardens, and to start new gardens where none exist. Further, there are plans to implement C4P Healthy Living Program activities at a Chicago-area community hospital.

How to Start a Healthy Living Program

There is a need for creative approaches in the US healthcare system to engage patients in preventive care where they live and to promote a sense of health and overall well-being. Building a Healthy Living Program with all or a subset of its components may seem daunting to a hospital or clinic;

however, from the perspective of the C4P program, it is possible to do this with minimal resources. First, it is important to clearly define the target population. Programming is most beneficial to patients with complex medical and social problems, and particularly for those with specific healthy eating, physical activity, and social engagement needs. Implementing a simple screening tool that is completed with some regularity would be helpful. On the other hand, too narrow a focus on such a population may result in too small a population to engage at scale and a dearth of more active individuals who can serve as program ambassadors. These are tradeoffs for each new program that must be vetted during the scale-up process.

Once the target population has been identified, the frequency and content of Healthy Living Program events can be determined. One to two of these events each month are conducted by the C4P program, but this frequency can be flexible based on patient and site needs. The complement of team members that staff the activities can be tailored. Involving members of the clinical team, even in a limited way, can be valuable. In addition, having a fairly stable team of engaged staff emphasizes the relational continuity of the C4P model.

Designing and executing an evaluation plan is important. Begin by identifying the target outcomes and design tools that will allow measurement of progress and impact. Simple statistics like attendance are an important start, but recognize that a program can have a large impact on a small number of individuals and that the percentage of eligible individuals who attend is not nearly as important as the number of individuals who attend and the impact the program has on them. While a randomized trial can provide strong evidence of the impact of an intervention, observational approaches and other mechanisms such as pre-post surveys and patient feedback forms are more practical and informative for early stages of program development. In pursuing goals of better engaging and activating patients in their care, increasing knowledge of techniques to eat healthier, and exercises to increase physical activity, the scope of opportunities that can be pursued, even with limited resources, and also conducive to iterative experimentation, are extremely valuable. Programs and funding sources will find it worthwhile to encourage continuing pragmatic evaluation for new programs, while reserving more rigorous approaches for more mature programs.

References

1. Centers for Medicare & Medicaid Services. National health expenditure data. https://www.cms.gov/Research-Statistics-Data-and-Systems/Statistics-Trends-and-Reports/NationalHealthExpendData/NationalHealthAccountsHistorical.html. Accessed 25 Jan 2020.
2. Papanicolas I, Woskie LR, Jha AK. Health care spending in the United States and other high-income countries. JAMA. 2018;319:1024–39.
3. Raghupathi W, Raghupathi V. An empirical study of chronic diseases in the United States: a visual analytics approach to public health. Int J Environ Res Public Health. 2018;15(3):E431. https://doi.org/10.3390/ijerph15030431.
4. Sagner M, Katz D, Egger G, et al. Lifestyle medicine potential for reversing a world of chronic disease epidemics: from cell to community. Int J Clin Pract. 2014;68:1289–92.
5. Herskind AM, Mcgue M, Holm NV, et al. The heritability of human longevity: a population-based study of 2872 Danish twin pairs born 1870-1900. Hum Genetics. 1996;97:319–23.
6. Said MA, Verweij N, van der Harst PVD. Associations of combined genetic and lifestyle risks with incident cardiovascular disease and diabetes in the UK biobank study. JAMA Cardiol. 2018;3:693–702.
7. Khera AV, Emdin CA, Drake I, et al. Genetic risk, adherence to a healthy lifestyle, and coronary artery disease. N Engl J Med. 2016;375:2349–58.
8. Institute for Health Metrics and Evaluation. Measuring what matters, 2017. http://www.healthdata.org/results. Accessed 25 Jan 2020.
9. Popkin BM. The nutrition transition and its health implications in lower-income countries. Public Health Nutr. 1998;1:5–21.
10. Danaei G, Rodríguez LAG, Cantero OF, et al. Observational data for comparative effectiveness research: an emulation of randomised trials of statins and primary prevention of coronary heart disease. Stat Method Med Res. 2011;22:70–96.
11. Imamura F, O'Connor L, Ye Z, et al. Consumption of sugar sweetened beverages, artificially sweetened beverages, and fruit juice and incidence of type 2 diabetes: systematic review, meta-analysis, and estimation of population attributable fraction. BMJ. 2015;351:h3576. https://doi.org/10.1136/bmj.h3576.
12. Nakanishi S, Yamane K, Kamei N, et al. The effect of polymorphism in the intestinal fatty acid-binding protein 2 gene on fat metabolism is associated with gender and obesity amongst non-diabetic Japanese-Americans. Diab Obes Metab. 2004;6:45–9.
13. Heron M. Deaths: leading causes for 2016. Natl Vital Stat Rep. 2018;67:1–77.
14. GBD 2017 Risk Factor Collaborators. Global, regional, and national comparative risk assessment of 84 behavioural, environmental and occupational, and metabolic risks or clusters of risks for 195 countries and territories, 1990–2017: a systematic analysis for the Global Burden of Disease Study 2017. Lancet. 2018;392:1923–94.
15. Micha R, Peñalvo JL, Cudhea F, et al. Association between dietary factors and mortality from heart disease, stroke, and type 2 diabetes in the United States. JAMA. 2017;317:912–24.
16. Mozaffarian D, Hao T, Rimm EB, et al. Changes in diet and lifestyle and long-term weight gain in women and men. New Engl J Med. 2011;364:2392–404.
17. Li R, Xia J, Zhang X, et al. Associations of muscle mass and strength with all-cause mortality among US older adults. Med Sci Sports Exerc. 2018;50:458–67.
18. Morland K, Roux AVD, Wing S. Supermarkets, other food stores, and obesity. Am J Prev Med. 2006;30:333–9.
19. Leung CW, Laraia BA, Needham BL, et al. Soda and cell aging: associations between sugar-sweetened beverage consumption and leukocyte telomere length in healthy adults from the National Health and Nutrition Examination Surveys. Am J Public Health. 2014;104(12):2425–31.
20. Office of Disease Prevention and Health Promotion. Healthy people 2020, food insecurity. https://www.healthypeople.gov/2020/topics-objectives/topic/social-determinants-health/interventions-resources/food-insecurity. Accessed 25 Jan 2020.

21. Chetty R, Stepner M, Abraham S, et al. The association between Income and life expectancy in the United States, 2001–2014. JAMA. 2016;315:1750–66.
22. Umberson D, Montez JK. Social relationships and health: a flashpoint for health policy. J Health Soc Behav. 2010;51(suppl):S54–66.
23. Cudjoe T, Roth D, Szanton S, et al. The epidemiology of social isolation: National Health and Aging Trends Study. J Gerontol B Psychol Sci Soc Sci. 2020;75(1):107–13.
24. Wilson RS, Krueger KR, Arnold SE, et al. Loneliness and risk of Alzheimer disease. Arch Gen Psychiat. 2007;64:234–40.
25. Alcaraz KI, Eddens KS, Blase JL, et al. Social isolation and mortality in US Black and White men and women. Am J Epidemiol. 2018;188:102–9.
26. National Institute on Aging. Social isolation, loneliness in older people pose health risks. https://www.nia.nih.gov/news/social-isolation-loneliness-older-people-pose-health-risks. Accessed 25 Jan 2020.
27. Centers for Medicare & Medicaid Services. Innovation center home. https://innovation.cms.gov/. Accessed 25 Jan 2020.
28. Meltzer D, Manning WG, Morrison J, et al. Effects of physician experience on costs and outcomes on an academic general medicine service: results of a trial of hospitalists. Ann Int Med. 2002;137:866–74.
29. Wasson JH. Continuity of outpatient medical care in elderly men. A randomized trial. JAMA. 1984;252:2413–7.
30. Tingley K. Trying to put a value on the doctor-patient relationship. The New York Times. https://www.nytimes.com/interactive/2018/05/16/magazine/health-issue-reinvention-of-primary-care-delivery.html. Accessed 25 Jan 2020.
31. Meltzer DO, Ruhnke GW. Redesigning care for patients at increased hospitalization risk: the comprehensive care physician model. Health Aff. 2014;33:770–7.
32. Meltzer D, Cursio J, Flores A, et al. Effects of a Comprehensive Care Physician (CCP) Program on patient satisfaction, health status, and hospital admissions in Medicare patients at increased risk of hospitalization: initial findings of a randomized trial. Academy Health; 2018. https://academyhealth.confex.com/academyhealth/2018arm/meetingapp.cgi/Paper/23609. Accessed 25 Jan 2020.
33. Noice T, Noice H, Kramer AF. Participatory arts for older adults: a review of benefits and challenges. The Gerontologist. 2013;54:741–53.
34. Cohen GD, Perlstein S, Chapline J, et al. The impact of professionally conducted cultural programs on the physical health, mental health, and social functioning of older adults. The Gerontologist. 2006;46:726–34.
35. Perlstein S. Really caring: why a comprehensive healthcare system includes the arts. Health Advocacy Bull. 1998;6:1–4, article 1.
36. HealthLeads. Resource library. https://healthleadsusa.org/resource-library/. Accessed 25 Jan 2020.
37. Smith LP, Ng SW, Popkin BM. Trends in US home food preparation and consumption: analysis of national nutrition surveys and time use studies from 1965–1966 to 2007–2008. Nutrition J. 2013;12:45. https://doi.org/10.1186/1475-2891-12-45.
38. Gallagher M. Examining the impact of food deserts on public health in CHICAGO. 2006. https://www.marigallagher.com/2006/07/18/examining-the-impact-of-food-deserts-on-public-health-in-chicago-july-18-2006/. Accessed 25 Jan 2020.
39. Monlezun DJ, Leong B, Joo E, et al. Novel longitudinal and propensity score matched analysis of hands-on cooking and nutrition education versus traditional clinical education among 627 medical students. Adv Prev Med. 2015;2015:656780. https://doi.org/10.1155/2015/656780.
40. Raber M, Chandra J, Upadhyaya M, et al. An evidence-based conceptual framework of healthy cooking. Prev Med Rep. 2016;4:23–8.
41. Dietary Guidelines for Americans 2015–2020, 8th ed. http://health.gov/dietaryguidelines/2015/guidelines/. Accessed 25 Jan 2020.
42. Garvin E, Branas C, Keddem S, et al. More than just an eyesore: local insights and solutions on vacant land and urban health. J Urban Health. 2012;90:412–26.
43. Cooking Matters. Who we are. http://cookingmatters.org/who-we-are. Accessed 25 Jan 2020.

The Role of Physical Infrastructure on Health and Well-Being

Norma A. Padrón

Introduction

The intertwined relationship of the built environment and public health spans centuries and is one of the several targets of lifestyle medicine. The 1842 *Report on the Sanitary Condition of the Laboring Population of Great Britain* [1] used statistical information to inform how the high mortality of the city's poor could be abated or eliminated by drainage, proper cleansing, and ventilation – an infrastructure that was not equally accessible by the rich or the poor. Similar reports in the United States, in states such as Massachusetts and New York stressed the connection between health and the physical infrastructure. Since both public health and urban planning have evolved and relied on data and causal evidence, it is now widely understood that physical infrastructure (cities, public spaces, and the design of living quarters) plays an important role in a community's ability to thrive socially and economically.

The intellectual trajectory and the impetus to understand the role of physical infrastructure have been shaped for over more than a century. The nineteenth-century Institutes of Medicine Report on the Future of Public Health [2] referred to as the "Sanitary Awakening" brought—what at the time were—revolutionary ideas about the causes of disease and social responsibility. This report, and its resulting impact, effectively cemented the initial public perspective on the role of public infrastructure on health and underscored the need to form public boards, agencies, and institutions involved in the planning and maintaining of the cities' infrastructure and resources in order to protect the health of citizens. To a large extent, it represents the philosophical and intellectual foundation of today's organizational structure across key public agencies and local public health departments.

Social and economic complexities, as well as the rapid population growth of urban cores over the past century, have made it clear that cities and communities need an intentionally multisectoral approach to the design and understanding of physical infrastructure to ensure equitable and sustainable well-being. With this in mind, health systems, local public health departments, and community-based organizations continuously develop models of care and access to health services that take into account the impact (both positive and negative) of local infrastructure on individual and community health.

There are several key interdisciplinary concepts that relate the role of the local physical environment and infrastructure to health outcomes (Fig. 6.1). These concepts include the built environment, environmental health, social determinants of health (SDOH), and urban planning, which directly and indirectly shape the lifestyles and well-being of communities. There is now a broad consensus across academia, policy, and care delivery that the physical environment interacts with social circumstances, ultimately having a substantial impact on lifestyle and well-being. Therefore, it is important that as data and evidence accumulate, research efforts to improve individual and community lifestyles and well-being should take into consideration these interactions and feedback loops. This chapter aims to present an overview of key concepts, insights and available data, and resources on the role of the physical environment as a driver of health and how lifestyle medicine as a field can address current challenges and opportunities.

Environmental Health

According to the American Public Health Association, environmental health is the branch of public health that focuses on the relationships between people and their environment, promotes human health and well-being, and fosters healthy and safe communities [3]. The current frontier research and practice of environmental health focuses on the impact of air pollution, water and sanitation, chemicals, occupational

N. A. Padrón (✉)
American Hospital Association, Center for Health Innovation, Chicago, IL, USA
e-mail: Norma.padron@anthem.com

© Springer Nature Switzerland AG 2020
J. I. Mechanick, R. F. Kushner (eds.), *Creating a Lifestyle Medicine Center*, https://doi.org/10.1007/978-3-030-48088-2_6

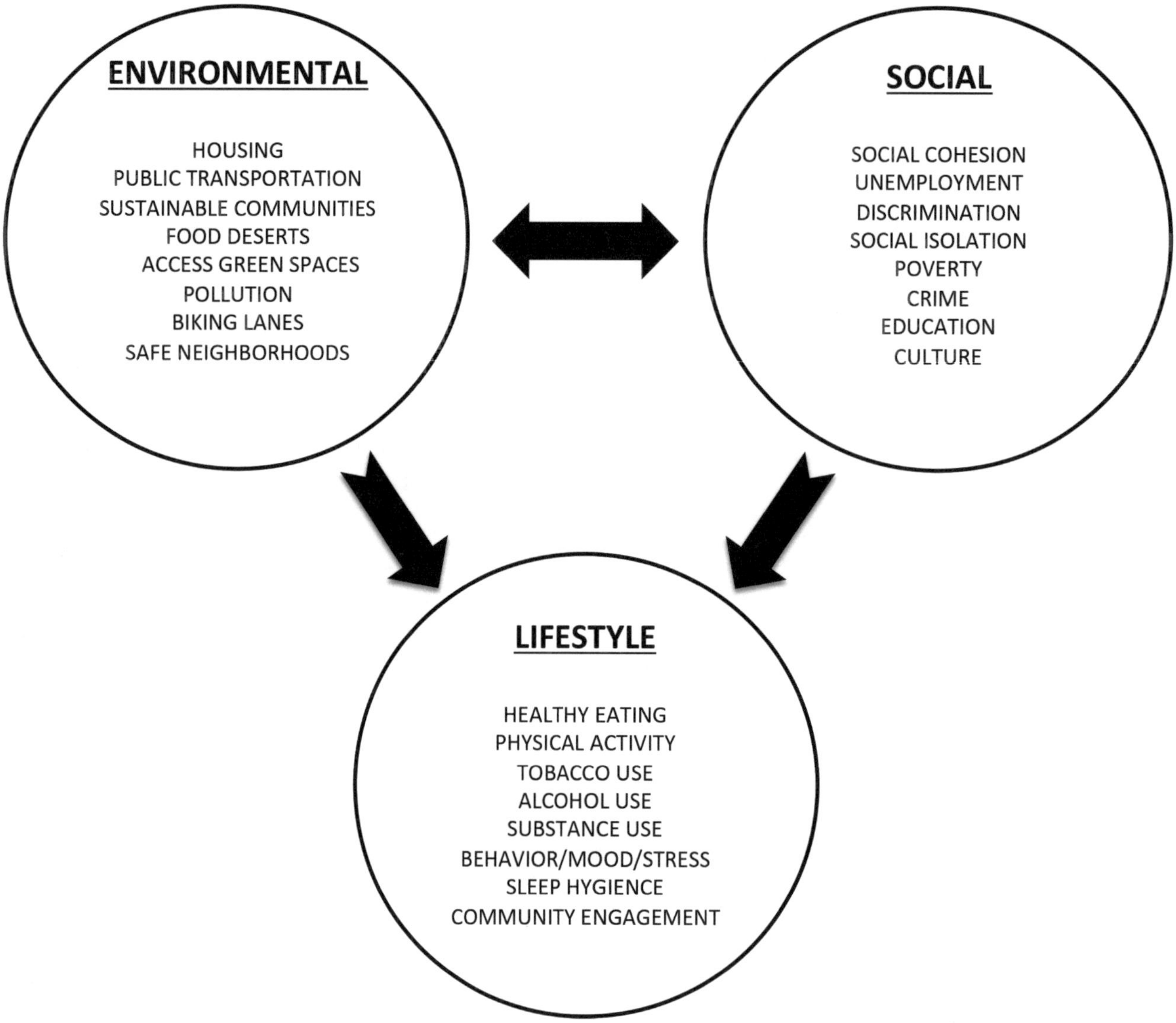

ENVIRONMENTAL

HOUSING
PUBLIC TRANSPORTATION
SUSTAINABLE COMMUNITIES
FOOD DESERTS
ACCESS GREEN SPACES
POLLUTION
BIKING LANES
SAFE NEIGHBORHOODS

SOCIAL

SOCIAL COHESION
UNEMPLOYMENT
DISCRIMINATION
SOCIAL ISOLATION
POVERTY
CRIME
EDUCATION
CULTURE

LIFESTYLE

HEALTHY EATING
PHYSICAL ACTIVITY
TOBACCO USE
ALCOHOL USE
SUBSTANCE USE
BEHAVIOR/MOOD/STRESS
SLEEP HYGIENCE
COMMUNITY ENGAGEMENT

Fig. 6.1 Environmental, social and lifestyle factors that determine health

risks, agricultural practices, and other factors, such as the built environment and community noise.

According to the 2016 World Health Organization report *Preventing Disease Through Healthy Environments: A Global Assessment of the Burden of Disease from Environmental Risks*, 12.6 million deaths, representing 23% of global deaths (and 26% of deaths among children under 5 years of age), are due to modifiable environmental factors [4]. There is variation in the burden across low-income and developed countries, and of course, even within countries. Hence, the strategies to address, prevent, and ameliorate the effects from environmental exposures need to be designed, deployed, and evaluated at a local level in order to be effective. This continuous work relies on local public health departments and surveillance data from federal agencies like the Centers for Disease Control and Prevention, Food and Drug Administration, and others, as well as healthcare delivery systems. For example, the California Department of Public Health maintains an environmental health investigations branch that actively collaborates with local environmental experts, as well as health delivery systems to monitor and address the community's health impact from wildfires (https://www.cdph.ca.gov/Programs/CCDPHP/DEODC/EHIB/EES/pages/wildfire.aspx [Accessed 26 Jan 2020]).

Environmental impacts on health are uneven across age and socioeconomic status and have lasting impacts on health and well-being. There is extensive evidence of the vulnerability of toxic chemicals in utero and in infants. A seminal study using data from the Environmental Protection Agency Toxic Release Inventory Program and the Vital Statistics Natality and Mortality files found that reductions in cadmium, toluene, and epichlorohydrin releases during the 1990s account for about 3.9% of the overall decrease in infant mortality in the United States [5].

Similarly, policies that aimed at improving the living conditions of those near highways (generally lower income families) by reducing exposure to pollution from cars can have substantial and lasting positive impacts on health outcomes. A study of data from a policy change introducing the use of EZ-Pass in New Jersey found that among the roughly 30,000 births to mothers living within 2 kilometers of a toll plaza, there were 255 premature and 275 low-birth-weight births averted, resulting in an estimated $444 million savings on healthcare spending from the reduced pollution [6].

Overall, the efforts to safeguard and improve environmental conditions are intrinsically complex, as they require a multisector, multiagency effort across surveillance and data-gathering efforts, policy design, and a coordinated deployment of strategies and evaluation. According to the US Healthy People 2020 plan, developed by several federal agencies and experts, a set of 10-year objectives for improving the health of all Americans focuses on six themes for environmental health initiatives:

1. Outdoor air quality
2. Surface and ground water quality
3. Toxic substances and hazardous wastes
4. Homes and communities
5. Infrastructure and surveillance
6. Global environmental health [3]

Each of these themes has a direct and indirect connection to lifestyle, as they shape choices and opportunities for individual and medical health prevention, and health management and access. These and similar implications from the environment should be at the forefront of the design of effective local lifestyle and health promotion.

The local nature of the impact of the environment and health and the increasing availability of big data drive some of the most recent research in the field of environmental health such as the research on the "exposome," a term coined in 2005 [7]. This is an area of study focusing on a scientific and comprehensive approach to the totality of an individual's exposures to environmental and societal stressors (including the microbiome), from preconception to death, on human health. Exposome research continues to evolve and includes a conceptualization of macro-level exposures (e.g., air and water pollution, built

environment, climate change, noise, and social support) and its implications on individual and community health. According to the National Institute for Occupational Safety and Health, genetics accounts for only about 10% of chronic disease, with the remaining causes derived from environmental factors [7].

Another area at the frontier of environmental health is the adverse effect of climate change on human health. The multiagency scientific assessment on the impacts of climate change on human health in the United States contains seven key areas of findings [8], which shape and drive all aspects of lifestyle and well-being:

1. Climate change and human health
2. Temperature-related death and illness
3. Air-quality impacts
4. Extreme events
5. Vector-borne diseases
6. Water-related illness
7. Food safety, nutrition, and distribution

Indeed, some cities have already begun incorporating planning and training to address microclimates (areas of significant temperature variation within cities) such as New York City which in 2017 launched a $106 million initiative termed *Cool Neighborhoods NYC*, a comprehensive resiliency program aimed at reducing heat-related health impacts and deaths in heat-vulnerable neighborhoods, strengthening social networks, and providing climate risk training for home health aides [9].

There are also mechanisms that relate to environmental factors but have indirect repercussions on health and lifestyle medicine. One of these is food safety. There is some evidence that changes in rainfall patterns and temperature may aggravate food safety across the production process [8]. Some of these impacts on food safety may be gradual, so there should be a strong emphasis in local surveillance and public health communication. These impacts may be in the form of local outbreaks, which are hard to predict and require timely action for containment and prevention. For example, recent research using longitudinal data on all US states and the District of Columbia has found a positive association between farmers' markets and foodborne illnesses [10]. Specifically, researchers found that there was an increase in total outbreaks and cases of norovirus and *Campylobacter* [10]. Together, the data and evidence, as well as the national and international policy agenda, highlight the need to ensure that environmental considerations are taken into account in the design, implementation, and evaluation of lifestyle medicine strategies at the individual and community levels.

The Built Environment

The built environment has a profound impact on well-being by determining the choices available for maintaining and improving lifestyles [3, 11–13]. The built environment – human-modified places such as homes, schools, workplaces, parks, industrial areas, farms, roads, and highways – is a human's most important habitat. These places can influence the management of chronic disease by affecting physical activity and the natural environment, as well as through individual and community perceptions of health and joy from physical activity and social connectedness. The study of the built environment and its impact on health lie within the field of environmental health which include research on the connection of health outcomes and housing, urban development, urban planning and design, land-use and transportation, industry, and agriculture.

The development of meaningful measures and instruments to design interventions, programs, and delivery models is necessary for research on the built environment. Some steps in this direction have been taken. For example, the Centers for Disease Control and Prevention's Built Environment Assessment Tool measures the core features and qualities of the built environment that affect health (https://www.cdc.gov/nccdphp/dnpao/state-local-programs/built-environment-assessment/index [Accessed 22 Feb 2020]). This tool focuses on five core features:

1. *Built environment infrastructure* –road types, curb cuts and ramps, intersections and crosswalks, traffic control, and public transportation
2. *Walkability* – access to safe, attractive sidewalks and paths with inviting features
3. *Bikeability* –the presence of bike lanes or bike path features
4. *Recreational sites and structures* –playgrounds, parks, and public squares
5. *Food environment* –access to grocery stores, convenience stores, and farmers' markets

In the context of assessing and understanding the built environment in rural communities, many favorable components can be scarce or nonexistent and so adressing the root causes of limited access to healthy environments is intrinsically complex. However, this does not mean that the built environment cannot be evaluated, monitored, and, wherever possible, improved, in rural settings. The *Inventories for Community Health Assessment in Rural Towns (iChART)* is a tool developed in 2013 to understand the features of the built environment that influence active living and physical activity [11]. These features include community design, transportation infrastructure, safety, aesthetics, and recreational

facilities and the goal of the tool is to assess and develop opportunities for healthy lifestyles that are contextually appropriate to rural settings [11]. Similarly, models that aim to understand the impact of physical infrastructure on communities, should incorporate contextual data and information on socio-economic disparities at the local level in addition to population density. There are substantial disparities in leisure-time physical activity by race/ethnicity and socioeconomic factors in large part, due to the lack of recreational resources (such as playgrounds or public spaces) [14, 15]. The field of lifestyle medicine continues to make strides in the development of models of community health that incorporate local conditions and that aim to be culturally and contextually relevant to local populations. An example of this is the Community-Engaged Lifestyle Medicine framework created at the University of Texas Rio Grande Valley School of Medicine and General Preventive Medicine and Public Health, defined *as the practice of preventing chronic disease and promoting health lifestyle behaviors* via *collaborative multi-stakeholder, and community engaged delivery of lifestyle medicine in diverse, low-income populations* [16]. Lifestyle Medicine models that successfully incorporate the built environment generally include three key factors: First, a deep understanding of the local physical infrastructure resources (which as we noted, may vary across rural-urban environments); second, an aim to be culturally appropriate; and third, a feedback look to communicate progress and effectiveness back to the participating individuals and communities.

Lifestyle medicine and behavioral models that take into account socioeconomic disparities are more likely to be relevant and actionable in addressing risk factors, including tobacco and e-cigarette use, alcohol use, poor nutrition, and inactivity as the social dynamics to which the vulnerable and low-income groups are exposed increased both their exposure and impact from adverse circumstances.

Due to the multiple factors that encompass the built environment, assessing it and understanding how it may be improved or changed to effect positive change in a community's health require access to local and current (real time) data. Therefore, many cities and states across the country have created their own built environment assessment tools. An example of this hyperlocal effort is in Harris County, Texas, where the local public health department has a unit focused on the built environment (The Harris County Public Health Built Environment Unit). This unit developed the Environmental Scan Tool to collect and analyze data at the street segment level on pedestrian, bicycle, and drainage infrastructure, which is then used with other available data assets at the county level to better understand the built environment (http://publichealth.harriscountytx.gov/Resources/Built-Environment-Toolkit [Accessed 7 Dec 2019]).

In another example, Philadelphia developed interactive, open source, and open data dashboards leveraging geospatial data to understand the connection of the built environment at a hyperlocal level with health outcomes. The City of Philadelphia Community Health Explorer leverages publicly available data and information from local agencies and departments and provides information on factors such as walkability, access to parks, and access to healthy foods, among other key factors (https://healthexplorer.phila.gov/ [Accessed 7 Dec 2019]).

Despite the consensus in academic, policy, and practice circles of the relevance of the built environment, the use of these measures in the context of public health (and not for urban planning) is still relatively new. Therefore, one of the challenges to overcome is the large degree of variability in the operationalization of these measures, such as population density and access to recreational facilities [12]. The convergence of these metrics with technological advances to gather and analyze data (including the use of drones and sensors) allows for better reliability and accuracy.

The role of the built environment on physical activity and other healthy lifestyle habits is well established [3, 11–13]. Incorporating considerations of the built environment and conditions that patient populations and communities face into the design and planning for care delivery models and population health strategies remains a nascent area. It is not uncommon to hear that "our zip codes determine our health more than health care" and there is a broad acknowledgement in public health and medicine that geography is a significant determinant of healthcare use [17].

Urban Planning and Design for Health

According to the United Nations' *World Urbanization Prospects*, 55% of the world's population live in urban areas, a proportion that is expected to increase to 68% by 2050 [18]. Moreover, according to the US Census Bureau, 62.7% of the US population lives in cities [19]. Of course, cities have been at the epicenter of human settlement and development for millennia, so these demographic and social trends are not surprising. Increasingly, there is attention from a variety of stakeholders, including healthcare delivery systems, payers, and public health departments, to urban design and planning and how they can lead to healthy lifestyles and healthy communities.

Indeed, the design (and redesign) of cities and living enclaves can encourage healthy lifestyles through a wide set of strategies. This is both a tremendous opportunity and challenge experienced at a global scale. The 2016 series on urban design, transport, and health, published in the *Lancet* as *City Planning and Population Health:*

A Global Challenge identified seven regional and local interventions:

1. Destination accessibility
2. Equitable distribution of employment
3. Managing demand by reducing the availability and increasing costs of parking
4. Designing pedestrian-friendly and cycling-friendly movement networks
5. Achieving optimum levels of residential density
6. Reducing distance to public transport
7. Enhancing the desirability of active travel modes (e.g., creating safe attractive neighborhoods and safe, affordable, and convenient public transport) [20]

Though the fields of urban planning, design, and engineering are fundamentally concerned with the development of safe and sound infrastructure, the fields of medicine and public health are connected with current epidemiologic trends and urban design. For example, landscaping can support environmental and health efforts, such as conservation of water, wildlife habitat, and access to respite and recreation [21]. The intrinsic complexity of urban design and planning grows as it seeks to achieve alignment of demographic, social, and economic trends with the development of newer technologies for the design, construction, and development of infrastructure. Many cities have adapted "healthy urban planning" across the world, and there are successful examples in Europe [22, 23]. Indeed, the field of public health continues to actively engage and acknowledge the impact of urban design and planning on health [24].

These efforts point to an optimistic outlook. The concept of a "smart city" is the one that has evolved since the 1990s due to the rapid evolution of civic technology, broadly defined as the tools and technologies to enable the basic functions of cities. However, according to Albino et al. [25], the common denominator of the wide set of definitions of smart cities encompasses certain key dimensions:

- A networked infrastructure that enables political efficiency and social and cultural development
- An emphasis on business-led urban development and creative activities for the promotion of urban growth
- Social inclusion of various urban residents
- Social capital in urban development
- The natural environment as a strategic component of the future

It is therefore evident that the tenets of a smart city inherently promote a healthy (or healthier) lifestyle and take into account human well-being. Furthermore, it is crucial to ensure that the concepts, frameworks, and models developed by efforts around the *smart city* continue to evolve; the fields of practice and research on population health, community health, and lifestyle medicine are actively engaged; and each of these activities do not remain siloed.

In addition to urban planning and design, there is also an interest to incorporate more generally design principles into medical education. For example, the School of Design at Stanford offers a "Design for Health" course (https://dschool.stanford.edu/classes/design-for-health-fall [Accessed 26 Jan 2020]) and the Medical School at Jefferson University (https://www.jefferson.edu/university/skmc/programs/scholarly-inquiry/tracks/design.html [Accessed 16 Feb 2020]) offers a pathway for medical students to train in human-centered design, biomedical design, and design thinking. Similar medical training programs exist at the University of Virginia School of Medicine and their UVA Medical Design Program (http://uvamedical.design/ [Accessed 16 Feb 2020]) and at the University of Texas at Austin, Dell Medical School (Design Institute for Health; https://dellmed.utexas.edu/units/design-institute-for-health [Accessed 16 Feb 2020]).

In addition, some international architecture firms have now opened executive positions for medical experts (such as the newly created role of Chief Medical Officer at HOK Architects), and various health systems have created executive roles for designers (such as the Cleveland Clinic and its new role of Chief Design Officer). These efforts to "cross-pollinate" fields of research and practice will undoubtedly work toward reducing silos and increasing understanding and evidence of the strategies that may positively impact lifestyle medicine.

Social Determinants of Health

The built environment, environmental health, and health outcomes are inextricably embedded in the design and implementation of public policies and investments in housing, public transportation, open spaces, and infrastructure, including water, roads, energy, and connectivity. SDOH refers to the social, economic, and environmental (non-medical) factors that have an impact on health outcomes. Examples of individual- or group-level SDOH include gender, race/ethnicity, education, employment status, poverty, housing, and living conditions, such as crime, pollution, or other environmental factors [26]. As the evidence on the impact of these nonmedical factors on population impact accumulates, there is a strong interest in effecting positive change via policies aiming to improve upstream factors. These are policies geared to improve population health through improvements on the SDOH.

The public policy discourse has focused on the SDOH in part due to the worrisome trends in the United States, which has some of the lowest health outcomes among developed countries, despite substantial and increasing expenditures in healthcare [27–29]. The convergence of data availability and rigorous evidence have motivated concerted efforts to develop policies and strategies that can address, prevent, or encourage social, economic, or behavioral factors that promote health, and may result in a reduction of health expenditures [30].

Methodologically, SDOH are generally assessed by leveraging geospatial data on factors such as income and poverty levels, unemployment, average education (by census tract or county), and other public data at available levels of aggregation (generally census tract, county, or state). Despite the increased availability of relevant data, the systematic incorporation of insights from these data, into the design, implementation, and evaluation of strategies to advance health, remains scarce. Hence, there is a significant gap between the availability of SDOH data (that, though imperfect, is substantial) and the current strategies used by local, state, and federal public health departments, as well as health systems and healthcare professionals. Some models, such as the Area Deprivation Index by Singh et al. [31–33], recently extended by Kind et al., aim to focus on the development of composite indices that can serve as actionable lenses to address socioeconomic disadvantage and differing dimensions of poverty. More recent work has continued the development of multivariate indices focusing on the quantification of neighborhood-level dimensions such as *socioeconomic advantage* (poverty, health insurance status, educational level), *limited mobility* (physical mobility disabilities and aging populations), *urban core opportunity* (generally dominated by population-dense areas), and *mixed migrant cohesion and accessibility* [34]. Crucially important to the sustained impact from the efforts to quantify SDOH is the communication and accessibility of these data to the field of public health and medicine and to the general public. An example is the recently launched SDOH Atlas https://sdohatlas.github.io/ (Accessed 12 Feb 2020), which presents information, data, and an interactive map to facilitate interaction and familiarity with the data. Similar examples are listed in Table 6.1. There is an opportunity for the use of data-driven tools to enable the design of patient-centric strategies that are more effective and more holistically take into account the SODH.

There remain some challenges in the understanding and quantification of SDOH. In particular, some key dimensions do not have a standard definition. For example, food and housing insecurity definitions vary across public policy, medicine, and public health studies [35, 36]. Not having clear definitions on these crucial aspects of SDOH represents an obstacle to design and enable strategies to address them. Access to safe and stable housing, affordability, and gentrification have been shown to have a negative impact on health [36, 37] and should therefore be clearly defined when

Table 6.1 Available sources of data to advance research and strategic development across key infrastructure dimensions*

Infrastructure dimension	Available sources of data	Online access
Transportation	*National Household Travel Survey* Shows the travel behavior of Americans: travel modes, commuting habits, and long-distance trips	https://nhts.ornl.gov/
	PolicyMap Shows everything from transportation to demographics, incomes, housing, lending, quality of life, economy, education, and health across the United States	https://www.policymap.com/maps
	WalkScore Ranking of cities and neighborhoods by walkability, including bike scores and data chart of walk, bike, and transit scores by city/state	https://www.walkscore.com/
Physical activity	*Food Environment Atlas* Statistics on food environment indicators and community access to healthier food options. Indicators include restaurant availability, food assistance, state food insecurity, food prices and taxes, local foods, health and physical activity, and socioeconomic characteristics	https://www.ers.usda.gov/foodatlas/
	Neighborhood Atlas Ranks locations in states from least disadvantaged to most disadvantaged. The Atlas shares measures of disadvantage including education, health systems, non-profits, and government agencies	https://www.neighborhoodatlas.medicine.wisc.edu/
	Physical Activity Reports, Data and Surveillance Data and reports on the proportion of US adults meeting aerobic and muscle-strengthening physical activity guidelines by state	https://www.cdc.gov/physicalactivity/data/surveillance.htm
	Assessing Place-Based Access to Healthy Food: The Limited Supermarket Access (LSA) Analysis Report prepared by Reinvestment Fund showing the LSA figures by state, race/ethnicity, and income disparities	https://www.reinvestment.com/wp-content/uploads/2018/08/LSA_2018_Report_web.pdf
	Healthy Food Access An interactive map – simply select an area on the US map and add any of the *indicators* to include them on the map	https://www.healthyfoodaccess.org/access-101-research-your-community
Recreation and social connection	*ParkServe* Ranks cities according to a Parkscore rating based on access, acreage, investment, and amenities. Compares cities to the national average of percent of residents within a 10-minute walk of a park	https://www.tpl.org/parkserve
Cities and health outcomes	*The SDOH Atlas* Interactive maps, visualizations, and data on the quantification of neighborhood-level social determinants of health. It focuses on leveraging large, open data to better understand (at the neighborhood level) socioeconomic advantage, economic mobility, mixed-immigrant cohesion and accessibility, and opportunities available in urban cores	https://sdohatlas.github.io/
	500 Cities Project: Local Data for Better Health City and census tract-level small area estimates for chronic disease risk factors, health outcomes, and clinical preventive service use for 500 largest cities in the United States. Features an interactive map and compare cities report	https://www.cdc.gov/500Cities/
	Atlas of Inequality Massachusetts Institute of Technology Lab data in NYC and Boston areas, which categorizes visits to various places in the city by income	https://inequality.media.mit.edu/
Environment	*Environmental Atlas* Tool created by Environmental Protection Agency with geospatial data, maps, and research among many variables. This interactive *map* has many tools by which you can compare different variables like health and economic outcomes, landscape, water supply, population distribution, commuting and walkability, along with other variables	https://enviroatlas.epa.gov/enviroatlas/interactivemap/
	The Housing and Transportation Index An affordability index showing cost of housing and transportation at the neighborhood level. Can access comparison maps or enter a location and find metrics and average costs of housing, transportation, job access, average greenhouse gas consumption per household, etc.	https://htaindex.cnt.org/
	National Environmental Public Health Tracking Network Data explorer where you can narrow your data around specific variables such as community design and select indicators and measures across the United States by state/county	https://ephtracking.cdc.gov/DataExplorer/#/

(continued)

Table 6.1 (continued)

Infrastructure dimension	Available sources of data	Online access
Additional resources	*Health Impact Assessments and Other Resources by PEW* Includes links to all types of data resources, reports, and data needed for planning and local public health strategies	https://www.pewtrusts.org/en/research-and-analysis/data-visualizations/2015/hia-map?sortBy=relevance&sortOrder=asc&page=1
	Community Commons Includes toolkits, data sets, and other resources across different public health topics	http://www.communitycommons.org/collections/Maps-and-Data

*All of the online access websites on this table were accessed 12 Jan 2020

incorporated into approaches to lifestyle medicine and the prevention and management of chronic conditions.

Without a doubt, the physical infrastructure, environmental conditions, and SDOH determine – to a large extent – the health of individuals and communities. Therefore, lifestyle and well-being strategies can, and should, be designed with these factors in mind, so that available resources can be leveraged and correctly proportioned to advance community health.

Health in All Policies

The key idea behind the concept of *Health in All Policies (HiAP)* is that health outcomes are determined by a multidimensional set of factors and these factors are, in turn, determined by multiple sectors (public, private, nonprofit, and academia) across local and national policies [38–40].

The HiAP approach underscores the essential collaborative nature across disciplines, sectors, and fields of research and practice to leverage – and wherever needed, improve – the physical environment and infrastructure for individual and community health. In one example, the 2012 Minnesota Department of Health worked with its Healthy Minnesota Partnership to change the narrative around health and develop a HiAP approach for eliminating health disparities and achieving health equity (https://www.health.state.mn.us/communities/practice/healthymnpartnership/index.html [Accessed 22 Feb 2020]). Similarly, the state of California HiAP program works with more than 20 state agencies and departments to ensure that health impact and outcomes are taken into considerations across the design and implementation of all policies (http://sgc.ca.gov/programs/hiap/ [Accessed 7 Dec 2019]).

New models of developing and sustaining partnerships across sectors continue to be developed and evolve. However, the HiAP framework has propelled several efforts for interagency and multisector collaboration that has and will continue to have an impact on individual and community health outcomes. Key stakeholders in healthcare delivery and access including health systems, payers, and healthcare professionals can engage in the HiAP framework at the local level to better understand and design care services for their populations.

Given the current policy, technical features, and economic landscape, the HiAP framework needs to include a more holistic approach to the design and implementation of HiAP strategies. In particular, some areas of opportunity include a more proactive involvement with multidisciplinary training of medical and public health students, an approach to locally coordinated campaigns to drive participatory design and implementation science leveraging publicly available data, and active engagement with community-based organizations to drive individual and community-level healthy lifestyles driven by empathy and evidence-based research.

Table 6.1 presents a set of resources available to advance the HiAP approach as well as research and strategic development across key infrastructure dimensions such as transportation, physical activity, recreation and social connection, cities and health outcomes, environmental health, and others.

Conclusion

Local infrastructure, environmental conditions, urban planning, SDOH, and the built environment play a large role on individual and communities' experiences and connections to their social, family, and work networks. The visible infrastructure of roads, parks, and housing has a strong impact on the less visible and personal factors of social circumstances and health behaviors. Together, these factors promote or hinder social support or isolation, as well as access to healthy foods and recreation, and impact all aspects of lifestyle and behavior. Therefore, these are key aspects to consider for lifestyle medicine strategies. For lifestyle medicine approaches to be most effective, they must take into account the physical infrastructure, which may be a barrier or enabler of healthy lifestyles and even, within a specific geography, be an enabler for some and a barrier to others.

Through user-centric design, taking into account the physical infrastructure and leveraged data, prevention and healthy lifestyle strategies and initiatives can help achieve the prevention of chronic disease and promote health. In order to achieve this, local governments, public health departments, healthcare delivery systems, and community-based organizations can collaborate through local ecosystems to disseminate available resources and proactively engage local communities. It is crucial that intentional efforts around communication and participatory design are part of the local approaches to community health. One of the most successful accomplishments of the collaborative efforts of public health and preventive medicine has been the introduction of smoke-free legislation (limiting indoor and outdoor spaces where cigarette smoking is permitted) which has resulted in gains to life expectancy and adult and child health [41]. Now, the question arises as to what are similarly impactful changes to our physical infrastructure that could help reduce extant stark disparities in health?

The familiarity with the phrase *your zip code determines your health* can serve as an anchor to activate multisector stakeholders, including federal and state agencies, as well as the public, private, and nonprofit sectors, to improve local infrastructure and the environment. Ultimately, the SDOH need to be addressed with systematic and sustained efforts. As several aspects of the fields of public health, lifestyle medicine, and urban planning and design are converging due to the increased availability of data and technology, it is clear that training, research, and practice across these fields dismantle the silos in which they still currently operate.

References

1. UK Parliament. 1842 report on the sanitary condition of the labouring population of Great Britain. https://www.parliament.uk/about/living-heritage/transformingsociety/livinglearning/coll-9-health1/health-02/. Accessed 7 Sept 2019.
2. Institute of Medicine. The future public health. Chapter 3: a history of the public health system. Washington, DC: National Academies Press; 1988. p. 56–72.
3. Srinivasan S, O'Fallon LR, Dearry A. Creating healthy communities, healthy homes, healthy people: initiating a research agenda on the built environment and public health. Am J Public Health. 2003;93:1446–50.
4. World Health Organization. Preventing disease through healthy environments: a global assessment of the burden of disease from environmental risks. Available: www.who.int/quantifying_ehimpacts/publications/preventing-disease/en/. Accessed 10 Nov 2019.
5. Currie J, Schmieder JF. Fetal exposures to toxic releases and infant health. Am Econ Rev. 2009;99:177–83.
6. Currie J, Walker R. Does living along a busy highway increase premature births? Chicago: MacArthur Foundation; 2015.
7. Centers for Disease Control and Prevention. Exposome and exposomics – NIOSH workplace safety and health topic, November 9, 2018 www.cdc.gov/niosh/topics/exposome/default.html. Accessed 10 Nov 2019.
8. Herrera M, Anadón R, Iqbal SZ, et al. Climate change and food safety. In: Selamat J, Iqbal SZ, editors. Food safety: basic concepts, recent issues, and future challenges. New York: Springer International Publishing; 2016. p. 149–60.
9. The City of New York. Cool Neighborhoods NYC. https://www1.nyc.gov/assets/orr/pdf/Cool_Neighborhoods_NYC_Report.pdf. Accessed 22 Feb 2020.
10. Bellemare MF, Nguyen N. Farmers markets and food-borne illness. Am J Agric Econ. 2018;100:676–90.
11. Seguin RA, Lo BK, Sriram U, et al. Development and testing of a community audit tool to assess rural built environments: inventories for community health assessment in rural towns. Prev Med Rep. 2017;7:169–75.
12. Brownson RC, Hoehner CM, Day K, et al. Measuring the built environment for physical activity: state of the science. Meas Food Phys Act Environ. 2009;36(Suppl 4):S99–S123.
13. Hills AP, Farpour-Lambert NJ, Byrne NM. Precision medicine and healthy living: the importance of the built environment. Prog Cardiovasc Dis. 2019;62:34–8.
14. Moore LV, Diez Roux AV, Evenson KR, et al. Availability of recreational resources in minority and low socioeconomic status areas. Am J Prev Med. 2008;34:16–22.
15. McKenzie TL, Moody JS, Carlson JA, et al. Neighborhood income matters: disparities in community recreation facilities, amenities, and programs. J Park Recreat Adm. 2013;31:12–22.
16. Krishnaswami J, Sardana J, Daxini A. Community-Engaged Lifestyle Medicine as a framework for health equity: principles for lifestyle medicine in low-resource settings. Am J Lifestyle Med. 2019;13:443–50.
17. Rising KL, Karp DN, Powell RE, et al. Geography, not health system affiliations, determines patients' revisits to the emergency department. Health Serv Res. 2018;53:1092–109.
18. United Nations. World urbanization prospects – Population division. https://population.un.org/wup/. Accessed 10 Nov 2019.
19. U.S. Census Bureau Population Trends in Incorporated Places: 2000 to 2013. Current Population Rep 2015; March 25–1142.
20. Giles-Corti B, Vernez-Moudon A, Reis R, et al. City planning and population health: a global challenge. Lancet. 2016;388:2912–24.
21. Jackson LE. The relationship of urban design to human health and condition. Landsc Urban Plan. 2003;64:191–200.
22. WHO City Action Group on Healthy Urban Planning. Healthy urban planning in practice: experience of European cities, 2017. http://www.euro.who.int/en/health-topics/environment-and-health/urban-health/publications/2003/healthy-urban-planning-in-practice-experience-of-european-cities.-report-of-the-who-city-action-group-on-healthy-urban-planning. Accessed 10 Nov 2019.
23. Barton H, Grant M. Urban planning for healthy cities. A review of the progress of the European Healthy Cities Programme. J Urban Health Bull NY Acad Med. 2013;90(Suppl 1):129–41.
24. Shanahan DF, Lin BB, Bush R, et al. Toward improved public health outcomes from urban nature. Am J Public Health. 2015;105:470–7.
25. Albino V, Berardi VU, Dangelico RM. Smart cities: definitions, dimensions, performance, and initiatives. J Urban Technol. 2015;22:3–21.
26. Singh GK, Daus GP, Allender M, et al. Social determinants of health in the United States: addressing major health inequality trends for the nation, 1935-2016. Int J MCH AIDS. 2017;6:139–64.
27. Braveman P, Egerter S, Williams DR. The social determinants of health: coming of age. Annu Rev Public Health. 2011;32:381–98.
28. McGinnis JM, Williams-Russo P, Knickman JR. The case for more active policy attention to health promotion. Health Aff (Millwood). 2002;21:78–93.
29. Murray CJL, Atkinson C, Bhalla K, et al. The state of US health, 1990-2010: burden of diseases, injuries, and risk factors. JAMA. 2013;310:591–608.
30. Adler NE, et al. Addressing social determinants of health and health inequalities. JAMA. 2016;316:1641–2.

31. Singh GK, Siahpush M. Increasing inequalities in all-cause and cardiovascular mortality among US adults aged 25-64 years by area
socioeconomic status, 1969-1998. Int J Epidemiol. 2002;31:600–13.
32. Singh GK. Area deprivation and widening inequalities in US mortality, 1969-1998. Am J Public Health. 2003;93:1137–43.
33. Singh GK, Azuine RE, Siahpush M, et al. All-cause and cause-
specific mortality among US youth: socioeconomic and rural–
urban disparities and international patterns. J Urban Health.
2013;90:388–405.
34. Hu J, Kind AJH, Nerenz D. Area deprivation index predicts
readmission risk at an urban teaching hospital. Am J Med Qual.
2018;33:493–501.
35. Frederick TJ, Chwalek M, Hughes J, et al. How stable is stable?
Defining and measuring housing stability. J Community Psychol.
2014;42:964–79.

36. Kushel MB, Gupta R, Gee L, et al. Housing instability and food
insecurity as barriers to health care among low-income Americans.
J Gen Intern Med. 2006;21:71–7.
37. Cutts DB, Meyers AF, Black MM, et al. US housing insecurity and the health of very young children. Am J Public Health.
2011;101:1508–14.
38. McQueen DV, Wismar M, Lin V, et al. Intersectoral governance
for health in all policies – structures, actions and experiences. Rev
Direito Sanitário. 2013;14:264–7.
39. Collins J, Koplan JP. Health impact assessment: a step toward
health in all policies. JAMA. 2009;302:315–7.
40. Wernham A, Teutsch SM. Health in all policies for big cities. J
Public Health Manag Pract. 2015;21(Suppl 1):S56–65.
41. Hawkins SS, Hristakeva S, Gottlieb M, et al. Reduction in emergency department visits for children's asthma, ear infections, and
respiratory infections after the introduction of state smoke-free legislation. Prev Med. 2016;89:278–85.

Preventive Medicine and Problem-Solving in Populations

Scott Kahan

Abbreviations

DALY   Disability-adjusted life years
HIPPA   Health insurance portability and accountability act
QALY   Quality-adjusted life years
YPLL   Years of productive life lost

Introduction

"Preventive medicine" should not be conflated with "clinical prevention" or "clinical preventive services." What is often interpreted as preventive medicine – such as referral for screening colonoscopy for colon cancer prevention, prescribing a statin or aspirin therapy to prevent adverse cardiovascular events, or administering a vaccine to prevent infectious diseases – are individual-level, clinical preventive healthcare services. Clinical preventive services, however, are only a small part of the broader field of preventive medicine, a medical specialty that focuses on improving the health of individuals and populations [1]. Some examples of relevant populations include a census of patients managed by a team of healthcare professionals, groups of workers covered by a self-insured employer, persons living in a specific region or geographic area, or a community or society as a whole. In addition to the provision of clinical preventive services, some examples of preventive medicine practices include the following:

- Epidemiologic research and surveillance to generate knowledge about important health issues
- Consensus-building and guideline development to inform evidence-based practice and policymaker decisions

S. Kahan (✉)
National Center for Weight and Wellness; Faculty, Department of Health Policy & Administration, Johns Hopkins Bloomberg School of Public Health, Washington, DC, USA

- Training of the healthcare workforce to support appropriate and efficient provision of recommended clinical preventive services
- Generation of healthcare policies to improve access to healthcare
- Analysis and interpretation of epidemiologic trends, health services research, and economic data to inform prioritization of treatment options
- Cost-effectiveness analysis for healthcare and community interventions
- Communication with policymakers and payers to influence science-informed healthcare policies

As the name implies, preventive medicine emphasizes chronic disease risk reduction. Preventive medicine overlaps with and is closely related to lifestyle medicine – indeed, the seminal publication identifying physician competencies for lifestyle medicine was conceptualized and led by the American College of Preventive Medicine [2]. In addition to managing health and risks for individuals, preventive medicine especially focuses on population approaches for risk reduction, which can have an outsized impact on prevention and health improvement outcomes [3]. Consider, for example, a treatment course that results in 5% improvement in blood pressure over a year for a given patient. While likely clinically meaningful, it is also likely that both clinician and patient would be frustrated with the modest outcome, and the patient may even require further intensive treatment. However, a community-, organization-, or practice-wide intervention leading to a 5% reduction in mean blood pressure across the population would be heralded as an immense success. Many people with hypertension would achieve normalized blood pressure and/or reduction or discontinuation of corresponding medications, and even those who did not have hypertension may still achieve small improvements in blood pressure and other benefits (Fig. 7.1). Additionally, substantial financial savings would be expected, and in some cases the structures and processes put into place as part of

© Springer Nature Switzerland AG 2020
J. I. Mechanick, R. F. Kushner (eds.), *Creating a Lifestyle Medicine Center*, https://doi.org/10.1007/978-3-030-48088-2_7

Fig. 7.1 The impact of
population-level interventions
versus individual treatments
on risk reduction. Compared
with targeting high-risk
individuals (**a**), which can be
challenging and costly, a
population-wide program that
yields a relatively small mean
improvement across the
population leads to many
fewer individuals at higher
risk and has the potential to
benefit everyone (**b**). The
X-axis on these curves
could represent blood
pressure, body mass index,
cholesterol, etc

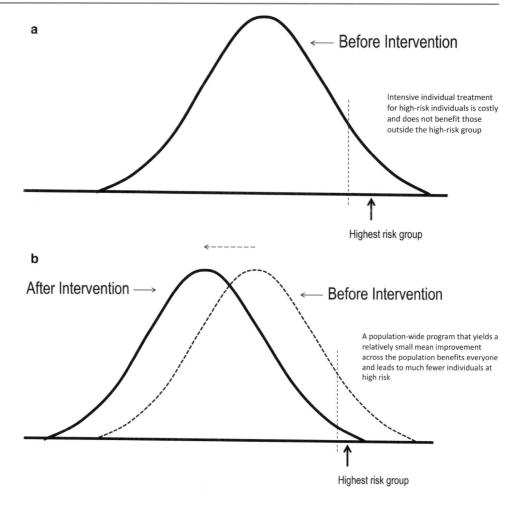

the intervention could positively impact other aspects of the population or future interventions. For example, as a by-product of a program aimed at increasing physical activity in older individuals by improving access to walking paths in the community, the walking paths could be utilized by the whole of the community long after the program has ended.

Since lifestyle medicine addresses many of the behavior-related diseases that are among the most prevalent and costly health issues twenty-first century for the US and most global populations [4], lifestyle medicine practitioners and leaders will benefit from developing an orientation and proficiency in understanding population-level strategies for solving broad, behavior-related, public health problems. Moreover, because the census of patients in a Lifestyle Medicine Center is itself a relevant population, preventive medicine principles can inform the creation and implementation of Lifestyle Medicine Centers.

Using a systematic framework to address health problems and risk reduction in populations – large or small – can help guide strategic assessment and management of the problem. This is analogous to the structured, patient-focused evaluation used in medical practice to diagnose and treat patients: beginning with the patient's chief complaint, the clinician progresses through a series of targeted questions on the history

of present illness, past medical history, lifestyle and social history, and review of systems, followed by a physical examination, laboratory testing, and so forth, ultimately developing a differential diagnosis, prioritized set of treatments, and (hopefully) resolution of the patient's health issue. A similar "workup" can help understand the nature of health problems and risk factors in populations and devise and implement targeted strategies to reduce health risks and improve the health of the population. This process includes defining the problem, measuring the magnitude of the problem, understanding the key determinants of the problem, devising a set of prioritized programs, interventions, or policies to target the problem, and evaluating the effectiveness of the chosen approach.

Define the Problem

How a problem is conceptualized impacts how it will be approached. For example, in a clinical setting, if obesity is interpreted as an issue of deficient nutrition knowledge, the clinician would offer advice, provide patient education materials, or refer to a dietitian. If, instead, obesity is interpreted as the patient's lack of interest or "willpower," the clinician might sternly warn the patient about impending health consequences to scare or "shame" the patient into action – or avoid the topic entirely. If obesity is instead understood as a physiological problem, the clinician may initially recommend pharmacotherapy or even a bariatric procedure; or if defined as a psychological issue, then immediate referral for psychotherapy may be offered.

A clear and specific description for a population health problem – the problem definition – will influence how the problem will be interpreted, investigated, and treated. In the case of childhood under-vaccination, if the problem is framed in terms of the morbidity and mortality associated with an infectious disease outbreak, intervention would focus on treating affected patients, which may or may not include sufficient attention to increasing immunization coverage within the population. If defined as inadequate vaccination, then maximizing immunization coverage would be indicated, even if outbreaks are not occurring. Alternatively, if the problem is understood as being driven by inadequate access to healthcare, the approach would focus on policies aimed at social determinants and access to care – putting to the side the problem of immunization per se, with the expectation that vaccination rates would improve passively.

The problem definition should be as specific and targeted as possible, with clearly reasoned and researched descriptions with respect to the problem and population of interest. A poorly defined problem increases the likelihood of painting a misleading picture of seriousness and the true burden of the issue in specific populations. If defined too generally, the interpretation of the problem may mask discordant trends in high-risk subgroups. A cursory assessment of smoking rates, for example, could be interpreted as a problem nearly solved: substantially decreased tobacco use is one of the greatest achievements of the twentieth century, having plunged more than 50% since mid-century, with several states and localities near or under 10% adult smoking prevalence, and daily tobacco use down by nearly 90% in adolescents – levels once thought to be unreachable [5]. However, these impressive numbers disguise many concerning trends. Nearly 40 million American adults still smoke and rates of smoking initiation are increasing in many subgroups. In populations with serious mental illness, such as schizophrenia and bipolar disorder, several studies show that smoking approaches 75–85% prevalence [6–8]. Though tobacco-related mortality among men in the USA has been declining, deaths in women continue to increase [9]. Use of alternate tobacco options, such as hookahs, which may have more serious health effects than traditional cigarettes, and e-cigarettes, for which health concerns are mounting, may have unintended consequences and it is still unclear whether they will ultimately lower tobacco-related health consequences or serve as gateways to addiction. Moreover, tobacco epidemics are still increasing in much of the rest of the world.

It is all too common for researchers, practitioners, policymakers, advocates, the media, and other stakeholders to over- or underemphasize attention, resources, or funding for a problem in the face of unclear, inconclusive, or contradictory data. Thus, how we specifically define the issue informs how to understand the nature of the problem and sets the stage for solving the problem. If defined too vaguely, too broadly, too narrowly, or otherwise inaccurately or ineffectively, progress will be limited.

Measure the Magnitude of the Problem

Characterizing the size and scope of the problem, the population(s) affected, the frequency and distribution of the health condition (or risk factor or behavior), the severity in affected groups, and patterns of change have enormous implications for understanding and addressing the problem – as well as garnering public attention, political support, and investments toward research and interventions. Collecting relevant data and measuring magnitude informs:

- Understanding of the size of the disease or epidemic and parameters that define the population at risk
- Comparisons of frequency and change within and among populations
- Identification of subgroups with highest frequency, those at highest risk, and those that may be disproportionately affected
- Insights into changes in rates that occur over time
- Associated behaviors or risk factors
- Advocacy for funding and resources to investigate and/or address the problem
- Targeting of resources to specific affected populations

Measurement must be carefully thought out and tailored to the population(s) of interest, as using the wrong measures, such as overly narrow or broad indicators, or insufficient range of measures may mischaracterize the problem. The measurement process should correspond to the problem definition. For example, immunization status as defined by up-to-date vaccinations by entrance into first grade, a traditional indicator, may suggest substantially higher vaccination rates than other measures, such as age-appropriate immunization rates or being up-to-date by 2 years of age. Similarly, flawed interpretations of the magnitude of obesity can mislead researchers, advocates, and policymakers into thinking this is less of an emergent issue. Even though the prevalence of obesity as defined by a body mass index >30 kg/m^2 has leveled off, severe obesity continues to increase at an alarming pace – especially in lower socioeconomic groups – and rates of obesity-related comorbid conditions, complications, and costs continue to rise [10].

Common sources of data for measuring magnitude include public health surveillance systems (such as the Behavioral Risk Factor Surveillance System [11]), vital statistics (e.g., birth and death certificates), disease registries, and surveys). Frequently used measures are described in Table 7.1 and include the following:

- Incidence, which is ideal for measuring the occurrence of disease in a population over a specified period but is often not available. Incidence may be estimated by

Table 7.1 Common measures of disease burden

Measure	Description	Notes
Incidence	Measures the occurrence of a disease or risk factor in a specific population over a specified period of time	Often not easily available. May be estimated by reported diagnoses, case reports, reported deaths, and other means
Mortality	The number of deaths from a disease, risk factor, or exposure in a specific population over a specified period of time	Often used in lieu of incidence because mortality rates may be easier to obtain. However, mortality rates may only be reasonable surrogate measures when the disease is relatively fatal and preventing premature death is a primary outcome of interest (as opposed to problems, in which compromised function or quality of life are most relevant)
Prevalence	The total number of persons who have a disease or health condition in a specific population and at a specific period of time	Typically used for planning interventions and allocating resources.
Category-specific rates	Characterized an issue by "person," "place," or "time," such as rates of a disease or risk factor stratified by age, gender, and ethnicity (person); locality or region (place); or changes over a specified period (time)	These may help to identify subgroups at increased risk and prioritize populations to be targeted for intervention
Intermediate indicators	Examples include the percentage of persons who report exercising at least 3 days weekly, the proportion of women 50 years or older who are screened annually for breast cancer, changes in knowledge or attitudes about a given health behavior, or reported intentions to change a behavior	Especially useful when incidence is difficult to assess directly or when lengthy periods of time would limit data collection (such as needing years or decades for mortalities to accrue)
Indictors of quality-of-life and functional outcomes	Years of productive life lost (YPLL) or Disability-adjusted life years (DALY)	These take into account the impact of compromised function and disability

reported diagnoses, case reports, reported deaths, and other means.

- Mortality rates, based on the number of deaths from the disease of interest during the same period, are often used in lieu of incidence rates because these may be easier to obtain. However, mortality rates may only be reasonable surrogate measures when the disease is relatively fatal and preventing premature death is a primary outcome of interest, as opposed to problems in which compromised function or quality of life is most relevant.
- Intermediate indicators are especially relevant when incidence is difficult to assess directly or when lengthy periods of time would limit data collection (such as needing years or decades for mortalities to accrue). Examples include the percentage of persons who report exercising at least 3 days weekly, the percentage of women 50 years or older who are screened annually for breast cancer, changes in knowledge or attitudes about a given health behavior, or reported intentions to change a behavior.
- Prevalence, the total number of persons who have a disease or health condition at a specific period of time, is typically used for planning interventions and allocating resources.
- Category-specific rates, which help to identify subgroups at increased risk and prioritize groups to be targeted for intervention, characterize the issue by "person, place, and time." For example, diabetes rates may be stratified by age, gender, and ethnicity ("person"); locality or region ("place"); and changes over time ("time").
- Other common measures of disease burden focus on quality of life and functional outcomes such as years of productive life lost (YPLL), which describes reductions in productive lifespan, and disability-adjusted life years (DALY) and quality-adjusted life years (QALY), which take into account the impact of compromised function, quality-of-life, and disability (Table 7.1).

Identify Key Determinants of the Problem

Understanding the variables central to the development and growth of population health problems influences how they will be addressed. This is similar to the clinical management approach in medicine, in which knowledge of risk factors, etiology, and the natural course of a disease impacts the treatment strategy. When a patient presents with signs and symptoms of an infection, for example, a clinician would investigate the type of infection (which, among other things, influences whether to prescribe an antibiotic), the time course of the infectious process (which may influence a decision to quarantine the patient if infectious), and likelihood of re-infection or secondary infection (in which case chemoprophylaxis may be indicated).

Unlike clinical diseases, however, which often have a single etiology and a relatively small number of contributing factors, population health problems are more likely to be multifactorial, with multiple intersecting influences, of which only some may be causally linked to the outcome of interest. Determinants of population problems – especially unhealthful behaviors and behavior-related conditions – tend to cluster into several categories, including individual factors (e.g., biological and behavioral), interpersonal factors (e.g., relationship dynamics and social interactions), structural factors (e.g., laws, policies, and built environment), social norms, political factors, and economic settings.

Not all determinants are equally important. Those that appear to be central to understanding and addressing the problem are "key determinants," in that they are critical to the problem itself, recognition of the problem, or approaches for solving the problem, or they may predispose to, enable, or reinforce the problem or associated determinants of the problem.

- Key determinants are usually, but not always, causally related to the problem or outcome of interest. For example, unaffordability or minimal access to fruits and vegetables is often a key determinant for poor nutritional intake and risk for obesity and diabetes, despite not directly causing these outcomes.
- Not all causal factors are key determinants, as they may not be modifiable or may not be highly effective or cost-effective to address. For example, genetic factors strongly influence the risk for obesity, yet no current treatments are able to modify genetics to cause weight loss (claims of some commercially hyped genetic testing kits notwithstanding).
- Predisposing factors, such as knowledge, attitudes, beliefs, values, and preferences, motivate or support a behavior or outcome. Enabling factors are often environmental or structural factors that facilitate a behavior or outcome. Examples include nutrition labeling and access to counseling. Reinforcing factors are the positive (e.g., rewards) or negative (e.g., punishments) consequences of a behavior, such as peer approval or disapproval, social support, and enforcement of laws and regulations.
- Proximal ("downstream") variables, such as behavioral cues and prices, often have direct effects on the outcome of interest, but may not strongly influence the outcome, as in the case of nutrition knowledge, which is often necessary but not sufficient to cause behavioral change. Distal ("upstream") factors may afford more leverage for solving or preventing large health problems; examples of distal factors include social and economic policies, access to health care, social norms, and socioeconomic factors.

A conceptual framework is a diagram that helps visualize and integrate information about the nature of the problem, frame research questions to investigate the problem, and identify opportunities for prevention or intervention. Key determinants are organized into a conceptual framework to highlight their relationships, interactions, relative importance, and linkages with the outcome(s) of interest. Unlike theoretical models, which are derived from singular theories, conceptual frameworks are often informed by multiple theories, as well as empirical findings and professional experience. Conceptual frameworks may broadly depict the overarching complexity of a problem or narrowly focus on a specific aspect of a larger problem [12]. A notable example of a broad framework is an ecological model (Fig. 7.2a), which illustrates how health outcomes and behavioral patterns are influenced by numerous overlapping factors at multiple levels of influence, ranging from individual factors to societal policies and social norms [12]. Ecological models have been adapted to inform countless population health problems. For example, the Foresight Obesity System Map (http://www.visualcomplexity.com/vc/project.cfm?id=622 [Accessed 26 Jan 2020]) is an expansive model that organizes hundreds of factors and dependencies that influence weight regulation and obesity [13]. In contrast, a policy to require nutrition labeling on fast food restaurant menus may be guided by a narrow framework that illustrates the factors involved in overconsumption of fast food and opportunities for intervention (Fig. 7.2b) [14].

Identify and Prioritize Strategic Interventions

Defining the problem, measuring its magnitude, and identifying key determinants and appreciating their interactions via a conceptual framework will inform opportunities for research, prevention, and intervention. In contrast to clinical medicine, in which singular, curative treatments based on the biological basis of the disease may be available, population health solutions will more likely require multiple, overlapping strategies targeting several key determinants. Effective interventions, programs, or policies usually target those determinants that are most central, modifiable, and/or cost effective to address. Strategies should be informed by what has previously been attempted, whether successful (to build on) or not (to learn from prior challenges). Several principles inform intervention design and choice, including levels of prevention, level of passivity, and categories of intervention.

Risk reduction strategies are often categorized as primary, secondary, or tertiary prevention. Primary prevention refers to preventing the development of a disease or disability before it occurs; secondary prevention refers to early identification of disease, often before the onset of overt signs and

Fig. 7.2 Examples of conceptual frameworks that depict relationships, complexity, or specific aspects of a health problem. Figure 7.2**a** is an ecological model, which illustrates how health outcomes and behavioral patterns are influenced by several overlapping levels of influence, ranging from individual (person) factors to societal policies and social norms [12]. Figure 7.2**b** is an example of a conceptual model that is narrowly focused on a specific aspect of a larger problem. To inform a proposed policy requiring nutrition labeling on fast food restaurant menus, Figure 7.2b illustrates the determinants of caloric intake and factors involved in overconsumption of fast food when dining in fast food restaurants [14]

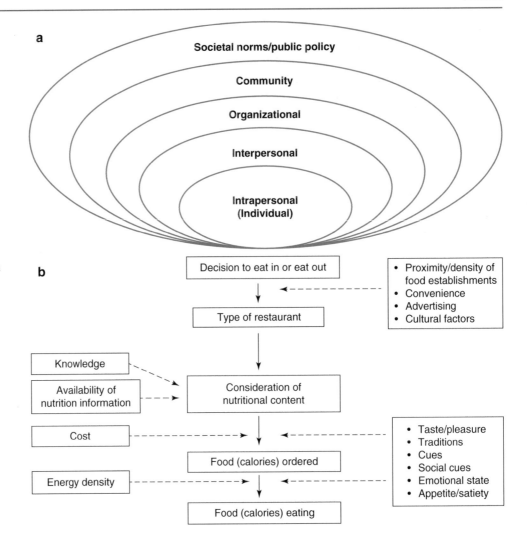

symptoms or early enough to prevent recurrence; and tertiary prevention refers to managing an existing disease after diagnosis to mitigate or cease its progression (Table 7.2). Two additional levels of prevention include primordial prevention, which refers to addressing the conditions that underlie the risk for an exposure or disease, and quaternary prevention has been referred to as protecting from medical harm, such as avoiding or discontinuing treatments that may cause more harm than good [15].

Interventions fall along a continuum of "passivity." Active strategies require a person to act in some way (or avoid an action) in order to achieve benefit or protection. For example, an active strategy to prevent childhood injury would be to hawkishly oversee a child at all times. Passive strategies afford protection without action by the individual, such as eliminating lead-based paints or asbestos in building materials, banning *trans*-fats in restaurant foods, or supplementing grains with folic acid to minimize neural tube defects. Few strategies are purely active or passive. For example, incorporating childproof caps on medication containers affords some passive protection but still optimally requires active

parental attention, and requiring seat belts in all cars still requires that each individual straps them on. In general, the effectiveness of interventions improves as the need for individual action decreases.

Population-level interventions tend to be educational, technological, or regulatory in nature. The "4 E's" describe categories of intervention approaches: Educational, Engineering, Enforcement, and Economic [14]. Educational methods usually attempt to influence knowledge, attitudes, beliefs, and self-efficacy and include a range of approaches from one-on-one counseling to widespread social marketing campaigns. Engineering solutions aim to facilitate behavioral change or prevent adverse outcomes by technological innovation, such as seatbelts, shatterproof windshields, or backup cameras. Enforcement includes policies, mandates, regulations, and laws to guide behavioral changes, prevent negative outcomes, or protect bystanders, such as traffic control regulations and speed limits, requirements for child safety seats in cars or safety helmets when bicycling, bans on marketing of tobacco products or smoking in public places, regulations against junk food marketing during children's television

Table 7.2 Levels of Prevention

Level of Prevention	Description	Examples
Primordial	Addressing the conditions that underlie the risk for an exposure or disease	Addressing social determinants of health, promoting education and modeling healthful behaviors, adjusting the built environment to support safe physical activity, iodination of table salt to prevent severe hypothyroidism
Primary	Preventing the development of a disease or disability before it occurs	Vaccination, counseling to alter risky behaviors such as tobacco use and unhealthful nutrition intake
Secondary	Early identification and treatment of disease, usually before the onset of overt signs and symptoms	Clinical screening such as mammography and blood pressure testing, chemoprevention such as statin use and antihypertensive treatment
Tertiary	Managing an existing disease after diagnosis to mitigate or cease its progression and minimize limitations on quality of life and disability	Interventional treatments such as coronary artery stenting, chemotherapy, rehabilitation, screening for disease complications
Quaternary	Protecting from medical harm, such as treatments that may cause more harm than good [15]	Avoiding unnecessary medical interventions, refraining from treatments that have not been adequately evaluated, informed consent and discussion with patients regarding false-positive results, medication adverse effects, and polypharmacy

shows, and so forth. Economic incentives and disincentives persuade adoption of healthful, safe, or productive practices (such as access to clinical preventive services without copays or cost sharing, rewards for implementing electronic health records in medical practices, and subsidies or reduced insurance premiums for those who sign up for an exercise facility) or avoidance of dangerous or unhealthful behaviors (such as taxation of tobacco products, penalties for Health Insurance Portability and Accountability Act (HIPPA) violations, and severe penalties for driving under the influence of alcohol).

A range of strategic options should be considered in order to maximize the likelihood of achieving the intended outcome(s). It is tempting to quickly anoint a favored intervention without fully considering other options and without evaluating the relative strengths and drawbacks of each. This would be akin to reflexively prescribing an antibiotic without a thorough workup or a rush to surgery in the absence of sufficient presurgical planning. Upon identifying potential options, prioritize those most likely to be effective by assessing their relative utility, acceptability (cultural, political, and social), effectiveness, efficiency, and potential for unintended

consequences (or benefits), among other factors. Successful strategies are rarely singular; for example, the impact of seatbelts, a technological innovation, may not have been as transformative for automobile safety if not combined with educational approaches (e.g., educating the public about the importance of using seatbelts when driving and "buckle-up" social marketing campaigns) and policy interventions (e.g., regulations requiring all cars to include seatbelts and laws to enforce seat belt use).

Evaluate the Impact of Interventions

The process of monitoring programs and policies is necessary in order to evaluate the progress, effectiveness, impact, and opportunities for improvement, as well as to inform future interventions and opportunities to replicate successful programs in other populations. Evaluation is often an afterthought, although progressively more attention has been devoted to this process. Four aspects of program evaluation are formative evaluation, process evaluation, summative (outcome) evaluation, and cost-effectiveness evaluation [14, 16].

Formative evaluation includes qualitative (e.g., focus groups and direct observation) and quantitative (e.g., surveys) methods to assess what factors influence the success of the intervention. This process should be planned and initiated as early as possible to guide program design and implementation. Formative evaluation may include gathering data on the epidemiology of the health or behavioral problem to be addressed, the population of interest and individuals who are most affected, barriers to change, sources to inform program development, channels of information to reach target groups or individuals in the population, and other key insights. Formative evaluation continues throughout the intervention to solicit participant input and reactions to the program, assess public support for the program, enhance understanding of findings, and inform ongoing decision-making.

Process evaluation assesses on-the-ground progress to document how the program is being implemented and may point to needed mid-course corrections. Some important aspects of process evaluation include assessing that key pieces of the program are put into place in the manner intended, participant recruitment, and that the intervention reaches target groups with sufficient levels of exposure.

Summative evaluation measures the outcomes of the intervention. Randomized controlled trials, group-randomized trials (in which whole groups, rather than individuals, are randomized to intervention or serve as controls), quasi-experimental trials (such as when a group or individuals are alternately assigned to an intervention, thus serving as their own controls), and observational studies are designed to assess outcomes. Behavior change programs frequently utilize intermediate outcome indicators, such as changes in knowledge, perceptions, self-efficacy, intentions to change behavior, and specific behavioral goals. This is because longer term outcomes, such as actual changes in morbidity or mortality are often not realistic to evaluate, due to the lengthy time frames that would be needed to observe these changes. In some cases, studies can be designed to assess longer-term outcomes – such as those showing that aggressive anti-smoking and nutrition policies initiated in the early 2000s in New York City contributed to reductions in cardiovascular disease mortality over the next decade [17]. In addition to monitoring behavioral or health outcomes, the evaluation process may be able to prove that the achieved outcome(s) was causally related to the intervention.

Cost-effectiveness quantifies the costs per unit of change and may include cost-benefit evaluation (benefits are calculated based on financial savings), cost-effectiveness analysis (benefits are calculated based on health improvements, such as lives saved or life years saved), and cost-utility analysis (in which health improvements are adjusted for quality of life limitations, such as disability-adjusted life years). Data on cost-effectiveness can be especially valuable for negotiating with policymakers and payers.

Conclusion

This chapter describes an overview of a problem-solving process to address population health problems and health risk reduction. Lifestyle medicine practitioners and leaders will benefit from developing an orientation and proficiency in population approaches to broad, behavior-related, public health problems. Core steps in the problem-solving framework include defining the problem, measuring the magnitude of the problem, understanding the key determinants of the problem, devising a set of prioritized programs, interventions, or policies to target the problem, and evaluating the effectiveness of the chosen approach. Applying the principles of preventive medicine can be especially valuable for the design and implementation of Lifestyle Medicine Centers, as the census of patients can be approached both as individuals and as a unique population for which population medicine concepts can be applied. Examples include identifying protocols for primary and secondary prevention to inform the center's clinical operations, implementing evidence-based practices and monitoring for potential overdiagnosis or polypharmacy to minimize risks of medical harm and improve cost-effectiveness, engaging in community advocacy to support interventions for primordial prevention, and coordinating a disease or treatment registry to inform population assessment and data mining.

References

1. American College of Preventive Medicine. About preventive medicine. https://www.acpm.org/about-acpm/what-is-preventive-medicine/. Accessed 26 Jan 2020.
2. Lianov L, Johnson M. Physician competencies for prescribing lifestyle medicine. J Am Med Assoc. 2010;304:202–3.
3. Rose G. Sick individuals and sick populations. Int J Epidemiol. 1985;48:71–9.
4. Bennett JE, Stevens GA, Mathers CD, et al. NCD Countdown 2030: worldwide trends in non-communicable disease mortality and progress towards Sustainable Development Goal target. Lancet. 2018;392:1072–88.
5. U.S. Department of Health and Human Services. The health consequences of smoking: 50 years of progress. A report of the surgeon general. Atlanta: U.S. Department of Health and Human Services, Centers for Disease Control and Prevention, National Center for Chronic Disease Prevention and Health Promotion, Office on Smoking and Health; 2014.
6. Center for Behavioral Health Statistics and Quality. Behavioral health trends in the United States: results from the 2014 National Survey on Drug Use and Health. HHS Publication No. SMA 15-4927, (NSDUH Series H-50). Rockville: SAMHSA; 2015. Retrieved from http://www.samhsa.gov/data/. Accessed 26 Jan 2020.
7. Ziedonis D, Hitsman B, Beckham JC, et al. Tobacco use and cessation in psychiatric disorders: National Institute of Mental Health report. Nicotine Tob Res. 2008;10:1691–715.
8. Heffner JL, Strawn JR, DelBello MP, et al. The co-occurrence of cigarette smoking and bipolar disorder: phenomenology and treatment considerations. Bipolar Disord. 2011;13:439–53.
9. Thun MJ, Carter BD, Feskanich D, et al. 50-year trends in smoking-related mortality in the United States. N Engl J Med. 2013;368:351–64.
10. Trust for America's Health. The state of obesity: 2019. Better policies for a healthier America. Section II: obesity-related data and trends. 2019. https://www.tfah.org/report-details/stateofobesity2019/. Accessed 26 Jan 2020.
11. Center for Disease Control and Prevention. Behavioral risk factor surveillance system. https://www.cdc.gov/brfss/index.html. Accessed 26 Jan 2020.
12. Glanz K, Kahan S. Chapter 2: conceptual framework for behavior change. In: Kahan S, Fagan PJ, Gielen AC, Green LW, editors. Health behavior change in populations. Baltimore: Johns Hopkins University Press; 2014. p. 9–25.
13. Vandenbroeck P, Goossens J, Clemens M. Tackling obesities: future choices – obesity system atlas. UK Government Office for Science. https://assets.publishing.service.gov.uk/government/uploads/system/uploads/attachment_data/file/296290/obesity-map-full-hi-res.pdf. Accessed 26 Jan 2020.
14. Kahan S. Obesity prevention and interventions. In: Lawrence R, Kahan S. Problem solving in public health. Baltimore, MD: Johns Hopkins Bloomberg School of Public Health. 2012.
15. Martins C, Godycki-Cwirko M, Heleno B, et al. Quaternary prevention: reviewing the concept. Eur J Gen Pract. 2018;24:106–11.
16. Fowler CC, Kahan S. Program planning for behavior change programs. In: Kahan S, Fagan PJ, Gielen AC, Green LW, editors. Health behavior change in populations. Baltimore: Johns Hopkins University Press; 2014. p. 64–89.
17. Ong P, Lovasi GS, Madsen A, et al. Evaluating the effectiveness of New York City health policy initiatives in reducing cardiovascular disease mortality, 1990–2011. Am J Epidemiol. 2017;186:555–63.

Clinical Service Line Strategies in Lifestyle Medicine

8

Daniel K. Zismer

Abbreviations

CHS Community health system
CSL Clinical service line
HCP Healthcare professional
SLT Social learning theory

Setting the Stage

Definition of Terms

In a survey conducted in 2012, 85% of community health systems (CHSs) reported they would launch clinical service lines (CSLs) as a strategy to differentiate their services from competitors, while improving the clinical outcomes and health status of patients served [1]. Here, a CSL is defined as follows:

> A grouping of related clinical services and programs dedicated to an identified constellation of related diagnoses and conditions, designed and directed to produce and deliver a superior course of care, over time, based upon evidence-based best practices for defined clinical populations.

Clinical service lines are a deliberate and intentional strategy born of the belief that a comprehensive, integrated, and coordinated approach to care, and the patient experience, will enhance the potential for superior clinical outcomes, and improved management of total costs of care. Likewise, well-designed and executed CSL strategies are believed to be more effective as a means to engage the patient (and the family support system) as active and activated contributors to the continuum of care and related clinical outcomes and health status of patients served.

Directed and managed CSLs represent a potentially productive strategy for integrated healthcare systems. Clinical service line models are applied to deliver efficacious and efficient management of chronic diseases, including the incorporation and integration of lifestyle medicine services programming as integral and intrinsic components. Lifestyle medicine can be defined in different ways. Lifestyle medicine is the nonpharmacological, nonsurgical/nonprocedural management of chronic disease. However, lifestyle medicine can also be described as an evidence-based approach to prevent, treat, and reverse lifestyle-related chronic diseases [2]. Integrated healthcare systems are the type and nature of the organization that houses and sponsors CSLs. A sponsoring integrated healthcare system can be corporately organized, owned, and controlled in various ways. The entity can exist for the purpose of operating as a CHS, as a specialized integrated group of physicians, or as an organizational grouping of different HCPs [3]. Healthcare professionals within a CSL may be employed by the sponsoring health system. Alternatively, HCPs may operate as teams of employed and independent members, all functioning in concert with other affiliated clinical and administrative partners under a common unifying CSL model and brand.

What makes healthcare systems and their CSLs integrated is more about shared beliefs, culture, and philosophy of mission, vision, and values than an overarching corporate design and ownership. Successful integrated healthcare systems are designed with a focus on the whole patient and are operated with the goal to deliver superior and durable outcomes. People, skill sets, competencies, resources, and assets are aggregated, organized, branded, and provided to enable such a vision and mission. Shared beliefs, at the integrated health system level, translate to each of the operating CSLs within the health system (Table 8.1) [4].

D. K. Zismer (✉)
Professor Emeritus and Chair, Division of Health Policy and Management, School of Public Health, University of Minnesota, Minneapolis, MN, USA

Co-Chair and Chief Executive Officer, Associated Eye Care Partners, LLC, Stillwater, MN, USA
e-mail: daniel.zismer@castlingpartners.com

© Springer Nature Switzerland AG 2020
J. I. Mechanick, R. F. Kushner (eds.), *Creating a Lifestyle Medicine Center*, https://doi.org/10.1007/978-3-030-48088-2_8

Table 8.1 Translating shared beliefs into clinical service lines in an integrated health system

1. Superior patient outcomes are best designed and delivered from a holistic philosophy of care.
2. An interdisciplinary team approach to care is required.
3. Patients and their related support systems must be activated and actively engaged with the care team and the care process.
4. The status of patients' health must be considered and appreciated within a framework of mind, body, and spirit status of balance.
5. The healthcare team must accept and internalize a commitment to a long-term relationship with those served.

Potential leaders and HCPs in a Lifestyle Medicine Center will need to understand the principal challenges in the design, delivery, and management of complex CSLs:

- *Challenge 1 – Increased Accountability:* CSLs are generally focused on patients with chronic disease conditions promising integrated, coordinated care, over time. Such CSL "brand promises" create an accountability for health systems and affiliated HCPs that differs from the more-conventional, less-integrated models of specialized and episodic medical care.
- *Challenge 2 – Creating a Shared Belief System:* the clinical model necessarily brings to bear a more expansive roster of expanded and specialized HCPs, all of whom are required to work together to organize and deliver care according to a shared belief system, unified vision, and common mission.
- *Challenge 3 – Managing Expectations:* well-managed outcomes extend beyond clinical results to include patients' and their support systems' expectations for the care management experience.
- *Challenge 4 – Defining Value:* the value proposition of CSLs, as evaluated by external parties, especially third-party payers, will extend beyond clinical outcomes to efficiencies of care and total costs of care [5].
- *Challenge 5 – Financial:* few health systems have the financial wherewithal, or the clinical services depth and capabilities, to deliver all services required to care for all the needs of the patients served by a CSL. Consequently, CSLs often need to work with tertiary and quaternary referral centers to provide for a complete and ongoing, comprehensive and coordinated care model.
- *Challenge 6 – Geographic Reach:* CSL strategies often link together several locations of service over a defined, regional geography, offering patients multiple points of access for initial visits and ongoing care. Patients move around and within the geographic reach and services delivery map defined by the CSL.

Clinical Conditions Amenable to Clinical Service Line Strategies

A public health view of opportunities is required for the process of selecting clinical conditions for application in CSLs. About 75% of US healthcare dollars, or $3.8 trillion, is spent annually on the management of chronic diseases and conditions [6]. Multiple studies on the efficiency and productivity of the annual US healthcare budget, dating as far back as the early 1980s, demonstrate that an estimated one-third of this total spending has only an insignificant impact on the health status of the afflicted and even causes harm to some [7]. Specifically, for an estimated one-third of patients treated by the US healthcare system annually, this interaction demonstrably contributes to iatrogenic conditions and mortality, with a significant cause being the nature and function of the health services delivery model [8]. This finding affirms the need for innovation in health services delivery.

The principal mission of CSLs is superior clinical outcomes delivered safely with an exceptional patient experience to effectively manage chronic disease conditions over time. Accordingly, the CSL is designed to engage and activate patients as participants in their own care, with due consideration for the whole of the person. Processes of care are designed for efficiencies and efficacies, with total costs of care effectively managed and the convenience of the patients and support systems in mind.

As US health systems consider CSLs as opportunities for strategy, they logically focus on chronic diseases, which consume a disproportionately high number of health care dollars. These disease states include cardiovascular and stroke; orthopedic and connective tissue disease; women's services; neurological, neurovascular disease, and movement disorders; diabetes; cancer; traumatic brain injury; and autoimmune diseases.

CSLs as a strategy enable the more integrated health systems, whether organized community-based not-for-profits, governmental systems, large multispecialty medical group practices, or for-profit hospitals, to differentiate clinical programs, such as lifestyle medicine programs, in crowded and competitive markets. CSLs lend well to creative branding, as they tend to focus brand positional strategies on messaging designed for users and not the HCPs. For example, a CSL specializing in cardiovascular disease may be positioned simply as the "Regional Heart Center," connoting specialization in comprehensive heart diseases services with some geographic reach, or the "International Diabetes Center," implying global reach and deep experience.

Effective design, deployment, and management of comprehensive CSLs create business models that aggregate,

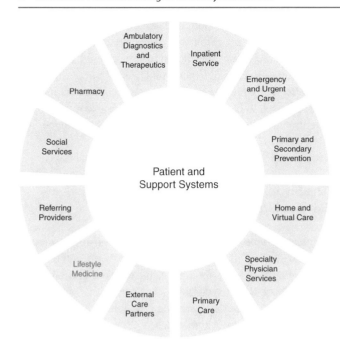

Fig. 8.1 Clinical service lines and application to patient care

Table 8.2 Distinguishing characteristics of effective clinical service lines

Brand positioning
Intake process
Registration process
Information management
Control by patient
Interaction with patient
Support services
Referring provider involvement
Administration
Team captain

coordinate, and deliver a diverse portfolio of integrated, interdisciplinary services. This creates an expandable base of revenues that provides management opportunities to use program size, scope, and scale as a competitive advantage in complex and competitive healthcare markets (Fig. 8.1).

The Anatomy of a Clinical Service Line Strategy

Clinical service lines are organized to deliver a comprehensive, integrated approach to the management of identified chronic conditions, delivered by an interdisciplinary team of HCPs at multiples sites, to patients over long periods of time. The principal clinical goal is optimized health status with care efficiency and cost being well managed. The principal patient care goal is effective engagement and activation as a partner in the care management process. The principal business goal is the efficient acquisition of patients who become loyal, satisfied patients. CSL models exhibit identifying strategic, functional, and patient experience characteristics in common (Table 8.2).

There exists an encompassing, effective, and efficient brand positioning strategy that establishes distinguishing and differentiating value propositions for priority markets. The brand strategy effectively connects the CSL value propositions with potential users. Target markets are defined in

various ways based upon an identified chronic condition. A principal goal of the brand strategy is to correctly position the value propositions of the CSL in the mind's eye of those to be served. In addition, the brand strategy answers the important question of "why you [the target market] should come to us."

The CSL also establishes multiple portals of entry that are easily contacted and accessed by those served. The intake process efficiently directs patients to the first, best point of contact, based upon the first, best response to clinical impressions of referring HCPs and/or patients' presenting expressions of wants and needs.

The registration process not only gathers, synthesizes, and systemizes demographics and the required patient information, but it also sets the expectations for the first contact and experience. This includes expectations, concerns, and questions about the first visit and CSL contact. Likewise, patients are pre-introduced to the HCP who will start them on their journey as a patient of the CSL and team. Patients are prepared for their initial visit with understandings of the mission, philosophy, values, care model, and methods of the team, as well as how the CSL provides for a sense of community for those who are cared for over time. Expectations of their participation as a patient in the CSL are established early on and are reinforced over time. Along the way, the value of a team approach for effective management of chronic disease and related environmental factors becomes a distinguishing characteristic of a CSL.

The system of care is connected by a unifying and integrated format of information management. Patients have a single point of contact to help them navigate the CSL during each encounter, which is consistent and familiar over time. Information system outputs extend to the patient and can include clinical health status, administrative information, and access to other portions of their electronic health record. Control over access for routine, episodic, and urgent visits also rest in the patient's control. However, encouraging appropriate interactions with patients to optimize care rests with the CSL. This includes ongoing routine encounter recalls, special alerts on diagnostic test results, tailored health education opportunities, and patient-focused provider reports.

Participation in related support services is encouraged with the goals of engagement, activation, and effective self-management of heath and health status. A broad portfolio of services is provided, such as special education sessions, patient and family support groups, contacts for acute problems and concerns, sources for patients and families for continuous education about their clinical condition, and ongoing methods of self-help. HCPs who are peripheral to the direct care provided by the CSL are kept informed about the current care and services available. This includes primary care and specialist physicians outside the control boundaries of the CSL.

Administrative matters, such as services billing and third-party payer matters, are managed by CSL-supporting personnel and related systems. There should be a single point of contact to manage patients' needs regarding services costs and payment methods. Patients must see the CSL as an advocate for related financial matters. Lastly and most importantly, there must be an identified team captain or navigator for all patients active within the CSL.

Lifestyle Medicine and Clinical Service Line Design and Operations

Positioning Lifestyle Medicine

The totality of all health care consumed by the US population accounts for an estimated 20% contribution to the health status of the population, with lifestyle, genetics, and environmental factors exerting far more influence, in the aggregate [9]. Included in the ambit of lifestyle medicine are the comparatively obvious factors such as diet and exercise. But there are also the less obvious factors, such as patients' reactions to intrinsic and extrinsic stressors, emotional and psychological states, perceptions of inherent abilities to exert control over personal health, and perceived value of participation in the management of health. These last two factors affect a patient's interactions with a CSL, especially the lifestyle medicine components.

Clinical service lines present opportunities to engage users as both patient and customer. Managers and HCPs within CSLs need to appreciate the fundamental differences between the healthcare delivery that is episodic in purpose and nature versus that focused on chronic disease management. Active and long-term participation in chronic disease management requires a comprehensive understanding of how the tenets of lifestyle medicine integrate with CSL programming to create a satisfying outcome for patients,

HCPs, and related support staff. Likewise, it is important to understand how specific types of patients will interact with the CSL care model and its philosophy, based on psychological, emotional, and experiential factors. Successful CSLs will effectively prepare patients for a specialized philosophy and approach to care. Successful CSLs are also guided by an intentional culture that is decided, designed, deployed, and directed by CSL leadership.

The Social Psychology of Effective Clinical Service Lines

Clinical service lines are organisms within organizations. They are intentionally designed to behave differently from conventional models for delivering medical specialty services. There is a psychology to the effective design and management of CSLs, described here within an established social psychological framework.

By design, CSLs create enduring communities of care for two types of affinity groups: patients and HCPs, along with their respective support systems. These communities operate from a unified purpose, belief system, value set, goals, incentives, and culture. Thus, CSLs are considered as defined social units with a stated mission and identified society to serve. There is a distinctive social psychology of CSL design, operations, and leadership.

The discipline of social psychology is defined as the study of how a person's feelings and actions are affected by the presence of other people and all internal and external factors that pertain. Patients interact with CSLs and expect valuable outcomes and benefits. Expectations of benefits will vary from patient to patient. For instance, some patients will hope for and even expect full recovery from their condition, while other patients will simply hope for a fulfilling life despite their condition. The success of a CSL is, to a great extent, dependent upon how patients are engaged through the social psychology of the CSL and related diagnoses. The social psychology and resultant belief system of a CSL create the framework for how HCPs and staff interact with patients, patients' support systems, and each other. This framework determines how patients are managed through therapeutic processes over time and influences how patients think, behave, and react to their engagement with their clinical condition and the CSL. Ultimately, the social psychology of the CSL shapes patients' total self-view of where they are, what and who they have become, and their outlook of what life ahead may hold in store.

Rotter's social learning theory (SLT) provides a robust, social psychological framework for designers of CSLs. Julian B. Rotter (1916–2014) was an American psychologist who predicated his theory of social psychology on the premise that an individual's personality does not exist independent of their environment, and people are motivated to seek positive stimulation. Rotter's SLT holds that a person's behaviors (including health behaviors) are a function of their expectations for rewards of sufficient value, and a person's behaviors and personality are shaped by experiences and interactions with their environments.

Rotter's more basic formula for behaviors and related outcomes, and here attitude is a behavior, postulates that behavior (and the potential for behavior) is a function of a person's expectation for a reward that is of sufficient value (Fig. 8.2) [10]. Expectations for a specific reward and the value of that reward can both work together and separately to influence behavioral outcomes. A third environmental factor can work separately or together, as well, with one or both of the other two to affect behavioral outcomes. This factor of the model pertains to what is happening situationally or chronically within the person's environment, at levels levels sufficient to affect how the other two factors, individually or together, affect the the potential for behavior patterns and behavior change.

How can Rotter's SLT be applied to a patient within a CSL? In the example of a cardiovascular CSL, a 65-year-old CAUCASIAN female is being treated for diastolic heart failure. She reports shortness of breath and fatigue. She has obesity and type 2 diabetes, which she believes are genetically determined and not due to her health behavior decisions. She is recently widowed, lives alone, and has two adult children who live out of the state. She was diagnosed with clinical depression by a psychologist who saw the patient shortly following admission to the CSL. A battery of cardiovascular diagnostics demonstrated diffuse cardiovascular and pulmonary vascular diseases. The treatment plan consists of multi-vessel coronary artery bypass grafting, along with significant weight loss and regular exercise. With this plan, she is told that her life can be prolonged and the progression of her diastolic dysfunction can be managed better than it has been to date.

In the context of Rotter's SLT, the patient is asked to endure a major surgical procedure, followed by a significant lifestyle change, to presumably gain an unknown number of years of life with no assurance of a positive perceived change of quality of life. The psychologist and other members of the lifestyle medicine team apply Rotter's SLT to tailor the treatment plan to the patient. First, the patient's attitudes are reviewed.

1. She does not appreciate how her own health behaviors have contributed to her current state of health. The expectations variable is construed as a person's health locus or control [11]. Those who are more internally oriented believe their health behavior decisions affect their health status, whereas those who are more externally oriented believe their personal health status to be more a result of luck, fate, or factors beyond their control.
2. She does not expect that if she survives the surgery, the reward value presented by what is perceived to be a radical and near impossible lifestyle change will produce rewards at levels greater than the sacrifices needed to achieve the goals presented.
3. Lastly, given her depressed state, coupled with her personality and environmental circumstances, the prospects of the prescribed surgery, long recovery, and required lifestyle change are daunting, at best.

The lifestyle management team for the cardiovascular CSL develops an approach to help the patient confront these attitudes and see through the unapproachable decision to have coronary artery bypass surgery, including arranging transitional care following the surgical event, and through the cardiac rehabilitation that follows. An affiliated psychiatrist can work with the CSL clinical pharmacist to coordinate the patient's antidepressive medication regimen with the expected post-surgical cardiac and ongoing heart failure medications. The patient is offered and encouraged to take advantage of a heart failure support group, which includes opportunities for a tailored approach to nutrition and weight

$$B = f(E x + R v + \psi)$$

$\psi =$ Situational state, including intervening environmental factors—real or perceived.

$Rv =$ Reward value. Behavior is affected by perceived value of the reward available. Value affects an individual's likelihood to engage in the behaviors required to attain the reward.

$Ex =$ Expectancy for a reward (tangible or intangible). Expectancy can be affected by an individual's locus of control (specific or general); an individual's expectation for their ability to exert personal control over an outcome.

Description: Julian Rotter's social learning theory defines the causality of behavior (including related attitudes and emotions) as a function of an individual's expectancy for a valued reward, plus situational factors and circumstances operating within the related environment. Change to one or all factors can affect behavior or behavior potential of an individual.

Example: An individual might ascribe value to receiving a promotion on the job, but expectancy for it is low and the company might be at risk for sale. So, the individual's expectancy for that valued promotion is sufficiently low, predicting that efforts to go "above and beyond" to achieve the desired reward are unlikely.

Fig. 8.2 Rotter's social learning theory explained. (Reprinted with permission by Phys Leadership J, 6(3)). Figure 1, page 2, American Association for Physician Leadership®, 800-562-8088, www.physicianleaders.org

loss, and is enrolled in a regular exercise program offered for patients with similar needs provided on the main campus of the health system. Individual counseling sessions are scheduled providing talk therapy to address her depression, including video check-in sessions with family members. Social services begin to interact with family that is out of state to establish needed family support. The underlying therapeutic path follows the SLT theoretical framework with a multispecialty, multidisciplinary, holistic approach and several key elements:

1. To help the patient establish a sense of control over their health and health behaviors
2. To help the patient appreciate and connect the reward value derived from exchanging old health behaviors for new ones
3. To help the patient accommodate to and cope with uncontrollable environmental and situational stressors
4. To encourage ongoing participation in appropriate support group activities
5. To engage, educate, and prepare her children on how to support her as she begins her care regimen

Rotter's SLT is not as much a therapeutic method as it is a way of operations for a CSL. Larger-scale CSLs operating with an interdisciplinary care model, caring for large numbers of patients, served by several sites, and interacting with hundreds of referral sources and multiple contributing CSL partners, require a way of thinking (and psychology) that applies to the care of patients and the functionality of the CSL at the HCP level, all at the same time.

Within the CSL, HCPs must learn to trust that the efficacy and efficiency available from CSL model exceed those available from their more traditional and conventional models of specialty medical care delivery. In Rotter's SLT terms, HCPs must expect that the reward value of the model for patients and HCPs will be superior to alternative models, at levels that are sufficient to warrant the time, effort, and periodic disruptions endured along the way.

The Practicalities of Clinical Service Line Strategy Management

Clinical service line models of care organization and delivery provide sponsoring health systems opportunities to differentiate services in crowded and competitive markets. To achieve such an end, strategic plans are required that effectively position and connect value propositions and CSL potential with the mind's eyes of the target clinical user groups, related referral sources, and strategic third-party payers. Lifestyle medicine can play a central role in distinguishing CSLs through the application of certain strategic and management goals.

1. Create a CSL programmatic design and system of service delivery that competitors will be challenged to replicate.
2. Create multiple CSL open doors across the system of care, with superior "first touch" and ongoing access, coordinated for patients and referring HCPs.
3. Create predictable patient demand flow rates and services volumes sufficient to meet operating economics and financial requirements of the clinical model, including all direct and indirect operating and capital asset expense rates. In other words, a sufficient and reliable flow of the right patients.
4. Create an appropriate capital asset base, staffing model, and clinical and programmatic services offerings across strategic, geographic locations.
5. Create a unifying brand strategy for execution across sites to reach key referral sources and potential patients.
6. Identify and engage the key professional referral sources (other HCPs) in the mission, vision, and strategy of the CSL, including how each can participate in the care of their patients referred and benefit from the CSL care model and program design.
7. Create appropriate service demand for the current patient base of the health system.
8. Establish ongoing direct-to-markets brand awareness campaigns emphasizing ease of access, comprehensive and specialized personalized care, and care coordination across all sites of service.
9. Ensure ongoing referral source education, including marketing the value of the CSL method of care delivery.
10. Most importantly, differentiate with lifestyle medicine programming. This creates an emotional connection to potential patient candidates in terms of comprehensive, personalized, whole person care, well-coordinated team approach to care, respect for the uniqueness of every patient cared for, availability of HCPs and programs that recognize and appreciate that well-being is more important than absence of disease, and understanding that loved ones require care along with the patient. Such brand promises not only create honest and sincere emotional connections with patients, but they also present a barrier to entry and competition for other HCP groups and health systems ill-equipped to deliver on such a strategy.

Case Vignette #1: Community Health System's Heart and Vascular Center – A Cardiovascular CSL Strategy

Community Health System (CHS) leaders have been employing cardiologists and heart surgeons at an accelerating rate. This is largely due to physicians' concerns for mounting economic pressures in the marketplace, such as downward pressures by payers on price, service volumes, and total costs of care. Another factor is the reduction in financial productivity of private practice engendering younger physicians' willingness to trade the uncertainties of independent practice for the perceived securities available from employment by large health systems.

The CHS takes stock of its existing model of integrating cardiovascular medical and surgical specialists as employees. The findings cause CHS leaders, physicians, and administrators to conclude that a reorientation of mission, vision, philosophy, culture, clinical model, and strategy will provide a unique approach to mounting competing threats. The strategic plan begins with the collective reorientation of shared beliefs as summarized below [12].

1. But for some repairable genetic or acquired clinical anomalies, cardiovascular disease represents a chronic health condition for most people. Patients with related diagnoses require integrated and well-coordinated, efficacious, cost-effective care, over long periods of time, provided by a well-orchestrated team approach to care.

2. To date, a physician-centric practice model dominates. The philosophy of employing physicians has been based on letting each decide how they wish to practice, care for patients, interact with referring physicians, peers, other colleagues, and staff and permit each to work from differing economic incentives established by individualized compensation plans and employment agreements. Patients are viewed as belonging to individual physicians. Physicians decide how ancillary professional staff are to interact with their patients. This approach is affirmed by patients, who expect and want a coordinated team approach to care, relying on the guidance of a physician they identify with as being the leader of an interdisciplinary care team.

3. The majority of new patients derive from physician referrals to individual cardiologists. The referral network is composed of independent primary and secondary care physicians in smaller, independent practices and physicians employed by the CHS. The average age of the independent referring physicians is 56 years. However, the total number of referring independent physicians has been reduced by 40% over the past 7 years due to retirements and employment by competing health systems.

Therefore, the CHS will need to employ more referring physicians who must be prepared to work interactively with a range of health system-based CSLs where they become an engaged and activated partner. Eventually, the growing proportion of new patients will result from self-referrals within and across CSLs.

4. While clinical outcomes are reported according to industry standards, patient experience scores are less structured and uniform in nature. Perspectives on the physician/patient experience vary. Complaints generally demonstrate dissatisfaction with access, hand-offs from HCP-to-HCP, lab and procedure results follow-up, inconsistencies in information transfers, inadequate education, and simply not knowing what comes next in the care process. Patients expect, want, and deserve a more accessible, integrated, and well-coordinated experience with each encounter. HCP and support staff must understand how the design and performance of the CSL affect patient engagement and satisfaction.

5. Most patients present with lifestyle and health behavior patterns that interact with their disease state. Many patients lack the knowledge, skill sets, and outcome expectations required to change health behavior patterns, including attitudinal and emotional responses to their disease state and response opportunities. A healthcare milieu that prepares, activates, and empowers patients to become knowledgeable and engage participants in their care and well-being is required.

6. The health care regimen and programmatic enhancements required to meet the revised mission, expectations, and opportunities will significantly alter the existing operating delivery model and related economic and financial performance, as compared with the existing model of cardiovascular services delivery. In order to meet these financial performance requirements at the health system level, marketing efforts will need to positively affect the following:
   - New patient volumes that have increasing clinical complexity
   - Stimulation of appropriate services demand from the existing patient base
   - Positively shift the payer mix
   - Ensure clinical complexity is well-matched to provider training and skill sets

With the establishment of this new system of shared beliefs, administrative leadership and clinicians can address the new CSL culture. Healthcare organizational culture affects patient experience and potential for engaging with HCPs, support staff, and the clinical model. The CSL culture will affect patient adherence with treatment and care recommendations [13], as well as potential to change health behaviors.

Fig. 8.3 Clinical service line strategic plan performance "score card". *Abbreviation*: *RVU* relative value equivalent

For Accounting Period #2, Current FY _____

Strategic Performance	Site 1	Site 2	Site 3
New Patients	⬆	▬	⬇
Provider Referrals	⬆	⬇	⬇
Case Mix	▬	▬	⬆
Net-Operating Revenues	⬆	▬	⬇
Contribution Margin	⬇	⬇	⬇
Clinical Outcomes Index	▬	▬	▬
Patient Experience	⬇	⬆	⬆
Provider and Staff Culture	⬆	⬆	⬇
Total Costs of Care Index	⬆	▬	⬇
Provider Productivity (wRVU's)	⬆	⬇	⬇

Performance Indicators:

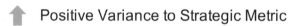 Positive Variance to Strategic Metric

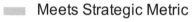 Meets Strategic Metric

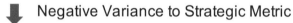 Negative Variance to Strategic Metric

The CHS embarks upon a mission of culture shift. Leadership, especially physician leadership, is charged with moving the fulcrum of culture from individual physician specialists practicing an idiosyncratic philosophy of disease management, to a shared CSL vision, mission, and strategy [14, 15]. A snapshot of this new cardiovascular CSL strategy is provided below.

1. Successful differentiation of the CSL, from competitors, as perceived by potential and existing patients, existing and potential referring physicians, and local, regional, collaborative community health systems and participating third-party payers.
2. Extend the CSL brand and care model to controlled and affiliated regional health system partners, including the installation of required care model support systems, such as an integrating foundation of information technologies.
3. Effectively reposition the CSL with existing patients.
4. Effectively reposition the CSL with existing referral sources.
5. Effectively reposition the CSL for general and regional awareness.

The strategy of CSLs must be actively managed, with results that are identifiable and quantifiable. The perfor-mance metrics are dictated by the strategic goals and objectives of a CSL, during a specific strategy cycle (Fig. 8.3). The effective repositioning of the conventional specialty care delivery models to CSL strategies is challenging and potentially expensive. The goal is differentiation based upon a compelling value proposition that is unavailable from other HCPs of similar specialty care. Effective strategy requires the successful positioning of all potential sources of referral, third parties who pay for care, and most importantly, the end-users: patients and their support systems.

The Business and Financial Management of Clinical Service Lines

Various financial terms need to be defined in this discussion of CSL business management.

- *Clinical models* are the constellation of clinical services and identified sub-programs that compose the whole of the CSL clinical portfolio.
- *Gross charges* are billed to payers and based on a health system price list (charge master).

- *Net operating revenue* represents the estimated cash collections generated for services provided and billed to patients or after contractual adjustments if billed to responsible third-party payers.
- *Direct operating expense* refers to all expenses required for providing direct clinical care to patients.
- *Indirect operating expense* structure refers to supporting services, such as accounting, billing and collections, information systems, human resources support, facilities, and other hard assets costs, insurances, taxes, and cost of capital.
- *Contribution margin* is reflected as a ratio, and in absolute dollars. It is the remainder of net operating revenue minus all direct operating expense. Contribution margin is often the single best indicator of CSL financial performance trends.
- *Net operating margin* is the remainder of net operating revenue minus all direct operating expenses and all indirect operating expenses.
- *Investment capital* for CSLs is typically required for areas of ongoing need: facilities to house services and programs, clinical services technologies, capital required to fund the start-up and expansion of CSL programming (referred to as working capital), replacement capital, and ongoing capital investments required to maintain hard assets needs in support of the whole of the CSL.
- *Per-unit economics* refers to the relationship between resource inputs, services outputs, and economic scalability. With every CSL subcomponent, there is formula of resource inputs and outputs.

A lifestyle medicine programming within CSLs is composed of HCPs delivering individual units of service directly to individual patients. With each unit of service, there is a prescribed requirement of resource inputs such as hours of professional time, units of related clinical products, and other identifiable and accountable direct and indirect operating expenses. Likewise, there is always an expected financial return for each unit of service provided. These per-unit relationships, in the aggregate, dictate the financial performance of the programmatic CSL sub-components such as lifestyle medicine programming. For example, a unit of lifestyle medicine counseling, as provided by a clinical social worker, is delivered at an expected net operating revenue rate of $100.00. The wage and benefit rate of this HCP is $45.00. Therefore, the contribution margin available to the CSL to cover all other related direct and indirect operating expenses, and net operating margin requirements, is $55.00. However, if the identified service can be provided equally well to five patients in a group counseling delivery model, the direct operating expense structure remains constant and the net operating revenue potential and contribution margin is scaled up by 500%. The obvious question here relates to the extent to which individual

lifestyle medicine counseling sessions can be translated to group counseling sessions.

All CSLs are an aggregation of complementary clinical services and programs. Clinical service lines produce a more complex operating revenue structure, generated by a range of programs and HCPs. Inasmuch as CSLs typically deliver services from multiple sites, facilities, and geographic locations, management of operating revenues and the related accounting across the CSL is a challenge. Most health services delivery organizations are not well equipped to reliably perform CSL operating revenue and cost accounting.

In contrast, CSL business models are by design more horizontal than vertical. The CSL model interacts with the business model to produce a resultant set of operating economics that drives overall financial performance. These sub-components operate interactively to create the financial performance signature of each CSL operating within a health system. A principal responsibility and challenge for CSL leaders is to understand how these CSL sub-components actually interact. In the CHS example previously described, the CSL provides a broad array of clinical services ranging from comprehensive cardiac interventional and surgical services to cardiology diagnostics, ongoing management of chronic heart, vascular, and pulmonary diseases, acute and emergent care, regional outreach, lifestyle medicine for chronic conditions, clinical research, and postgraduate training. The whole of the CSL must operate at a 30% contribution margin to meet its full financial performance requirements. Cardiovascular care serves as a significant financial contributor to the health system's financial performance overall. This CSL accounts for an estimated 40% of the total net operating margin of the health system. As such, the financial performance of the cardiovascular CSL matters to the overall financial performance of the health system.

Individual service offerings within the CSL operate with unique operating, economic, and financial signatures. Each produces unique revenue and expense structures and requires capital investments at varying levels and time intervals. When all programs and services within the portfolio operate in balance, the financial performance meets requirements of the sponsoring health system (i.e., a 30% contribution margin). When the portfolio is out of economic balance, the financial performance suffers. For example, if volumes for surgical and interventional cardiology services are low with respect to business plan expectations, financial margins underperform, placing the financial performance of the whole CSL at risk.

There is an art and science to the effective economics management of CSLs. Leaders and managers need to develop an intimate understanding of the operating economics signature created by the composition of the CSL clinical model, which drives business model performance. The business model drives operating economics, and the operating economics drives financial performance (Fig. 8.4). The effective management of operating economics for CSLs is based on a foundation of management principles that represents the recipe for economic success. The extent to which leaders and managers adhere to these principles will dictate the level of CSL performance success achieved.

- *Principle #1:* The clinical service portfolio is designed to balance economic performance potential. The size, scope, and economic scaling of each service are managed individually to create a net operating financial result sufficient for the CSL to meet its financial contribution obligations to the sponsoring health system.
- *Principle #2:* Each individual clinical service component will have value that extends beyond financial, strategic, and brand values. The total value of each service is evalu-

$$\sum_{1 \text{ (CSL sub-component)}}^{n \text{ (CSL sub-components)}} (x - y)$$

The consolidated contribution margin performance of a clinical service line (CSL) is the summation of the contribution margin performance of its programmatic sub-components over a defined accounting period. Here x = net operating revenues of the CSL program sub-component and y is the aggregate of direct operating expenses. Contribution margins of CSL program sub-components can range from the positive to negative during a defined accounting period.

Fig. 8.4 Calculation of the consolidated contribution margin potential for clinical service lines

ated for its contribution to the mission and strategy as well. Specific programmatic sub-components of a CSL can produce low or even negative operating economic and financial returns, but they provide strategic value that outweighs the financial. For example, lifestyle medicine can be a programmatic differentiator.

- *Principle #3:* Internal operating economic incentives must align to best serve the mission and financial requirements of the CSL. This particularly applies to internal incentives that affect HCP practice and total productivity in the CSL business model. The HCP compensation design, for example, must align the incentives that drive the mission, strategic plan, and financial requirements of the CSL. Compensation incentives alignment should be a focus of CSL leaders and managers.
- *Principle #4:* Human resources represent the largest component of the operating expense structure of virtually all CSLs. Human resources require optimized productivity leverage within and across CSL programmed components. The total annual, human resource spend of a CSL can be as much as 60–62% of the total operating expense budget. Figure 8.5 demonstrates an unproductive application of primary care physicians and APCs were interchangeable, i.e., physicians and APCs were doing the same work. Physicians were not applying their capacity productively to more complex patients. APCs were paid a salary and physicians were paid on a productivity-based compensation model: a fixed rate per work relative value units (WRVU) produced.
- *Principle #5:* Economic productivity and financial performance are optimized with patients acquired into the CSL and remaining loyal to the CSL over the long term. It costs more to acquire a patient than it does to retain one.

Fig. 8.5 Physician and assistant practice clinicians shared vs. exclusive services. *Abbreviations*: MD medical doctor, APC assistant practice clinician (also referred to as advanced practice provider)

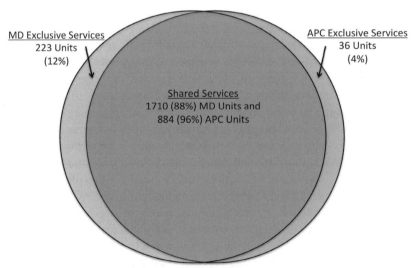

MD Exclusive Services
223 Units
(12%)

APC Exclusive Services
36 Units
(4%)

Shared Services
1710 (88%) MD Units and
884 (96%) APC Units

The size of the spheres indicates the relative number of units of service performed. The vast majority (88% of MD and 96% of APC services) of services are shared, meaning that these services are at some point performed by both MDs and APCs in this practice. Similarly, only 12% of MD and 4% of APC services are exclusive to those providers

Those who lead CSLs can benefit by understanding the difference between two important and basic terms of business management as they relate to CSLs: efficiency and productivity. For CSLs, efficiency, especially operating cost efficiency, generally refer to the reductions of operating cost with output being held constant. For example, the number of eye surgeries produced per day remains the same, but the operating costs per surgery are reduced. However, productivity (specifically, economic productivity) on the other hand, generally refers to the production of increasing outputs produced on a relatively fixed cost structure. For example, eye surgeons produce 15 surgeries per day from one operating room. Direct costs are equal per case produced. Management implements a plan to reduce cost per case. The total number of cases performed is produced more cost-efficiently. Alternatively, management, working with the eye surgeons, determines a path to producing five incremental surgical cases per day. Here, the number of units produced, on a relatively fixed cost structure, increases by 33%. Now, the operating room has become more productive and more cost-efficient. Dyad leaders of CSLs are encouraged to learn how to apply such business and clinical care management acumen to opportunities to improve both operating efficiencies and productivities in CSLs.

Case Vignette #2 – Heart Failure Programming and Lifestyle Management

The heart failure program of the cardiovascular CSL focuses on existing patients and direct referrals from primary care and specialty physicians, internal and external to a community-based integrated health system. In addition to the expected clinical services offered by cardiologists and cardiac surgeons, a cornerstone of the program is lifestyle medicine programming, offering a wide range of services to reduce the development of additional heart failure risk factors and complications. The whole of the CSL is driven by a total of a 200,000 work relative value equivalents produced annually by all cardiologists. Of these, 30,000 (15%) are provided to patients with heart failure diagnoses. The related lifestyle medicine services provided to these heart failure patients require three full-time equivalents of specialized non-physician HCPs. With the existing clinical model, these HCPs are at full-service capacity. The new business plan calls for a 25% increase in heart failure patients by the beginning of year 2 of program expansion. This calls for lifestyle medicine components of the heart failure programming to be quickly scaled up by two additional full-time equivalents. The financial performance of the lifestyle medicine component of the heart failure program will produce

a negative contribution margin by an estimated, aggregate amount of $225,000 over the next 24–36 months and will thereafter operate at a fully accounted 30% negative net operating margin. While not a profitable component of the heart failure program, the availability of the lifestyle medicine programming is a notable heart failure program differentiator and patient satisfier. Furthermore, lifestyle medicine HCPs have proven to be enhancers to clinical outcomes and serve as an accessible front door for HCP-referred and self-referred patients.

Health system leadership will no doubt become concerned with the projected financial losses due to the lifestyle medicine programming expansion for heart failure patients. What is not fully appreciated in the related financial analyses are the associated strategic, economic, and financial values that loyal heart failure patients provide to the CSL. Over a lifetime, each heart failure patient consumes a significant amount of ongoing diagnostic and treatment services at financial margins that more than compensate for the accounted financial losses directly attributed to lifestyle medicine programming expansion within the CSL (Fig. 8.6). So, the negative financial performance of heart failure programming must be weighed together with the other non-profitable services provided to heart failure patients.

The Art of Leading in CSLs

By definition, CSLs present an interdisciplinary model as the preferred approach to the effective management of chronic disease. Clinical service lines more typically exist as strategies of integrated health systems. They are usually led by a clinician working in partnership with an administrative professional in what is referred to in the industry as a dyadic leadership team. Figure 8.7 presents a schematic of a CSL dyad leadership model: a physician and administrative leadership team.

Clinical service lines, by their very nature and design, do not fit the conventional models of healthcare organization and management. They operate more horizontally than vertically and dyad leaders of CSLs must be equipped to operate within a matrixed management model, meaning, the program components of the CSL are necessarily linked to and interact with other support services and clinical programs that are positioned within the organization but are controlled and managed by leaders who do not operate within CSL (e.g., leaders of hospital inpatient services, clinical imaging services, discharge planning, surgical services, and pharmacy). Consequently, the art of leadership of a high-performing CSL requires leaders of the CSL to operate a program with a defined mission, vision, strategy,

Fig. 8.6 Financial contribution margin analysis of services

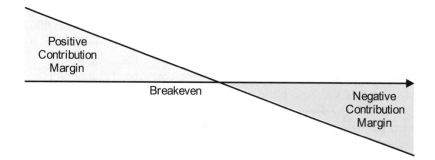

Clinical service lines, within integrated health systems, will produce varying financial and operating economic signatures. Financial contribution margin performance will vary across CSL's. The consolidated contribution margin (produced by all CSL's, in the aggregate) must produce a satisfactory, consolidated financial outcome. Subpar financial performance by a specific CSL may be compensated for by its strategic or clinical services value contributions to the whole of the integrated health system strategy.

Fig. 8.7 The dyadic management model for the integrated community health system

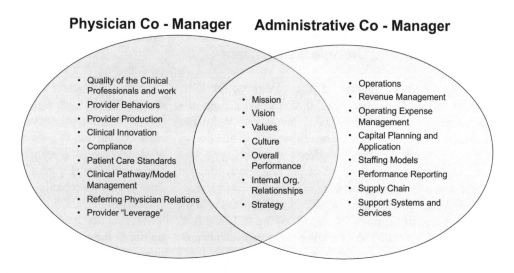

and clinical and business models, within a larger, more conventional, and complex vertical health system organizational design.

A veteran physician clinical service line leader once observed that the style required of a CSL leader is more like that of a stage play director than that of a conventially trained and practiced leader/manager in other industries. The design of a successful CSL culture is based on a shared belief system that is also, by design, unconventional when compared with that of more traditional approaches to health care delivery. This shared belief system is composed of CSL elements that convert behaviors of providers and patients.

References

1. Zismer DK, Wegmiller DC. Clinical service lines: mapping the future of community health. Minneapolis: C-Suite Resources Report; 2012.
2. American College of Lifestyle Medicine. https://lifestylemedicine.org//. Accessed 1 Feb 2020.
3. Zismer DK, Cerra FB. High functioning, integrated health systems: governing a learning organization. A Governance Institute White Paper, Summer 2012, The Governance Institute, https://www.governanceinstitute.com/. Accessed 1 Feb 2020.
4. Zismer DK. Managing strategic risk effectively requires shared beliefs. Special ed: Boardroom Press; 2019, https://www.governanceinstitute.com/. Accessed 1 Feb 2020.

5. Zismer DK, Schuh D. Clinical service line strategy, managing the risks of geographic expansion. Healthc Financ Manage. 2016;70:50–6.

6. Sisko AM, Keehan SP, Poisal JA, et al. National health expenditure projections, 2018–27: economic and demographic trends drive spending and enrollment growth. Health Aff. 2019;38:491–501.

7. Berwick D, Nolan TW, Whittington J. The triple aim and cost. Health Aff. 2008;27:759–69.

8. Mafi J, Russell K, Bortz B, et al. Low-cost, high-volume, health services contribute to unnecessary health spending. Health Aff. 2017;36:1701–4.

9. Magna S. Social determinants of health 101 for health care: five plus five. NAM Perspectives. Discussion Paper, National Academy of Medicine, Washington, DC; 2017, https://doi.org/10.31478/201710c.

10. Zismer DK. Framework to gauge physician burnout. Am Assoc Phys Leadership 2019; May/June: 50-54.

11. Strickland B. Internal-external expectancies and health-related behaviors, 1978. J Consult Clin Psychol. 1978;46:1192–211.

12. Zismer DK. The social psychology of clinical service line management. A model and method for dyads to understand and manage the inevitable "situational disorders." Leadership Coaching Corner, Castling Partners, April 12, 2017, https://www.castlingpartners.com/leadership-coaching-corner/2017/4/3/the-social-psychology-of-clinical-service-line-management. Accessed 1 Feb 2020.

13. Zismer DK. An argument for the integration of healthcare management with public health practice. J Healthc Manag. 2013; 58:253–7.

14. Zismer DK, Utecht BJ. Part one: culture alignment, high-performing healthcare organizations, and the role of the governing board, culture and culture alignment – the foundation of a board's culture game plan. E-Briefings, The Governance Institute 2018;15. https://www.keystoneculturegroup.com/2018/03/01/culture-alignment-high-performing-healthcare-organizations-and-the-role-of-the-governing-board-part-one/. Accessed 1 Feb 2020.

15. Zismer DK, Utecht BJ. Part two: culture alignment, high-performing healthcare organizations, and the role of the governing board, setting a culture of high performance and the responsibility of governing boards. E-Briefings, The Governance Institute 2018; 15. https://www.keystoneculturegroup.com/2018/05/01/culture-alignment-high-performing-healthcare-organizations-and-the-role-of-the-governing-board-part-two/. Accessed 1 Feb 2020.

Business Plans for a Lifestyle Medicine Center

Marc Braman and Joe Raphael

Abbreviations

ACO	Accountable Care Organization
DO	Doctor of Osteopathic Medicine
DPC	Direct primary care
HCP	Healthcare professional
LCSW	Licensed clinical social worker
LMFT	Licensed marriage and family psychotherapist
MD	Medical Doctor
PhD/PsyD	Doctor of Psychology
RDN	Registered dietitian nutritionist

Introduction

Realistically, sustainable healthcare systems must pervasively and successfully diagnose and manage causes of disease. Lifestyle medicine focuses on treating the lifestyle causes of the majority of modern diseases, from primary prevention through active disease treatment. However, a major challenge to the development and survival of Lifestyle Medicine Centers is navigating from the current problematic payment structure to one with appropriate payment for improved levels of care and overall health.

Healthcare professionals (HCPs) empowering patients to transform illness to long-term wellness is the essence of lifestyle medicine (Fig. 9.1). However, healthcare business and operational systems are geared for pharmacotherapy and procedures, not for behavior change or other structured lifestyle interventions. Therefore, while the clinical application

of lifestyle medicine may be highly rewarding, the business side of the value equation impairs lifestyle medicine implementation and is disheartening to many HCPs.

Healthcare will continue to evolve, both from medical knowledge and from socioeconomic standpoints. Changing payment structures, the Internet, and technology are rapidly reshaping the landscape and dynamics of health. Very slowly moving healthcare behemoths are not keeping up with the expectations of consumers/patients, while continuing to dominate and control financially and operationally. Political upheaval maintains a dynamic of chaos. Despite these challenges, lifestyle medicine has a tremendous opportunity to rewire healthcare on the business side, with a sound business plan playing a critical role.

The Lifestyle Medicine Practice Business Plan

The business basics of a lifestyle medicine practice have been reviewed by Braman [1] and Raphael [2] and details will be provided here for those tasked with developing a Lifestyle Medicine Center or Clinical Service Line. An evidence-based, rational approach to the business of lifestyle medicine is necessary to have successful, sustainable services. A proper business plan is a necessary component of this operational success, but typically requires more effort than initially anticipated. Conceptually, drafting a business plan is easy. Navigating the complexities of the current healthcare jungle to a successful outcome is not.

Foundations

Need for a Sound Business Plan to Support a Lifestyle Medicine Center

Business operations support effective lifestyle medicine care delivery. Core clinical concepts of effective lifestyle medi-

M. Braman (✉) · J. Raphael
Lifestyle Medicine Pro, LLC, Salem, OR, USA
e-mail: mbraman@lifestylemedicine.pro; jraphael@lifestylemedicine.pro

© Springer Nature Switzerland AG 2020
J. I. Mechanick, R. F. Kushner (eds.), *Creating a Lifestyle Medicine Center*, https://doi.org/10.1007/978-3-030-48088-2_9

WHOLE HEALTH - TREATMENT

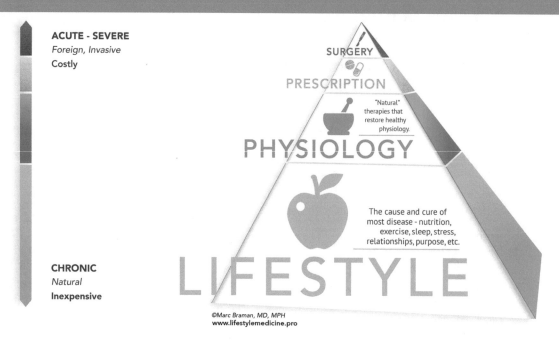

Fig. 9.1 Universal model of rational healthcare∗. (∗Data indicate that 60–90% of modern disease is a product of lifestyle factors. Lifestyle medicine is about "treating the cause" of disease versus managing or minimizing symptoms and consequences with medication or procedures. Published with the kind permission of © Marc Braman, MD 2020. All Rights Reserved)

cine in clinical practice include, but are not limited to, the following:

1. Practice person-centered care vs. typical behavior-centered care: understanding behaviors is a relatively superficial product of the deeper generative aspects of a person.
2. Prioritize enjoyment of life and healthy "connectedness" as the primary objectives to achieve positive behavior change.
3. Recognize that time spent with the patient is a critical ingredient for success.
4. Healthcare professionals and nonprofessional staff must genuinely care about patients and each other.
5. Healthcare professionals and staff personal lifestyles matter and their lifestyle should be healthy.
6. Deep, whole-person, and comprehensive care (e.g., mind-body and spiritual) is required.

Therefore, a successful business plan serves to enable quality clinical lifestyle medicine care in an immersive, high-touch, and safe environment for patients that can endure the challenges of an adverse healthcare environment.

The current business of healthcare is geared for the rapid delivery of pills and procedures as the engines of financial success. To sustainably deliver a different approach requires a deeper-than-average understanding of the business of healthcare. This is not just knowing how care is normally delivered,

but also understanding the principles of the care processes to achieve reimbursement in new models. For instance, a Lifestyle Medicine Center should be in tune with the changing dynamics of society. Smartphone apps, artificial intelligence, online patient communities, wearable technologies, etc., are all part of our rapidly evolving ways of life. Technology empowers patients and alters the traditional HCP-patient relationship. Prevailing attitudes toward foods and physical activity, socioeconomic pressures that limit the purchasing power for pills and procedures, and a generally higher level of stress in daily living are important factors of our current context. Business plans that lead to sufficient financial security for a Lifestyle Medicine Center nurture the ability to adapt to societal changes in order to improve the health of patients.

The two realms of deep expertise – business and lifestyle medicine -- need to be interwoven to achieve sustainable delivery of high-quality clinical care. This process must not fundamentally compromise effective clinical care, while tweaking the care delivery process to mesh with reimbursement requirements. Rather, the successful integration of business and lifestyle medicine both enables short-term sustainability and lays the groundwork for large-scale healthcare transformation. Outcome-based reimbursement and similar payment models based on standards and performance have great potential for lifestyle medicine. But to get to that future, lifestyle medicine needs to be clinically excellent and highly efficacious in hard number terms. Lifestyle medicine must be managed operationally at a high standard to realize a future of appropriate reimbursement for critical interventions that improve health.

Healthcare is not a normal business operation. A conventional business is a straightforward sale of a product or service that people pay for directly. The successful business pays for expenses from revenue generated, keeps the profit, and continues the cycle. However, hospitals and many other medical facilities, in general, are not a product of this revenue cycle; they are a product of subsidization, grants, private donations, and other sources in a robust fundraising effort, coupled with management styles that engender wasteful consumption of resources – the latter motivated by philosophical conflicts among fiscal responsibility, non-evidence based interventions, and ethical standards of compassionate care. As a fundamental concept, Lifestyle Medicine Centers should be developed and operated based on novel and more enlightened models, more akin to normal, healthy, value-based business dynamics.

Healthcare Culture in Conflict

The business of lifestyle medicine requires an understanding of the business of medicine as a whole, its historical context, present cultural state, and future direction. Historically, healthcare services were provided by individual HCPs and directly paid for by patients, in money or in-kind (other services or products). Over time, healthcare services became more sophisticated and expensive. Third-party payers entered the picture, intermediating services and payments, obfuscating direct relationships and self-correcting marketplace forces in most cases at a population scale. Whereas clinical services were the dominant factor and payment was secondary, this dynamic has inverted. Now, financial activities (prior authorizations, pharmacy benefit managers, expansion of non-covered services, etc.) dominate the mission of providing clinical care.

Another complicating variable is that HCPs have increasingly become employees of medical institutions instead of independent clinicians. The burden imposed by heightened healthcare regulation and involvement of third-party payers has made private practice much more onerous, with loss of autonomy and increased burnout. Primary care is the control point for much of healthcare, but the lack of proportionately valued reimbursement has led private primary care practices to succumb to acquisition by hospitals, healthcare systems, and even third-party payers. Consequently, private primary care practices with autonomy to provide a better kind of care have become a rare commodity. These events have aggravated the situation, and now healthcare systems manage the flow of care primarily for business purposes.

Misaligned incentives compromise the impact of lifestyle medicine. For example, current payment systems reward interventions (e.g., pharmacotherapy and procedures) for symptoms and consequences of disease-producing lifestyles, while indirectly displacing services that prevent and treat disease by addressing the cause. In another example, in the early days of the Ornish program, an academic medical center about to adopt this program considered how traditional interventional cardiology revenues might be threatened and then abruptly abandoned this lifestyle medicine initiative (authors' experience).

There is a general lack of training in lifestyle medicine for HCPs. According to Adams et al. [3], 71% of medical schools fail to meet the National Academy of Sciences recommendations for 25 hours of nutrition education for medical students. Moreover, only 8 hours of physical activity education is provided in US medical schools [4]. Foster et al. [5] found that over 51% of family physicians felt inadequately trained to prescribe weight loss plans to patients with obesity. Misperceptions also exist within the medical world that lifestyle factors should be relegated to either population health or public health or that they are not bona fide medical interventions for individual patients. With nutrition and other aspects of lifestyle medicine being de-emphasized or even virtually abandoned by professional medicine, confusion is rampant, creating a growing opportunity for quackery, profiteering, and other forms of inappropriate medical care.

Payers

"He who pays the piper calls the tune."

Payer dynamics are key drivers in healthcare and, more specifically, lifestyle medicine. Most healthcare is not paid for directly by the patient but instead by a third-party payer. As a result, there is no real marketplace for most of the healthcare provided today.

> A real marketplace is the direct exchange of goods or services for monetary value. I sell apples for $1 each. You buy one. If you like the apple and thought it was worth $1, you will be back and we will do the exchange again. If the apples are good or not, or the price is too high or too low, natural marketplace forces will correct the transactions to an equilibrium of value between buyers and sellers. There are direct cause and effect relationships. This is NOT the case in healthcare. There is no consistent relationship between cost and value in healthcare, and there is some evidence of an inverse relationship [6].

It is also true that those referred to as "payers" (e.g., health insurers) are not true payers but instead middlemen managing the flow of dollars for the true payers. The real payers are typically either employers or the government (i.e., taxpaying citizens), since they ultimately provide the dollars paying the insurance premiums. This deconstruction of natural cause and effect business relationships has produced hidden dynamics and adverse clinical and administrative effects. The business incentive structures vary and are unknown to most in the system. In some arrangements, many insurers make a profit based on a percentage of dollars flowing through them, which is a perverse incentive for cost control. In other arrangements, these middlemen make more money as more care is denied. Rational measures for controlling costs from a medical perspective (e.g., lifestyle medicine: "treating the cause") rarely align with the financial drivers of those who control the dollars and thus the care.

Lifestyle Medicine Business Planning

Many HCPs and staff are disconnected from the charges being billed, as well as the reimbursements received. Contemporary lifestyle medicine requires that everything possible is known and managed. A lifestyle medicine practice business plan is a thorough process that makes the intangibles tangible, and the unknowns known, to the greatest extent possible. Then, one can either manage the pieces involved to create a sustainable practice or stop the process before investing additional amounts of money, time, energy, and other resources.

The vast majority of HCPs, and even those in management positions, have little realization of how much work is involved in creating a proper business plan for a lifestyle medicine practice [7]. Hence, a common fundamental mistake in Lifestyle Medicine Centers or Clinical Service Lines is inadequate business planning. A proper business planning process is conceptually the exploration of poorly defined territory and the creation of a map for a successful journey. One must understand the details of the map, preferred route, and alternate routes, if one is to navigate the course successfully. This map concept allows for better understanding and engagement with a very complex environment and set of circumstances.

The initial Practice Map framework configures all the pieces and functional relationships together in one place at a basic level (Fig. 9.2). Clinical operations are often referred to as "front office" and business and adminis-

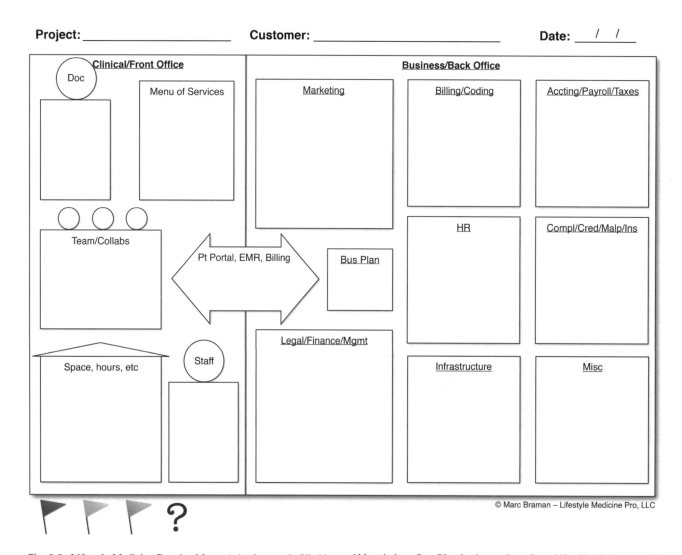

Fig. 9.2 Lifestyle Medicine Practice Map∗. (∗As the map is filled in, the following color-coded flags can be positioned: *Red Flag* critical issue to be resolved in the short term; *Yellow Flag* non-critical issue to be resolved in the short to medium term; *Green Flag* resolved element (or strength), and *Question Mark* more information needed.

Abbreviation: *Bus Plan* business plan, *Compl/Cred/Malp/Ins* compliance, credentialing, malpractice, and insurance, *EMR* electronic medical record, *HR* human resources, *Mgmt* management, *Misc* miscellaneous. Published with the kind permission of © Marc Braman, MD 2020. All Rights Reserved)

trative operations are often referred to as "back office." There are significant numbers of variables, and complexity varies significantly between instances. For any given situation, addressing each of these areas to the depths necessary is critical. Generally speaking, the best starting point is the front office and the clinical services to be delivered. Color-coded flags and associated labels for identified issues are inserted into the map. Other pages of text describe the issues identified and approach to addressing them in outline form. Generally, red flags are critical issues that must be addressed for a basic function to occur; yellow flags are items that will need to be addressed but are not mission-critical in the short term; and green indicates issues that are resolved or may be strengths. Notice that the Business Plan element is at the center of everything.

The initial or internal Practice Map essentially addresses functions primarily within the walls of a typical center or practice. A "Big Picture" Map is the best way to capture the context and environmental dynamics that are so important (Fig. 9.3). What is the environment in which the center seeks to operate? Who are the players? What are they concerned about and how will that affect the center? What role does the Lifestyle Medicine Center play in the community? In the healthcare system, what and/or who is the Center relevant to? What forces are pushing the local healthcare system in what directions? Where is danger and where is opportunity? While the Practice Map is fairly standard in issues to be processed, the Big Picture Map is often unique and is adapted to the particular context. It is important to have team members experienced in the local healthcare environment to identify exposed or hidden dynamics.

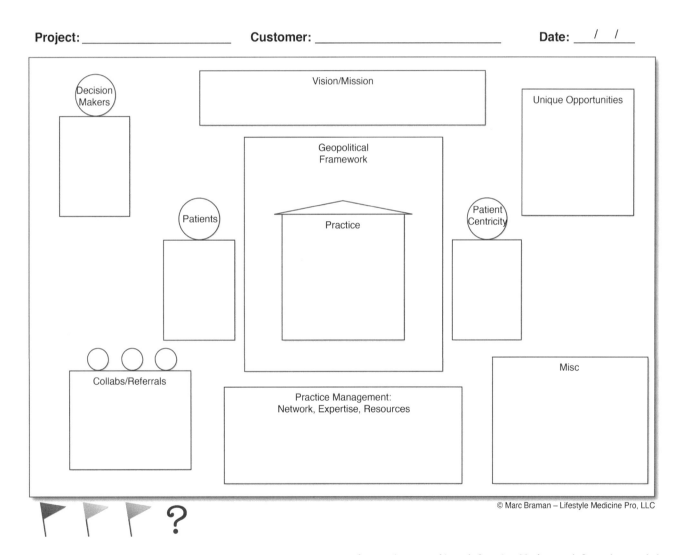

Fig. 9.3 Lifestyle Medicine "Big Picture" Map∗. (∗As the map is filled in, the following color-coded flags can be positioned: *Red Flag* critical issue to be resolved in the short term, *Yellow Flag* non-critical issue to be resolved in the short to medium term, *Green Flag* resolved element (or strength), and *Question Mark* more information needed. Published with the kind permission of © Marc Braman, MD 2020. All Rights Reserved)

Sources of Payment

Where Does the Money Come from?

The government is the single biggest payer for healthcare in the USA, though it is the citizens and businesses that pay the taxes. The government provides and pays for healthcare within limits, as long as requirements are satisfied. However, lifestyle medicine coverage is extremely limited and not well funded within health insurance policies. In the USA, health insurers operate in ways similar to the government, except there are many of them with a plethora of different plans, each with their own variations and quirks, and still requiring a significant staff commitment to track, navigate, and respond to the idiosyncrasies. If one adheres to the rules and invests in necessary operational machinery, then payments and funding for the center are fairly reliable. Depending on the center's infrastructure and extent of resources available, the extra work needed for billing–/collection-related activities might constrain core clinical activities.

The more direct the relationship between the true payer and the HCP, the more the opportunity to deliver ideal healthcare with minimal distraction. Direct Primary Care (DPC), where a patient pays an HCP a direct monthly fee, allows almost the entire focus to be on patient care and minimally on administration and has great potential for a high-quality lifestyle medicine implementation [8]. Other payment models include fee-for-service, membership, direct contracting between employers and healthcare systems, collaborative care management, chronic care management, outcomes-based reimbursement, patient-centered medical homes of various flavors, integrated systems, intensive lifestyle medicine programs, accountable care organizations (ACOs), and coordinated care organizations [9–13]. Unfortunately, there are still significant pressures toward increasing layers of bureaucracy and seemingly endless checklists and administrative paperwork with many of these payment models. Technology can be leveraged to help counter the detriment of these pressures, but this can detract from patient care. One promising payment model is a fully capitated arrangement that allows the care team to completely restructure themselves as a team, liberating time and energy for maximal efficiency and care for patients (e.g., https://www.iorahealth.com [Accessed on February 8, 2020]) [14].

What Gets Paid by Third-Party Payers?

Lifestyle medicine-related services that may be reimbursable in the USA include the following:

1. Standard fee-for-service office visits (consults, initial visits, and follow-ups)

2. Shared medical visits (standard fee-for-service office visits in group context)
3. Chronic care management monthly fees (usually modest but worthwhile if done efficiently)
4. Remote patient monitoring (relatively new but promising)
5. Common behavioral health services
6. A minority of dietitian services
7. Some other less consistently reimbursed mechanisms

Numerous other services and codes, some old and some new, are not reimbursed or reimbursed at unsustainable levels, and/or are not functional for other reasons (e.g., the Diabetes Prevention Program at the time of this writing).

Patients

Direct pay from patients is the simplest and consequently the most desirable. But it is also the most difficult to implement. Patients have either paid into a governmental system with the expectation that it would pay the bills or are employed by an employer who has promised that part of their remuneration would be healthcare coverage. For patients that have no coverage through third-party payers, they are often very reluctant to pay out-of-pocket for healthcare expenses, which are typically disproportionately larger than most of their other expenses. True marketplace forces have been dismantled and patients have become disenfranchised as consumers in this space. However, with increasing dysfunction and frustration with healthcare, some patients with enough incentive and initiative are starting to function as consumers again.

Academic Centers

For academic centers, funding from major donors, grants, or non-service-based monies is the norm for funding lifestyle-medicine-like centers. Unfortunately, most centers in this vein tend to become a "wellness center" that incorporates healthy living classes with aspects of integrative medicine such as yoga and/or tai chi, acupuncture, mind-body programming, sometimes Chinese medicine, and alternative medicine practices. These centers serve relatively small numbers of patients without providing as a core service durable lifestyle medical care that adequately changes the lifestyle causes of chronic disease as an inherent part of healthcare as a whole. Nevertheless, these centers can have a public relations appeal for the academic center. Wellness centers per se often expend an inordinate amount of money and resources on what impacts very few patients. Medical centers have various pressures to give back to the community or do things that seem popular, and this may check that box for them.

There is tremendous potential for lifestyle medicine centers-of-excellence development in academic settings. In fact, some hospital systems have established lifestyle medicine departments by combining reimbursed elements such as physical therapy, rehabilitation programs, dietitian services, and medical fitness center memberships under one umbrella. The challenge is matching the Lifestyle Medicine Center's overhead to revenues in the current reimbursement paradigm, and then collaborating in an active paradigm transformation to value-based constructs (in which lifestyle medicine is properly valued). It is very difficult to engage two polar opposite reimbursement paradigms at the same time.

Bundling

In various contexts and in various ways, lifestyle medicine elements are often bundled into other services. One example is a dietitian working in a specialty prostate cancer treatment center, where their services are free to the patient. The center covers this cost from other revenues because it is the right thing to do based on the evidence, even though they are not paid for this aspect of evidence-based medicine. In another example, a practice may pay a pharmacist and an exercise physiologist to participate in a shared medical visit session without direct reimbursement for their services by another party. The practice pays them directly and does not bill for their services, but factors it into the practice's service delivery. While such situations are reflective of what is best for patients and based on good evidence, there must be ongoing efforts to deter free services being the norm and to establish all lifestyle medicine services as valuable and paid at appropriate levels.

Who Gets Paid?

Whom the third-party payers pay is another critical component of the developing business model for Lifestyle Medicine Centers and Clinical Service Lines. Depending on the practice and the team, this can vary significantly. Physicians almost always get paid as long as they stick to the common service codes. Behavioral health professionals typically get paid with reasonably good consistency. Dietitian services are much more inconsistent and depend on the medical conditions at issue relative to specific payers, meaning government or various insurers. The physical therapist typically gets paid well for their services, but formal physical therapy is often not necessary, and if included, difficult to integrate into other services. Other staff have very limited ability for reimbursement for their services, but they may in some circumstances

perform functions under a physician's direction that would be reimbursable by third-party payers. Otherwise, staff services and functions must be accounted for or factored in other ways. A very important part of a proper business plan is mapping out the details of who gets paid, by which payer, and for what things that are part of the Lifestyle Medicine Center's services. A high level of proficiency in coding and billing as applied to less conventional delivery is crucial.

Do Programs Get Covered?

The short answer is "no," at least not as such. The long answer is "occasionally" or kind of. In the USA, Dr. Dean Ornish spent 17 years to get an act of Congress passed to cover a heart disease reversal lifestyle program at sustainable levels [15]. But even this is bound up with restrictions and limitations that keep it functionally hamstrung. This secondary prevention cardiovascular program remains significantly different from the usual pharmacological and procedural care plan such that it is difficult to mobilize interested cardiologists and referral patterns into being readily accessible to patients.

The Diabetes Prevention Program is technically covered, but the requirements for development, operation, and reimbursement are so onerous that it is essentially not possible by many HCPs passionate about lifestyle medicine. A sponsoring hospital or health system must dedicate significant resources to provide free services for a prolonged time as part of the development process. By the time the program is approved, reimbursement is limited and vague, and indications are that it would not even be financially sustainable.

A Summary Process for Approaching a Lifestyle Medicine Business Plan

The following list provides the basic actions for developing a lifestyle medicine business plan.

1. Start with the patient: understand the patient population wants and needs.
2. Specify in writing exactly what success looks like in detail – what you will achieve for patients.
3. Develop a list of potential revenue sources for the lifestyle medicine-related services (e.g., third-party payers, true payers, direct or patient pay, or customized or special arrangements [ACO, advanced patient-centered medical homes, etc.]).
4. Obtain tangible, real-world data and match by using a table or matrix of the center's services and current procedural terminology codes, payer mix, reimbursements, and reimbursable HCP types (e.g., physician

(Doctor of Medicine [MD] or Doctor of Osteopathic Medicine [DO]), registered dietitian nutritionist [RDN], and behaviorist).

5. Consider other payment options for services where reimbursement cannot be obtained from traditional sources (e.g., employers as other true payers, an ACO for a specific program and conditions, and other sources of patients with out-of-pocket payment capabilities).

6. Identify and engage the best lifestyle medicine and healthcare management/leadership experience available.

Types of Centers or Clinical Service Lines

Lifestyle medicine practices extend across the spectrum in terms of type, from solo practitioner to a freestanding center to a clinical service line in a multidisciplinary academic health system, and in terms of specialty, from primary care to a lifestyle medicine specialist. The vast majority of HCPs will incorporate lifestyle medicine aspects into practices in some other specialty, while only a small number will be dedicated lifestyle medicine specialists in bona fide Lifestyle Medicine Centers or Clinical Service Lines. There are several configurations where lifestyle medicine has the greatest potential to shine clinically and financially.

Lifestyle Medicine-Based Direct Primary Care

This structure provides freedom to focus on the patient and their health, and nothing else. The challenge is combining the dynamics of effective lifestyle medicine with this business model. In this model either the patient or the employer pays a HCP or practice directly for primary care services on a monthly recurring membership-type basis. The scope of care is defined and often includes 24/7 access to a HCP who knows them, common lab tests at HCP cost or with basic labs included, imaging at HCP cost, and most common pharmaceuticals greatly discounted or at HCP cost. Lifestyle medicine is founded on positive relationships and personal caring, and the DPC model delivers on this in spades. A patient still needs insurance or wrap-around coverage for their healthcare needs beyond primary care. DPC practices are typically small, not standardized, and may find limitations from not being part of a larger network or system. "Concierge" practices are similar but are typically geared for the affluent, while DPC is geared for the general population. In comparison, most of the "patient-centered medical home" and similar models seek to functionally integrate more disparate pieces of the current systems, but are so bogged down in mechanics, pro-cess, and paperwork that the patient gets lost, and they still use a "pills-and-procedures" focused approach that can never achieve healthcare's full potential.

Lifestyle Medicine Center

A Center has tremendous potential to demonstrate real integration of "treating the cause" into healthcare delivery. The structure may be represented as a Department, Specialty, Clinical Service Line, or free-standing facility. While the potential to demonstrate a superior type of evidence-based care is great, the barriers are also great. Healthcare is chronically financially diseased and most personnel in administration and operations are constantly overwhelmed with sustainability challenges and the repeating tsunamis of "quality metrics," inspections, acquisitions, funding changes, and other hurdles. This often results in a narrow bandwidth for growth and innovation. In fact, any new or different venture may prove to be an impediment for the present round of survival. However, when quality lifestyle medicine actually becomes one of the basic metrics for institutional survival, then the C-suite (executive level managers) can be serious about building and implementing Lifestyle Medicine Centers. The ways in which services are combined are almost unlimited and should be guided by the needs of an institution and those they care for. The key is to truly deliver a fundamentally different kind of care while still integrating with some of the conventional elements of modern healthcare.

Lifestyle Medicine Specialist Practice

The vast majority of healthcare operations do not have the time or resources to build a true, dedicated Lifestyle Medicine Center. However, a Lifestyle Medicine Center should be an important part of the healthcare space since chronic diseases, with lifestyle drivers, are overwhelming, and current guideline-based approaches and quality metrics fail to provide effective implementation strategies and tactics. Therefore, one or more HCPs, functioning as lifestyle medicine specialists, can serve patients, busy primary care practices, larger sponsoring healthcare systems, and even larger population-based efforts.

A lifestyle medicine specialist practice may include any or all reimbursed HCP types, but is typically best anchored with a physician formally educated in lifestyle medicine. Designing and implementing a lifestyle medicine program for patients are often the most effective ways of delivering these services, but many program formats are not, or are poorly, reimbursed, and thus is a significant limiting factor for success. Fortunately, newly reimbursed services such as chronic care management and remote patient monitoring can create some new opportunities. One very tangible example is some primary care practices designating one of their own HCPs as the group's lifestyle medicine specialist.

Lifestyle Medicine Programs

Intensive programs, whether local or live-in, are the most powerful formats for a rapid, often dramatic, change in health status for patients. Yet, these programs are plagued by major problems related to lack of payment, the difficulty of patients taking a large block of time off, and lack of follow-up and systems for maintenance. From medical and patient perspectives, local and high-quality lifestyle medicine programs are needed. But, this does not yet mesh with the majority of existing payment models. Ideally, these programs can be conducted in various types of clinical practices, delivered by competent lifestyle medicine HCPs as a basic part of mainstream care. The programs should not be farmed off to disinterested or ill-equipped HCPs, or irrelevant contexts, leaving them functioning as optional, bolt-on accessories. Overall, there are creative ways to maximize programmatic delivery with acceptable reimbursement. This endeavor is more complex, requires a deep understanding of both clinical lifestyle medicine and billing, and should incorporate a portion of the services to be directly paid.

Lifestyle Medicine for Self-Insured Employers

The imperatives for self-insured employers who are considering different products with a lifestyle medicine component for their employees include reduced risk of injury due to poor physical condition, healthcare costs, presenteeism, and increased work productivity. The premise is that chronic disease risk factors can be prevented or mitigated, leading to better health. Some major employers (e.g., Cummins, Inc. [16]) have made major investments in shifting their whole care continuum toward lifestyle medicine foundations. Others cover lifestyle medicine-based DPC services for their employees. Employers simply picking from the standard menu of insurance options have limited control over the actual care they are paying for. They are simply wishing upon a star for an actual benefit on employee lifestyle as a result of their insurance product selection. Increasingly,

employers are starting to find, often from sheer necessity, that they are able to find creative means of securing better care for a better price for their employees. This may require extra work for employers, but there are indications that it is worth it [17, 18].

Typical Lifestyle Medicine Team Members

Lifestyle Medicine Centers vary in the number of team members and in how many work in the same space versus in different locations. Team member types typically include the following:

1. Clinicians (MD, DO, nurse practitioner, or other advanced practice providers) with either a dedicated lifestyle medicine specialization or another certified specialty (e.g., endocrinology, obesity medicine, diabetes medicine, cardiology, or internal medicine) along with individual emphasis in lifestyle medicine
2. Practice/operations manager
3. Relevant administration personnel, particularly in larger centers
4. RDN
5. Behavioral health professional (PhD/PsyD/LMFT/LCSW)
6. Exercise professional (e.g., licensed exercise physiologist)
7. Coaches with skills and training in facilitating behavior change
8. Other support and operations staff (e.g., certified diabetes educator, supervisors, medical assistants, nurses, telemetry personnel)

Team dynamics will vary, but in general team members should be personally passionate about lifestyle medicine and the mission of the practice, program, and/or center.

Lifestyle Medicine-Related Services

There are many service types that can be effective and sustainable, as well as customizable, based on the specific lifestyle medicine mission statement.

1. Individual HCP office visits (MD/DO, behaviorist, RDN, others)
2. Group visits of different types and reimbursements
3. Chronic care management

 4. Remote patient monitoring
 5. Telehealth
 6. Intensive lifestyle programs
 7. Cardiac rehabilitation
 8. Lifestyle medicine-based direct primary care
 9. Direct to employer services
10. Health risk assessments
11. Classes on various health topics (e.g., stress management/burnout, and exercise)
12. Cooking schools
13. Smart grocery shopping tours
14. Medical nutrition therapy
15. Technology-based services and programs
16. Condition-specific services (e.g., tobacco/nicotine dependence, insomnia, diabetes, depression)
17. Facilitated healthy communities/networks
18. Medical fitness centers

Common Pitfalls

The most common pitfall is often committed by well-intentioned healthcare professionals who "don't know what they don't know", and is manifest as approaching lifestyle medicine as a typical healthcare service. These HCPs are not aware of the need for a proper business planning process for a different kind of healthcare. Other pitfalls relate to financing, such as not having sufficient start-up funding. Sponsoring health systems may set up a Lifestyle Medicine Center or Clinical Service Line, but unless there is a tangible plan for sustainable funding and reimbursement, these centers will likely experience a series of stressful leaps from grant to grant or donation to donation. The changes in health administration or system budgetary pressures can easily provoke the end of such fragile entities. In addition, taking on too much overhead, especially at the outset, should be avoided. Lifestyle medicine does not generally support fancy shiny buildings. Many Lifestyle Medicine Centers fail because there is no realistic way for lifestyle medicine to pay for what is considered to be typical medical overhead. Also, not treating lifestyle medicine like a hard-core business process is problematic. A lifestyle medicine entity needs to be approached diligently from a business standpoint to avoid eventual disillusionment. Lastly, accounting management is critical and it is important to work with the accounting department from the beginning. The amount of overhead being assigned to lifestyle medicine operations is one of the most important financial aspects. It is also critical to

plan from the beginning how the system will value and account for the impact of the lifestyle medicine services. For example, successfully managing a patient with diabetes and stage 5 chronic kidney disease requires a substantial amount of work and resources, and the center may receive just enough revenue to cover expenses. But, hundreds of thousands of dollars in the system can be saved with a capitated payment model, or lost with a fee-for-service payment model.

Additional Opportunities

Lifestyle Medicine Centers provide many opportunities to improve the health of individual patients and populations, as well as serving other roles in the urban infrastructure or a sponsoring health system. There are additional opportunities that are not always apparent, but can be discovered and acted upon with appropriate environmental assessment. They include the following:

1. Direct contracting with employers.
2. Contracting for services or programs relative to lifestyle-related high-cost conditions or patient populations.
3. Developing a center-of-excellence within a system or facility.
4. Where systems, HCPs, or practices have to deal with bureaucratic checkboxes that may relate to lifestyle medicine, there may be opportunities to improve other programs (e.g., weight loss as a prerequisite for orthopedic surgery, or assistance meeting lifestyle medicine quality metrics for other chronic diseases, such as obesity, type 2 diabetes, hypertension, or hyperlipidemia).
5. Increasing consumer demand in a setting where there are more empowered patients in the context of increasing distrust of healthcare; consider working with administration and/or the marketing department.

Prescription for Action

Creating an initial, basic Practice Map is the first organizational step. The basic dynamics are forced to become apparent in this process if done well. Those in leadership, stakeholders, and participants involved start to learn what it will take to be successful in implementation. The second step is then making informed decisions regarding moving forward with a proper business plan process. The business plan should be designed by those with clinical and busi-

Table 9.1 Sample profit and loss statement

Income/Expenses	Notes
Operating Revenue/Income	
Sales	
Services	
Other	
Total income	
Operating expenses	
Accounting	
Rent	
Continuing education	
Wages	
Training	
Insurance	
Bank charges	
Advertising	
Electricity	
Motor vehicle	
Telephone	
Software/subscriptions	
Total expenses	
Profit/loss	

Table 9.2 Sample balance sheet

Company name	$ Amounts (current ± prior year)		$ Amounts (current ± prior year)
Assets		*Liabilities & equity*	
Bank accounts		**Current liabilities**	
Savings		Accounts payable	
Checking		Accrued wages	
Total		Line of credit	
		Total current	
Accounts receivable			
Accounts rec.		**Long-term liabilities**	
Total		Notes payable	
		Mortgage	
Fixed assets		Total, long term	
Vehicles			
Furniture		**Total liabilities**	
Equipment			
Building		**Owners equity**	
Land		Common stock	
Total		Retained earnings	
Total assets		**Total liabilities and owners equity**	

ness expertise in lifestyle medicine specifically, internally or externally, to the sponsoring organization as needed. If the decision is made to implement the business plan, the third step is to commit resources for the project.

The fourth and final step is utilizing the initial Practice Map as the stepping off point to implement and engage people, processes, space, referral networks, metrics, and other details. The following example outlines a sample business plan for a Lifestyle Medicine Center (Appendix 9.1. Business Plan Implementation Sequence (Sample – Transitioning To Fiscal Sustainability)). The context for this lifestyle medicine business plan is the transition from a completely medical-center-funded program to a sustainable fee-for-service center. This medical center was in the midst of testing new capitated-style integrated delivery models, while still having to survive with fee-for-service. The full plan is about 60 pages, and with relevant appendices is about twice that amount. The unique business plan structure is created for a primarily clinician user audience. In general, business plans should be adapted for greatest usability of those responsible for implementing them. A staged or phased approach is often best. Healthcare processes move relatively more slowly than those in other sectors. Therefore, the order of implementation is particularly important for timely realization of operations. In this example, the center could go from a very large annual operating deficit to breakeven in roughly 12 months based on fairly conservative estimates with methodical implementation. Existing clinical services delivery would need to be modi-

fied to a modest degree, and much work needed to be done on the fundamentals of operations for documentation and billing purposes. The annual budget for approximately six staff would be roughly $750,000. Other expenses would need to be organized and determined. Further business planning examples and tools are provided in Appendix 9.2. Aspects of a Business Plan for a Lifestyle Medicine Center, and Tables 9.1 and 9.2.

Conclusion

Successful Lifestyle Medicine Centers must have a higher-than-typical level of clinical and healthcare business expertise to succeed in providing a "treat the cause" care plan within a "pills and procedures for symptoms and consequences" business paradigm. This expertise needs to be integrated into a thorough business and operational planning process, utilizing a proper business plan as the primary tool. In sum, sustainable lifestyle medicine practices are possible today.

Glossary of Financial Terms

Audits Consider internal and external audits, not limited to compliance, performance, and stakeholders.

Bad Debt Money one is owed that one does not get paid for.

Financial Planning Financial analysis of a new business, new program, and/or long-range plan to support analysis of strategic opportunities and establish budget guidelines for profit, cost, and capital investment.

Goal Setting and Budgeting Forecasts demand measures, compiling operations, financial and capital budgets to support strategic decisions, coordination of activities, and setting performance goals.

Managerial Accounting Prepares cost and revenue for monitoring and improving support for HCP teams with resource and output data.

Operational Measures Consider measures other than financial, e.g., provider satisfaction, absenteeism, retention, and spending ratios.

Operating Revenues and Rates Provide historical and comparative forecasts to centers and service lines, address operating budgets, suggest guidelines that specify operational expectations for each year, and improve competitive position or mission achievement.

Pricing Structures Cash, preferred provider organization contracts (negotiated fees), diagnosis-related groups, single-price contracts, contracts with penalties or bonuses for utilization or quality targets (group incentives), and payment independent of incidence or actual cost of treatment (capitation).

Process Improvement Reports performance against budget providing activity-based cost analysis and guidance with intent to exploit opportunities to improve competitive position.

Standard Reports Balance sheet, income, or profit and loss statement, statement of use of funds, and change in fund balances.

Appendix 9.1. Business Plan Implementation Sequence (Sample – Transitioning to Fiscal Sustainability)

1. *Executive summary*
2. *Transition to sustainability: Phase 1 (3–6 months)*
   (a) Objective: to get paid for services already being provided at the Lifestyle Medicine Center
   (b) Hire and orient a Medical Practice Manager as soon as possible
   (c) Hire and orient a Medical Director
   (d) Hire and orient a Program Director (modified/combined position)
   (e) Identify and implement a billing system
   (f) Identify and implement accounting system
   (g) Establish and standardize charting
   (h) Clinical documentation: Subjective-Objective-Assessment-Plan format
   (i) Credentialing with payers
   (j) Initiate an Electronic Medical/Health Record
3. *Transition to sustainability: Phase 2 (5–9 months)*
   (a) Clarify initial "Menu of Services"
   (b) Consider potential future services for "Menu of Services"
   (c) Conditions and services – prioritized initiation of service lines
   (d) Additional services implementation strategy
   (e) Identify and develop strategic alliances with various medical specialties
   (f) Diabetes Prevention Program (as may be important to organization)
   (g) Annual Wellness Visits
   (h) Group visits (with standard office visit codes)
   (i) Chronic Care Management
   (j) Telemedicine
4. *Transition to sustainability: Phase 3 (12 months or more)*
   (a) Strengthen the current payer mix
   (b) Continually assess referral base satisfaction
   (c) Further strategic alliances with community HCPs
   (d) Achievable goals should be set for reimbursements
   (e) Customer service assessment
   (f) Lifestyle Medicine Center branding and recognition
   (g) Reevaluation of basics
5. *Implementation of clinical operations (items identified that needed substantial guidance in implementation for clinical, operational, and/or financial considerations)*
   (a) Sample operational flow
   (b) Program fee
   (c) Shift of terminology
   (d) Lifestyle Vital Signs
   (e) Shared Medical Appointments
   (f) Medication Management Protocols
   (g) Annual Wellness Visits
   (h) Specific contract with state Medicaid
   (i) Medical Center system-wide metrics opportunities
   (j) Population health
   (k) Diabetes Prevention Program
   (l) Chronic Care Management
   (m) In-clinic patient flow

(n) Sample patient flow in first week of patient engagement

(o) Classes

(p) Potential memberships

6. *Financials*

(a) Estimated revenue generation based on expected reimbursements per HCP type/department from initial planned services and programs

(b) "Incident to" billing guidance

(c) The bottom line is achieving financially sustainable lifestyle medicine services

(d) Take Away Message: Average patient charges in first 2 months of program

(e) Payer mix

(f) Examples of billing

(g) Core units of best professional services

(h) Situation coding, billing guidance, and examples

(i) Miscellaneous services and procedure codes

(j) Sample Medicaid fee schedule for typical office visits

(k) Financial projections

(l) Additional clinical services

(m) Adding staff

(n) Classes and other non-medical services accounting

(o) Offering Lifestyle as Medicine services to employees

(p) Financial projections

(i) General framework

(ii) Use in practice for those implementing

(iii) Focus on most important items

(iv) Additional items

(v) Non-patient care items separated in accounting

(q) Revenue explanations

(r) Expenses explanations

(s) Personnel – when to add relevant staff

(t) Year 2 implementation

(u) Titles of staff – guidance and considerations

7. *Marketing*

(a) Market overview

(b) Market segmentation

(i) Referred patients

(ii) Client/Patient mix and Decision Markers (Consumer/Corporate)

(iii) The Center's employees

(iv) Target market

(c) Marketing to the Sponsoring Medical Center's audiences

(d) Competition

(e) Naming and branding

(f) Inherent marketing (word of mouth, quality services, and satisfied customers)

(g) Community health activities

(h) More conventional marketing possibilities

(i) Website and Social Media

8. *Keys to success*

(a) Educating how lifestyle medicine aligns the Lifestyle Medicine Center and sponsoring Medical Center's vision, mission, and values

(b) Measure clinical outcomes consistently.

(c) Celebrate patient champions

(d) Consistent internal and external lead generation

(e) Create and demonstrate a sustainable operational model

(f) Employ consistent, credible, caring staff who embody the Lifestyle Medicine Center's mission, vision, and values

(g) Employ the right clinical and operational leadership

(h) Create sustainability

9. *Qualities to demonstrate in practice*

10. *Organizational profile*

(a) What is Lifestyle as Medicine?

(b) Name and company profile

(c) Staff

(d) Description of organization

(e) Mission statement

(f) Vision statement

(g) Values

(h) Current services included

(i) Sample Class Calendar (rotating)

11. *Business plan work list*

12. *Appendices*

Appendix 9.2. Aspects of a Business Plan for a Lifestyle Medicine Center

1. Your Business History

(a) Your business was developed in (year)

(b) Your business type (limited liability company, privately owned, etc.)

(c) Your business leadership (describe experience in 1–3 sentences; include specialty, duration, and why your leadership is important to your business)

(d) Your business goals (what is your business trying to accomplish in 1–2 sentences; what problem is your business addressing)

2. Concept (what is your 1–2 sentence tag line)
3. Strategic Statement (Executive Summary)
   (a) Mission statement
   (b) Vision statement
   (c) How your mission and vision intend to position your business (list 1-, 3-, and 5-year intentions)
   (d) Purpose of your business plan (e.g., business X intends to establish a Lifestyle Medicine Center serving the community by [enter date] targeting [list services])
4. Critical Success Factors
   (a) Some complete a Strengths, Weaknesses, Opportunities, and Threats (SWOT) analysis here; others address the type of leaders, services, stakeholders, decision makers, financial commitments/debts, patient-driven factors, interoperability clinically and operationally with referrals or records, or obstacles
5. Clinical
   (a) The services to be rendered (primary care, specialist, health transformation, etc) or conditions to be addressed (diabetes, cardiovascular disease, hypertension, tobacco dependence, etc) by what provider types (MD/DO, RDN, Behaviorist, etc) via what formats or structures (one-on-one office visits, group visits of different types by different provider types, program, hybrid, telemedicine, other)
6. Financial
   (a) Follow the Generally Accepted Accounting Principles to complete the following:
      (i) Balance Sheet, Income Statements, Cash Flows, Cost per Patient
      (ii) Operating and Profit Margins
7. Security/Safety/Technology/Legal
   (a) Moral agency and standards of care (e.g., Clinical Laboratory Improvement Amendments [CLIA], Department of Homeland Security [DHS], Emergency Medical Treatment and Labor Act [EMTALA], Federal Bureau of Investigation [FBI], Genetic Information Nondiscrimination Act [GINA], Health Insurance Portability and Accountability Act [HIPPA], Occupational Safety and Health Administration [OSHA], Stark Law, and the US Department of Justice [DOJ])
      (i) Patient portal, electronic medical/health record, billing (see practice map in Fig. 9.2)
      (ii) To consider – interoperability, access, and content
      (iii) Consider – tele-, video-, and remote use and monitoring

8. Standards of Care
   (a) Intensive induction, tapered consolidation, ongoing sustainability by educating, equipping, and empowering to treat, reverse, and prevent the root cause of chronic disease
9. Marketing
   (a) "4 P's" (Price, Product, Place, Promotion), population demographics, differentiate marketing from sales cycles, identify target markets, tools, and target audience within a market
10. Front Office
    (a) Personnel – who do you have, who do you need, and when do you need them
    (b) Schedules – when will services be offered
    (c) Collaborations
    (d) Resources – understanding rules and roles, informed consents, releases, and patient flow
11. Back Office
    (a) Forms, billing, profit and loss, accounting, electronic medical/health record, credentialing, insurance, CLIA, etc.

References

1. Braman M, Edison M. How to create a successful lifestyle medicine practice. Am J Lifestyle Med. 2017;11:404–7.
2. Raphael J. Applying the business of lifestyle medicine. Am J Lifestyle Med. 2017;11:227–9.
3. Adams K, Butsch W, Kohlmeier M. The state of nutrition education at US medical schools. J Biomed Educ. 2015:357627. https://doi.org/10.1155/2015/357627.
4. Stoutenberg M, Stasi S, Stamatakis E, Danek D, Dufour T, Trilk J, Blair S. Physical activity training in US medical schools: preparing future physicians to engage in primary prevention. Phys Sportsmed. 2015;43:388–94.
5. Foster G, Wadden T, Makris A, et al. Primary care physicians' attitudes about obesity and its treatment. Obes Res. 2003;11:1168–77.
6. Hussey P, Wertheimer S, Mehrotra A. The association between health care quality and cost: a systemic review. Ann Intern Med. 2013;158:27–34.
7. Comber S, Crawford KC, Wilson L. Competencies physicians need to lead – a Canadian case. Leadersh Health Serv. 2018;31:195–209.
8. Rubin R. Is direct primary care a game changer? JAMA. 2018;319:2064–6.
9. Sunaert P, Bastiaens H, Nobels F, et al. Effectiveness of the introduction of a chronic care model-based program for type 2 diabetes in Belgium. BMC Health Serv Res. 2010;10:207. https://doi.org/10.1186/1472-6963-10-207.
10. Doherty R, Medical Practice and Quality Committee of the American College of Physicians. Assessing the patient care implications of "concierge" and other direct patient contracting practices:

a policy position paper from the American College of Physicians. Ann Intern Med. 2015;163:949–52.

11. Eriksson M, Hagberg L, Linholdm L, et al. Quality of life and cost-effectiveness of a 3-year trial of lifestyle intervention in primary health care. Arch Internal Med. 2010;170:1470–9.

12. Mechley AR, Dysinger W. Intensive therapeutic lifestyle change programs: a progressive way to successfully manage health care. Am J Lifestyle Med. 2015;9:354–60.

13. Larson E, Sharma J, Bohren MA, et al. When the patient is the expert: measuring patient experience and satisfaction with care. Bull World Health Organ. 2019;97:563–9.

14. Paul DP III, Brunoni J, Dolinger T, et al. How effective is capitation at reducing health care costs? Paper presented at the 41st annual meeting of the Northeast Business & Economics Association. New Jersey: West Long Branch; 2014.

15. Centers for Medicare & Medicaid Services (CMS). Decision memo for Intensive Cardiac Rehabilitation (ICR) Program-Dr. Ornish's program for reversing heart disease (CAG-00419N); 2010.

16. Shurney DW. Cummins' vision: improved health through lifestyle medicine innovation. Am J Lifestyle Medicine. 2018;12:46–8.

17. Torinus J. The company that solved health care. Dallas TX: Ben Bella Books; 2010.

18. Torinus J. The grassroots health care revolution. Dallas TX: Ben Bella Books; 2014.

Resource Listed

Griffith JR, White KR. The well-managed healthcare organization. Health Administration Press. AUPHA Press. 2012.

Immersive Physical Environment: Office Interiors and Preparedness

10

Altaf Engineer

Abbreviations

HCP   Healthcare professional
IPE   Immersive physical environments
VR   Virtual reality

The Immersive Physical Environment

Immersive physical environments (IPE) bring the user to a perceptual experience of representation of environments in virtual reality (VR) from an inside perspective, giving a sense of presence. Virtual reality is a term coined by Jaron Lanier in the 1980s and defined as a "representation of scenes or images of objects produced by a computer system, which gives the sense of its real existence" [1]. In the 1960s, Morton Heilig created a projector for visible images in three-dimensional chambers or rooms [2]. The immersive experience, due to recent technological advances, was first available when Oculus Rift glasses appeared and cameras that captured images at 360 degrees were developed in 2012 [3]. With these special glasses, the user connects to a world that is virtually created.

Using external accessories, such as helmets, glasses, and positioners, creates a feeling of disconnection from the real world. Once users wear the glasses, they find themselves completely immersed in an environment that stimulates the visual and aural senses. The user can transition from being the spectator to being the protagonist of a situation who is living the experience. This makes it easier to assimilate and remember information. Immersive environments also allow the user to move while interacting with VR.

A. Engineer (✉)
University of Arizona CAPLA, School of Architecture and UA Institute on Place, Wellbeing, and Performance, Tucson, AZ, USA
e-mail: aengineer@email.arizona.edu

Spatial and Temporal Awareness

By incorporating external VR accessories, the user is automatically in the immersive VR. Ideally, the experience should feel like a soft transition similar to walking through a threshold. The scale of objects, dimensions, depth, senses of proximity, closeness, danger, and feelings of relief or security should be perceived.

The immersive physical environment must transmit a sufficient representation of space-time. If this relationship is not close to reality, both the design narrative and the user-experience lose their effectiveness [4]. Therefore, it is necessary to experience vision at 360 degrees. One of the most popular techniques to make this possible is to have users couple a mobile device with goggles, which causes the sensation of immersion in the moment and place [5]. The vision, or the possibility of having 360 degree vision, allows for the sensory adjustment necessary to recognize a real space. Peripheral vision and the anticipation of the appearance of objects are essential to experience a virtual space as if it were real.

Spatial awareness can be manipulated with controls within the virtual environment (Fig. 10.1) [6]. For example, users can select their real height or a different one, and a successful immersion depends on consistency. Natural dimensions, i.e., dimensions of the human body and proportion of the ergonomics, are as crucial as the appearance of the surrounding objects. The user is exposed to fixed spaces where the image is presented from a single point of view or to a continuous sequence where the user can opt to move through virtual spaces. For both alternatives, there are visual capacities that can offer a range of 180 degrees or even 360 degrees. Another dimension of awareness of space, commonly in the area of architectural design and construction, is the bird's-eye view that allows for a visual of everything from above (Fig. 10.2).

Fig. 10.1 User testing immersive environment∗. (∗Image showing a user testing an in-progress, design of an immersive environment in virtual reality to get a better perception of time and spatial awareness. User feedback of this experience may help in making better design decisions before actual construction)

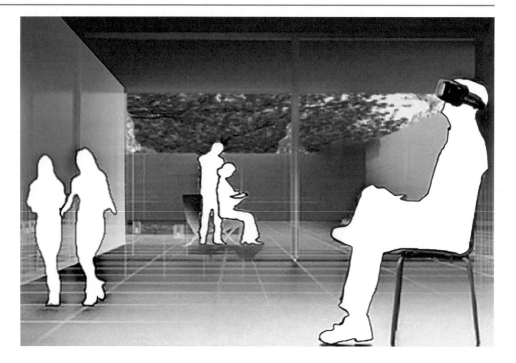

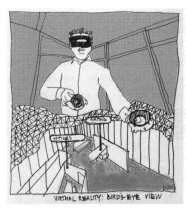 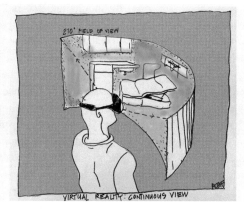 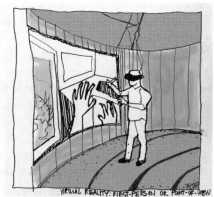

Fig. 10.2 Views in virtual reality∗∗. (∗Left panel: bird's eye view; center panel: continuous view; and right panel: point-of view in virtual reality)

Virtual Reality

Virtual reality through a screen will always have the user with one foot in the real world. In other words, people who are experiencing the virtual world through a screen are still aware of their presence out of the screen. The main attraction of IPEs is the ability to live within them. As mentioned before, the immersion is subject to the adequate recreation of the elements and its relationship with the user [7]. However, it is still unreal. There remain unanswered questions, such as "are virtual objects real?" or "are virtual events as meaningful to the user as actual events?" For example, when accumulating points for certain actions during a video game, one could question, "Does the user feel that hurting someone or breaking an object during the immersion are real events?" Seeking answers to such questions will help immersive

reality better create stronger bonds with the virtual world. This reflection will help in the successful advancement of Lifestyle Medicine Center design protocols.

Interacting with virtual space is an opportunity to provide better health services and, therefore, the immersion should respect the value of the events and objects. Ultimately, the success of this field depends on multidisciplinary teams deciding on the construction of better spaces to save them from failure and unsustainability [8].

The most crucial difference between IPE and the real world is the awareness of the user. The immersion is a consensual act where the user is conscious of being plugged in and geared. The user is usually well aware that both environments are different. Needless to say, there are situations where the virtual world offers such a relieving escape from reality that people may choose to accept the recreated reality as their preferred version. By understanding the benefits of the IPE for the sustainability of architectural models, healthy relationships between VR technology and users are possible. Following are the other considerations to keep in mind:

- Innovation may eventually reach a hyperrealist effect where there will be no noticeable difference between VR and actual reality; until then, immersive experience users will still be attached to external devices, and images may still have failures in their representations;.
- The successful use of IPE depends on the ability to represent the desired environment with enough clarity for the expected outcome to happen.
- Users must receive adequate orientation and training so they stay focused on the objective of the exercise.

These considerations point out the need for more progress and innovation, but at the same time, the design field is ready to use what is available to start including these cost-effective processes. This is in contrast to current design practices that are primarily based on two-dimensional plans and screen-sized (or paper-sized) renderings. Therefore, IPE to visualize representations close enough to real design scenarios is an attractive strategy.

In architecture, the design process should expose the user to a sensory experience rooted in a way that human cognition can structure the information. Most of the processes are unconscious, implying a relationship with the environment shaped by a mentally constructed idea, which may prove to be a challenge for innovation in IPE. However, mentally constructed ideas may facilitate the use of an immersive virtual world because users can provide naturally developed inputs.

Changing the Perception of the Physical World

In simulated reality, there is a connection that the architect or designer imagines to make the function and form a collaborative process between body and mind. Spatial immersion incorporates awareness and the sense of ownership of the place, which allows for better and more critical improvements. The designer can become a user, the user a designer, and the user can be in the role of another user. Even investors and consultants can experience the design and user processes.

Generally speaking, people are equipped to interact in IPEs. The production and consumption of video games and apps for furnishing interiors, or taking pictures and applying filters for choosing new wall colors, are all available to designers. Currently, digital images through photography are available that allow manipulation of objects or images both manually and with predesigned accessories. The critical dif-

ference between these methods and immersive reality is the positioning of the user in space.

The design process using VR entails the inclusion of a series of objects according to the following four broad categories:

1. *Structural* – basement, foundation, and vertical and horizontal elements necessary for a generic shape of the space to be built.
2. *Elemental* – walls, roof, ceiling, stairs.
3. *Utilitarian* – window, doors, toilets, ventilation systems, and essential furniture that the user interacts with actively.
4. *Decorative* – paintings, curtains, and vegetation; these elements will provide realism to the place and even some design solutions for visual or comfort improvement; according to this description, color and textures may be added to this category as well.

The design of a building does not always develop in its construction. This can result in unsuccessful designs that are built, but then modified for improvement, or demolished and rebuilt, with both efforts at great cost. Hence, the potential of incorporating an immersed reality to save time and money is immense. The capability of recreating images that suggest the real existence of a space and its components allows transcendence beyond the use of unidirectional models. The architectural narrative may have the possibility of involving scenarios of multiple interactions of the user and the space in different settings, such as the following:

1. Single user interacting with multiple layouts.
2. Multiple users interacting with a single layout.
3. Single user interacting with a single layout.
4. Multiple users interacting with multiple layouts.

This experience can be enhanced by adding background noise, light simulations, and the ability to include the elemental, utilitarian, and decorative elements. These improvements cannot only improve space, but the surrounding site as well. One scenario of how the user-layout expertise can be useful when there is excess daylight coming in through south-facing windows in the Northern hemisphere is shown in Fig. 10.3. In this scenario, certain environmental variables, such as the following, can be analyzed in order to make design adjustments:

1. The wall dimensions, color, texture, heat absorption coefficient, and wave intensity of the materials exposed to the light that enters through the window in question.
2. The multiple positions in which the user is exposed to this source of light, the ergonomic measures of the user, the reflection of the sun on the different surfaces, and the surface textures and colors that are related to the experience and possible solutions.

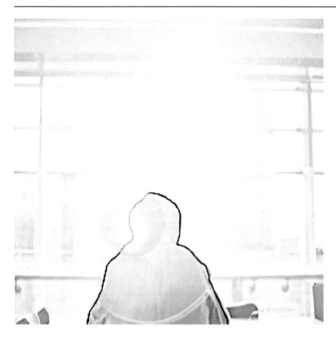

Fig. 10.3 Visual discomfort from excessive glare∗. (∗Image showing how excessive glare from sunlight through windows creates visual discomfort. Spaces such as these can be analyzed by computer simulations and redesigned for optimal comfort)

3. The objects outside the window, their opaqueness, and their change of appearance with changing user position.
4. The sun angles at different hours of the day and seasons of the year.

Upon understanding this scenario, possible solutions need to be recreated. This scenario is more of a reflection that can have a positive impact on the return of investment and the cost-benefits of IPE.

At this point, the use of IPE brings the possibility of a virtual *charrette*. A simplistic description of a design charrette is that it is an intensely focused activity intended to build consensus among participants, develop solutions, and motivate stakeholders to be committed to pursuing the goals of, in this case, a Lifestyle Medicine Center [9]. A charrette is designed to be an in-person interaction and is led by a facilitator. The attendees are the design specialist, stakeholders, members of the community as potential users, and other decision-makers or influencers of the decision-making process, such as lawyers, accountants, or technicians. For a virtual space, some conditions can be eliminated and then substituted with digitized attributes. The charrette idea can be deconstructed through the lens of an immersive experience. In Table 10.1, a direct contrast is made between the characteristics of a traditional design charrette and an immersive design "shar-ette". Charrette is a contemporary term and "shar-ette" is the original term in French that refers to a small cart that transported students and their architectural projects to the l'Ecole des Beaux-arts in Paris. Since most students were using every precious second to finish or improve their projects, in the

Table 10.1 Design charrette vs. immersive design 'shar-ette'∗

	Design charrette	Immersive design shar-ette
Location	A room	IPE: Virtual creation of the actual space to be designed
Tools	Markers, papers, boards	Computer, IPE gear, video or audio recorder
Resources	Literature, blueprints, building schedule, guidelines, and multiple speakers from specialized fields	All the resources will be implemented in the IPE. Specialists may also record their own interaction with the IPE to get their advice or guidance
Steering committee	Owner, facilitator, project manager, one stakeholder, one member of the community	Owner, project manager, VR specialist, notetaker
Participants	25–50 (more usually results in less productivity)	Any number
Time	Subject to availability and multiple scheduling conflicts	The time may or may not be a major determinant since some people would participate longer than others. Also, specialist or specific users can be invited to many sessions if needed

aCharrette: meeting in which all the project participants collaboratively design solutions. Abbreviations: *IPE* immersive physical environments, *VR* virtual reality

end, shar-ettes became a place for intense brainstorming sessions [9]. Using this interactive technique, multiple participants in an immersive experience may be recorded and their feedback annotated. The host (i.e., a computer, hard drive, cloud, or server) is essentially the cart of the shar-ette, and the many interactions are the contributors to the results.

Lifestyle Medicine Architecture

Current Codes and Requirements of a Health Center

The criteria to design any health center start from the basics of good maintainability and high reliability. Shorter distances between key areas of attention to patients are recommended. Facilities must also have the following elements, regardless of the residential or outpatient therapeutic programs that apply:

1. Toilet facilities in a ratio of at least one toilet and one lavatory for every 15 occupants in the case of outpatient treatment programs [10].
2. At least one room for every 15 potential patients or users of the clinic, allowing private interviews with users or with users and their families.
3. "Living rooms," i.e., waiting areas that provide comfortable sitting and natural and artificial lighting for multiple uses including group therapy or recreational activities

4. Outdoor areas for recreation, patios, terraces, or gardens.
5. Air-tight containers for the temporary storage of health-care waste in three categories:
   (a). Regulated (as indicated by the World Health Organization): infectious, hazardous, and radioactive.
   (b). Non-regulated: general waste.
   (c). Recycling which is optional but highly desirable.
6. A safe space to keep cleaning supplies.
7. Rooms for the preparation and consumption of food as needed.
8. A first-aid kit area or room.
9. Other spaces required for specialized programs.

In general, all healthcare facilities must have walls, floors, and ceilings in a good state of conservation and maintenance. In addition, these facilities should have surfaces that are free of moisture or leaks, sanitary installations including fixtures and fittings in a good state of operation, natural and artificial lighting, mechanisms for heating that are safe for the users and the staff, especially those who are overweight/obese or disabled/handicapped, and a maintenance plan for the equipment and the facilities.

Elements of Lifestyle Medicine Facilities

Physical Rehabilitation

Physical rehabilitation (including physical therapy) is the set of corrective measures to restore the disabled patient's independence to the highest capacity possible. As part of the medical assistance responsible for developing functional and psychological capabilities of the individual, rehabilitation activates the mechanisms of compensation to enable a dynamic and autonomous existence.

The physical spaces needed are specific to the diagnosis, evaluation, prevention, and treatment of disability to facilitate, maintain, or return the patient to the highest degree of functional capacity and independence possible. Space should allow for natural and mechanical movements of both the physical exercise of a person and the therapeutic staff as needed. It is important to note that good or bad performance of physical movements should be expected and planned for, not only those natural body movements that we all are familiar with. The people receiving this kind of care are at risk of losing or altering proper motion either temporarily or permanently and, thus, the role of this space is also to provide a relaxing environment to have physical rehabilitation and not to obstruct the progress of the patient.

There are various design concerns and implications in the layout of a physical rehabilitation area (Fig. 10.4). At first glance, this physical rehabilitation area may be adequate since it is clean and visually pleasing. The concerns from the architect or designer may be around the aesthetics and other issues, such as efficiency of the air circulation and distribution of light. However, focusing solely on these issues may actually exclude crucial user needs, such as transferring into a wheelchair, not directly facing doctors who are working on the computer, and having no seating accommodation for a companion. All these concerns should be appropriately addressed in the design.

Nutrition, Gym, and Cooking Demonstration Rooms

Basic requirements for nutrition and weight loss facilities include a private office for a doctor or nutritionist, an area for the interview and physical examination, a scale with

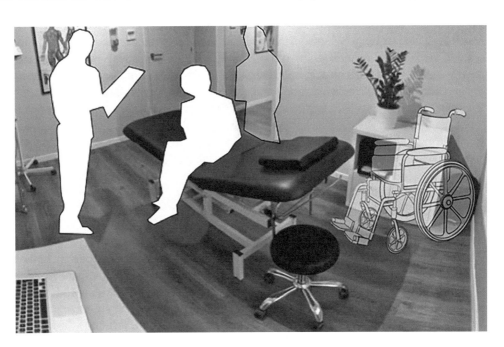

Fig. 10.4 A typical physical therapy office space

stadiometer, and weight and height charts. Additionally, a larger gathering room for demonstrations and testimonials, and a kitchenette or culinary cart for demonstrations should be provided. This innovative element of Lifestyle Medicine Centers brings the opportunity to demonstrate the preparation of food and sharing of information and insights about nutrition in a more visual and practical way. The type of health concerns addressed in these spaces includes weight loss, diabetes, and high blood pressure. They are also used for education on sport nutrition, vegetarian and veganism, and allergies. These demonstration rooms can help inspire people to make lifestyle changes and make otherwise difficult processes easy, and even entertaining. Therefore, these spaces should also allow for counseling, workshops, and team activities. Due to cooking activities, these rooms have to follow the same recommendations for a kitchen, which accounts for a balance of hard and soft surfaces that can be 100% sanitized, a sink with potable water, stove or electric range, safe garbage disposal, and an air supply that ensures air exchange of a minimum of 100 cubic feet per minute or a direct opening to the exterior which provides natural ventilation as recommended by the American Society of Heating, Refrigeration, and Air-Conditioning Engineers.

Substance Abuse and Medication Management

Substance abuse treatment and care of people who are experiencing withdrawal symptoms require treatment and rehabilitation rooms that must have infrastructure free of structural risks for users and the staff working in them. Patients should be accommodated in rooms for 15–25 people in units with excellent acoustics that provide privacy for conversations. Both individual and group conversations need comfortable sitting areas with peaceful settings and neutral colors and textures. They should also be free of smells that may trigger anxiety or cravings and allow interaction with games, food, and even pets. The characteristics of the space may include homelike features, natural beauty, and special attention to the scale of the area in a relationship to the user. One example of why the scale of a room matters is that when the volumes of spaces are too big, then the emptiness and echoes disturb the experience; alternatively, when the volumes of spaces are too small, then the occupants feel crowded. Decisions should be based on the needs of users exposed to specific treatments and the environmental features and surroundings required. A more specific example is when patients are experiencing anxiety due to withdrawal symptoms, and that anxiety is exacerbated by certain colors, noises, or crowded spaces.

Stress Management: Acupuncture Rooms, Meditation Rooms, and Outdoor Spaces

Stress management spaces, which also form a part of substance abuse treatment, should be clean, intimate spaces that allow for lying on the floor as well as providing chairs, beds, and/or pillows. Acoustics are critical since very low voices and sounds, as well as silence, are part of the therapies. Appropriate storage of clinical materials (e.g., acupuncture needles) requires controlled, secured, and clean space. Adjustable natural and artificial light, and access to views to the outside, is also crucial. Colors and textures in surfaces play a role in the relaxation process and are crucial elements to consider in design, ideally tested with users and specialists in pilot studies.

Immersive Physical Environments Applied to Lifestyle Medicine Centers

Creating Virtual Reality Scenarios

The number of structural, elemental, utilitarian, and decorative objects in Lifestyle Medicine Centers continues to increase as technology advances. New medical, therapeutic, and experimental procedures provide spaces with updated specialized objects that, at least during a transitional period, share the space with the older ones. What would be different once the design process is open to an immersive experience? A virtual charrette, as described earlier, would create awareness of unused objects, misused space, and accessibility issues.

Lifestyle Medicine Centers do not generally serve emergencies as hospitals or other clinics with the obvious exception in medical fitness and cardiac rehabilitation programs. Lifestyle Medicine Centers should emphasize customer service with routine activities that involve cashiers, receipts, transactions, claims, and emotional tensions. As in any healthcare space, these centers have paperwork, laughter, conversations, arguments, and coexistence of patients who are in recovery with others that are in the process of deterioration. Some patients arrive with enthusiasm, while other patients arrive in anxiety or solitude. This is consistent with the tenet that lifestyle medicine aims to optimize health for all patients across the spectrum of wellness-to-illness.

For each step in any healing process, space provides opportunities for different user interactions. Embodiment and involvement in design increase awareness and presence. In some cases, the user can be replaced by a virtual replica, even one with different physical characteristics if needed. These virtual replicas in the form of an avatar, i.e., a graphical representation of a user, can modify actions and alert the user to any design deficiencies [11].

Workflow

The workflow in healthcare facilities reveals physical relationships among multiple functions that ultimately determine the configuration of the spaces. The flow diagrams in Figs. 10.5 and 10.6 show movement and communication of functions, people, procedures, and safety. The physical configuration of the healthcare facility and its logistical sys-

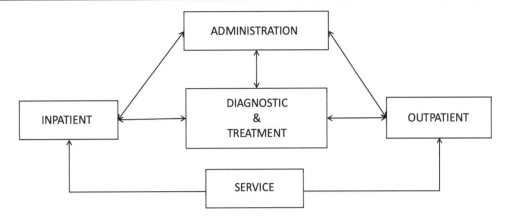

Fig. 10.5 Recommended workflow for spaces in healthcare facilities

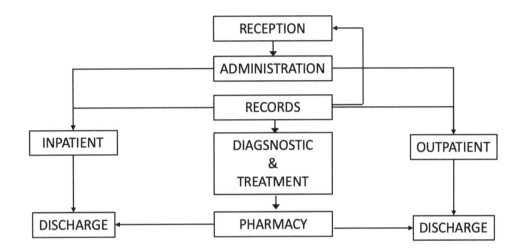

Fig. 10.6 Recommended clinical workflows in hospitals

tems are inextricably intertwined. The site restraints, climate, surrounding facilities, budget, and available technology also influence the configuration. The implementation of new alternatives generated by new medical procedures, such as immersive reality, will eventually change the configuration. Preparedness, adaptive spaces, and a bundled generation of alternatives where technology and sustainability merge are essential [12].

All units must have ventilation, natural lighting, colors, and subtle textures, which have a positive impact on mood. The versatility of the spaces is a determining factor for the design of an efficient health center. Another primary design requirement is accessibility. The different offices of the Lifestyle Medicine Center may have architectural barriers that do not correspond to its requirements. In the design of a healthcare building, stakeholders should be aware that any person, regardless of age or level of ability, should easily be able to perform the following actions:

- Wandering (navigate to another space).
- Apprehension (e.g., catch or grab something for personal safety).
- Location (identification of the self in a precise place).

- Communication (exchanging information necessary for the development of an activity).

All of these actions are directly related to activities. The workflow in these facilities begins with the appointment of the patient in person or remotely, i.e., via phone or electronically. Once the patient is present to be attended, there is a pre-interview, after which the person receives information and is subject to the primary auscultation, e.g., weight, blood pressure, temperature. These initial steps are part of a preventive service to not only confirm or establish a record of individual health but also assess the physical or psychological state at that time to guide priority of the attention. These steps may be annoying and tedious to some personnel. Therefore, a better workflow should operationalize efficiently the following functions:

1. Streamline patient flow, which improves the level of service.
2. Welcome patients as they come or allow them to wait comfortably and accommodate proper signage.
3. Keep staff organized and in control of their responsibilities, which contribute to the quality of medical care.

4. Have clear access to the routine circulation of the staff and evacuation routes.
5. Have interior design solutions, which are scalable and adaptable to increases in volume, patients, emergencies, and contingencies.
6. Maintenance that is easy and effective.

Any disruption of the above functions can cause distractions, fatigue, and interruptions, which can interfere with the care of the patient. Workflows consolidate various working tools into a single system to reduce unnecessary inefficiencies, establishing a work order and rules of interaction for employee groups. One must remember that these workflows must allow for traumatic moments, alarming scenarios, and need to minimize infections by avoiding disturbing sensations and physical exposures.

Mobility solutions, with or without the use of immersed reality, help optimize the care of the patient and strive to be more efficient. However, patient-caregiver relationships have evolved to a state in the current healthcare climate that at times can be distant, cold, rude, and frankly counterproductive. The effective use of design and operation based on virtual spaces optimizes complicated workflows, while eliminating most risks for staff and patients and allowing humanistic and compassionate solutions.

Staff

Roles and functions of different types of healthcare professionals (HCPs) in lifestyle medicine follow the same workflow and hierarchy as any healthcare system, which focuses on patients with different chronic diseases. According to the Patient Navigator Training Collaborative (https://patientnavigatortraining.org/ [Accessed on February 15, 2020]), a state-of-the-art manual for collaborative healthcare environments, lifestyle medicine team members include:

- Physicians.
- Advanced practice providers (e.g., nurse practitioners and physician assistants).
- Nurses.
- Pharmacists.
- Medical technologists, assistants, and technicians.
- Therapists and rehabilitation specialists.
- Emotional, social, and spiritual support professionals.
- Administrative and support staff.
- Community health workers and patient navigators.
- Primary care clinician and appropriate consultants.

Lifestyle medicine patient encounters, especially the initial encounter when the diagnosis is first evaluated, involve many more people than just the physician. An example time sequence of events follows [13]:

1. The front desk staff schedules the appointment, finds the medical record, makes a reminder call, greets the patient, and verifies insurance information.
2. A nurse or medical assistant records the patient's weight (and other anthropometrics), vital signs, and other metrics (e.g., glucose), escorts the patient to an exam room, and records the reason for the visit and other routine information (e.g., new allergies and medications).
3. The physician or advanced practice provider examines and interviews the patient to develop a diagnosis and care plan.
4. If a lab or radiology test is necessary, a technician or other HCP performs the test.
5. Test results are discussed with the patient by members of the team.
6. Treatments are implemented with inclusion of other HCP team members, such as a pharmacist.
7. Finally, medical billing experts interact with the patient regarding pertinent financial aspects of the encounter, and for patients whose treatment requires follow-up, the administrative staff schedules necessary appointments.

Population Served

Lifestyle Medicine Centers rely on medical evidence to prevent and treat chronic disease, based on the underlying cause of illness and not just symptoms. Potentially, lifestyle medicine can serve up to 80% or more of all patients in the USA since most of the attention provided by hospitals, specialty clinics, and research care is the result of, or at least contributed by, unhealthy lifestyles [14].

Lifestyle medicine patients have to be particularly and actively involved in their care. Patient participation depends on motivational principles, including comfortable and welcoming spaces. Many causes of health problems that result in chronic disease are linked to vicious cycles. For example, inadequate sleep can lead to fatigue, fatigue to inactivity, inactivity to overeating, each of these to obesity and depression, leading to metabolic syndrome, type 2 diabetes, sexual dysfunction, mood disorders, and cardiovascular disease, which ultimately disturbs sleep hygiene [15]. In an ideal world, treatments would be supported by adequate and sustained public health efforts that offer not only temporary relief while being in the sessions but also a set of tools and new behaviors that support the necessary lifestyle changes outside of the Lifestyle Medicine Center. Therefore, the more the center has a welcoming, home-like appearance, the easier the patients can be engaged and activated for change.

Routine Clinical Equipment

The design of a clinic, or any functional space for that matter, should account for all the required equipment. The ugliness and bulkiness of an instrument can adversely change

Table 10.2 Routine clinical equipment requirements

Equipment	Size	Type of connection	Level of mobility
X-ray equipment	Large appliance	Electric	Fixed or mobile
Centrifuge	Small appliance	Electric	Mobile
Lab microscope	Small appliance	None	Mobile
Stretcher	Large tool	None	Mobile with wheels
Surgical table	Large furniture	None	Fixed or mobile with wheels

the patient experience. Noise and visual pollution may result from cramped and cluttered quarters, and the ultimate goal of healing will be unreachable. Routine clinical equipment should be organized and sorted in charts to show specific space requirements in a room, helping overall design decisions. First, the size and type of equipment (appliance, tool, chart, etc.) must be included. Second, the equipment should be sorted by the type of connection each piece needs, whether it be electric, water, gas, computer/data, or none, which can help with room location and organization. Last, the mobility for each piece of equipment – whether the equipment is fixed or mobile, with and without wheels – should be listed. Table 10.2 shows a sample chart with five pieces of equipment. Such organizing charts are crucial in the early stages of design of Lifestyle Medicine Centers.

Routine Miscellaneous Equipment

Miscellaneous equipment or large, medium, and small appliances (e.g., lab refrigerators, ventilators, computer equipment, exam tables, wheelchairs, oxygen tanks, and hospital beds) are usually in the way of the natural flow of people. Nonetheless, they are typically necessary and have to be accommodated. Many pieces of equipment are connected to data and electric outlets, and in most cases, they are attached or located beside the patient in the room. These considerations to create a less-intrusive environment with strategic equipment placement can be very challenging. Clustering and decentralizing equipment in this regard may be helpful. Having a place to store the equipment while it is not in use is ideal. A chart similar to the one shown in Table 10.2 should be used to categorize, organize, and sort the requirements of each piece of equipment so that suitable spaces to store and locate them when in use can be planned for in advance.

Handicap Accessibility

An important healthcare facility design feature is accessibility. Architectural barriers in the design of a Lifestyle Medicine Center should be avoided. The space must suit the spatial needs of any person, regardless of age or level of ability, to access and perform actions of wandering, apprehension, location, and communication. Examples of the

types of physical disability to consider for these actions are as follows:

1. Physical impairment.
2. Short or tall stature, cachexia and obesity.
3. Elderly and frail.
4. Cognitive dysfunction and developmental/psychiatric disorders.
5. Other special needs (bleeding diathesis, seizure, dysautonomia, etc.)

Architectural design considerations for these types of disabilities vary and require attention. Compliance with current rules of accessibility lists conditions for non-discrimination, which require the design to pay attention to the welcoming appearance of every space. Generally, a functional space has no edges or rough floors where people with disabilities can get hurt. Doors, steps, stairs, and access to the use of furniture should be available to all. Bathrooms should allow for appropriate levels of privacy and space with toileting, showering, and robing/disrobing as needed, as well as acceptable levels of cleaning and collection of items.

Furniture, Décor, and Artwork

The most used decorations and accessories for healthcare facilities are pictures, paintings, plants, coffee tables, toys, figurines, sculptures, panels, curtains, carpets and area rugs, lighting fixtures, and seasonal décor. The role of these accessories is to comfort the patient during the stay. Plants and area rugs, for example, contribute to cleaning the air and controlling acoustics respectively.

A feeling of being at home is key during healing processes and tends to lower stress. According to Jennifer Silvis, a specialist in healthcare design, the use of bright colors in patient rooms is disturbing, unpleasant, and make people agitated [16]. Vibrant bright colors are welcome in children areas and areas where one wants to keep moving. Another important consideration is to coordinate colors so the combination is soft, and not psychedelic. Cold and warm colors have different effects on people. Cold colors are calming and are characterized by the minimum or complete absence of red and yellow. Warm colors are more vibrant and tend to have more yellow and red hues. Neutral colors such as beige and wooden tones bring balance and tranquility, and work well alongside both cold and warm colors.

Safety and Emergency Management

The fundamental questions about safety and emergency plans are related to whether injuries or death to patients or staff will occur should the equipment or systems (interconnected pieces of equipment) fail [17]:

1. Would the failure of the system or equipment be likely to cause major injury or death to patients or caregivers?
2. Would the failure of the system or equipment be likely to cause minor injury to patients or caregivers?
3. Would the failure of the system or equipment be unlikely to cause injury, but discomfort to patients?
4. Would the failure of the system or equipment have no impact on patient care?

Failures of the system include any interruption to the routine of the facility. They could be natural disasters, chemical spills, infection exposure, leaks, fractures of building elements, fire, and many others.

It is recommended that instead of basing safety and emergency procedures on assumptions, plans for Lifestyle Medicine Centers should include a risk assessment of what would happen to patients or caregivers if the system was lost or compromised with the existing or planned conditions. The administrative requirements, which generally include policies and preventive maintenance requirements, should also apply to new and existing facilities, systems, and equipment. Again, the safety and emergency preparedness plans are a response to the real conditions of the building. An immersive experience where the site is virtually created may help allocate, distribute, manage, and create emergency scenarios for better planning in advance.

Operations, Management, Maintenance, Cleaning, and Utilities

General guidelines for healthcare facilities include having proper ventilation. All structural, elemental, functional, and decorative elements of the building and spaces should avoid excessive moisture (to prevent mold). Facilities must have easy-to-clean areas (asepsis) and smooth angles and corners. Ideally, cleaning routines are scheduled every day and recorded by the maintenance staff. Sanitation should be required more than once a day in bathrooms, laboratories, and other spaces where fluids are handled. Other areas should be sanitized with a different frequency depending on specific needs. Cleaning staff should be available at all times for urgent situations (spills, breakage, fecal and urinary incontinence, vomiting, bleeding, etc.). It is desirable to have a janitorial room with enough space for cleaning supplies, tools, and equipment as well as an all-purpose utility sink. A janitorial room in every floor (in case of a multistory building) or at reasonable distances is also desirable to avoid disruption of the work and patient flow as well as to attend to emergencies faster. The rule of thumb is to always have one of these rooms close to the service entrance of the building or by the stairs, or near the restrooms.

Improving Physical Spaces

Area, Volume, and Relationships of Spaces

Health centers should have spaces in which surfaces and heights of elements allow for sightlines or views from one point inside the facility to an element that gives directionality, orientation, or information, such as views to nature, sunlight, art, or a television screen. This, along with fresh air and good ventilation, brings comfort to the users. The design specifications for carrying out the functional program of a Lifestyle Medicine Center should have optimal ratios between the floor area and the number of users. Guidelines and policies have minimum requirements for operations; however, in order to realize the goals of a Lifestyle Medicine Center, design relationships between users and space should go over and above these requirements. Basic safety codes that encompass fire protection include the Life Safety Code and the Heath Care Facilities Code that regulate fire prevention, emergency procedures, smoke detection, and panic management. These codes not only cover installation, operation, testing and maintenance of the facilities, materials, equipment, and appliances, but also have recommendations for staff training and user preparedness. The distances between, and distributions of areas by function, within the building also need attention. Emergency exit corridor widths must consider door sizes, locations of sprinklers, and fire alarms. Their proximity to very crowded spaces and placement away from fuel or easily combustible materials is crucial. Emergency escape routes need to be designed after considering the distance between the farthest place of the building and the exit, obstacles, work and patient flows, and vertical circulation.

Centralization Versus Decentralization of Functions

Strategies are necessary for clinical processes that rely on machines and other elements that are easy to access or control. Healthcare involves multitasking and efficiency, which require highly organized staff, materials, and procedures. Some concerns retrieved from visitors' online reviews describe that a perception of clutter exists when many people and objects are interacting within an insufficient space. To succeed, this requires a level of coordination among staff and HCPs, and that can be physically and mentally intensive and exhausting.

Compact treatment rooms may improve performance only if the necessary devices for the treatment have enough space to operate. Good design will allow both users and devices to perform efficiently. Some suggestions for meeting this design goal are as follows [18]:

- *Centralize:* Cluster all the devices and accessories that are used for the same purpose in the same area of the room or space, or store them in wall closets to keep them organized and safe.

- *Integrate:* Remove unnecessary barriers such as walls or unused furniture when possible.
- *Decentralize:* Optimize routes for machines and people to move in and out as needed and share spaces within the facility.

Acoustics

Optimal acoustics in a Lifestyle Medicine Center includes noise control and wayfinding through an echolocation effect. It is difficult to understand and separate different noises in places with bad acoustics. While this is true for anyone, people who use hearing aids are especially sensitive to background noise, such as ventilation equipment, chairs being dragged across the floor, and weights banging in the gym.

In order to listen to conversation, sound in an enclosure must have a very short resonance. Acoustic walls are needed to absorb and direct sound, especially in waiting rooms. For staff, as well as people with visual impairments, excellent acoustics can be of great help since it is a wayfinding tool [19].

Good acoustics require insulation in walls, ground, roof, windows, and doors to attenuate outside noise. Despite the importance of this environmental feature, noise pollution is one of the most disregarded problems that happen in indoor and outdoor spaces in Lifestyle Medicine Centers. Some effective acoustical materials are sound absorbing panels made up of glass and mineral fibers that can be suspended from the ceiling to increase speech intelligibility, or wall panels made up of or glass and natural fibers to reduce echoes [20].

Sightlines

Clear wayfinding and signage naturally guide users through a building. Patients, visitors, and staff all need to know where they are, what their destination is, and how to get there and return. A patient's sense of independence and confidence is encouraged by making spaces easy to find, identify, and use without asking for help. Building elements such as colors, textures, patterns, as well as artwork and signage should all give cues [12].

The following design considerations could measurably improve patient outcomes.

- Include sound and braille in posters and signage to make them inclusive and accessible. All of them should be illuminated in such a way that they do not produce glare, and the characters of the labels should be clear, with vivid and contrasting colors and large letters with enough separation provided between them.
- Hallways must be identified through edges, color contrasts, and textures. All the flooring must be non-slip and without protrusions, which may cause tripping. Different

textures can distinguish the difference between different spaces. They must be non-reflective and their color must contrast with the walls.
- The sounds produced by floor and wall finishes as one walks should be carefully considered since some individuals who are visually impaired touch walls and floors with their sticks to identify the location of obstacles.

Air Quality

Air quality includes controlled airflows for optimal natural ventilation, mechanical ventilation, odor management, and pollution control (to manage volatile organic compounds, semi-volatile organic compounds, and cross-contamination). Poorly designed, maintained, and operated ventilation systems elevate the risk of infections. The techniques applied to control contaminants in healthcare facilities consist of (1) control by dilution through the ventilation with clean air, (2) purification of the air by physical filtration (passive system), and/or (3) the use of systems to dilute active contaminants, such as ultraviolet radiation or photocatalysis [19].

Air conditioning must ensure the control of temperature and humidity within ranges of comfort and must minimize odors, prevent uncontrolled dispersal of pollutants, and protect against environmental contaminants. Strategic allocation of natural and strictly expert-guided planning of ventilation systems is also required [19]. The guidelines for odor control recommend avoiding contact with materials and plants that provoke allergies. Specific allergens include formaldehyde, isocyanate (found in insulation, adhesives, and paints), nickel, dust, mold, tobacco smoke, environmental pollution, perfumes, animal dander, pollen, birch, and bushes and other non-coniferous plants with strong fragrances (jasmine, hyacinths, lilacs, chrysanthemums, etc.).

Daylight and Electrical Lighting

Light is associated with well-being and health. A diagram and careful analysis of the solar path will assist the design and positioning of windows, skylights, and other openings, admitting sunlight (directly or indirectly) throughout the year. This allows collective strategies that may admit ample natural light wherever feasible and using color-corrected lighting sources in interior spaces, including ones that simulate natural daylight [12].

Lighting installation must consider two aspects: aesthetics and technology. The aesthetics, while mostly qualitative, must ensure a comfortable visual environment and pleasant atmosphere where light and shadow are well organized. The technological aspect is quantitative and ensures that the lighting levels for activities in each place are satisfied. Lighting levels for various spaces in the Lifestyle Medicine Center, as well as the glare index (index for discomfort due to visual glare) and color-rendering index (ability of light to reveal colors), have to be considered during the lighting design process.

Thermal Comfort

Thermal comfort is a subjective evaluation of how comfortable a certain place feels based on the body's transfer of heat. Thermal comfort is closely related to thermal stress, which is also subjective. Both thermal comfort and thermal stress rely on the relationship between environmental elements (e.g., air and objects) that hold heat and the human. The environmental factors that must be taken into consideration for optimal thermal comfort are air temperature, radiant temperature, air velocity, and humidity.

The built (man-made) environment uses air dynamics to condition indoor and outdoor spaces. Typically, ventilation systems can control the air temperature, velocity, and humidity. However, most ventilation systems are generic and fail to consider properties of building materials and accessories, such as radiation (the capability of retaining heat and transferring it to air). Radiation (electromagnetic waves transferring energy) accounts for 75% of the total of heat transfer in a building, while conduction (transfer of heat by direct contact) and convection (transfer of heat by motion of matter) account for the remaining 25%. The effectiveness of the system is determined by the emittance (ability to emit temperature) of materials and placement of insulation (materials that slow down heat transfer). To prevent offsets between the thermal quality of different spaces, walls, and interior partitions of the thermal envelope, designers and decision-makers should follow guidelines suited to the climatic zone in which the building is located [21].

Assurance of Effective Design

The use of advanced VR, although shown in science fiction movies for decades (e.g., The Matrix, Ender's Game, Ready Player One), is still a new field. Its effectiveness in designing IPE needs to be established by controls, which include isolating the system from external factors that are not part of the evaluation. There is much debate in this area, but isolation from external factors is necessary so that the evaluation is fair. Design has become more complex as technology advances, and the options are endless. Sometimes, there are too many options along with market pressures, leading to standardization, as well as some level of dehumanization. Social behavior research now includes algorithms to guess user preferences based on social media and web searches data. In general, people lack the ability to control their environments according to personal needs. The immersive design shar-ette may be impractical or unfeasible at times, but it can work very effectively as a tool to obtain better results based on experiences of different types of users and stakeholders. Since IPE are still not commonly used, all the parameters to

measure their effectiveness are preliminary. In practice, it is still challenging to prevent designs based on IPE from being affected by external factors such as privacy, misuse of data and technology, computer failure, lack of participants, inadequate interpretation, market pressures, and others. However, there is a set of preliminary assessments that measure the effectiveness of design processes in IPE [22].

1. *Prediction* vs. *Feedback*: to predict a design, convert it into IPE, test it with users, decision-makers, stakeholders, and analyze the feedback.
2. *Cost-benefits*: to account for the costs of technology, software, programming, designing, animation, and other expert areas implicated in the creation of IPE, use per session, and the collection and interpretation of data; also to account for the costs of a traditional design process, with modifications, delays, construction, demolition (when those demolitions are the product of bad design), and failures in systems; and then to compare the costs of IPE with the traditional design process.
3. *Engagement*: organize a site visit to existing facilities (one that needs to be renovated or a similar, existing facility as the one to be constructed) with users, decision-makers, and stakeholders. Collect comments, recommendations for improvements, and other valuable feedback. Take a similar sample of participants into an IPE and collect the same set of observations. The key is to identify whether the participants are more engaged when the building is not built, as compared to being in an existing building.
4. *Commitment*: designers, architects, planners, contractors, subcontractors, investors, and consultants from the design side and facilities manager, staff, administrators, physicians, and nurses from the Lifestyle Medicine Center will compare their decisions in both an actual built environment and an IPE. The key is to observe whether these participants feel more committed to their job when knowing that their opinions are considered before construction happens.

Responses to Health and Wellness

Harmonious environments are a result of natural responses to a person's needs, which are desirable for any person, but crucial for those in medical treatment. Including users' voices into the design process is an approach that connects the person with the healing process. IPE may sometimes serve as treatments themselves. Healing processes have been tied to practicing yoga or other practices that involve the control of the functions of the body, organs, and energies to heal. Immersive technologies can make people aware of their healing process and influence their recovery. Now, there is a real possibility of incorporating personal needs and expectations into Lifestyle Medicine Centers by digitally recording experiences from users that are in search of their wellness.

Therapeutic Environments

Therapeutic environments and their design include envisioning the facilities from their interiors, surroundings, and views. Patient safety protocols, equipment, crowded spaces, internal corridors, and similar elements that tie the user to being in an institutional setting commonly add to stress. For a Lifestyle Medicine Center, a therapeutic environment must provide home-like experiences while maintaining safe conditions. Design alternatives, such as IPE can help create this balance. Knowledge of how equipment and procedures work, especially those machines that are heavy or require connection to power or to the patient, requires attention.

Environmental Stress Strategy

The success of a well-designed space will reduce or eliminate environmental stressors, provide positive distractions, enable social support, and give a sense of control. Providing views of the outdoors from wherever possible or photo murals of nature scenes is helpful where outdoor views are not available and using familiar and culturally relevant materials wherever it is consistent with sanitation procedures and other functional needs all help provide a stress-free environment. Some examples sanitation concerns when using culturally relevant materials include, for example, using porous materials such as adobe that are difficult to clean and sanitize. However, there are other strategies to make comfortable environments for patients, such as using cheerful and varied colors and textures. It is important to keep in mind that some colors are inappropriate and can interfere with proper assessments of health, for example, patients' pallor and skin tones when the specialist needs to observe skin color during diagnosis. Particular colors or color combinations may disorient older or impaired patients due to their reflectivity or contrast. Some patients and staff, and particularly some psychiatric patients, may find some certain color combination to be disturbing [12]. The inclusion of elements that establish a calming mood and motivational experience in the IPE is key. The ability to get accurate feedback from the design process based on immersive experience depends on how realistic the experience is.

Visitors' Experiences

Approximately 50 Google reviews of lifestyle medicine were found and studied after using the search terms "Lifestyle Medicine Center" in Google and checking search results (reviews) randomly. Reviews of top Lifestyle Medicine Centers across the USA revealed feedback about the quality of the attention by the staff or physician as the first concern. The next most discussed topic is waiting time, and the third

is the condition of the facility. Although the feedback regarding attention and time is key for the design process, the quality of facilities is also very important. It is worth reflecting about how proper design may solve or alleviate concerns. The comment "Long wait but great service" provides insight that people can wait for long periods, but a comfortable place to stay must be provided. Other comments that relate to facility conditions are as follows:

"Very nice and clean facility."

"Best place for physical."

"Clean, friendly staff and different choices on menu to choose from."

"All round great office, great staff, great Dr, great experience!"

"I have never seen such dingy and run down rooms, and especially the bathrooms."

"Horribly rude staff, super slow service, and dirty restrooms!"

"Very knowledgeable and a pleasant experience."

"Friendly environment and good customer care and services!"

A larger and more systematic review of comments is required to make sound conclusions; however, a short preliminary study of Google reviews indicates that visitors may be very aware of the quality of the surrounding environment and design in Lifestyle Medicine Centers. Good service in these facilities includes not only aspects of medical care but also the design features. The design process is responsible for providing the overall mindset of staff. For users, visitors, and companions, the waiting time and buildup of stress require that they enter facilities that are conducive to relaxation.

Performance of the Clinical Staff.

There is an expected increase of productivity in healthcare facilities through better design practices. Noise reduction, access to daylight, appropriate lighting, safe "off-stage" areas for respite, proximity to other staff, and proper use of technology, supplies, and charting have mostly been focused on the patient and patient's family. However, these factors also have potential benefits for staff and caregivers in terms of satisfaction, effectiveness, and staff retention.

Core Recommendations

Decision-Making

IPE and VR may be used to assess the impact of user input toward design.

1. Consider creating immersive design shar-ettes for collecting voices that can be recorded digitally to obtain better results based on living experiences from all types of users and stakeholders [9].

2. Plan an introductory session for participants to get familiarized with the technology and stay focused on the objective of the exercise.
3. Add layers of awareness into virtually created or recreated environments where users can identify unused objects, misused space, accessibility issues, and any other design deficiencies [23].

Cost Control

Projected savings from a cost-benefit analysis may include savings on treatments, patient satisfaction, productivity, and operational-construction costs.

1. Compare the costs of technology, software, programming, designing, animation, and other expert areas required in the creation of IPE, the amount of use per session, and the collection and interpretation of data with the costs of a traditional design process, its modifications, delays, construction, demolition (when those demolitions are the product of bad design), and failures in systems.
2. Create an architectural narrative that makes participants value the importance of their input in the cost of the project.
3. Consider emergency preparedness or contingency plans not only for safety but also for unnecessary expenses or misuse of elements.

Engaging Stakeholders

More productive and efficient design shar-ettes and working sessions can be developed.

1. Inspire people to commit to the goals of the project by highlighting the importance of their decisions and help them identify better or different ways to perform their responsibilities based on what they experience in the IPE.
2. Develop the capability, as a design team, to represent the desired environment with enough clarity for expected outcomes to happen from all kinds of users and stakeholders.
3. Inspire ownership of the place to allow for better and more critical improvements. The designer could become a user, the user a designer, or the user could be in the role of another user; even investors and consultants could experience design and use the spaces.
4. Base safety and emergency plans on simulations of real conditions of the building. An immersive experience where the site is virtually created may help allocate, dis-

tribute, manage, and create emergency scenarios for better planning.

Incorporating Individual Input into Participatory Virtual Spaces

There are enhanced opportunities of comparing and contrasting multiple design solutions at once. The immersive design shar-ette is an intensely focused activity intended to build consensus among participants, develop solutions, and motivate stakeholders to be committed to pursue the goals of a Lifestyle Medicine Center. Design guidelines need to be considered when creating an IPE for a Lifestyle Medicine Center.

1. Provide a relaxing environment to have adequate therapy and not obstruct the progress of the patient in physical rehabilitation, nutrition treatment, substance abuse control, and stress management.
2. Respect workflows and safety procedures.
3. Address accessibility to provide adequate freedom for performing actions of wandering, apprehension, location, and communication.
4. Provide proper ventilation and access for deep cleaning in all areas.
5. Attend centralization and decentralization needs for staff, materials, and procedures.
6. Provide good acoustics, sightlines, wayfinding, air quality, lighting, and thermal comfort.

Conclusions

For Lifestyle Medicine Centers, stakeholders and users should be key decision-makers in architectural and interior design processes, but most often they are not consulted until significant planning is done. The IPE opens a virtual threshold bringing participants into decision-making and an active interaction with the building without actually constructing it. The sense of presence empowers investors, contractors, designers, future staff, and potential patients by giving them voice and accountability.

Innovative approaches are necessary to advance strategies for sustainable built environments, and avoid unnecessary expenses for mistakes or high costs of failed projects. The integration of state-of-the-art VR tools is key for the development of design and construction. Collaboration and communication between all the participants can be enabled by taking advantage of computational systems and programs to collect firsthand data from vivid experiences in immersive spaces. For current and future patients, some of their most personal, healing moments may occur inside Lifestyle Medicine Centers, and they deserve spaces that connect them to the best care and help them heal in the best way possible. Staff working in the facility requires a building that allows them to perform at their highest level, while also improving their own health and wellness. Family members and visitors should step into spaces that inspire comfort and joy.

References

1. Gifreu-Castells A, Zambrano V. Educational multimedia applied to the interactive nonfiction area. Using Interactive Documentary as a New Model for Learning. Proceedings of Edulearn14 Conference, 2014, Barcelona, 1306–1315. ISBN: 978–84–617-0557-3/ISSN: 2340–1117.
2. Grau O. Virtual art: from illusion to immersion, chapter 4. Cambridge MA: MIT Press; 2003. p. 140–91.
3. Owen T, Pitt F, Raney Aronson-Rath R, et al. Virtual reality journalism. Columbia J Rev. 2015; https://www.cjr.org/tow_center_reports/virtual_reality_journalism.php.
4. De la Pena N, Weil P, Llobera J, et al. Immersive journalism: immersive virtual reality for the first-person experience of news presence. Presence Teleop Virt Envir. 2010;19:291–301.
5. Domínguez E. Going beyond the classic news narrative convention: the background to and challenges of immersion in journalism. Department of Communication, Universitat Pompeu Fabra, Barcelona, Spain. Front Digit Humanit .2017; https://doi.org/10.3389/fdigh.2017.00010.
6. Kotlarek J, Lin I, Ma K. Improving spatial orientation in immersive environments. SUI'18 proceedings of the symposium on spatial user interaction. 2018:79–88. https://doi.org/10.1145/3267782.3267792.
7. Rubio-Tamayo JL, Barrio MG, Garcia-Garcia F. Immersive environments and virtual reality: systematic review and advances in communication, interaction and simulation. Multimodal Technologies Interact. 2017;1:21. https://doi.org/10.3390/mti1040021.
8. Geydarian A, Carneiro JP, Gerber D, et al. Immersive virtual environments versus physical built environments: a benchmarking study for building design and use-built environments explorations. Automation Construction. 2015;54:116–26. https://doi.org/10.1016/j.autcon.2015.03.020.
9. Lindsey G, Todd JA, Hayter SJ, et al. A handbook for planning and conducting charrettes for high-performance projects, 2nd Edition. NREL (National Renewable Energy Laboratory) 2009; September, https://www.nrel.gov/docs/fy09osti/44051.pdf.
10. Maurer R. Bathroom business: OSHA's restroom rules. Better Workplaces Better Word. May 25, 2015, https://www.shrm.org/resourcesandtools/hr-topics/risk-management/pages/osha-restroom-rules.aspx.
11. Yee N, Bailenson J. The proteus effect of transformed self-representation on behavior. Hum Commun Res. 2007;33(3):271–90. https://doi.org/10.1111/j.1468-2958.2007.00299.x.
12. Carr RF. Hospital. Whole Building Design Guide, 2017, https://www.wbdg.org/building-types/health-care-facilities/hospital.
13. Patient Navigator Training Collaborative, Module 3: Healthcare Team. Introduction to the healthcare system; 2011, http://www.patientnavigatortraining.org/healthcare_system/module3/1_index.htm.
14. Ford ES, Bergmann MM, Kröger J, et al. Healthy living is the best revenge: findings from the European prospective investigation into Cancer and nutrition-Potsdam study. Arch Intern Med. 2009;169:1355–62.
15. Egger GJ, Binns AF, Rossner SR. The emergence of "lifestyle medicine" as a structured approach for management of chronic disease. Med J Aust. 2009;190:143–5.
16. Silvi J. Healing hues: choosing paint colors for healthcare. Healthcare Design. 2012. Available from: https://www.healthcaredesignmagazine.com/architecture/healing-hues-choosing-paint-colors-healthcare/.
17. Koffel WE, Lathrop JK, Gilyeat SS, et al. Fire protection requirements for health care facilities – an overview of NFPA 99. Fire Protection Engineering 2015, https://www.sfpe.org/page/FPE_2015_Q1_4/Fire-Protection-Requirements-for-Health-Care-Facilities%2D%2D-An-Overview-.htm.
18. Ahearn DJ. One dozen essential elements of a great office design – part 2. Dental Economics 2002; May, https://www.dentaleconomics.com/articles/print/volume-92/issue-5/features/one-dozen-essential-elements-of-a-great-office-design-part-2.html.
19. Calogiuri G, Litleskare S, Fagerheim KA, et al. Experiencing nature through immersive virtual environments: environmental perception, physical engagement, and affective responses during a simulated nature walk. Front Psychology. 2018;8:2321. https://doi.org/10.3389/fpsyg.2017.02321.
20. Ceilings and Interior Systems Construction Association. Acoustics in Healthcare Environments 2010; October, http://www.cisca.org/files/public/Acoustics%20in%20Healthcare%20Environments_CISCA.pdf.
21. Health and Safety Executive. The six basic factors, http://www.hse.gov.uk/temperature/thermal/factors.htm.
22. McAllister J. Four ways virtual reality can help is design and create better healthcare facilities. Becker's Health IT & CIO Reports. November 14, 2017, https://www.beckershospitalreview.com/healthcare-information-technology/four-ways-virtual-reality-can-help-us-design-and-create-better-healthcare-facilities.html.
23. Fisher C. Immersive virtual environment creates behavior change in the physical world. BMED Report; 2011: April, http://www.bmedreport.com/archives/25986.

Immersive Non-physical Environment: High-Touch and Human Resources

11

Janet H. Johnson

Abbreviations

APP   Advanced practice provider
EHR   Electronic health records
HCP   Healthcare professional
QOL   Quality of life

High-Touch Models

The term "high-touch" is difficult to define since it is utilized in multiple settings and with multiple components. High-touch starts with centering on the patient experience within the context of interactions among patients, health care professionals (HCP), and staff on the care team. The high-touch experience is particularly relevant for Lifestyle Medicine Centers and influences patients' willingness to engage the healthcare system [1]. Consequently, in order to improve quality of care and decrease costs, the Affordable Care Act and the Center for Medicare and Medicaid have encouraged a wide range of initiatives to design novel high-touch models (Table 11.1).

One model is a "direct patient contracting practice." The premise of this innovative construct is based on the idea that access and quality of care will be improved without third-party payers. These constructs are referred to as "concierge", "boutique," "cash-only," "retainer," "patient-centric," "direct primary care," "specialty care," or "high-touch primary care." In lieu of traditional insurance arrangements, patients are promised a more personalized and accessible care – "high touch" [2]. Typically, these patients pay a subscription fee (on a monthly or yearly basis) that covers all primary care services and gives unhurried, same day, round-the-clock accessibility by a primary care HCP with a limited panel of patients.

High-intensity models are defined by the National Institute of Health Care Reform as "…care provided by a multidisciplinary team for patients with complex conditions. The end result is to improve care and lower health care cost" [3]. This type of high-intensity care model is in fact high-touch and promotes frequent direct person-to-person interaction. The result is to optimize care by focusing on methods to improve adherence to treatment plans and behaviors that prevent disease and complications. Since there are multiple interactions, there are limitations on how to measure effective outcomes of high-touch primary care. Nevertheless, it has proved to be a cost-effective strategy [4].

A high-intensity, high-touch model can provide some or all of the following services:

1. A preventative cardiovascular program
2. On-site medication dispensing
3. Small patient panels

Table 11.1 High-touch models[a]

Ambulatory intensive caring unit
Care guides
Concierge
Community health advisors
Direct patient contacting practice
Electronic health record patient portal
Health through early awareness and learning
High-intensity
High-touch care
Patient-centered care
Patient navigators
Patient/team-based combination care
Team-based care
Warm handoff

[a]Patient portals are hybridized high-tech/high-touch

J. H. Johnson (✉)
The Mount Sinai Hospital, Marie-Josée and Henry R. Kravis Center for Cardiovascular Health at Mount Sinai, New York, NY, USA
e-mail: Janet.johnson@mountsinai.org

© Springer Nature Switzerland AG 2020
J. I. Mechanick, R. F. Kushner (eds.), *Creating a Lifestyle Medicine Center*, https://doi.org/10.1007/978-3-030-48088-2_11

4. More time allotted per visit
5. More frequent visits
6. Electronic health records (EHR) portal for patient access to lab results, other tests, and messaging
7. Courtesy transportation
8. Walk-in hours

Theories that explain a decrease in healthcare cost with these models point to a culture of accountability and trust that develops between the patient and the HCP. These positive interactions can result in positive behavior modification. More frequent HCP visits can bring about better adherence with lifestyle recommendations and therefore improved outcomes. For example, positive behaviors improve engagement and glucose monitoring, which translates into better glycemic control, decreased diabetes complications, and improved overall health. High-touch models also allow more timely diagnosis of problems in an ambulatory setting and facilitated preventive care [4].

Encouraging use of the EHR portal to view lab results and medical records, request medication refills, and ask non-emergent questions can be empowering and activate the patient for positive change. This is another form of high-touch/high-tech interaction where messages sent through a patient portal provides a system of timely human contacts with an electronic interface, and can be more efficiently utilized than just making rushed telephone callbacks.

Another innovative model is "high-touch care" [5]. This provides a highly supportive experience where patients are encouraged to play a more active role in their own healthcare. High-touch care integrates HCP and staff, in a multidisciplinary team approach to directly interact with ("touch") patients and provide many different services. An Advance Practice Provider (APP), such as a Nurse Practitioner (NP) or Physician Assistant (PA), can monitor the patient and assist in diagnosis, management, and follow-up. A Registered Dietician Nutritionist (RDN) and/or healthcare coach can also be consulted for nutrition, lifestyle, and behavior changes. A registered nurse (RN) can contribute further counseling about lifestyle change as well as medication education, safety, and adherence. A cognitive behavioral therapist can also be involved to focus on therapies (short and long term) that facilitate measurable changes in quality of life.

Team-based care offers many potential advantages, including increased access to care. This results in more coverage hours, shorter wait times, and expanded services that are essential to providing patient education, behavioral health, self-management support, and care coordination, all contributing to a high-quality care delivery system. For the team, these activities and successes yield increased job satisfaction and a workplace culture. This nurtures a pervasive attitude for staff to perform to the fullest scope and intensity of their job responsibilities. A diverse team can also supply more services for the patient. For instance, this phenomenon brought about by a larger care team might initiate and then support new administrative projects, such as quality improvement, data-driven protocols, and data-mining for research publications ("scale-up"), as well as support more sites over a larger geography ("scale-out") [5].

Patient-centered care is relationship based. In this high-touch model, the patient feels known and respected. Patients are involved and engaged in their care, and knowledgeable about their medical condition. The patient and HCP are at the center of the plan. Providing this high-touch type of care is increasingly perceived as "the right thing to do" and supported by research that links patient-centered care to positive outcomes [6]. Implementation of this model is associated with improved physician-patient communication, relationships, patient satisfaction, recall of information, adherence, recovery, and improved health outcomes [6]. A patient/team-based combination care model also has a patient-centered approach to planning and delivery methods (Fig. 11.1).

Healthcare plans institute implementation strategies to enable HCP to spend more time with needy patients. Specifically, the Ambulatory Intensive Caring Unit (A-ICU) model enables physicians to spend more time with patients having more comorbidities (Fig. 11.2). This tactic is achieved by ensuring the physical presence of appropriate personnel at the site of care [7]. This approach uses multiple high-touch HCP to coordinate care for these potentially high-cost patient members. The A-ICU differs from the usual disease management model because it is not conducted remotely (over phone or electronically) but with all critical caregivers present and interacting in-person in the treatment clinic. The key features and core activities of an A-ICU are:

1. Transfer of care to a stand-alone team
2. Comprehensive initial intake, which consists of a 60-minute intake with both an HCP and social worker, together developing a patient-centered, goal-based plan
3. Interdisciplinary team reviews
4. Transitions of care coordination/tracking
5. Built in counseling
6. Navigation of social services
7. On-demand availability
8. Pharmacy education
9. Chronic disease management [7]

By using multi-disciplinary teams with reduced panel size and increased flexibility, this intervention model promises to enhance self-efficacy through counseling, health education, and linkages to social services/case management [8]. The net effect is to improve care quality and reduce utilization for patients with multi-morbid chronic medical and social problems [8].

Lay healthcare workers or "Care Guides" provide a new type of high-touch care. This human resource focuses on

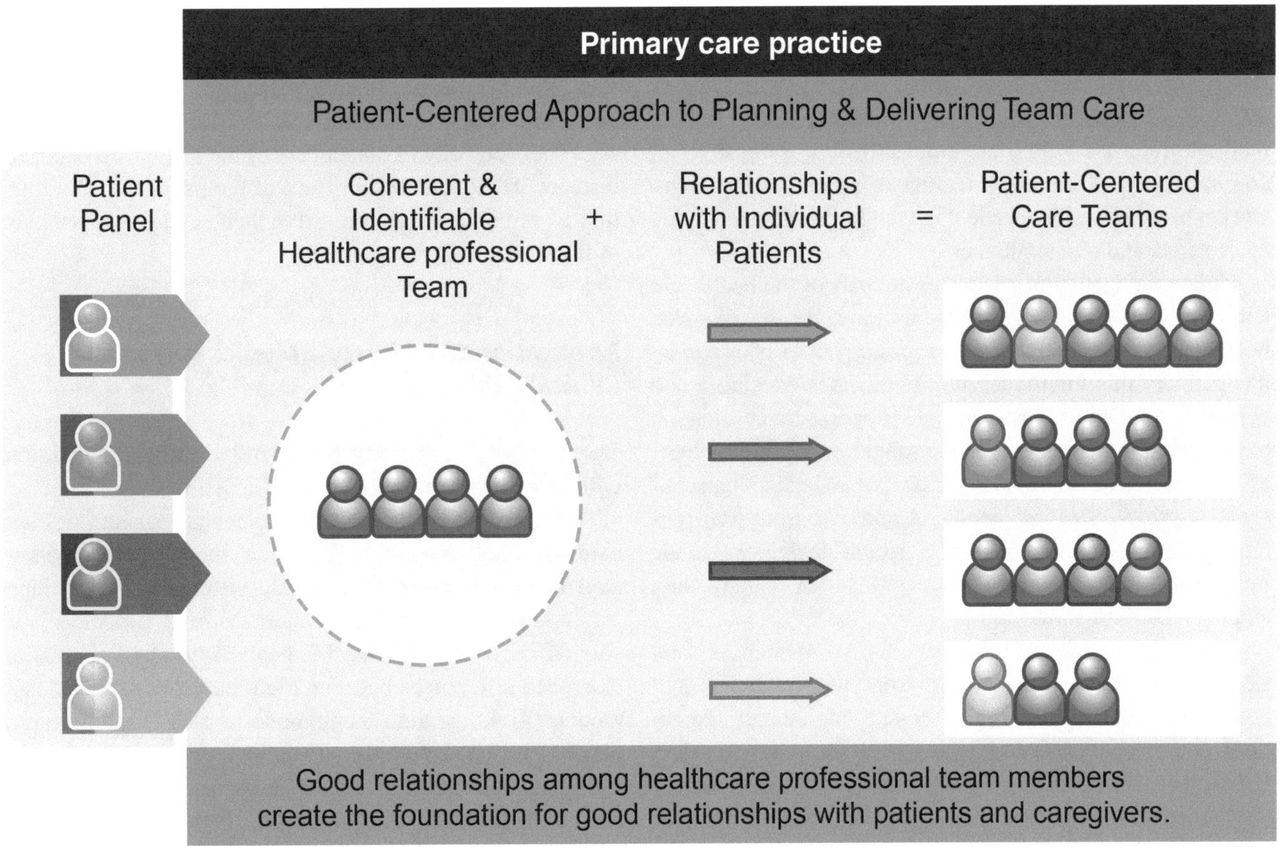

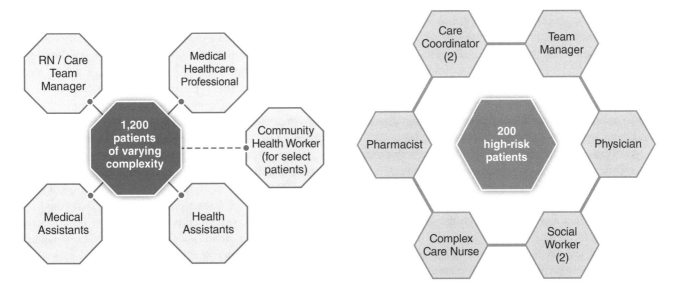

Fig. 11.1 Conceptual blueprint for the provision of patient-centered team-based care∗. (∗Developing good relationships with patients is a key component of high-quality care. Team members actively seek and appropriately respond to patients' preferences and values, which in turn assist patients in attaining their health goals. Patients seek care at a primary care practice that is committed to a patient-centered team-based approach. When they experience a united healthcare professional team with good relationships among its members, it is considered as coherent, that is, a well-functioning team that works collaboratively to meet the healthcare needs of the patient [6])

Fig. 11.2 Comparison of a "usual care" team and SUMMIT ambulatory intensive care unit model∗. (∗Panel A. The Usual Care Team operates within the clinic and consisting of primary care physicians, care team managers (usually a licensed practical nurse), medical assistants, and health assistants who handle clerical and phone communication duties. Patients have referral access to on-site non-medical services. Panel B. The Summit Ambulatory-Intensive Care Unit primary care model is a clinic team of co-located multi-disciplinary staff with reduced panel size and flexible scheduling. Staffing consists of 2 half-time physicians (1.0 full-time equivalent) with board certification in addiction medicine, 1 complex care nurse, 2 care coordinators, 2 licensed clinical social workers, 1 pharmacist, 1 team manager, and 1 quality analyst. All team members have additional training in motivational interviewing, patient goal setting, and palliative care principles [8])

interpersonal relationships and improves patient experience and engagement with patient education, communication, family input, and team building [9]. The person serving as a Care Guide can identify barriers to high quality care and facilitate referrals within the clinics, healthcare system, or community. The Care Guide facilitates interdependent teamwork when they visit the patient in their home, assisted living apartments, and nursing homes.

Patient navigators or advocates are part of the healthcare team and function to help patients navigate the complex healthcare systems of today. The primary role of a patient navigator in this high-touch model includes educating and connecting patients to resources and support services. Patient navigators are involved in the coordination of medical care, as well as scheduling appointments, assisting financial/social services, tracking outcomes, and accessing transportation. The potential benefits of a patient navigator include improved health outcomes, increased patient satisfaction, and decreased no-show rates [10].

The HEAL (Health through Early Awareness and Learning) project is designed to work with churches and health ministries to relay health messages to their congregations about early cancer screening [11]. Originally, Project HEAL began in Maryland with three early cancer detection projects. Researchers tested this concept in preventive medicine through faith-based partnerships carried out in 26 African American churches. This project works with health ministries to educate, empower, and connect with their congregation and has expanded to include a broader range of health topics with other faith-based organizations. This high-touch program provides training materials so that leaders in the church, Community Health Advisors, learn to teach health education workshops to their members about multiple topics. The Community Health Advisors use scripture and religious spiritual themes to teach the health message. This model is based on the theory of empowerment and the belief that every community has people that others turn to naturally for advice. Some healthcare institutions have adopted this model to promote cultural competency in settings characterized by many ethno-cultural patient populations.

A "warm handoff" is a type of high-touch that occurs during the transfer of care between two members of the health care team, where the handoff occurs in front of the patient, family, and/or patient navigator. This essentially brings the patient and the family into the team structure as illness details, management plans, and other relevant information are discussed. The warm handoff affords the patient an opportunity to correct any misinformation, ask questions, and participate in the care plan. The term warm handoff originated in customer service where it is used to describe referrals that ensure that the customer is connected to someone who can provide what he or she needs. In healthcare, this typically means that one member of the healthcare team introduces another team member to the patient, explaining why the other team member can better address a specific issue with the patient, and emphasizing the other team member's competence [12]. In this strategy, the warm handoff can occur between any two members of the healthcare team, for instance, HCP and staff in front of the patient. In short, the first team member reinforces the value and trustworthiness of the second team member.

Application to a Lifestyle Medicine Center: Clinical Evidence

The notion of high-touch is relatively recent and therefore clinical evidence in the Lifestyle Medicine Center is generally lacking. However, there are some data relating primary care visits that incorporate high-touch models with hypertension diagnosis, cardiovascular risk factor control, and diabetes control. A retrospective cohort study of two models of care ($N = 5695$) used in a Medicare Advantage population examined differences between high-touch and standard care models [4]. In the high-touch model, the HCP had a smaller panel of patients and each patient had a higher frequency of HCP encounters [4]. The study compared patients' healthcare utilization and hospitalization between both models using a propensity score-matched analysis of the Charlson Comorbidity Index of disease burden for different ages and genders [4]. Both models provided onsite medication dispensing and an EHR system portal that is accessible to patients [4]. The traditional care model delivered care at a frequency consistent with usual marketplace benchmarks [4]. This included a multispecialty practice, preventative care, access to care that includes walk-in hours and urgent care, close primary care physician follow-up, and urgent care on weekends and holidays [4]. However, the standard care model did not offer courtesy transportation and did not have transitional care teams [4].

The high-touch primary care allowed frequent contact at an average of 189 minutes with their PCP, with the goal of preventing or delaying complications of chronic conditions [4]. There was substantial improvement in both healthcare costs and utilization of services in the high-touch model system [4]. Patients receiving this high-touch care saw their PCP more often (8.7 versus 3.8 visits; $p < 0.01$), and the mean number of hospital admissions was 50% lower for the high-touch model group ($p < 0.01$) [4]. In addition, patients receiving high-touch care were up to 41% more likely to use preventive medicines ($p < 0.01$) [4].

High-touch team-based care is a strategy that is implemented at the health system level to enhance patient care by having two or more HCP working collaboratively with each patient. In cardiovascular disease prevention, a collaborative multidisciplinary team works to educate patients, identify risk factors for disease, and prescribe and modify treatments. This collaboration results in continuous discussion with updates [9]. These teams, which are applicable to lifestyle medicine, include primary care and specialist physicians, nurses, pharmacists, community paramedics and health workers, dietitians, and others.

Various organizations, such as the American Medical Association and the Agency for Healthcare Research and Quality, have developed guidelines to help healthcare systems and practices implement this strategy as part of their policies and protocols [13, 14]. A systematic review of studies (2003–2012) revealed that team-based care, compared with traditional care models, was associated with significantly improved systolic and diastolic blood pressure levels (overall median reductions were 5.4 mmHg and 1.8 mmHg, respectively) and improved patient adherence with hypertensive medication [15]. Team members supplemented the activities of the primary care HCP by providing support and sharing responsibility for hypertension care, such as medication management, patient follow-up, and helping the patient adhere to their blood pressure control plan, including monitoring blood pressure routinely, taking medications as prescribed, reducing sodium in the diet, and increasing physical activity [15]. Team-based care has also been found to be effective for diverse patient populations, including those with different racial and ethnic groups, low income, and multiple comorbidities [14].

The 10-year health and economic impact of a nationwide program of team-based care for hypertension is estimated to produce a net cost savings to Medicare of $5.8 billion (in 2012 US dollars) [5, 6]. This model also estimates an overall national savings of $25.3 billion in averted disease costs, which offsets an estimated $22.9 billion cost for this intervention. In addition, costs for patient time over this period are estimated at $15.8 billion, but are largely offset by an estimated $11 billion in productivity gains [16].

Another ongoing study on high-touch involves the A-ICU model. Participants in the SUMMIT ambulatory primary care model study [8] receive care from a clinic-based team consisting of a physician, complex care nurse, care coordinator, social worker, and pharmacist, with reduced panel size and flexible scheduling. The emphasis with this high-touch model is on motivational interviewing, patient goal setting, and advanced care planning [8]. The primary outcome will be total inpatient hospitalizations at 6 and 12 months after study enrollment [8]. It is expected that the results of this study will contribute to an evolving literature on intensive primary care interventions that addresses a research gap (a need for more real-world research studies that include control populations) and a practice gap (a focus on high-cost–high-need patients with high rates of homelessness and substance use) [8].

Patient portals in EHRs have been studied as a high-touch–high-tech tool for enhancing patient experience and improving quality of care in primary care practices. In one study, patients participating in a nurse-led care coordination program received personalized training to use the portal to communicate with the care team [17]. Patient portals have the potential to assist care coordination programs by improving patients' self-management and ultimately their care. Portals can decrease the fragmentation of multiple services by having information housed in one place. These portals foster patient participation by encouraging communications with the HCP and other team members. As a result, team members become more proactive by preemptively reaching out to patients and identifying early symptoms. As this tool is integrated in the new environment of nurse-led coordination in primary care, it could be used as a resource to increase patients' self-efficacy for managing chronic disease by scheduling their own appointments, asking questions earlier instead of waiting for follow-up appointments, and viewing test results, prompting more interest in their own care. This can result in better health outcomes, reduced unnecessary and high-cost healthcare visits, administrative costs, and efficiency for the HCP. By teaching patients to take responsibility for their own health and coaching them on how to sustain this positive behavior, the quality of care for chronic conditions can improve.

In another study, of 94 patients enrolled, 74 participants used the patient portal and were followed up for 7 months to assess their experience, and for 12 months to assess healthcare utilization [17]. By combining the high-touch of the care-coordinator and the high-tech of the EHR patient portal, functional status improved significantly [17]. Emergency room visits/1000 patients were reduced by 21% in the users group [17]. The percentage of patients with one or more hospital admissions was reduced by 30% among users, and hospital admissions per 1000 patients were reduced by 38% [17].

"Enhancing Diabetes Care through Personalized, High-Touch Case Management" is a program operated by the Rio Grande Valley Accountable Care Organization Health Providers, in Texas [18]. This program provides a multidimensional patient-focused model that uses a team-based approach to coordinate care across HCP through a site-based care coordinator, a centralized EHR system, and adherence to best practices in diabetes using a checklist [18]. This high-touch model showed improvement above the national average in 32 out of the 33 Quality Measures for Diabetes Care [18]. This included improvements in the number of patients with hemoglobin A1c <8%, low-density lipoprotein <100 mg/dL, blood pressure <140/90, tobacco non-use, and aspirin use [18]. The percentage of patients utilizing the service with poorly controlled hemoglobin A1c (>9%) dropped to less than 5%, while the national average is around 20% [18].

In diabetes care, the goals of a high-touch approach are to educate patients about their disease, initiate and motivate sustainable lifestyle changes, and facilitate adherence with published diabetes management protocols. In particular, diabetes care coordinators work with patients with uncontrolled diabetes, employing frequent high-touch contacts, with check-ins on patient status, blood glucoses, lifestyle changes, and medication needs. Other high-touch projects include weekly clinics for those still poorly controlled, where a nutritionist and diabetes educator are available after each of their HCP encounters. The high-tech part of this high-touch model corresponds to chart alerts if any quality measures are out of range. Communication is a critical high-touch element in diabetes care, particularly for those with missed appointments, poor glycemic control, poor adherence, or high risk for complications.

Wellness Coaching programs provide high-touch based on interpersonal relationships. One such high-touch program is based out of Mayo Clinic and incorporates the 5 Es of patient counseling:

1. *Engage*: build a trusting relationship with the individual
2. *Explore:* assist individuals in identifying their values and desires
3. *Envision*: facilitate a personal vision for wellness
4. *Experiment*: enhance self-confidence for wellness and transform values and goals into action
5. *Evolve*: facilitate and promote long-term positive lifestyle changes [19]

In a single-arm cohort study design, 100 employees completed the 12-week wellness coaching program where most were overweight or obese [19]. The primary aims of this study were to examine potential improvements in quality of life (QOL), depressive symptoms, and perceived stress level after 12 weeks of in-person wellness coaching [19]. Significant differences in mean score from baseline to 12-week follow-up were found for overall QOL, five domains of QOL, depressive symptoms, and perceived stress level ($p < 0.0001$) [19]. No significant differences were found between 12 and 24 weeks, suggesting that any improvements made were maintained through the 24-week follow-up visit [19].

Creating an Optimal Lifestyle Medicine Team

A team is a collection of individuals who are interdependent in their tasks but share responsibility for outcomes, who see themselves and who are seen by others as an intact social entity embedded in one or more larger social systems, and who manage their relationships across organizational boundaries [20]. The use of the term "health care team" is often vague with no uniform members. It is reasonable to propose that how the health care team functions can influence the

ways in which a patient experiences that team, participates in the care plan, and adheres with recommendations. Teams should be inter- or multidisciplinary and include all HCP and staff members. There are certain characteristics of a successful interdisciplinary team (Table 11.2) [21–23].

High-touch patient care requires different approach styles to induce behavior and lifestyle changes. One approach that is successful for the HCP is motivational interviewing [24]. This method helps patients identify and resolve ambivalence about changing their behavior, typically by exploring their personal perspectives as well as perceived barriers. Motivational interviewing can be utilized when the patient is unsure about a change in behavior. The strategies of motiva-

Table 11.2 Ten characteristics of a successful interdisciplinary team∗

1. *An identified leader* is assigned who relays the role and purpose of the team
2. *A set of values* or mission statement should be formulated that clearly provides direction for the team's service. These values need to be portrayed for every team member. Each team member demonstrates a commitment to the vision, both initially and consistently throughout the team's life
3. *A team culture* and interdisciplinary atmosphere of trust is important for valued contributions. Team members need to understand and respect each other's roles and how they impact patient care. Different skill sets of each team member can complement each other to provide the best care. There is an intensity of goal sharing from the same framework and swift meshing of ideas and plan of care. Clear team goals help focus development of strategies for achievement
4. *Appropriate processes* and infrastructures need to be in place to uphold the vision of the service. It is necessary to periodically review the system and ability to change based on the needs of the service. The infrastructure occupies a shared physical space in order to facilitate access, discussion, and sociability. Communications among the team, referral systems, and patients should be streamlined
5. *Quality benchmarks* should be established. Outcome results should be shared with the team on a regular basis. Feedback is used to improve the quality of care
6. *Good communication* is fundamental on all levels. This includes the ability to speak freely and safely within a team context. Conflict management skills must be developed in each team member
7. *Adequate staffing* is necessary to provide an appropriate mix of skills, competencies, and personalities to meet the needs of patients and enhance smooth functioning. Collaborative decision-making is an effective team process
8. *Recruitment* of staff who demonstrates interdisciplinary competencies, including team functioning, collaborative leadership, communication, and sufficient professional knowledge and experience. New staff must have cultural competency to work with a diverse population mix
9. *Role interdependence* is encouraged, while respecting individual responsibilities and autonomy, with flexibility to cover other roles when needed, within certain boundaries
10. *Personal development* is accomplished through advanced training, rewards, recognition, and opportunities for career development

∗See references [21–23]

tional interviewing are more about convincing than dictating, more supportive than argumentative.

There are four steps in the motivational interviewing process [25]. The first step is *engagement*, or "activation for change." A relationship is built that is based on empathy with the patient, through interested questioning and support of autonomy. Questions should be open-ended so the patient can provide more information. As needed, confirm with the patient that change is difficult and that the patient may be going through difficult situations and commend positive behaviors and even minor improvements. The second step is *focusing*. Encourage the patient to evaluate issues based on the present situation. Motivation for change is enhanced when clients perceive differences in what their life is and what they want it to be. The idea is to help the patient concentrate on how current behaviors differ from ideal behavior and what is hampering goal attainment. The third step is *evoking* or having the patient discover goals or aspirations, understand the problems reaching these goals, and what would assist attaining them. Use of reflective listening and summarizing the discussion can be useful in this step. The fourth step is *planning*. This involves solidifying commitment to change by reinforcement, and then deciding on an action plan.

Shared decision-making is another high-touch approach to support behavior change. Shared decision-making is a method where the HCP and patient make decisions together using the best available evidence. The HCP provides the options of test, procedures, and treatment or management plans. The risk/benefit ratio of each is discussed [26]. With this method, the HCP's role is to help patients become well informed, help them develop their own personal preferences for available options, and provide professional guidance where appropriate. In a high-touch practice, this is not a one-time decision to have surgery or a procedure, but an ongoing process in making lifestyle changes.

With shared decision-making, it is understood that the HCP has achieved the first step of building a trust relationship with the patient. Next are the three steps of shared decision-making. First, to explain the need to consider alternatives as a team ("team talk"). Second, to describe the alternatives in more detail ("option talk") using decision support tools when possible and appropriate. Third, to help patients explore and form their personal preferences ("decision talk"). Generally, shared decision-making and motivational interviewing have been applicable in distinct situations. Clinicians may benefit from drawing on both approaches to maintain a patient-centered orientation in real-world situations (Fig. 11.3).

Fig. 11.3 The relationship of shared decision-making and motivational interviewing*. (*Interdependent processes of shared decision-making and motivational interviewing can be incorporated in counseling for chronic conditions, such as diabetes, as well as for behavioral changes, such as weight loss [24])

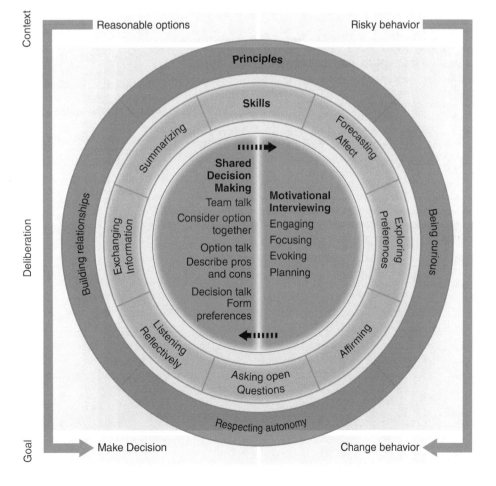

References

1. Kushner RF, Sorensen KW. Lifestyle medicine: the future of chronic disease management. Curr Opin Endocrinol Diabetes Obes. 2013;20:389–95.
2. Doherty R. Assessing the patient care implications of "concierge" and other direct patient contracting practices: a policy position paper from the American College of Physicians. Ann Intern Med. 2015;163:949–52.
3. ChenMed. Concierge care for low-income seniors: how high-touch care improves outcomes and reduces costs, 2017. www.chenmed.com. Accessed Oct 9 2019.
4. Ghany R, Tamariz L, Chen G, et al. High-touch care leads to better outcomes and lower costs in a senior population. Am J Manag Care. 2018;24:e300–4.
5. Kresser C. Patient communication: how to provide high-touch care without burning out, 2017. https://kresserinstitute.com/patient-communication-provide-high-touch-care-without-burning/. Accessed 23 Feb 2020.
6. Agency for Healthcare Research and Quality, U.S. Department of Health and Human Services. Creating Patient-centered Team-based Primary Care, AHRQ Publication No. 16–0002-EF, March 2016. www.pcmh.ahrq.gov/page/creating-patient-centered-team-based-primary-care. Accessed 10 May 2019.
7. California Health Care Foundation. How ambulatory intensive caring units can reduce costs and improve outcomes, May 2011. www.chcf.org/publication/how-ambulatory-intensive-caring-units-can-reduce-costs-and-improve-outcomes/. Accessed 10 May 2019.
8. Chan B, Edwards S, Devoe M, et al. The SUMMIT ambulatory-ICU primary care model for medically and socially complex patients in an urban federally qualified health center: study design and rational. Addict Sci Clin Pract. 2018;13:27. https://doi.org/10.1186/s13722-018-0128-y.
9. Krypel K, Hutchison M. How Lay Health Care Workers Can Add High Touch To High Tech, June 2015. www.healthaffairs.org/do/10.1377/hblog20150611.048452/full/. Accessed 10 May 2019.
10. Mailloux C, Halesey E. Patient navigators as essential members of the healthcare team: a review of the literature. J Nurs Patient Care. 2018;3:1. https://doi.org/10.4172/2573-4571.1000122.
11. Holtr C, Tagai E, Scheirer M, et al. Translating evidence-based interventions for implementation: experiences from project HEAL in African American churches. Implement Sci. 2014;9:66. https://doi.org/10.1186/1748-5908-9-66.
12. Agency for Healthcare Research and Quality. Implementation quick start guide warm hand off. www.ahrq.gov/sites/default/files/wysiwyg/professionals/quality-patient-safety/patient-family-engagement/pfeprimarycare/warmhandoff-quickstartfull.pdf. Accessed 23 Feb 2020.
13. Community Preventive Services Task Force. Cardiovascular disease: team-based care to improve blood pressure control. the guide to community preventive services website, April 2012. www.thecommunityguide.org/findings/cardiovascular-disease-team-based-care-improve-blood-pressure-control. Accessed 23 Feb 2020.
14. Center for Disease Control and Prevention. Promoting Team-Based Care to Improve High Blood Pressure Control. www.cdc.gov/dhdsp/pubs/guides/best-practices/team-based-care.htm. Accessed 23 Feb 2020.
15. Stephen S. Team-based care a step in the right direction for hypertension control. Am J Prev Med. 2015;49:e81–2.
16. Dehmer SP, Baker-Goering MM, Maciosek MV, et al. Modeled health and economic impact of team-based care for hypertension. Am J Prev Med. 2016;50(suppl 1):S34–44.
17. Sorondo B, Allen A, Fathima S, et al. Patient portal as a tool for enhancing patient experience and improving quality of care in primary care practices. EGEMS. 2016;4:1262. https://doi.org/10.13063/2327-9214.1262.
18. Center for Health Policy at Brookings. Enhancing diabetes care through personalized, high-touch case management. www.brookings.edu/wp-content/uploads/2016/06/Rio-Valley-ACO.pdf. Accessed 10 May 2019.
19. Clark M, Bradley S, Jenkins S, et al. The effectiveness of wellness coaching for improving quality of life. Mayo Clin Proc. 2014;89:1537–44.
20. Hoff T, Prout K, Carabetta S. How teams impact patient satisfaction: a review of the empirical literature. Health Care Manage Rev. 2019; https://doi.org/10.1097/HMR0000000000000234.
21. Nancarrow S, Booth A, Ariss S, et al. Ten principles of good interdisciplinary team work. Hum Res Health. 2013;11:19. https://doi.org/10.1186/1478-4491-11-19.
22. Sangaleti C, Schveitzer MC, Peduzzi M, et al. Experiences and shared meaning of teamwork and interprofessional collaboration among health care professionals in primary health care settings: a systematic review. JBI Database System Rev Implement Rep. 2017;15:2723–88.
23. Mickan SM, Rodger SA. Effective health care teams: a model of six characteristics developed from shared perceptions. J Interprof Care. 2005;19:358–70.
24. Elwyn G, Dehlendorf C, Epstein RM, et al. Shared decision making and motivational interviewing: achieving patient-centered care across the spectrum of health care problems. Ann Fam Med. 2014;12:270–5.
25. Miller WR, Rollick S. Motivational interviewing: preparing people for change. 3nd ed. New York: Guilford; 2012. ISBN 9781609182274.
26. Elwyn G, Laitner S, Coulter A, et al. Implementing shared decision making in the NHS. BMJ. 2010;341:c5146. https://doi.org/10.1136/bmj.c5146.

Planning, Constructing, and Operating a Clinic Gym

Karl Nadolsky, Spencer Nadolsky, and Yoni Freedhoff

Abbreviations

ABCD   Adiposity-based chronic disease
HCP   Healthcare professional
T2D   Type 2 diabetes

Introduction

With the goal of developing an optimal Lifestyle Medical Center, a recurring theme is that a prescription for exercise should be viewed as a first-line medicine (Fig. 12.1). Exercise is defined by the American College of Sports Medicine (www.acsm.org/ [Accessed on February 24, 2020]) as a type of physical activity consisting of planned, structured, and repetitive bodily movement done to improve and/or maintain one or more components of physical fitness. Therefore, it is imperative to provide a space, opportunity, guidance, supervision, and support to tactically implement this strategic target. Though exercise is a core lifestyle medicine intervention for all chronic diseases, a good example for context is obesity. This pathophysiological state is a chronic relapsing progressive disease of abnormal or excessive adiposity that impairs health [1]. Obesity, narrowly defined by the body

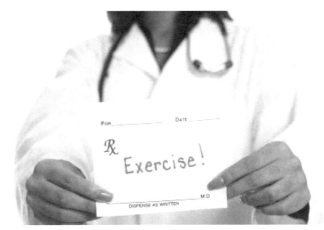

Fig. 12.1 Exercise as a medical prescription

mass index, is a complex disease for which exercise, physical activity, and fitness represent central components of lifestyle change for all modalities of preventive medicine.

More specifically, clinical practice guidelines recommend aerobic activity, resistance training, and non-exercise physical activity to increase the energy deficit to lose weight, but also as part of a comprehensive approach to adiposity-based chronic disease (ABCD), defined more broadly in terms of adipose tissue amount, distribution, and function, to improve glycemic control, cardiometabolic risk, cardiorespiratory fitness, weight maintenance, strength, and mortality [2–6]. Therefore, physical activity as a component of lifestyle change emerges a first-line therapeutic recommendation for type 2 diabetes (T2D) management [7–9], T2D prevention [10], dyslipidemia [11–13], hypertension [14], and overall cardiovascular risk [15]. Pragmatically, motivating patients with obesity or ABCD to adhere to a physical activity prescription is a formidable hurdle, which can be overcome through the use of a medically oriented fitness center embedded in the medical clinic. In addition to the obesity setting, a physical activity prescription, initially under the supervi-

K. Nadolsky (✉)
Michigan State University College of Human Medicine, Spectrum Health Medical Group, Department of Diabetes & Endocrinology, Grand Rapids, MI, USA
e-mail: karl.nadolsky@spectrumhealth.org

S. Nadolsky
UCSD, Preventive Medicine, Family Medicine, San Diego, CA, USA
e-mail: snadolsky@ucsd.edu

Y. Freedhoff
Department of Family Medicine, University of Ottawa, Bariatric Medical Institute, Ottawa, ON, Canada
e-mail: drfreedhoff@bmimedical.ca

sion of medical staff, is necessary for cardiac rehabilitation, following events or other cardiogenic disease [16], and pulmonary rehabilitation or therapy of chronic obstructive pulmonary disease and other chronic respiratory diseases [17]. Bone health and prevention or treatment of osteoporosis to decrease fall and fracture risk can also be a target for an exercise prescription within a medically supervised fitness center. Weight-bearing and resistance training are basic parts of therapy for bone strength and fracture risk reduction, along with balance training for fall prevention, and therefore should be first-line recommendations [18, 19]. In addition to bone health, exercise remains first-line therapy for osteoarthritis including aerobic and resistance training [20–23]. Fibromyalgia remains a very frustrating clinical syndrome for both patients and healthcare professionals (HCP), confounded by controversy and regarded as having only modest benefit with medications. Exercise remains a first-line therapy in the treatment plan for patients with fibromyalgia including a personalized graded combination of resistance and aerobic training [24]. Physical therapy is a comprehensive type of exercise or movement evaluation and prescription that differs from a general exercise prescription. Physical therapy is used to specifically help patients regain or improve their physical abilities, whereas a general exercise prescription is used to improve overall fitness and health. Physical therapy is an important adjunctive component to recovery from sports injuries, musculoskeletal surgeries, and joint replacements. Sarcopenia/frailty, well-being, mental health, and cognition are other important aspects of health that improve with a supervised exercise prescription.

Adherence is another important challenge with the routine prescription for exercise, even when appropriate education is provided. Following initial efforts to motivate patients, the next step to actualize participation is physically navigating patients into the structure where a physical activity prescription can be implemented. Integrating an efficient, yet comprehensive and inviting fitness program within a Lifestyle Medicine Center is a key strategy in breaking down this barrier to entry. A medical fitness program also provides sufficient opportunity to engage patients in education on exercise in a safe and supervised environment, as well as ingrain why physical activity is so important, as well as guide performance in a variety of exercise training options. Consequently, patients will develop a decreased fear of exercise, especially resistance training. This fear or aversion to participation in a gym has been termed "gymtimidation" and refers to a large proportion of people who view working out with others in a gym unnerving. Incorporating exercise in a medical fitness program also increases patient contact with HCPs, leading to improved adherence, and reinforcing a support structure.

Incorporating a gym into a Lifestyle Medicine Center affords many opportunities to customize programs for a wide variety of patients, based on evidence-based guidelines. Not all Lifestyle Medicine Centers cater to the same patient population. Some programs target specific disease states but can still include a variety of services and approaches. For example, a structured program that focuses on lifestyle therapy for ABCD can incorporate elements of T2D prevention or therapy, such as certified diabetes prevention program protocols. Patients with type 1 diabetes could also benefit from lifestyle optimization but are often hindered by the fear of hypoglycemia with exercise. Providing structured and monitored exercise therapy, along with the education and experience accrued over time, can nurture confidence for those patients, so they can flourish in the gym environment [25]. Moreover, use of continuous glucose monitoring devices under the supervision of a diabetes educator, exercise physiologist, and/or physician in the gym could be a powerful facilitator. Other specialized medical fitness programs could include osteoporosis prevention/treatment, cardiac/pulmonary rehabilitation, neurodegenerative disease, and physical therapy. Customization of a medical fitness program and a physical gym in the Lifestyle Medicine Center also include recognition of other comorbidities, lifestyle medicine needs, cultural adaptations, and sensitivities to various biases and stigmas. For example, patients come from a variety of ethnic backgrounds comprised of different ancestries, anthropometrics/body compositions/physical appearances, cultures preferences, and genetic variations affecting prescribed lifestyle medicine therapy.

Designing the Physical Space

There are several important decisions to make prior to designing and building a fitness center or gym. First, to clarify the clinical target, population, and endpoints, all within the strategic plan of the parent Lifestyle Medicine Program. Second, to clarify the budget and financial goals of the enterprise so decisions and operations can be fiscally responsible, and also consistent with the business plan of the Lifestyle Medicine Center. Third, to provide ample consideration to future expansion as the program succeeds and needs to "vertically" scale up (add new service lines and/or resources to an existing site), "horizontally" scale out (add new geographic sites), or both, based on overt demands, marketing and performance indicators, new/revised strategic/business plans, or even unexpected changes in the health care landscape.

Waiting Room

The waiting room for the Lifestyle Medicine Center will likely also serve as the waiting room for the fitness or gym facility. From the moment patients walk into the medical office, they will know whether they have been considered in the design. Among the first things they encounter are the chairs. Though more expensive, ensuring the waiting room chairs are wide seated bariatric chairs is crucial since, as with the general population, the majority of patients will be overweight or obese. So too is ensuring that a fair percentage of those chairs also have arms for those who require the aid of pushing off chair arms to stand. One of the other items that will immediately be noticed is the reading material. Ensuring that assorted magazines and reading sundry do not promote rarely attainable body images or articles on fat diets or dietary supplements is easy enough. Travel, outdoorsmanship, photography, and science magazines are generally safe bets. Alternatively, a host of various new or used coffee table books can be purchased from the local bookstore. One thing, which should not be visible or within earshot of your waiting room, is your weight scale. Protecting the privacy of patient's weight is easy and worthwhile to safeguard. It was Mickey Stunkard, in his 1993 book *Obesity: Theory and Therapy* [26], who said it best:

> Here is a golden opportunity. As with any chronic illness we rarely have the opportunity to cure. But we do have the opportunity to treat the patient with respect. Such an experience may be the greatest gift that a doctor can give to (a person with obesity); it compares favorably with the modest benefits of our programs of weight reduction.

Examining and Physical Therapy Rooms

The overarching consideration in an examining room is equipment that is appropriate for patients with obesity and physical limitation. From blood pressure cuff sizes (e.g., thigh-sized cuff for use when needed on a larger arm and/or a quality wrist cuff), to adequately sized gowns and 100-inch measuring tapes for waist circumference, to wider than average examination room tables rated for higher weights and inclusive of a wide based platform to help a patient sit on the table which you've also placed a few inches away from the wall. All of these will protect not only a patient's comfort, but will also serve in building trust.

The weigh scale deserves special mention. It should provide a very wide based platform, ideally one that's not too high a step to reach, to ensure that a patient can comfortably stand on it as patients with very large thighs will not be able to utilize a small narrow platform scale. It certainly should be capable of weighing patients with weights up to at least 750 lbs. in order to avoid the horror of a patient receiving an error message rather than a weight. A scale that has arm handles for stability is also useful. A built-in stadiometer is nice, but not essential.

Long extended handled shoehorns are for patients that are asked to remove their shoes. If a bioimpedance scale is part of the routine, which requires the removal of socks, then having a reacher/grabber mobility aid visible and available is reassuring and necessary.

Hallways and Doorframes

Though most HCPs do not have the opportunity to design their offices and fitness facilities from the ground up, those that do should consider double width hallways so that two patients with obesity can walk comfortably by one another. This is also true of doorframes where it is important to keep in mind that bariatric wheelchairs, walkers, and scooters are often wider than an average sized doorway will allow, and typically require a minimum clearance of 36 inches.

Bathrooms

Bathrooms will be necessary not only in the clinic but also in the fitness area depending upon the size of the overall facility. If large enough to incorporate locker rooms, bathrooms should be included in that area along with showers. Grab bars and raised toilet seats (or installing the toilet on a raised platform) are a must. Toilets need to be floor mounted, or supported by a toilet jack, rather than wall mounted to avoid the risk of one breaking off the wall.

The Change Rooms and Showers

As with the hallways and doorframes, extra wide shower stalls with privacy curtains are preferred. The change room should also sport visible long-handled shoehorns and reacher/grabbers to help with shoes and socks. Seating in the change room can include the same chairs as the waiting room, but if incorporating benches, again ensure their weight rating, as well as height since a higher bench helps with standing up. Grab bars installed by the bench are also useful.

Building and Operating a Gym

The most fundamental aspects of a fitness center or gym are deciding upon the best and the most cost-effective and clinically effective exercise equipment, coupled with optimal space utilization and selection of ancillary equipment. Before choosing the equipment, it is important to consider budgetary concerns and decide whether to purchase (new or used) or lease exercise equipment. Purchasing provides the benefits of ownership (stability, control, financial, etc.) but also requires maintenance and more responsibility, while leasing can support initial efforts in deciding upon equipment satisfaction and/or maintaining the latest and greatest equipment.

Before deciding on what exercise equipment to focus on and invest in, thought must be given to ancillary equipment. There are necessities including places to sit, such as benches or chairs, and there are also luxuries like flat-screen monitors for videos or programs, and stereo systems. A small studio focused on individual or small groups of patients may require just one to two sturdy benches or several large chairs for rest, whereas large comprehensive centers will need many seatings dispersed strategically throughout the Center to accommodate larger numbers and potentially group education. Big flat-screen televisions have become nearly standard in high-quality gyms these days, but will range for a given Center depending upon size and patient population emphasis. Small television screens may be incorporated with aerobic machines for individual viewing; alternatively, larger screens may be incorporated into areas of aerobic equipment concentration for group viewing during exercise or rest. Televisions could also be used as instructional tools for group sessions.

Exercise Equipment

Several branded products are presented in this section with price estimates easily searched on dedicated vendor websites, such as www.amazon.com (Accessed on February 29, 2020). Although the inclusion of specific product brands is not intended as an endorsement to the exclusion of other brands, the descriptions and prices are intended as a logistical starting point for those interested in building a gym.

Aerobic exercise can be performed in many different ways; keeping an open mind and thinking "out of the box" will help develop a variety of potential activities for a wide variety of patients and preferences. It is vital to have many options to fit the needs of all the different patient capabilities and their barriers to aerobic activity. Integrating equipment into a portfolio of exercises should be consistent with the strategic and business plans for the Lifestyle Medicine Center.

Ambulation, via walking or running, is one of the most commonly recommended first-line physical activities for many chronic diseases. The limitations of patients (e.g., weight-related, traumatic injuries, balance and cognitive issues, etc.) bear on decision-making for designing optimal therapeutic programs to improve ambulation. There are many treadmill options, but due to the relatively large footprint, consideration must be directed to space allocations indoors and possibly outdoors. If the physical dimensions and other facility or property attributes permit, further consideration should be made to incorporate a track for walking or running (e.g., inside and outside options, railings and mandated protections for those with disabilities, and outdoor/natural trails). Treadmills provide the ability to control and adjust for many factors including speed and incline, while also providing support for balance and fatigue. Most high-quality treadmills have weight limits of over 300 pounds including the Sole F80 (about $600 on Amazon) and Life Fitness 95Ti (for patients up to 500 pounds, though pricier, and available on Amazon for under $2000).

Exercise bicycles are available in various types and are popular due to their ease of use, variable intensity, and usability even with physical limitations. Recumbent bicycles may be an ideal starting exercise for patients with severe obesity as they can accommodate larger patients comfortably though provide less of an overall workout. The Fitnex R70 cites a weight capacity of 400 pounds and includes several desired features to personalize workouts (less than $1900 on Amazon). There are also recumbent combination or hybrid machines, like an elliptical, which could be useful for patients not able to perform on a traditional elliptical. The ProForm Hybrid Trainer Pro (under $600 on its website) can provide patients with a fine full-body aerobic workout with the option of being recumbent, but may not be sufficiently durable with heavy use in a commercial gym (Fig. 12.2).

AirDyne bikes are a traditional favorite with the potential to provide full-body aerobic (or anaerobic) workouts to a diverse spectrum of patients ranging from the elderly with chronic pain to elite athletes. The Schwinn Airdyne Pro is a high-level bike with a capacity of 350 pounds and designed to increase resistance to match the force being exerted (Fig. 12.3). The drive belt system is durable and claims to be far quieter than most air bikes on the market (available on Amazon for around $1000 and other reasonable versions via www.SchwinnFitness.com for lower cost [Accessed on February 29, 2020]).

Rowing machines are a great option to include in a gym as they provide a broad spectrum of aerobic or anaerobic intensity for full-body exercise. These machines mimic rowing a boat, like the sport of crew, but are obviously stationary and

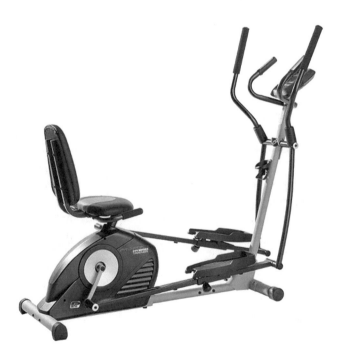

Fig. 12.2 Proform hybrid recumbent

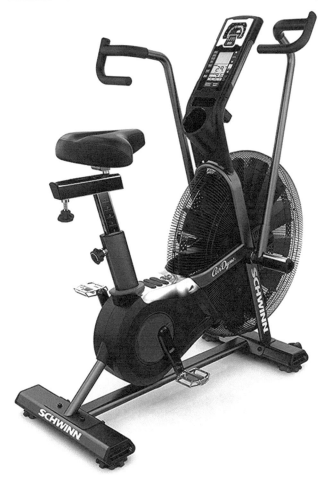

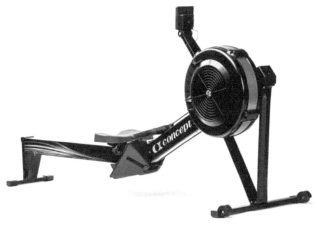

Fig. 12.4 Concept model series rowers

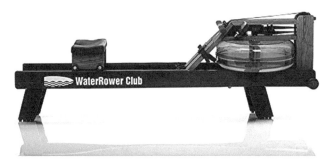

Fig. 12.5 Water rower club rower

Fig. 12.3 Schwinn Airdyne Pro

utilize a fan, water, or magnet to provide resistance. Their popularity has increased significantly over the past several years due to their versatility in promoting fitness for a broad clientele. The Concept Model Series Rowers are highly rated air-resistance rowers with varying options for height, 500 pound capacity, and accessories – available for under $1000 via Amazon or www.RogueFitness.com (Accessed February 29, 2020) (Fig. 12.4). Water rowers provide very smooth movement and add some aestheticity to the gym. The Water Rower Club Rower is available via Amazon for under $1300 (Fig. 12.5).

Ellipticals guide movements that mimic cross-country skiing and have become a popular machine in gyms because of their smooth, full-body exercise movement, and ease of use. They can be used for a very good warm-up or even intense interval training. Resistance, incline, stride length, and speed adjustments can fine-tune individualization. High-quality elliptical machines, such as the SOLE E35 (Fig. 12.6) and Nautilus 614, are available from Amazon and www.Nautilus.

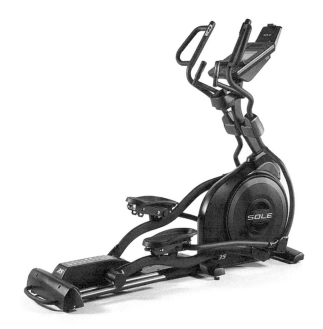

Fig. 12.6 SOLE E35 elliptical

com (Accessed on February 29, 2020) for under $2000 and $1000, respectively.

Arm ergometers are staple in physical therapy and rehabilitation clinics but are also useful to athletes for intense upper-body aerobic/anaerobic exercise, as well as beneficial for patients with significant lower body injuries or other limitations. They basically work in the same way exercise bikes work, but using only the arms and can be approached in a seat, standing, or even via wheelchair (Fig. 12.7).

Resistance Training Weights

Incorporation of resistance training is an important part of comprehensive fitness, though under-recognized due to a general lack of experience and knowledge by HCPs, despite the critical health benefits attained. Considering which free-weights, machines, or other apparatus to invest in is based on available expertise, vision of physical activity goals, and desired patient outcomes. There must be a balance found among space availability, efficiency and efficacy of the available exercises, and plans for supervision and patient access. Resistance training in commercial gyms, especially with personal trainers, is often overly complicated. So, in a clinical setting, this activity should be simplified to provide the fun-

damental education and benefits. Movement groups should include the basics in pushing, pulling, and leg exercises, with the ability to utilize major muscle groups and some isolated muscles. If using free-weights, the barbells, dumbbells, and accessory equipment must be study and be of high quality. This includes benches (often adjustable) and "racks" which can be used for squatting, bench press, or other exercises. There should also be a pull-up bar and adequate storage for the weights (Fig. 12.8).

Circuit training, described as rotating through different muscle group exercises with minimal rest, can be an effective plan for patients and essential programmatic component of a fitness center's offerings. Circuit training can be accomplished with a variety of machines, free-weights, and/or hybrids depending upon the preferences of the health care team and target population. Several machines can be utilized which have the basic components all-in-one. Dedicated machines that isolate each exercise can be placed in a more literal circuit for patients to move station to station. Free weights, especially dumbbells, may also be a good choice for incorporating circuit training, while also accommodating

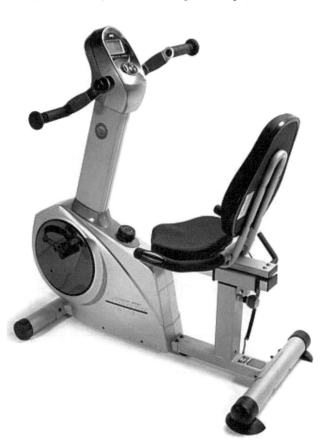

Fig. 12.7 Stamina elite total body recumbent bike

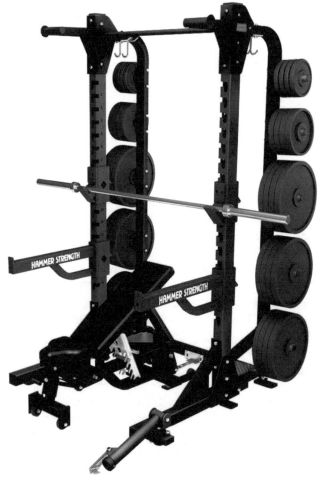

Fig. 12.8 Hammer strength elite half rack

the most patients in the least amount of space without movement (Fig. 12.9).

Life Fitness (www.LifeFitness.com [Accessed on February 29, 2020]) is a suggested source for resistance training equipment, ranging from a variety of effective multi-use machines that don't require a large amount of space to plate-loaded machines (coined "Hammer Strength") designed to move with the body's natural path of motion and are a favorite of elite athletes and those with physical limitations alike. Ideally, at least one machine or station for each basic movement can be included to cover fundamental upper-body movements and major muscle groups: a chest press for pushing forward, a shoulder press for pushing up, seated rowing machine for pulling back, and pull-down machine (similar to pull-ups) for pulling down (Fig. 12.10).

Ancillary exercises are often included in the multi-use machines to focus on triceps, biceps, and deltoids. A quality leg press machine can be extremely beneficial for a broad

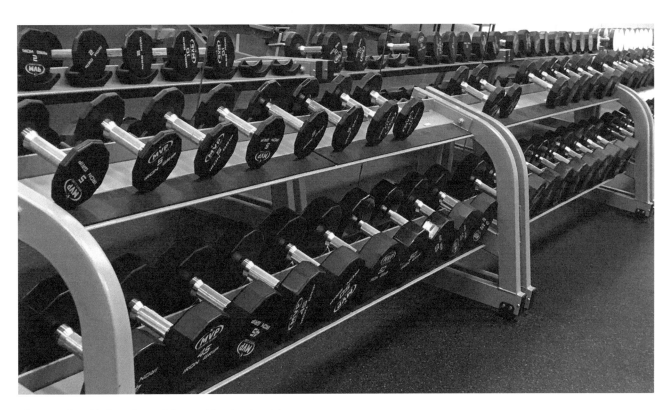

Fig. 12.9 Dumbbells as free weights used for circuit training

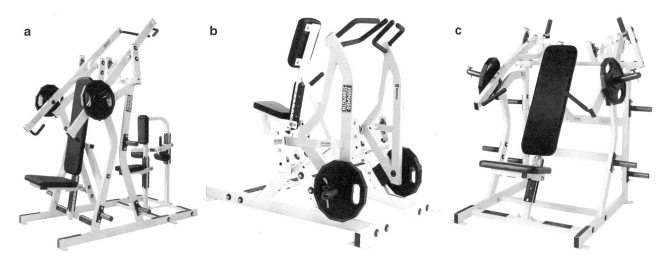

Fig. 12.10 Life fitness resistance training equipment∗. (∗Panel A: iso-lateral chest press and back pull-down; panel B: iso-lateral seated rower; panel C iso-lateral supine incline chest press)

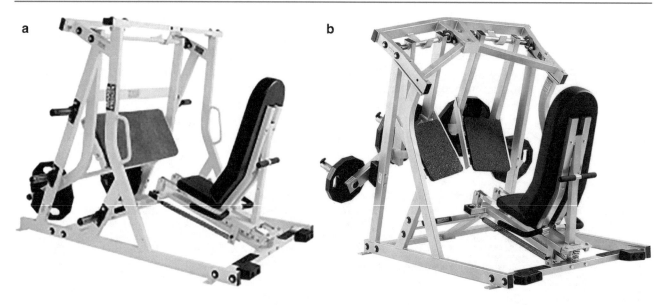

Fig. 12.11 Hammer strength leg press machines∗. (∗Panel A: leg press; panel B: iso-lateral leg press)

spectrum of patients and very useful for therapy of a variety of disease conditions or preventive measures, including metabolic health, bone health, functional capacity, and fall prevention. Hammer strength produces high-quality leg press machines (Fig. 12.11). Their Iso-Lateral Leg Press was designed based on the study of human movement and utilizes separate weight pendulums to engage independent diverging paths of motion for equal bilateral strength development and muscle stimulation variety. The seat and footplates are angled appropriately to reduce undesirable stress and tension, allowing this to accommodate the full spectrum of patients, from the elderly/frail to elite athletes.

Ancillary exercise equipment, including resistance bands and exercise balls, are relatively inexpensive and can be beneficial for teaching home exercises, physical therapy, balance training, and beyond (Fig. 12.12). These items can be purchased for a reasonable cost at a variety of sporting goods stores and even in the sporting goods section of larger general stores.

Miscellaneous Equipment

Flooring necessary for a gym may vary depending upon the space utilization. In a weight room, interlocking rubber mats are the most commonly used adjunctive flooring and are widely available at general stores or hardware stores at low cost, generally coming in about 24 × 24-inch sections.

Sanitation is vital for the health of patients with several options deployed in gyms ranging from "wipe stations," which must be refilled with pre-soaked tissue, or spray bottles and rags dispersed throughout the gym, which must be refilled with fluid and washed, respectively. If rags are utilized or other towels, lines, etc., then laundry services will need to be available in some capacity. First aid kits should be readily avail-

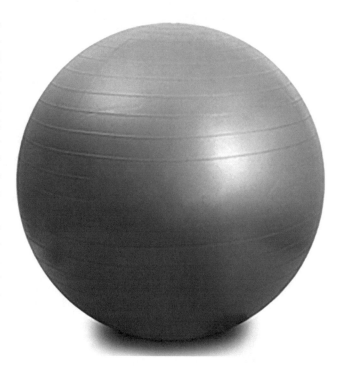

Fig. 12.12 Exercise ball

able throughout the facility. There should be fire-extinguishers monitored for expiration and smoke alarms monitored for battery life. Shower facilities require adequate drainage to avoid slip and fall accidents, and consideration should be given to mats in the locker room to reduce that risk. Access to hydration should be kept in mind via water fountains or perhaps bottled water and sports beverages for purchase. Commercial resources, such as https://zogics.com/facility (Accessed on February 29, 2020), provide the necessary or potentially beneficial equipment to include in the facility.

Size and Capacity

The Lifestyle Medicine Center gym facility can range in scale from a minimalist type of setting where one sees only barbells, to a comprehensive setting similar to a commercial gym (Table 12.1). Relevant decisions depend on considerations of cost, space, and practicality for patients. Equipment specifications and needs depend on the strategic plan and scale of the Center (Table 12.2). Barbells are an amazing universal tool for patients to learn strength training, but some patients may lack the functionality and strength to even begin with an empty barbell. Nevertheless, many weight training machines are appropriate for the majority of patients to use, despite their lack of strength, function, and experience in a gym, but these machines are relatively expensive and typically take up considerable space.

The design and operation of gym is based on the strategic plans of the Lifestyle Medicine Center or Clinical Service Line, within a sponsoring private practice, larger medical group, hospital or medical center, or expansive health system. If conceived and operated by a solo practitioner, there is more autonomy, but also financial burden and risk. If conceived and operated by a larger sponsoring organization, there may be more funds available, but also administrators

Table 12.1 Scales of gym size and comprehensiveness

Minimal or focused	Intermediate	Comprehensive
Small space <1000 square feet	Medium space 1000–10,000 square feet	Large space >10,000 square feet Some >100,000 feet
Individual or small group	Multiple rooms	Many individuals and large group sessions
Low cost	Many individuals and small group sessions	High cost
Solo or small group practice	Large group practice	Associate with medical system
Minimal equipment	Modest cost	Variety of modalities
Minimal personnel	Several modalities	Weight room
	Weight room	Aerobic room
	Aerobic room	Focused studios
	Focused studios	Track
	Rehabilitation	Pool
	Variety personnel	"Functional" area
	+/− personal trainers	Rehabilitation
	+/− physical therapists	Variety personnel
	Custodial staff	Personal trainers
	Maintenance	Physical therapists
	+/− child care	Custodial staff
	Financial	Maintenance
	+/− locker room	Child care
	Minimal luxuries	Financial
		Locker room
		Luxuries
		Televisions

Table 12.2 Exercise equipment based on gym size and comprehensiveness

Equipment	Minimal	Intermediate	Comprehensive
Aerobic	Few options Air resistance bike Treadmill Rowing machine Stair machine	Several options with higher quantity Air resistance bikes Treadmills Rowing machines Stair machines	Several options with high quantity to accommodate large numbers Air resistance and spin bikes Various treadmills Several stair machines Rowing machines Lap pool Track
Dumbbells	Adjustable dumbbells e.g., Powerblock Adjustable bench	Partial dumbbell rack 5's-50's lbs. 2–3 adjustable benches	Complete dumbbell rack from 5's-100's lbs. Several adjustable benches
Barbells	Barbells with 200 lbs. of plates	Barbells with 300 lbs. of plates and a squat stand and padded bench	Several barbells with 500 lbs. of plates, few squat racks and few padded benches (including incline)
Leg press	Air resistance bike	Standard leg press machine	Multiple types of leg press machines
Cable combination	Universal cable machine	Universal cable machine	Dual-sided universal cable machine
Major muscle group resistance machines	Singe hybrid or combo machine	Few hybrid or combo machines Some variety of specific movements	Multiple press and row machines Variety of specific movements
Focused muscle resistance machines		Hip thrust/ glute-raise station Combination leg extension and curl machine Combination hip abduction and adduction machine	Variety of hip-thrust/ glute-raise options Multiple leg extension and curl machines Multiple hip abduction and adduction machines
Miscellaneous	Efficient use of resistance bands for space and cost-effectiveness	Resistance bands Exercise balls	Resistance bands Exercise balls "Functional equipment" like tires for "flipping" and sleds for pushing
Pool		Perhaps a small exercise pool	Possibly a large pool for group water aerobics, laps, etc.

and other managers who share in the decision-making process, thus diluting an individual's (perhaps even the "champion's" or leader's) initial (and imaginative) concept.

One must also consider how the training will be set up. Will it be one-on-one training, group training, semi-private training, a combination of these depending on individual needs, or potentially a free gym where everyone comes and goes and trains as they please? These different scenarios depend on the lifestyle center's strategic plan, business plan, and resources. Commercial gyms usually have group classes, one-on-one training, and free gym where one is able to do whatever workout they please. Smaller boutique gyms oftentimes follow a semi-private training format where each individual is working on their own exercise but is overseen by one or two trainers during the entire workout. There are also personal trainer studios where it is all one-on-one with a trainer. Personal trainers may have a variety of experience and education with several potential "certificates" that are recognized by commercial gyms. Exercise physiologists have earned a bachelor's degree in exercise physiology and may have pursued further education, specialization, or certification beyond that degree.

With a typical solo practice, space is limited and a small 10 ft. × 10 ft. room may be all that is needed to do one-on-one private training for a patient with some of the minimal equipment listed above. This setup allows for a medical encounter preceding or after a quick workout with the HCP or staff all in one room, or a tailored combination of consult, examining, and/or workup rooms in close proximity.

In a group private practice, if the other physicians are on board, one could create a thriving gym clinic using an intermediate list of equipment mentioned above. Finding the space is usually the limiting factor in a busy clinic. The one small room idea as noted above is an option, but ideally a larger space is created for a better patient flow. A larger 30 ft. × 30 ft. room would allow for group or semi-private training throughout the day with one or two staff members. Patients could sign up for particular times of the week and come only during their scheduled time.

Another item to consider is that if the gym and Lifestyle Medical Center or Clinical Service Line are part of a large sponsoring healthcare organization, there is a dedicated cardiac and/or pulmonary rehabilitation program already established. Often these programs have not realized their full capacity, nor generating sufficient revenue, despite taking up a considerable amount of space with much of the equipment listed above. Physical therapy programs are also an option but are usually busier with less equipment. A well thought out discussion with hospital administrators, program supervisors, and other key decision-makers is a best, first step to jumpstart the planning process for a gym and medical fitness program. There are many examples of this process, but unfortunately the process and interest are not pervasive or standard.

Payment

In order for a gym to be financially viable, an appropriate business plan must be developed and implemented. In solo practice, where fitness training can be performed by the physician during the appointment, then the insurance can be billed based on time. Direct payment, or subscription-based, models are simpler because the prices of services are usually more transparent. Providing services which include physical therapy, rehabilitation, or others which are "billable" can subsidize personnel and equipment costs. This is in contrast to large commercial gyms that thrive on a premise that many will sign up and pay, but less will actually show up and exercise – a model that is antithetical to the chronic care model design to improve health for all patients.

Case Study

In 2004, the Bariatric Medical Institute opened in Ottawa, Ontario, Canada. This Institute is an inter-professional behavioral weight management program serving as a site that hosts medical, dietetic, and social work students, residents, and postdoctoral fellows. In addition, the Institute administers multiple lifestyle medicine activities, including a standard behavioral weight management program, a Ministry of Health funded program for parents of children with obesity, and a program for perioperative care for 20% of the city's bariatric surgical patients. An onsite fitness program is included from day 1 in all of these activities.

The gym space is in a converted warehouse with 30-foot ceilings and occupies roughly 1200 square feet, the bulk of which is an open area. The focus is on resistance training with free weights (primarily dumbbells), even though there is a treadmill (for fitness testing that monitors heart rate and heart rate recovery) and a functional trainer, who helps patients work on improving everyday activities. The decision to focus on resistance training is both evidence-based and practical. From an evidence-based perspective, the thought is that resistance training during active weight loss mitigates muscle loss and improves functional independence. Practically, the thought is that aerobic exercise is more familiar to patients and easy for them to obtain outside of the gym, that most would not have experience with weights, that small circuit type classes would be easily conducted with weights, and for those that are interested, used or new dumbbells and a weight bench, which are not particularly expensive, are introduced as potential items for a home gym.

The gym space purposely excludes mirrors based on anecdotal experience that this can make patients feel uncomfortable. Gym use in this example is currently restricted to patients with a minimum BMI of 27 kg/m^2 with comorbidities to maximize patient comfort and decrease potential anxiety, but this varies for different goals and clientele. There is a defibrillator, an Ambu bag with various oral airways, and a naloxone kit.

The dumbbells range from 3 lbs. (1.4 kg) to 70 lbs. (32 kg), and there are two class levels based on exercise intensities. Level 1 and 2 classes have 30- and 45-minute circuits, respectively. All of the classes are instructed by certified personal trainers who are comfortable with patients with obesity, as well as modifying exercises to accommodate various aches, pains, and disabilities. The fitness classes operate from as early as 6:15 am to as late as 8:00 pm, including Saturday mornings, with caps at 15 patients per session. If a particular class is getting too busy, then another class is added to the schedule.

When the Institute opened, there was no precedent to model after. Naturally, there were worries about attendance and interest. Even though attendance could have been better initially (only 30–40% of patients were taking advantage of their ability to attend 3 weekly fitness classes; based on a catchment area of at least 100 miles), those who did attend reported that the fitness program had the greatest impact on their health. These patients continued with the program for years, some as long as over a decade.

Along with the fitness program, trainers provide "learn to run" programs, assembling teams for charity runs and dragon-boating (small watercraft which use paddles), as well as leading a walking club. The gym also hosts multi-week workshops, which over the years have included self-defense, yoga, dancing, and even hula-hooping.

Lastly, HCPs themselves participate in healthy physical activities, training programs, and exercise, setting an example for the patients, as well as sustaining the high level of health among all who are part of the Institute. In this regard, physician personal behaviors can exact a beneficial effect on the overall success for patients.

Conclusion

Priority should be given to development and incorporation of a gym and fitness program into a Lifestyle Medicine Center to provide the greatest opportunity for patient success. Exercise is medicine for many chronic disease states but patient adherence remains a barrier to the desired outcomes. An on-site patient-oriented gym should improve utilization, education, and experience, thus removing or mitigating some barriers to engage in physical activity prescription. Diligence and thought are required when designing, constructing, and assembling a gym for details such as size preference, program development, cost, and available personnel. The goals and objectives laid out for the Lifestyle Medicine Center should be reflected in the development of the gym's strategic and business plans, influencing human resources, exercise equipment, and other building and operating requirements. These plans are necessary to realize both clinical endpoints and financial targets for sustainability. Scalability is critical, with great outcomes achieved over a wide variety of gym sizes and complexities.

There are six "Take-Home Points" for building a gym in a Lifestyle Medicine Center:

1. Development of a gym provides patients with the opportunity for learning and safely adhering to a physical activity prescription.
2. Size and capacity must appropriately reflect the desired patient population and utilization.
3. If constructing from scratch, take into consideration the patient population which may require some uncommonly considered building adaptations (wide hallways, toilet jacks, etc.).
4. Cost and fiscal considerations are critical to balancing patient participation and the economic health of the Lifestyle Medicine Center.
5. Exercise equipment options are vast and variable, but focusing on clinical needs, exercise fundamentals, cost, and safety can help guide the acquisition process.

Ancillary supplies and equipment, from sanitation to drinking fountains, are necessary while luxuries such as televisions should be considered (Table 12.3).

Table 12.3 Concluding points

Key considerations in development of a clinic gym	Concepts to consider	Section, table, or reference
Size	Likely the first issue to decide upon which will be based upon several factors ranging from desired patient volume, staff volume, financial expenditure, room available, equipment quantity, and program variety	Table 12.1. Scales of gym size and comprehensiveness

(continued)

Table 12.3 (continued)

Key considerations in development of a clinic gym	Concepts to consider	Section, table, or reference
Mission and vision	Target patient populations can range from very broad and inclusive to very specific or exclusive depending upon the clinic and medical specialties involved. Examples may include general health and fitness for the community to specific groups like obesity and cardiometabolic health, cardiac/pulmonary rehabilitation, bone health and osteoporosis therapy, fibromyalgia, and neurodegenerative or neurologic injury rehabilitation to orthopedic musculoskeletal rehabilitation Include personal interests and expertise as well as expected needs of the patient community in development	Introduction
Financial considerations	Know, understand, and review the budget with business advisors and/or the office manager or others involved in the clinic's economy. The budget needs to account for all of the potential costs including the space, renovations, exercise equipment, ancillary equipment, and operating expenses	
Exercise equipment	High-quality equipment is an important priority to provide patients May range from very simple and basic, utilizing space and minimizing actual machines to comprehensive aerobic and resistance machines of many varieties. Before purchasing or leasing, decide on the clinical goals and space utilization	Table 12.2
Ancillary equipment/facilities	Safety and sanitation must be a priority with special attention. Cleaning wipes or rags with laundry service, first aid kits, fire-extinguishers, smoke alarms, etc. shower facilities and locker room. Water fountains or perhaps bottled water and sports beverage for purchase	Miscellaneous section
Limitations and challenges	Financial: Cost to patients, payment methods, overhead Space, equipment, and supervision or ancillary staff	Payment section

References

1. Bray GA, Kim KK, Wilding JPH. Obesity: a chronic relapsing progressive disease process. A position statement of the world obesity federation. Obes Rev. 2017;18:715–23.
2. Garvey WT, Mechanick JI, Brett EM, et al. American Association of Clinical Endocrinologists and American College of endocrinology comprehensive clinical practice guidelines for medical Care of Patients with obesity. Endocr Pract. 2016;22(Suppl 3):1–203.
3. Jensen MD, Ryan DH, Apovian CM, et al. AHA/ACC/TOS guideline for the management of overweight and obesity in adults: a report of the American College of Cardiology/American Heart Association task force on practice guidelines and the Obesity Society. J Am Coll Cardiol. 2014;63(25 Pt B):2985–3023.
4. American Diabetes Association. 7. Obesity Management for the Treatment of Type 2 Diabetes: Standards of Medical Care in Diabetes-2018. Diabetes Care. 2019;41(Suppl 1):S65–72.
5. Mechanick JI, Hurley DL, Garvey WT. Adiposity-based chronic disease as a new diagnostic term: the American Association of Clinical Endocrinologists and American College of endocrinology position statement. Endocr Pract. 2017;23:372–8.
6. Frühbeck G, Busetto L, Dicker D, et al. The ABCD of obesity: an EASO position statement on a diagnostic term with clinical and scientific implications. Obes Facts. 2019;12:131–6.
7. American Diabetes Association. Obesity management for the treatment of type 2 diabetes: standards of medical care in diabetes – 2019. Diabetes Care. 2019;42(Suppl 1):S81–9.
8. Davies MJ, D'Alessio DA, Fradkin J, et al. Management of Hyperglycemia in type 2 diabetes, 2018. A consensus report by the American Diabetes Association (ADA) and the European Association for the Study of diabetes (EASD). Diabetes Care. 2018;41:2669–701.
9. Garber AJ, Handelsman Y, Grunberger G, et al. Consensus statement by the American Association of Clinical Endocrinologists and American College of endocrinology on the comprehensive type 2 diabetes management algorithm – 2020 executive summary. Endocr Pract. 2020;26:107–39.
10. American Diabetes Association. Prevention or delay of type 2 diabetes: standards of medical care in diabetes – 2019. Diabetes Care. 2019;42(Suppl 1):S29–33.
11. Jellinger PS, Handelsman Y, Rosenbilt PD, et al. American Association of Clinical Endocrinologists and American College of endocrinology guidelines for management of dyslipidemia and prevention of cardiovascular disease. Endocr Pract. 2017;23(Suppl 2):1–87.
12. Grundy SM, Stone NJ, Bailey AL, et al. 2018 AHA/ACC/AACVPR/AAPA/ABC/ACPM/ADA/AGS/APhA/ASPC/NLA/PCNA Guideline on the Management of Blood Cholesterol: A Report of the American College of Cardiology/American Heart Association Task Force on Clinical Practice Guidelines. Circulation. 2019;139:e1082–143.
13. Jacobson TA, Maki KC, Orringer CE, et al. NLA Expert Panel. National Lipid Association Recommendations for Patient-Centered Management of Dyslipidemia: Part 2. J Clin Lipidol. 2015;9(6 Suppl):S1–122.e1.
14. Martínez-Rueda AJ, Olivas-Martinez A, Vega-Vega O, et al. New 2017 American College of Cardiology/American Heart Association high blood pressure guideline. Hypertension. 2019;73:142–7.
15. Arnett DK, Blumenthal RS, Albert MA, et al. 2019 ACC/AHA guideline on the primary prevention of cardiovascular disease: executive summary: a report of the American College of Cardiology/American Heart Association task force on clinical practice guidelines. J Am Coll Cardiol. 2019;74:1376–414.

16. Price KJ, Gordon BA, Bird SR, et al. A review of guidelines for cardiac rehabilitation exercise programmes: is there an international consensus? Eur J Prev Cardiol. 2016;23:1715–33.

17. Spruit MA, Singh SJ, Garvey C, ATS/ERS Task Force on Pulmonary Rehabilitation, et al. An official American Thoracic Society/European Respiratory Society statement: key concepts and advances in pulmonary rehabilitation. Am J Respir Crit Care Med. 2013;188:e13–64.

18. Camacho PM, Petak SM, Binkley N, et al. American Association of Clinical Endocrinologists and American College of endocrinology clinical practice guidelines for the diagnosis and treatment of postmenopausal osteoporosis – 2016. Endocr Pract. 2016;22(Suppl 4):1–42.

19. Eastell R, Rosen CJ, Black DM, et al. Pharmacological Management of Osteoporosis in postmenopausal women: an Endocrine Society* clinical practice guideline. J Clin Endocrinol Metab. 2019;104:1595–622.

20. Brosseau L, Thevenot O, MacKiddie O, et al. Ottawa panel evidence-based clinical practice guidelines for therapeutic exercise in the management of hip osteoarthritis. Clin Rehabil. 2016;30:935–46.

21. Brosseau L, Taki J, Desjardins B, et al. The Ottawa panel clinical practice guidelines for the management of knee osteoarthritis. Part three: aerobic exercise programs. Clin Rehabil. 2017;31:612–24.

22. Brosseau L, Taki J, Desjardins B, et al. The Ottawa panel clinical practice guidelines for the management of knee osteoarthritis. Part two: strengthening exercise programs. Clin Rehabil. 2017;31:596–611.

23. Hochberg MC, Altman RD, April KT, et al. American College of Rheumatology. American College of Rheumatology 2012 recommendations for the use of nonpharmacologic and pharmacologic therapies in osteoarthritis of the hand, hip, and knee. Arthritis Care Res (Hoboken). 2012;64:465–74.

24. Fitzcharles MA, Ste-Marie PA, Goldenberg DL, et al. National Fibromyalgia Guideline Advisory Panel. 2012 Canadian guidelines for the diagnosis and management of fibromyalgia syndrome: executive summary. Pain Res Manag. 2013;18:119–26.

25. Riddell MC, Gallen IW, Smart CE, et al. Exercise management in type 1 diabetes: a consensus statement. Lancet Diabetes Endocrinol. 2017;5:377–90.

26. Stunkard AJ, Wadden TA. Talking with patients. In: Obesity: theory and therapy. New York: Raven Press; 1993. p. 356.

Wearable Technologies in Lifestyle Medicine

Jeffrey I. Mechanick and Shan Zhao

Abbreviations

A1C	Hemoglobin A1c
BMI	Body mass index
BP	Blood pressure
ECG	Electrocardiogram
HR	Heart rate
MARD	Mean absolute relative difference

Introduction

The traditional encounter model between patient and healthcare professional is evolving under the strong influences of chronic care models, economic constraints, and advanced technologies. Wearable technologies will be a cornerstone of early and sustainable preventive care to not only offset the consequences of chronic disease, but also as an effective tool to prevent chronic disease risk, progression, and consequences. Wearable technologies are electronic computing devices, capable of primarily functioning passively, attached and detached from the body freely, and commonly connected with the Internet. The incorporation of wearable technologies into the cloud has been recently referred to as the "Internet of Things" (IoT), and when specifically incorporating medical wearables, the "Internet of Medical Things" (IoMT). The coordination of smartphone applications, wearables, and point-of-care testing (e.g., in a Lifestyle Medicine Center) allows individual adaptations to activities of daily living [1]. Intelligent healthcare systems have been described utilizing Wireless Body Area Network concepts to link sensors with a hub in a reliable and scalable way, especially as integration becomes more complex with more and more wearables being used [2]. Sensor data can also be incorporated into electronic health records for both inpatients and outpatients [3]. Protected health information can be safeguarded using Integrated Circuit Metric technology, which provides authentication, confidentiality, secure admission, and symmetric key generation [4].

The purpose of wearable technologies in the setting of lifestyle medicine and prevention and management of chronic disease is to measure any clinical parameter, preferably a continuous parameter, that has value to the user, and in many cases, to provide context for interpreting that measurement. A major presumption is that the measurement is interpretable and actionable in a way that improves the user's health. This is particularly attractive in low-income countries, where measurements should be easy to perform and scalable, with open access and adaptability [5].

Wearable technologies are an indispensible implementation tool in lifestyle medicine. There are two broad categories of wearable technologies: those that monitor clinical parameters (e.g., activity with a step counter; certain vital signs, such as heart rate [HR], heart rhythm, and blood pressure [BP]; and laboratory values, such as interstitial fluid glucose) and those that monitor and intervene based on clinical parameters (e.g., cardioverter-defibrillator, ultrasound, and mobility assistance). Examples of wearables that measure movement, and posture; wearables related to exosuits with sensors for augmented movement and cardiac physiology; and wearables as mixed reality goggles are shown in Fig. 13.1. There are also wearables that detect environmental factors that comprise the human exposome (e.g., acoustic noise, temperature/heat, particle number counts, and geolocation) and impact health, though there are still problems with accuracy and interpretation of these variables [6].

J. I. Mechanick (✉)
The Marie-Josée and Henry R. Kravis Center for Cardiovascular Health at Mount Sinai Heart, and the Division of Endocrinology, Diabetes and Bone Disease, Icahn School of Medicine at Mount Sinai, New York, NY, USA
e-mail: jeffrey.mechanick@mountsinai.org

S. Zhao
Department of Anesthesiology, Icahn School of Medicine at Mount Sinai, New York, NY, USA
e-mail: Shan.Zhao@MountSinai.org

© Springer Nature Switzerland AG 2020
J. I. Mechanick, R. F. Kushner (eds.), *Creating a Lifestyle Medicine Center*, https://doi.org/10.1007/978-3-030-48088-2_13

Fig. 13.1 Examples of wearable technologies related to movement.* (∗(**a**) Fitbit Versa2™ (https://www.fitbit.com/shop/versa [accessed on December 21, 2019]); (**b**) Nike+ FuelBand SE™ (https://www.ebay.com/c/620182438 [accessed on December 21, 2019]); (**c**) Apple Watch Series 5 Nike™ (https://www.apple.com/apple-watch-series-5 [accessed December 21, 2019]); (**d**) Samsung Galaxy Watch™ (https://www.samsung.com/ [accessed on December 21, 2019]); (**e**) Seismic™ (http://www.meggrant.com/ [accessed December 21, 2019]); (**f**) BodyGuardian™ Heart (https://www.preventicesolutions.com/hcp/body-guardian-heart [accessed on December 21, 2019); (**g**) Microsoft Hololens 2™ ([accessed on December 21, 2019])

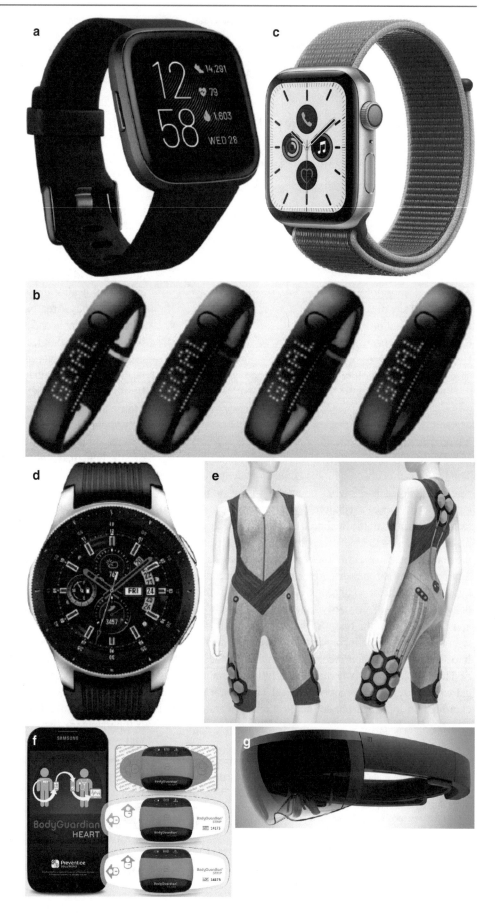

Clinical Scenarios

The value of wearable technologies becomes evident across levels of sophistication, clinical disorders, and endpoints (Table 13.1). These devices can provide simple chores, such as keeping a record of steps or calories, to inform conversations with the lifestyle medicine professional, to enable locomotion in a patient with paraplegia, to enable physical activity and to reduce cardiometabolic risk. There are also platforms, such as HealthSnap™ (www.healthsnap.io [accessed on December 22, 2019]), that capture, analyze, and present a broad range of lifestyle variables with many

Table 13.1 Examples of wearable technologies in healthcare[a]

Clinical target	Device	Description
Cancer	Optune™	Emits tumor-treating fields to treat glioblastoma
	Vivofit 2™	Correlates activity with behavior
Cardiovascular	Apple Watch™	HR/rhythm and energy expenditure
	BodyGuardian Heart™	Adhesive strips, mobile telemetry, cardiac event monitoring
	Fitbit Blaze™/ Charge 2™	HR/rhythm
	Garmin Forerunner™	HR
	Microsoft Kinect™	Correlates skin color with HR
	Phillips Actiwatch™	Measures mobility and sleep
	Preventice BodyGuardian™	ECG measures HR and respiratory rate
	Samsung Galaxy Gear™	HR/rhythm
	TomTom Spark™	HR
	ZioPatch™	ECG monitoring patch to detect AF
Diabetes	Dexcom™	Glucose sensor
	Freestyle Libre™	Glucose sensor
	Serenita™	Relaxation app measuring hemodynamics
Neurology	Empatica™	Wrist-worn detection of seizure counts
	ExoAtlet™	Exoskeleton used in multiple sclerosis
	iCalm™	Wrist-worn detection of seizure counts
	Nightwatch™	Wrist-worn detection nocturnal seizures, movement, HR
Nutrition	Healbe's GoBe 2™	Bioelectrical impedance detection of food intake
	SilkLab™	Tooth-mounted monitor for glucose, salt, and alcohol
	Styr life™	Voice-activated food logging
	The Bite Counter™	Wrist-worn device correlates with oral intake

Table 13.1 (continued)

Clinical target	Device	Description
Orthopedics	Fitbit™	Integrates physical activity with coaching sessions
	LUMOback™	Wearable back device provides posture information
	Micro-Motionlogger™	Correlates activity with clinical symptoms
	Primewalk™	Robotic power-assist locomotor for paraplegia
	ZetrOZ sam™	Provides low-intensity therapeutic ultrasound
Physical activity	ActiGraph™	Rest/activity monitor (e.g., fidgeting versus deskwork)
	ActivPAL™	Activity/incline monitor for sitting, standing, and stepping
	Bio2Bit Move™	Real-time muscle activity monitor
	Coffee WALKIE™	Wrist/waist-worn monitor
	Fitbit Flex™	Monitor with personalized predictors; reminders to exercise
	Seismic™	Powered garment with sensors to assist movement
	SenseWear Armband™	Monitors sleep, posture, and activity
Platform	HealthSnap™	Presents range of lifestyle variables
	Hololens™	Patient education and telemedicine
Sleep	SnoreLab™	Monitors snoring and provides analysis
	WatchPAT™	Monitors rest/activity, hemodynamics, and oximetry

[a]Devices listed are those that monitor clinical parameters with/without intervention. Smartphone apps are not included here. With some exceptions, specific device models are not provided since they frequently change over time. See Table 13.2 for expanded list of glucose sensors. Abbreviations: *AF* atrial fibrillation, *ECG* electrocardiogram, *HR* heart rate

derivative services. This is a rapidly changing landscape, and each Lifestyle Medicine Center will need to identify areas of interest and then consider how relevant wearables can be successfully implemented in their programs. The decision of whether to utilize a wearable device in patient care needs to be carefully considered, depending upon the patient population. Simpson and Mazzeo [7] found that health-tracking devices/applications might actually be detrimental in patients with eating disorders, serving as a reminder that these technologies are still, for the most part, in the development and early implementation stage. There are many other wearable technologies that may influence the implementation of lifestyle medicine, such as those related to obstetrics and neonatology, mental health, ostomy function, lymphedema, hearing and vision, and artificial kidneys, but describing a complete potpourri of devices is beyond the scope of this chapter.

Cardiometabolic-Based Chronic Disease

Cardiometabolic risks include obesity, dysglycemia, unhealthy eating patterns, physical inactivity, tobacco use, hypertension, hypercholesterolemia, poor sleep hygiene, unhealthy behaviors, and inflammation [8–11]. Wearable technologies that address cardiometabolic risk factors will be presented according to the evidence and three clinical scenarios: abnormal adiposity, movement, and sleep; dysglycemia; and cardiovascular disease (CVD).

Abnormal Adiposity, Movement, and Sleep

The mainstay of obesity management is to achieve an optimal body composition (adiposity amount and distribution) and decreased risk for obesity-related complications for a specific patient [8]. This is primarily, but not exclusively, accomplished through healthy eating and physical activity. Wearable technologies interrogate various nutritional and movement variables and can provide a cost-effective and durable adjunct to strategies and tactics delivered in the Lifestyle Medicine Center.

Manual reporting of food intake is generally unreliable [12]. Mobile, dietary self-monitoring, such as image analysis systems that identify foods and estimate portion sizes, can be a valuable tool [13, 14]. Turner-McGrievy et al. [15] found that the total number of days tracking at least two eating occasions per day correlated with improved adherence, highlighting the need for techniques to improve performance of these technologies. Recently, a voice-based mobile nutrition monitoring system has been developed that is based on speech and natural language processing, text-mining techniques, and a tiered matching algorithm that searches nutritional databases to provide a dietary composition monitoring function [16]. Weathers et al. [17] found that the use of The Bite Counter (a wrist-worn device that detects a rolling of the wrist that correlates with bites; http://icountbites.com/ [accessed on December 24, 2019]) is as effective as mental tracking for achieving eating goals. In another study by Shen et al. [18], bite-counting protocols have a sensitivity of 75% with positive predictive value of 89% for actual bites determined by video monitoring. Wearable technologies also support behavioral weight loss in patients with serious mental illnesses [19]. Nevertheless, in the Innovative Approaches to Diet, Exercise and Activity (IDEA) randomized, controlled trial ($N = 470$) of young adults (age 18–35 years) with a body mass index (BMI) between 25 and <40 kg/m^2, the use of wearable technologies compared with standard behavioral interventions resulted in less weight loss over 24 months [20]. The results are not fully explained by the authors and point out that more formal research studies into behavioral mechanisms in patients with abnormal adiposity, especially over longer periods of time, are needed to better understand the role for and mechanism of action of wearables [21].

In a study of patients with metabolic syndrome (central obesity 83.0%; hyperglycemia 54.7%; hypertension 90.6%; hypertriglyceridemia 83.7%; and low high-density lipoprotein cholesterol 54.7%), a 12-week intervention using a wrist- or waist-worn physical activity monitor (Coffee WALKIE +Dv.3™) improved engagement with regular walking and cardiometabolic risk factors, especially hypertension [22]. Using behavioral analytics, the system was able to provide personalized exercise predictors derived from Fitbit Flex™ output and smartphone assessment of daily stress experience and was associated with a 6.5% ($p = 0.04$) greater likelihood of exercising [23]. There are also wearable devices (e.g., Bio2Bit Move™) that perform real-time monitoring of muscle activity [24].

In a study by Kingsley et al. [25], there were large differences in activity intensity estimates among wrist-worn accelerometers, especially below moderate intensity levels (<3 metabolic equivalents or METs). In overweight/obesity, inclinometers (e.g., ActivPAL™ and ActiGraph™) are more error-prone for sedentary to upright transitions and stepping time, compared with sedentary behavior and standing time [26]. Moreover, in children, total activity counts are generally affected by moderate- and vigorous-intensity physical activity but can also be confounded by total wear time [27].

Sedentary behavior is generally any waking behavior in a sitting or reclining posture with <1.5 METs [28]. A preliminary study using the SenseWear Armband™ (for sleep and activity) and activPAL™ (for posture) devices can simultaneously measure sleep, posture, and activity [28]. Sedentary behavior varies according to occupation using device-measured movements, with office workers having the greatest, and laborers the lowest sedentary time; of note, higher BMI and BP correlate with sedentary time [29]. In a prospective cohort study using wrist-worn accelerometers ($N = 91,648$), Kim et al. [30] found that subjects with high levels of physical activity, lower sedentary or screen [TV viewing and computer use] time, and sleep times of 7 hours/ day were more physically active at 5.7 year follow-up. On the other hand, subjects with increased, compared with decreased, dynamic sitting (fidgeting and deskwork; assessed with a hip-worn accelerometer [ActiGraph GT3X™]) was associated with a lower BMI, smaller waist circumference, and lower risk for metabolic syndrome [31]. In addition, novel designs for smart shirts, integrating individual factors and machine learning algorithms, provide highly accurate information about sedentary behavior that is useful for designing active lifestyles, especially for frail, elderly people [32]. Future studies will need to discern how each component of sedentary behavior, and components of physically active lifestyles, contributes to sustainable health outcomes.

Obstructive sleep apnea is an obesity-related complication related to pulmonary function that compromises quality of life by reducing energy and wakefulness during the daytime, while also exacerbating problems with glycemic and weight control. Sleep quality (e.g., ratio of deep sleep to total sleep) estimated using an accelerometer, and correlated with data from pulse activity trackers, body weighing scales, and BP monitors, found that poor sleep quality was associated with being a male, young, having a fast heart rate, and having high BP, whereas increased total sleep was associated with increased weight [33]. Research is currently underway using wearable sensor data from electrodermal activity to more accurately measure sleep efficiency and quality [34].

The wrist-worn WatchPAT 200™ is a four-channel unattended home device that measures peripheral arterial tone, pulse oximetry, HR, and actigraphy (rest/activity cycles). Surges of sympathetic activity detected with this device correlate with apnea/hypopnea events [35]. This information can be useful in high-risk patients where polysomnography is not available [35]. In another study, Lin et al. [36] found that wearable piezoelectric thoracic and abdominal bands detect obstructive versus central sleep apnea with 81.8 ± 9.4% accuracy. The CBT-i Coach™ is a mobile app that has been shown to improve subjective sleep based on cognitive-behavioral therapy in patients with insomnia [37]. Obesity-related lung disease also includes an increased risk for asthma. A wireless wearable ultrasound sensor has been developed for early detection of asthma progression by measuring the FEV1/FVC ratio [38]. In patients with chronic obstructive pulmonary disease and mean BMI of 28.6 kg/ M^2, activity levels measured by a ActiGraph wGT3X-BT™ accelerometer for 7 consecutive days identified 3 behavioral constructs: [1] low-intensity movement associated with mobility, daily activities, health status, and BMI; [2] high-intensity movement associated with younger age and minimal self-care limitations; and [3] sleep associated with body adiposity and poor lung function [39].

Dysglycemia

The management of type 1 and type 2 diabetes includes lifestyle medicine, particularly medical nutrition therapy and healthy eating, as well as mitigation of other CVD risk factors that often includes pharmacotherapy. In patients with or suspected as having dysglycemia, especially as efforts are underway to mitigate cardiometabolic risk factors, capturing and visualizing glucose patterns and correlating them with eating patterns and physical activity provides a unique and valuable opportunity for motivation and lifestyle change. In fact, wearable glucose sensors are an integral part of single- and dual-hormone, closed-loop hormone (insulin ± glucagon) delivery systems that facilitate safe exercise and physical activity by reducing hypoglycemic episodes [40]. Various glucose-sensing technologies are available to increase patient engagement and motivation to improve glycemic control. Currently, there are some significant concerns about wearable glucose-monitoring devices: accuracy, bat-

tery life, burden to patients, comfort, confidentiality, cost, market stability, and standardization [41].

Many sensors are available. There is a curvilinear relationship between the mean absolute relative difference (MARD) and frequency of large (>20%) deviations in glucose determinations [42, 43]. This relationship is consistent across the full range of devices and manufacturers (Table 13.2) [42, 43]. Wrist-borne non-invasive glucose monitors use photoplethysmographic optical sensors and have a MARD in the 7.40–7.54%, which is at the lower part of the range for available glucometer models (5.6–20.8%) [44].

Wearable interfaces also provide measurements of glucose and alcohol in sweat that correlate with blood levels [45, 46]. In addition, a paper microfluidic device for integration into a silicone mouthguard has been developed to measure salivary glucose [47]. Many other paper-based electrochemiluminescence analytic devices, including 3-D origami devices, are suitable for wearing and available for detecting not only glucose but also metal ions, virulent DNA, pathogenic bacteria, and tumor cells [48]. Still other lab-on-skin devices can measure temperature, blood pressure, electromyography, electroencephalography, electrocardiography, hydration, blood oxygenation, wound care, lactate, and pH [49]. Cholesterol

Table 13.2 Current continuous glucose-monitoring sensors[a]

Device	MARD %	Calibrations	Lifetime days	Comments
Medtronic Enlite Sensor™	13.6	q 12h	6	Adjunctive only Acetaminophen Interference
Medtronic Guardian Sensor 3™	10.6 (abdomen) 9.1 (arm)	q 12h	7	Adjunctive only Acetaminophen interference
Freestyle Libre™	11.4	None	14	Scanning required
Freestyle Libre II™	n/a	None	14	Scanning required Improved sensors
Dexcom G4 Platinum™	9	q 12h	7	Adjunctive only
Dexcom G5 Mobile™	9	q 12h	7	Acetaminophen Interference
Dexcom G6™	10	None	10	Has "urgent low soon" alert
Senseonics Eversense™	11.4	None	90	Adjunctive only Inserted/ removed in doctor's office

[a]Adapted from Cappon et al. [43]. A full disposable Dexcom G7™ is anticipated in 2020–2021 with real-time monitoring, factory calibration, extended sensor life, with simple application, and significant cost reduction. Other models will be updated as well, especially with improved connectivity with insulin pumps, and Lifestyle Medicine Centers will need to keep pace with these advances. Abbreviation: MARD – mean absolute relative difference

monitoring is also important for cardiometabolic risk reduction and can be performed using organic electrochemical transistor-based sensors [50]. Electrochemical nose-bridge sensors on eyeglasses have been developed to detect glucose, lactate, and other analytes [51]. Even contact-lens biosensors are being developed for analysis of tear glucose levels in patients with diabetes [52]. Another area of active research is the development of wearables that measure foot temperature to provide a means of early detection of peripheral neuropathy and foot ulceration in patients with diabetes [53].

There are also various apps available to patients to store and analyze data from wearable glucose sensors, providing further incentives and motivation for patients: mySugr App™, Glooko™, and Livongo™. The use of these apps is associated with improved glycemic control (by hemoglobin A1c; A1C) according to a meta-analysis by Bonoto et al. [54]. Another type of app that has benefit in patients with diabetes is Serenita™. This is an interactive relaxation app based on acquiring a photoplethysmography signal from a mobile phone camera lens, measuring blood flow, HR, and HR variability, and providing feedback to the user, which in a clinical trial was found to reduce BP, A1C, and fasting plasma glucose [55].

Cardiovascular Disease

Mobile health technology involving apps and wearable devices guide patients to lead healthy lifestyles and reduce CVD risks [56]. Several devices have been developed and are currently available to enrich cardiovascular monitoring and guide lifestyle medicine interventions, particularly physical activity. These wearable devices can be sorted into heart rhythm and electrocardiography systems, HR monitors, daily activity monitors, hemodynamic technologies, remote dielectric sensing, and bioimpedance monitoring [57]. The Preventice BodyGuardian™ monitors heart and respiratory rates via single lead electrocardiogram (ECG) and Phillips Actiwatch Spectrum Pro™ monitors mobility and sleep and can be used to record physiological changes and pharmacological responses, though fit-for-purpose validation studies are needed for wide scale use [58].

Cardiac rehabilitation is a form of secondary prevention to avert a subsequent cardiac event. The Apple Watch™, Fitbit Blaze™, TomTom Spark™, and Garmin Forerunner™ measure HR with acceptable accuracy and can therefore be incorporated in cardiac rehabilitation sessions [59], though there may be overestimations in energy expenditure with the Apple Watch™, when compared against indirect calorimetry [59, 60]. In addition, three wrist-worn devices (Apple Watch series 2™, Samsung Galaxy Gear S3™, and Fitbit Charge 2™) accurately measure baseline and induced supraventricular tachyarrhythmia HRs [61]. There are many other wrist-worn devices measuring a wide range of biological signals. Interestingly, there is also an earlobe photoplethysmographic sensor that represents a less expensive alternative for detecting subclinical atrial fibrillation [62]. Overall, the selection of any device should be based on validation by clinical studies and a thorough understanding of shortcomings, such as decreased specificity for atrial fibrillation, inaccuracy for tachycardia, and decreased sensitivity for chronotropic incompetence in evaluation for bradycardia [63].

In patients who have had a transient ischemic attack or ischemic stroke, early and prolonged monitoring for paroxysmal atrial fibrillation using the ZioPatch™ (an ECG monitoring patch) is more cost-effective and superior in terms of detection rates, compared with shorter-duration Holter monitoring (16.3% vs. 2.1% [OR 8.9; 95% CI 1.1–76.0; $p = 0.026$]) [64]. In German patients, a wearable cardioverter-defibrillator provided an alternative to implantable devices for those with poor left ventricular function at risk for sudden cardiac death [65]. In the foreseeable future, devices of this type may allow for more patients to engage in structured secondary prevention programs.

Potential future wearable technologies are exciting, providing perspective and a realistic glimpse of what lifestyle medicine looks like on a population-based scale. These devices provide more detailed information about cardiovascular physiology, which can be correlated in real time with physical activity to optimize preventive strategies. Photoplethysmography is currently used for pulse oximetry, but by leveraging knowledge in waveform morphology and propagation theory, this technology can provide cuffless estimations of BP [66]. In fact, a wireless, wearable chest device has been developed that measures and analyzes HR and BP by detecting ECG, photoplethymography and ballistocardiogram signals, sending them via Bluetooth to a mobile phone and then to a server where offline MATLAB based operations are run [67]. Using another technology, chest vibrations that correlate with heartbeats are measured by seismocardiography, typically through the use of rigid accelerometers or non-stretchable piezoelectrical membranes, but moving forward, with ultrathin and stretchable e-tattoos [68]. However, even these innovations are challenged by difficulties with analysis, confounders, low sensitivity, and cost, paving the way for computing and analyzing second derivatives of pulse waveforms with the use of flexible, self-powered, ultrasensitive pulse sensors to detect a wider range of CVDs, including arrhythmia, coronary heart disease, and atrial septal defect [68].

By using a soft electro-mechanical-acoustic cardiovascular sensing tattoo, continuous BP readings can be derived based on the associations of systolic time intervals and systolic/diastolic BPs [69]. In patients with or at-risk for heart failure, a non-invasive, point-of-care skin patch sensor can monitor left ventricular fluid dynamics and stroke volume [70]. Clinical compensated versus decompensated heart failure status can be better predicted with wearable seismocardiography after exercise with the assistance of machine-learning algorithms [71]. Along these lines, lung fluid volume detection by remote dielectric sensing using a wearable vest can reduce rehospitalizations in patients with acute decompensated heart failure [72]. In a study by Lim et al. [73] of 233 normal volunteers that integrated data from wearable sensors, lifestyle questionnaires, cardiac imaging, and sphingolipid profiling, various risk categories could be determined, such as the extent that heart size is affected by exercise, or what chronic diseases may be more likely based on associations with specific sphingolipids.

One of the more interesting innovations lately is a wireless intraoral retainer that fits against the palate and contains hybrid electronics that quantify sodium intake in the management of hypertension [74]. There are even contactless innovations. The Microsoft Kinect™ device is a validated technology that reads small variations in skin color that correlate with HR measurements [75]. This device employs Eulerian Video Magnification, photoplethysmography, and videoplethysmography [75].

Orthopedics

There are various wearable technologies that can treat orthopedic and rheumatologic disorders, which ultimately serve to improve physical activity and lower risks for chronic disease. Many of these techniques can be incorporated in the physical therapy program in the Lifestyle Medicine Center or Clinical Service Line.

Diagnostic devices provide useful information to the lifestyle medicine team. Patients with lower back pain frequently report decreased ability to adhere with medical fitness recommendations. Integrating physical activity information booklets, coaching sessions (face-to-face and telephone-based), and an activity tracker (Fitbit™) with an Internet app can decrease care seeking in patients with lower back pain after inpatient and outpatient physiotherapy program completion [76]. Results from the Micro-Motionlogger™ actigraph correlate with four validated questionnaires related to clinical symptoms, as well as clinical measurements [77]. Lumbar spine and social life dysfunction correlate with actigraphy results, but there are also individual factors that correlate with sex, BMI, low back pain, and muscle mass [77]. Using the LUMOback™ wearable back device ($N = 15$), a more slouched lumbopelvic posture was associated with prolonged lower back pain [78], potentially providing personalized information that can improve well-being and greater participation with physical activities.

Wearable technologies can provide interventions that enable greater mobility. In a 6-week clinical trial ($N = 25$), Best et al. [79] found that daily multi-hour low-intensity therapeutic ultrasound (ZetrOZ sam™; with power controller, 2 ultrasound transducers, and specialized bandages) improved pain and strength in patients with chronic tendon injuries. Also, wearable pulsed electromagnetic fields pro-

vide pain relief and greater mobility in patients with knee osteoarthritis ($N = 66$) [80]. More sophisticated robotic devices can facilitate increased physical activity. For example, in patients with paraplegia, the Wearable Power-Assist Locomotor with conventional knee-ankle-foot orthoses (e.g., Hip and Ankle Linked Orthosis or Primewalk™) can improve energy efficiency and lower gait demand with locomotion [81]. The wearable exoskeletal device has also been shown to be safe, feasible, and associated with improvements in spatiotemporal and kinematic factors to enable locomotion and mobility in patients with spinal cord injury [82]. Fabric-based soft robotic gloves have also been used to assist hand function in patients with upper limb paralysis after spinal cord injury [83].

Many medical fitness programs in Lifestyle Medicine Centers need to address the challenges related to increasing physical activity in the geriatric and disabled populations, particularly when there are significant orthopedic concerns. The detection of disturbances in gait speed, positional transitions, and posture correlate with mortality, disability, and cognitive impairments [84]. Using accelerometry-measured physical activity using a hip-worn ActiGraph GT3X™, numbers of steps and duration of activity were correlated with lower CVD event rates in the elderly [85]. Unfortunately, estimating energy expenditure in the elderly based on accelerometer output is not as accurate as hoped for, across physical activity intensities and even with different equations [86]. In the elderly, robot-assisted gait devices (e.g., wearable hip assist) can stabilize the trunk [87] and spring-assist actuators can increase the required motor torque [88] for walking and other physical activities. There are even devices that can attach to walkers for positional feedback to improve adherence with guidelines, though posture was not improved [89].

Neurological

The literature on wearable systems, including sensors embedded in garments, to monitor and provide feedback on posture and movement in patients with a variety of neurological disorders is emerging and not yet conclusive [90]. For instance, fall prediction and prevention in the elderly and/or frail generally involves education, footwear advice, toileting, balance training, and exercise but can be enhanced using wearable motion and environment sensors [91]. Also, in a meta-analysis, Gordt et al. [92] found that wearable sensor training exerts a positive effect on static steady-state balance and gait parameters in patients with Parkinson's disease, stroke, peripheral neuropathy, and frailty. Specifically, in patients with Parkinson's disease, soft wearable sensors can detect signs, such as bradykinesia, and inform clinicians about disease progression to optimize therapy [93]. On-shoe wearable sensors can also provide important information with turning related to gain in patients with Parkinson's disease [94]. In patients with multiple sclerosis ($N = 18$), the exoskeleton ExoAtlet™ enabled or improved walking and maintenance of vertical posture [95]. In patients with seizure disorder ($N = 69$), certain multimodal wrist-worn devices (Empatica E3™ and E4™; MIT Media Lab iCalm™) detect seizure counts more accurately than other automated systems and self-reporting [96]; this can allow for correlation with various lifestyle factors to optimize overall care. In another study ($N = 28$), the Nightwatch™ combined HR and movement data to detect a broad range of nocturnal seizures [97].

Cancer

The role of lifestyle medicine in patients with or at-risk for neoplastic diseases is oriented toward prevention of risk at a population level (primordial prevention), prevention of disease in those at risk (primary prevention), prevention of disease progression in those with early, asymptomatic disease (secondary prevention), and prevention of suffering, further morbidity, and mortality in those with advanced disease (tertiary prevention). However, in patients with neoplastic disease, regardless of their staging or response to therapy, there still remains an imperative to prevent other chronic disease risks, progression, and complications. For instance, in patients fighting breast cancer, where the overwhelming focus of care is on tertiary prevention related to this primary diagnosis, the additional attention paid to preventing other chronic diseases, especially through lifestyle change, is often inadequate or completely neglected. With improved survivorships with cancer observed nowadays, this healthcare paradigm needs to be re-examined. The role of wearable technologies to concurrently improve lifestyle for prevention of cancer risk, development, and progression, as well as for other chronic diseases (e.g., cardiometabolic and neurodegenerative), is worthy of discussion and pragmatic implementation.

Healthy eating and physical activity are the core lifestyle medicine modalities, with wearable technologies playing an important role in the earlier primordial/primary/secondary prevention types. As an example, in postmenopausal women with stage I-III breast cancer who have completed primary therapy, the use of a Garmin Vivofit 2™ activity monitor with behavioral sessions was associated with more active lifestyles [98]. Among 42 colorectal cancer survivors, the use of a Fitbit Flex™ and reminder text messages was associated with increased motivation to exercise [99]. Activity monitors have also demonstrated efficacy for motivation and increased physical function in patients with advanced cancer ($N = 37$) [100]. Specifically, there were lower rates of patient-reported outcomes, as well as adverse events, hospitalizations, and mortality [100].

Implementation of Wearable Technologies

When building a Lifestyle Medicine Center or Clinical Service Line within a sponsoring healthcare system, a formal program should be developed that provides relevant wearable technologies to patients. The primary clinical endpoint of a Lifestyle Medicine Center is to decrease the risk for chronic diseases. This means that interventions will span a relatively long period of time and therefore benefits would need to be sustainable. One way to do this is through traditional educational [101] or more contemporary "robotic nudges" [102]. Wearable technology event nudges provide reminders, feedback, and planning prompts that direct human behaviors using intuition and reasoning in a certain direction over a long time, such as chronic disease self-management [103, 104].

From the outset, an expansive line of wearables should be explored that cover the full range of services offered in the Lifestyle Medicine Center. This would range from smartphone apps that monitor dietary patterns, to accelerometers, to more specialized devices for cardiopulmonary measurements or movement disorders with orthopedic or neurological conditions. As lifestyle medicine protocols are formulated within the Center, wearable technologies should be included to support these protocols. The clinical director and other assigned personnel in the facility should be familiar with the use of the devices and related operations, such as access to cloud-based data and troubleshooting protocols. Representatives from manufacturers should be invited to review the proper use of devices and apps with the healthcare professionals and staff in the Center. Personnel should be assigned to monitoring patient data and coordinating with Information Technology resources to incorporate, as easily as possible, data in the electronic health record. One could conceive a dedicated wearable technologies program within the Lifestyle Medicine Clinical Service Line, with trained personnel and a business model.

Not surprisingly, the economics of wearable technologies pose a significant obstacle to implementation by a Lifestyle Medicine Center, translating into decreased general use by patients. Many of these devices are expensive and not covered by insurance. However, many others are affordable and easy to obtain over the web, especially apps for smartphones already owned by the patient. Creative solutions should be considered by the Center's leaders, such as bundling resources and including one or more wearables for all users of the Center. Expenses for wearables that are distributed to all patients in the Center could be a line item in the total expenses as part of the business plan. Another option is to build a unique, dedicated app for the Center with startup funds or charitable donations.

References

1. Düking P, Achtzehn S, Holmberg HC, et al. Integrated framework of load monitoring by a combination of smartphone applications, wearables and point-of-care testing provides feedback that allows individual responsive adjustments to activities of daily living. Sensors. 2018;18:1632. https://doi.org/10.3390/s18051632.

2. Wang J, Han K, Chen Z, et al. A software defined radio evaluation platform for WBAN systems. Sensors. 2018;18:4494. https://doi.org/10.3390/s18124494.

3. Joshi M, Ashrafian H, Aufegger L, et al. Wearable sensors to improve detection of patient deterioration. Exp Rev Med Devices. 2019;16:145–54.

4. Tahir H, Tahir R, McDonald-Maier K. On the security of consumer wearable devices in the internet of things. PLoS One. 2018;13:e0195487. https://doi.org/10.1371/journal.pone.0195487.

5. Bell W, Colaiezzi BA, Prata CS, et al. Scaling up dietary data for decision-making in low-income countries: new technological frontiers. Adv Nutr. 2017;8:916–32.

6. Ueberham M, Schlink U. Wearable sensors for multifactorial personal exposure measurements – a ranking study. Environ Internat. 2018;121:130–8.

7. Simpson CC, Mazzeo SE. Calorie counting and fitness tracking technology: associations with eating disorder symptomatology. Eating Behav. 2017;26:89–92.

8. Mechanick JI, Hurley DL, Garvey WT. Adiposity-based chronic disease as a new diagnostic term: American Association of Clinical Endocrinologists and the American College of Endocrinology position statement. Endocr Pract. 2017;23:372–8.

9. Mechanick JI, Garber AJ, Grunberger G, Handelsman Y, Garvey WT. Dysglycemia-based chronic disease: An American Association of Clinical Endocrinologists position statement. Endocr Pract. 2018; 24: 995–1011. Cmbcd-1.

10. Mechanick JI, Farkouh ME, Newman JD, Garvey WT. Cardiometabolic-based chronic disease – adiposity and dysglycemia drivers. J Am Coll Cardiol. 2020; [In Press].

11. Mechanick JI, Farkouh ME, Newman JD, Garvey WT. Cardiometabolic-based chronic disease – addressing knowledge and clinical practice gaps in the preventive care plan. J Am Coll Cardiol. 2020; [In Press].

12. Livingstone MBE, Black AE. Markers of the validity of reported energy intake. J Nutr. 2003;133:895S–920S.

13. Hassannejad H, Matrella G, Ciampolini P, et al. Automatic diet monitoring: a review of computer vision and wearable sensor-based methods. Int J Food Sci Nutr. 2017;68(6):656–70.

14. Boushey CJ, Spoden M, Zhu FM, et al. New mobile methods for dietary assessment: review of image-assisted and image-based dietary assessment methods. Proc Nutr Soc. 2017;76:283–94.

15. Turner-McGrievy GM, Dunn CG, Wilcox S, et al. Defining adherence to mobile dietary self-monitoring and assessing tracking over time: tracking at last two eating occasions per day is best marker of adherence within two different mobile health randomized weight loss interventions. J Acad Nutr Dietet. 2019;119:1516–24.

16. Hezarjaribi N, Mazrouee S, Ghasemzadeh H, et al. Speech2Health: a mobile framework for monitoring dietary composition from spoken data. IEEE J Biomed Health Inform. 2018;22. https://doi.org/10.1109/JBHI.2017.2709333.

17. Weathers D, Siemens JC, Kopp SW. Tracking food intake as bites: effects on cognitive resources, eating enjoyment, and self-control. Appetite. 2017;111:23–37.

18. Shen Y, Salley J, Muth E, et al. Assessing the accuracy of a wrist motion tracking method for counting bites across demographic and food variables. IEEE J Biomed Health Inform. 2017;21:599–606.

19. Naslund JA, Aschbrenner KA, Scherer EA, et al. Wearable devices and mobile technologies for supporting behavioral weight loss among people with serious mental illness. Psychiatry Res. 2016;244:139–44.

20. Jakicic JM, Davis KK, Rogers RJ, et al. Effect of wearable technology combined with a lifestyle intervention on long-term weight loss: the IDEA randomized clinical trial. JAMA. 2016;316:1161–71.

21. Klasnja P, Hekler EB. Wearable technology and long-term weight loss. JAMA. 2017;317:317.

22. Huh U, Tak YJ, Song S, et al. Feedback on physical activity through a wearable device connected to a mobile phone app in patients with metabolic syndrome: pilot study. JMIR Mhealth Uhealth. 2019;7:e13381. https://doi.org/10.2196/13381.

23. Yoon S, Schwartz JE, Burg MM, et al. Using behavioral analytics to increase exercise: a randomized N-or-1 study. Am J Prev Med. 2018;54:559–67.

24. Mazzetta I, Gentile P, Pessione M, et al. Stand-alone wearable system for ubiquitous real-time monitoring of muscle activation potentials. Sensors. 2018;18:1748. https://doi.org/10.3390/s18061748.

25. Kingsley MIC, Nawaratne R, O'Halloran PD, et al. Wrist-specific accelerometry methods for estimating free-living physical activity. J Sci Med Sport. 2019;22:677–83.

26. Júdice PB, Teixeira L, Silva AM, et al. Accuracy of Actigraph inclinometer to classify free-living postures and motion in adults with overweight and obesity. J Sports Sci. 2019;37:1708–16.

27. Kwon S, Andersen LB, Grøntved A, et al. A closer look at the relationship among accelerometer-based physical activity metrics: ICAD pooled data. Int J Behav Nutr Phys Act. 2019;16:40. https://doi.org/10.1186/s12966-019-0801-x.

28. Myers A, Gibbons C, Butler E, et al. A novel integrative procedure for identifying and integrating three-dimensions of objectively measured free-living sedentary behaviour. BMC Public Health. 2017;17:979. https://doi.org/10.1186/s12889-017-4994-0.

29. Prince SA, Elliott CG, Scott K, et al. Device-measured physical activity, sedentary behaviour and cardiometabolic health and fitness across occupational groups: a systematic review and meta-analysis. Int J Behav Nutr Phys Act. 2019;16:30. https://doi.org/10.1186/s12966-019-0790-9.

30. Kim Y, Wijndaele K, Sharp SJ, et al. Specific physical activities, sedentary behaviours and sleep as long-term predictors of accelerometer-measured physical activity in 91,648 adults: a prospective cohort study. Int J Behav Nutr Phys Act. 2019;16:41. https://doi.org/10.1186/s12966-019-0802-9.

31. van der Berg JD, Stehouwer CDA, Bosma H, et al. Dynamic sitting: measurement and associations with metabolic health. J Sports Sci. 2019;37:1746–54.

32. Kantoch E. Recognition of sedentary behavior by machine learning analysis of wearable sensors during activities of daily living for telemedical assessment of cardiovascular risk. Sensors. 2018;18:3219. https://doi.org/10.3390/s18103219.

33. Fagherazzi G, Fatouhi DE, Bellicha A, et al. An international study on the determinants of poor sleep amongst 15,000 users of connected devices. J Med Internet Res. 2017;19:e363. https://doi.org/10.2196/jmir.7930.

34. Romine W, Banerjee T, Goodman G. Toward sensor-based sleep monitoring with electrodermal activity measures. Sensors. 2019;19:1417. https://doi.org/10.3390/s19061417.

35. Weimin L, Rongguang W, Dongyan H, et al. Eur Arch Otorhinolaryngol. 2013;270:3099–105.

36. Lin YY, Wu HT, Hsu CA, et al. Sleep apnea detection based on thoracic and abdominal movement signals of wearable piezoelectric bands. IEEE J Biomed Health Inform. 2016;21:1533–45.

37. Reilly ED, Robinson SA, Petrakis BA, et al. Mobile app use for insomnia self-management: pilot findings on sleep outcomes in veterans. Interact J Med Res. 2019;8:e12408. https://doi.org/10.2196/12408.

38. Chen A, Halton AJ, Rhoades RD, et al. Wireless wearable ultra-sound sensor on a paper substrate to characterize respiratory behavior. ACS Sens. 2019;4:944–52.

39. Orme MW, Steiner MC, Morgan MD, et al. 24-hour accelerometry in COPD: exploring physical activity, sedentary behavior, sleep and clinical characteristics. Int J COPD. 2019;14:419–30.

40. Castle JR, El Youssef J, Wilson LM, et al. Randomized outpatient trial of single- and dual-hormone closed-loop systems that adapt to exercise using wearable sensors. Diabetes Care. 2018;41:1471–7.

41. Schwartz FL, Marling CR, Bunescu RC. The promise and perils of wearable physiological sensors for diabetes management. J Diab Sci Technol. 2018;12:587–91.

42. Castle JR, DeVries JH, Kovatchev B. Future of automated insulin delivery systems. Diabetes Technol Ther. 2017;19(Suppl 3):S67–72.

43. Cappon G, Vettoretti M, Sparacino G, et al. Continuous glucose monitoring sensors for diabetes management: a review of technologies and applications. Diabetes Metab J. 2019;43:383–97.

44. Rodin D, Kirby M, Sedogin N, et al. Comparative accuracy of optical sensor-based wearable system for non-invasive measurement of blood glucose concentration. Clin Biochem. 2019;65:15–20.

45. Emaminejad S, Gao W, Wu E, et al. Autonomous sweat extraction and analysis applied to cystic fibrosis and glucose monitoring using a fully integrated wearable platform. Proc Natl Acad Sci U S A. 2017;114:4625–30.

46. Bhide A, Muthukumar S, Prasad S. CLASP (continuous lifestyle awareness through sweat platform): a novel sensor for simultaneous detection of alcohol and glucose from passive perspired sweat. Biosens Bioelectron. 2018;117:537–45.

47. de Castro LF, de Frietas SV, Duarte LC, et al. Salivary diagnostics on paper microfluidic devices and their use as wearable sensors for glucose monitoring. Analytic Bioanalytic Chem. 2019;411:4919–28.

48. Chinnadayyala SR, Park J, Le HTN, et al. Recent advances in microfluidic paper-based electrochemiluminescence analytical devices for point-of-care testing applications. Biosens Bioelectron. 2019;126:68–81.

49. Liu Y, Pharr M, Salvatore GA. Lab-on-skin: a review of flexible and stretchable electronics for wearable health monitoring. ACS Nano. 2017;11:9614–35.

50. Mak CH. Highly sensitive biosensor based on organic electrochemical transistors. Hong Kong, China: The Hong Kong Polytechnic University; 2015.

51. Sempionatto JR, Nakagawa T, Pavinatto A, et al. Eyeglasses based wireless electrolyte and metabolite sensor platform. Lab Chip. 2017;17:1834–42.

52. Tseng RC, Chen CC, Hsu SM, et al. Contact-lens biosensors. Sensors. 2018;18:2651. https://doi.org/10.3390/s18082651.

53. Martin-Vaquero J, Encinas AH, Queiruga-Dios A, et al. Review on wearables to monitor foot termperature in diabetic patients. Sensors. 2019;19:776. https://doi.org/10.3390/s19040776.

54. Bonoto BC, de Araujo VE, Godoi IP, et al. Efficacy of mobile apps to support the care of patients with diabetes mellitus: a systematic review and meta-analysis of randomized controlled trials. JMIR Mhealth Uhealth. 2017;5:e4. https://doi.org/10.2196/mhealth.6309.

55. Munster-Segev M, Fuerst O, Kaplan SA, et al. JMIR Mhealth Uhealth. 2017;5:e75. https://doi.org/10.2196/mhealth.7408.

56. Rehman H, Kamal AK, Sayani S, et al. Using mobile health (mHealth) technology in the management of diabetes mellitus, physical inactivity, and smoking. Curr Atheroscler Rep. 2017;19:16. https://doi.org/10.1007/s11883-017-0650-5.

57. Pevnick JM, Birkeland K, Zimmer R, et al. Wearable technology for cardiology: an update and framework for the future. Trends Cardiovasc Med. 2018;28:144–50.

58. Izmailova ES, McLean IL, Hather G, et al. Continuous monitoring using a wearable device detects activity-induced heart rate changes after administration of amphetamine. Clin Translat Sci. 2019;12:677–86.

59. Etiwy M, Akhrass Z, Gillinov L, et al. Accuracy of wearable heart rate monitors in cardiac rehabilitation. Cardiovasc Diagn Ther. 2019;9:262–71.

60. Falter M, Budts W, Goetschalckx K, et al. Accuracy of apple watch measurements for heart rate and energy expenditure in patients with cardiovascular disease: cross-sectional study. JMIR Mhealth Uhealth. 2019;7:e11889. https://doi.org/10.2196/11889. 10.2196/11889.

61. Hwang J, Kim J, Choi KJ, et al. Assessing accuracy of wrist-worn wearable devices in measurement of paroxysmal supraventricular tachycardia heart rate. Korean Circ J. 2019;49:437–45.

62. Conroy T, Guzman JH, Hall B, et al. Detection of atrial fibrillation using an earlobe photoplethysmographic sensor. Physiol Meas. 2017;38:1906–18.

63. Ip JE. Evaluation of cardiac rhythm abnormalities from wearable devices. JAMA. 2019;321:1098–9.

64. Kaura A, Sztriha L, Chan FK, et al. Early prolonged ambulatory cardiac monitoring in stroke (EPACS): an open-label randomised controlled trial. Eur J Med Res. 2019;24:25. https://doi.org/10.1186/s40001-019-0383-8.

65. Wäßnig NK, Günther M, Quick S, et al. Experience with the wearable cardioverter-defibrillator in patients at high risk for sudden cardiac death. Circulation. 2016;134:635–43.

66. Elgendi M, Fletcher R, Liang Y, et al. The use of photoplethysmography for assessing hypertension. NPJ Digit Med. 2019;2:60. https://doi.org/10.1038/s41746-019-0136-7.

67. Janjua G, Guldenring D, Finlay D, et al. Wireless chest wearable vital sign monitoring platform for hypertension. Cong Proc IEEE Eng Med Biol Soc. 2017:821–4. https://doi.org/10.1109/EMBC.2017.8036950.

68. Outang H, Tian J, Sun G, et al. Self-powered pulse sensor for anti-diastole of cardiovascular disease. Adv Mater. 2017;29:1703456. https://doi.org/10.1002/adma.201703456.

69. Ha T, Tran J, Liu S, et al. A chest-laminated ultrathin and stretchable e-tattoo for the measurement of electrocardiogram, seismocardiogram, and cardiac time intervals. Adv Sci. 2019;6:1900290. https://doi.org/10.1002/advs.201900290.

70. Alruwaili F, Cluff K, Griffith J, et al. Passive self resonant skin patch sensor to monitor cardiac intraventricular stroke volume using electromagnetic properties of blood. Cardiovasc Dev Syst. 2018;6:1900709. https://doi.org/10.1109/JTEHM.2018.2870589.

71. Inan OT, Baran Pouyan M, Javaid AQ, et al. Novel wearable seismocardiography and machine learning algorithms can assess clinical status of heart failure patients. Circ Heart Fail. 2018;11:e004313. https://doi.org/10.1161/CIRCHEARTFAILURE.117.004313.

72. Amir O, Ben-Gal T, Weinstein JM, et al. Evaluation of remote dielectric sensing (ReDS) technology-guided therapy for decreasing heart failure re-hospitalizations. Int J Cardiol. 2017;240:279–84.

73. Lim WK, Davila S, Teo JX, et al. Beyond fitness tracking: the use of consumer-grade wearable data from normal volunteers in cardiovascular and lipidomics research. PLoS Biol. 2018;16:e2004285. https://doi.org/10.1371/journal.pbio.2004285.

74. Lee Y, Howe C, Mishra S, et al. Wireless, intraoral hybrid electronics for real-time quantification of sodium intake toward hypertension management. PNAS. 2018;115:5377–82.

75. Gambi E, Agostinelli A, Belli A, et al. Heart rate detection using Microsoft Kinect: validation and comparison to wearable devices. Sensors. 2017;17:1776. https://doi.org/10.3390/s17081776.

76. Amorim AB, Pappas E, Simic M, et al. Integrating mobile-health, health coaching, and physical activity to reduce the burden of

chronic low back pain trial (IMPACT): a pilot randomised controlled trial. BMC Musculoskeletal Disord. 2019;20:71. https://doi.org/10.1186/s12891-019-2454-y.

77. Inoue M, Orita S, Inage K, et al. Relationship between patient-based scoring systems and the activity level of patients measured by wearable activity trackers in lumbar spine disease. Eur Spine J. 2019;28:1804–10.

78. Takasaki H. Habitual pelvic posture and time spent sitting: measurement test-retest reliability for the LUMOback device and preliminary evidence for slouched in individuals with low back pain. SAGE Open Med. 2017;5:2050312117731251. https://doi.org/10.1177/2050312117731251.

79. Best TM, Moore B, Jarit P, et al. Sustained acoustic medicine: wearable, long duration ultrasonic therapy for the treatment of tendinopathy. Phys Sportsmed. 2015;43:366–74.

80. Bagnato GL, Miceli G, Marino N, et al. Pulsed electromagnetic fields in knee osteoarthritis: a double blind, placebo-controlled, randomized clinical trial. Rheumatol. 2016;55:755–62.

81. Yatsuya K, Hirano S, Saitoh E, et al. Comparison of energy efficiency between wearable power-assist locomotor (WPAL) and two types of knee-ankle-foot orthoses with a medial single hip joint (MSH-KAFO). J Spinal Cord Med. 2018;41:48–54.

82. Sale P, Russo EF, Scarton A, et al. Training for mobility with exoskeleton robot in spinal cord injury patients: a pilot study. Eur J Phys Rehabil Med. 2018;54:745–51.

83. Cappello L, Meyer JT, Galloway KC, et al. Assisting hand function after spinal cord injury with a fabric-based soft robotic glove. J Neuroeng Rehabil. 2018;15:59. https://doi.org/10.1186/s12984-018-0391-x.

84. Buchman AS, Dawe RJ, Leurgans SE, et al. Different combinations of mobility metrics derived from a wearable sensor are associated with distinct health outcomes in older adults. J Gerontol A Biol Sci Med Sci 2019; glz160. https://doi.org/10.1093/gerona/glz160.

85. Cochrane SK, Chen SH, Fitzgerald JD, et al. Association of accelerometry-measured physical activity and cardiovascular events in mobility-limited older adults: the LIFE (lifestyle interventions and Independence for elders) study. J Am Heart Assoc. 2017;6:e007215. https://doi.org/10.1161/JAHA.117.007215.

86. Aguilar-Farias N, Peeters GMEE, Brychta RJ, et al. Comparing ActiGraph equations for estimating energy expenditure in older adults. J Sports Sci. 2019;37:188–95.

87. Lee HJ, Lee S, Chang WH, et al. A wearable hip assist robot can improve gait function and cardiopulmonary metabolic efficiency in elderly adults. IEEE Trans Neural Syst Rehabil Eng. 2017;25:1549–57.

88. Jung S, Kim C, Park J, et al. A wearable robotic orthosis with a spring-assist actuator. Conf Proc IEEE Eng Med Biol Soc. 2016;2016:5051–4.

89. Golembiewski C, Schultz J, Reissman T, et al. The effects of a positional feedback device on rollator walker use: a validation study. Assist Technol. https://doi.org/10.1080/10400435.2019.1637380.

90. Wang Q, Markopoulos P, Yu B, et al. Interactive wearable systems for upper body rehabilitation: a systematic review. J Neuroeng Rehabil. 2017;14. https://doi.org/10.1186/s12984-017-0229-y.

91. Nguyen H, Mirza F, Naeem MA, et al. Falls management framework for supporting an independent lifestyle for older adults: a systematic review. Aging Clin Exp Res. 2018;30:1275–86.

92. Gordt K, Gerhardy T, Najafi B, et al. Effects of wearable sensor-based balance and gait training on balance, gait, and functional performance in healthy and patient populations: a systematic review and meta-analysis of randomized controlled trials. Gerontol. 2018;64:74–89.

93. Lonini L, Dai A, Shawen N, et al. Wearable sensors for Parkinson's disease: which data are worth collecting for training symptom detection models. NPJ Digit Med. 2018;1:64. https://doi.org/10.1038/s41746-018-0071-z.

94. Haji Ghassemi N, Hannink J, Roth N, et al. Turning analysis during standardized test using on-shoe wearable sensors in Parkinson's disease. Sensors 2019; 19: pii: E3103. https://doi.org/10.3390/s19143103.

95. Kotov SV, Lijdvoy VY, Sekirin AB, et al. The efficacy of the exoskeleton ExoAtlet to restore walking in patients with multiple sclerosis. Zh Nevrol Psikhiatr Im S S Korsakova. 2017;117:41–7.

96. Onorati F, Regalia G, Caborni C, et al. Multicenter clinical assessment of improved wearable multimodal convulsive seizure detectors. Epilepsia. 2017;58:1870–9.

97. Arends J, Thijs RD, Gutter T, et al. Multimodal nocturnal seizure detection in a residential care setting: a long-term prospective trials. Neurology. 2018;91:e2010–9.

98. Lynch BM, Nguyen NH, Moore MM, et al. A randomized controlled trial of a wearable technology-based intervention for increasing moderate to vigorous physical activity and reducing sedentary behavior in breast cancer survivors: the ACTIVATE trial. Cancer. 2019;125:2846–55.

99. van Blarigan EL, Chan H, van Loon K, et al. Self-monitoring and reminder text messages to increase physical activity in colorectal cancer survivors (smart pace): a pilot randomized controlled trial. BMC Cancer. 2019;19:218. https://doi.org/10.1186/s12885-019-5427-5.

100. Gresham G, Hendifar AE, Spiegel B, et al. Wearable activity monitors to assess performance status and predict clinical outcomes in advanced cancer patients. NPJ Digit Med. 2018;1:27. https://doi.org/10.1038/s41746-018-0032-6.

101. Marcano-Olivier MI, Horne PJ, Viktor S, et al. Using nudges to promote healthy food choices in the school dining room: a systematic review of previous investigations. J School Health. 2019; https://doi.org/10.1111/josh.12861.

102. Borenstein J, Arkin R. Robotic nudges: the ethics of engineering a more socially just human being. Sci Eng Ethics. 2016;22:31–46.

103. Tagliabue M, Squatrito V, Presti G. Models of cognition and their applications in behavioral economics: a conceptual framework for nudging derived from behavior analysis and relational frame theory. Front Psychol. 2019;10:2418. https://doi.org/10.3389/fpsyg.2019.02418.

104. Möllenkamp M, Zeppernick M, Schreyögg J. The effectiveness of nudges in improving the self-management of patients with chronic diseases: a systematic literature review. Health Policy. 2019;123:1199–209.

Guidelines for Developing Patient Education Materials

Anne Findeis and Magdalyn Patyk

Abbreviations

ADA	Americans with Disabilities Act
AHRQ	Agency for Healthcare Research and Quality
AIDS	Acquired immunodeficiency syndrome
AV	Audiovisual
CDC	Centers for Disease Control and Prevention
CHAT	Conversational Health Literacy Assessment Tool
CMS	Centers for Medicare and Medicaid Services
CT	Computed tomography
HCP	Healthcare professional
HHS	US Department of Health and Human Services
HIV	Human immunodeficiency virus
HTML	Hyper text markup language
IS	Internet services or strategies
IT	Information technology
NIDDK	National Institute for Diabetes and Digestive and Kidney Diseases
NVS	Newest Vital Sign
PEMAT	Patient Education Materials Assessment Tool
RTF	Rich text format
SAHL	Short Assessment of Health Literacy
TOFHLA	Test of Functional Health Literacy in Adults

Lifestyle Medicine and Patient Education

The practice of lifestyle medicine embraces the tenet that certain lifestyle changes can lead to better health, reduce the risk of developing specific health problems, and help those with chronic illnesses manage their conditions with fewer complications, thus improving quality of life. Various strategies are used to achieve these goals, including counseling, motivational interviewing, and shared decision-making [1].

Patient education is integral to achieving health goals and may be described as a planned activity initiated by a healthcare professional (HCP) whose goal is to convey information, attitude, and skills, with the intention to change behavior, promote compliance with therapy and treatments, thereby improving overall health [2]. This planned activity includes the following [3, 4].

- Assessing:
  - Knowledge, attitudes, and beliefs related to the pertinent health topic
  - Learning priorities and concerns
  - Barriers to learning (such as physical, cognitive, psychosocial, and low literacy)
- Planning educational interventions by:
  - Utilizing information gathered during assessment
  - Setting mutually agreed upon measurable goals with specific attainable actions
- Implementing a plan, which:
  - Engages the learner(s)
  - Employs effective communication strategies, materials, and resources
- Evaluating learning outcomes, such as:
  - Knowledge, skill attainment, and problem-solving abilities
  - Goal attainment and adherence to behavioral changes

A key factor in goal achievement is patient engagement. Engaged patients are actively involved in managing their health and making decisions that lead to better outcomes. However, engaged patients must also have the knowledge, skills, ability, and willingness to do so [5]. The use of patient education materials plays an important role in acquiring the necessary knowledge and skills as well as promoting engagement. When used as part of an educational program, effective use of educational materials can help to promote

A. Findeis (Retired) (✉) · M. Patyk
Patient Education Department, Northwestern Memorial Hospital, Chicago, IL, USA

self-efficacy, which has been shown to correlate with positive attitudes and outcomes, including behavioral changes [6, 7]. Not only do these materials inform about specific health conditions, but they also help patients understand how to reduce the risks of developing certain diseases or their complications, make important healthcare decisions, learn new skills and problem-solving strategies to manage their health or medical condition, and monitor or track lifestyle changing behaviors.

Educational materials in lifestyle medicine that effectively individualize information are more likely to help patients understand the importance to their own care. This is particularly useful if materials are culturally relevant [8, 9]. Educational materials that also incorporate a multimodal approach invoking more than one of the senses (visual, auditory, or tactile) help engage those with different learning styles and have been found to improve recognition and memory [10]. Moreover, educational materials are most effective when they reinforce verbal explanations, rather than replace personal communication or relying strictly on memory [11]. Verbal information is often recalled incorrectly or even forgotten when patients experience the stress of a new diagnosis or a need for health-related behavioral change. This was found to be especially true among the elderly or those with low health literacy [12].

Patient Education and Health Literacy

Health literacy has been described as the degree to which one has the ability to obtain, process, and understand health information and services in order to make appropriate health decisions. Health literacy is necessary before one can become engaged in making health-related decisions, especially those that improve self-care behaviors [5].

It has been estimated that over 25% of US adults may have low health literacy and over 41% may have a poor understanding of numeracy [13]. Low health literacy has been associated with high rates of emergency room visits, hospitalizations, and even increased mortality [14]. Thus, enhancing health literacy has been the focus of developing patient educational materials since the Plain Writing Act was signed into law in 2010, requiring government developed materials to be written using simple, easily understood language [15].

Types of Health Literacy

Health literacy is comprised of several components, each of which contributes to comprehension of information and has implications for how educational information is not only developed but also delivered.

- "Aural" literacy refers to the ability to understand what is said. Those with limited literacy or health literacy were found to have difficulty accurately recalling verbal medical instructions [12]. Studies have linked low aural literacy not only to poor asthma management [16] but also to poor health outcomes [17].
- "Prose" literacy is the ability to understand written information. How well this is accomplished depends on how material is written and may be affected by the reader's educational background. Adults in the USA may read as low as 3 to 5 grade levels below their completed grade level [18].
- "Numeracy" refers to the ability to understand numerical concepts. This can affect perception of risk data, interpretation of food labels, and ability to engage in health management behaviors. Those with limited numeracy skills were found to be more readily influenced by how numbers are formatted and presented, and may over- or underestimate their significance. In one study, less numerate subjects perceived medication risks to be higher when frequency formats were shown; alternatively, percentage formats were perceived to be less risky [19]. Numeracy and reading comprehension do not necessarily correlate [20].
- "eHealth" Literacy is the ability to locate, comprehend, and evaluate online health information in order to make informed health decisions. Those that rate high in self-efficacy and eHealth literacy are more likely to be engaged in health-promoting behaviors and managing chronic conditions [21]. A 2016 analysis of health information-seeking behavior among adults in the USA indicated that those who were younger, had better internet skills, and were more educated were more likely to use the internet to seek out health information [22].

Assessing Health Literacy

Understanding health literacy among individual patients or patient populations can guide the HCP to select or develop appropriately designed patient education materials or teaching strategies. Both HCPs and researchers have long grappled with effective ways to assess health literacy and have used both formally validated tools and informal methods. Each has certain limitations and usefulness may vary. For example, anxiety for any reason, as well as the stress of taking a timed test or feelings of shame if dyslexia or other limitations to understanding verbal or written information are present, may adversely affect willingness to participate and impact the assessment [23, 24].

Validated Assessment Tools

Certain tools are more likely to be used by researchers yet may be useful to HCPs who wish to measure specific types of literacy. The Test of Functional Health Literacy in Adults (TOFHLA) measures numeracy and the ability to understand medical information [25, 26]. The TOFHLA can be purchased from Peppercornbooks.com. In addition, the Short Assessment of Health Literacy (SAHL) assesses understanding of medical terms and can be acquired free from ahrq.gov/professionals/quality-patient-safety/quality-resources/tools/literacy/index.html (Accessed on 7 Mar 2020). Other tools were developed for use primarily in the clinical healthcare setting. The Conversational Health Literacy Assessment Tool (CHAT) asks about health seeking, health promotion, self-care behaviors, and support [27]. Also, the Newest Vital Sign (NVS) primarily assesses numeracy by reading a specific food label and performing 6 math calculations. The NVS can be a valuable aid when counseling patients on diet modification and is available free in English and Spanish from https://www.pfizer.com/health/literacy/public-policy-researchers/nvs-toolkit (Accessed 3 Sept 2019).

Informal Assessment

Assumptions about literacy or health literacy cannot be based on appearance, verbal articulation, or information from forms. Instead, certain personal factors and behaviors may provide clues to health literacy (Table 14.1) [23]. Another assessment strategy is to use open-ended questions to elicit understanding, either before the teaching encounter to determine prior knowledge, attitudes, beliefs (e.g., "Tell me what foods you like that you think would be healthy for you.") or afterwards to determine understanding of new information (e.g., "Just to be sure I explained it clearly, tell me how much salt is in one serving as shown on this food label.").

Table 14.1 Factors affecting health literacy

Age greater than 65

Vision or hearing deficits

Less than a 12th grade education, or English as a secondary language

Poor reading skills. Patients may offer excuses when given written materials, for example, "I'll read it when I get home" or "I forgot my glasses"

Incomplete or inaccurate responses on health forms

Noncompliance with medications, appointments, testing, or referrals

Lack of knowledge about previous instructions such as medication regimens, diets, or care guidelines

Incorrectly answers healthcare-related questions or responds to questions in a way to avoid follow up questions

A lack of interest or focus during a teaching session; does not seek clarification

It is also important to point out that even well-educated patients can have trouble understanding or applying health information. When faced with a new diagnosis, a need to alter their lifestyle, or problems at home or work, patients may experience undue stress that impairs learning. Materials that effectively reinforce verbal information, and are easy to read and understand, can help offset this. It is also important to differentiate between low health literacy and a mental health disorder, cognitive decline, or developmental disability.

Patient Education Materials: What to Consider

Who Is the Intended Audience?

Identify the specific target patient population, if possible. This may include demographic, socioeconomic, ethnic and cultural background information, as well as patients with certain types of medical conditions. This may affect the type of educational material to be developed. For example, the young may respond more favorably to interactive videos or games. The elderly, or those with cognitive or literacy limitations, may have difficulty grasping complex information or using technologically advanced delivery modes.

What Type of Information Is Desired?

Identify the key topics to deliver for the specific target patient population. What purpose will these materials fulfill? What type of consequent behavioral changes will be incorporated into the educational programs?

What Resources Currently Exist to Meet Learning Needs?

It is very useful to first identify materials that are readily available. Many institutions use vendors who specialize in delivering health information on topics that may already meet the specific needs desired. Moreover, many of these materials are freely accessible on the internet. Table 14.2 lists common websites that contain content developed specifically for patients. Most include materials in Spanish and many offer resources in other formats, such as videos, podcasts, infographics, audio files, brochures for printing or ordering, and more.

Numerous mobile health applications (apps) that target health maintenance and disease management are also

Table 14.2 Internet resources for chronic diseases and health education[a]

Resource	Website	Key topics
American Cancer Society	www.cancer.org	Types of cancer, treatments, and support; healthy lifestyle tips
American Diabetes Association	www.diabetes.org	Aspects of self-management
American Heart Association	www.heart.org	Healthy eating, lifestyle, fitness, stress management, tobacco cessation
American Lung Association	www.lung.org/lung-health-and-diseases/lung-disease-lookup/	Asthma, chronic lung diseases, pulmonary, fibrosis, tobacco cessation
Anxiety and Depression Association of America	https://adaa.org	Management tips, support, and resources; concurrent disorders (e.g., post-traumatic stress disorders, substance abuse, eating disorders)
Centers for Disease Control	www.cdc.gov	Numerous health promotional topics, and prevention including tobacco cessation
HIV	www.hiv.gov http://hivinsite.ucsf.edu/	HIV and AIDS topics Lifestyle management
Liver Foundation	https://liverfoundation.org/for-patients/resources/	Various liver disorders, including non-alcoholic fatty liver disease
Medline Plus	www.medlineplus.gov	Wide variety of health and disease topics
National Cancer Institute	www.cancer.gov www.smokefree.gov	Prevention, treatment, screening, and research for all types of cancer Tobacco cessation
National Institute of Diabetes, Digestive and Kidney Disorders	www.niddk.nih.gov	Diabetes, kidney disease, crohn's, celiac diseases, irritable bowel syndrome, GERD
National Institute of Mental Health	https://www.nimh.nih.gov	*Healthtopics* covers a variety of disorders, treatments, resources, and support topics
Nutrition	www.nutrition.gov	Diet supplements, nutrition for AIDS, cancer, diabetes, digestive disorders, heart health, kidney disease, obesity; shopping, cooking, meal planning, food labels

[a]All websites accessed 26 Aug 2019. Abbreviations: *AIDS* acquired immunodeficiency syndrome, *GERD* gastro-esophageal reflux disease, *HIV* human immunodeficiency virus

Table 14.3 Mobile apps[a]

App name (manufacturer)	Key topics
Asthma MD (Dr. Sam Pejham & Asthma MD)	Asthma management system tracks asthma symptoms, triggers, medications, and peak flow meter use
Bellybio Interactive Breathing (Relaxline)	Tracks and graphs deep breathing to promote relaxation
FitBit	Wireless wearable activity and fitness monitor tracks heart rate, sleep quality, and personal activity metrics
Glucose Buddy (Azumio)	Diabetes management and monitoring tool tracks blood sugar trends, medications, and eating habits
My Fitness Pal	Tracks diet and activity; gaming elements motivate users; caloric and nutritional recommendations are based on weight loss goals
Quit Pal	Offers goal setting, motivational tips, and reminders to promote tobacco cessation; tracks progress, cravings, and milestones
Sleep Time (Azumio)	Tracks sleep movements and patterns to aid insomniacs

[a]Listing and discussion of commercial products should not be considered as an endorsement

of treatment options [29]. Apps have also been developed to support tobacco cessation [30] and promote positive changes in lifestyle improvement and health behavior [31]. In addition, food tracking apps can be valuable for those with diabetes or attempting to adhere to weight management programs [32, 33].

Mobile health apps combined with wearable technologies such as electronic tracking devices have facilitated the self-monitoring process and collation of data which help users see their real time progress towards goal attainment (Table 14.3). Electronic prompts ("nudges") remind users to engage in specific activities to improve adherence to their plan of care. These are important first steps; however, tracking alone may not be enough. Prompts to motivate and engage users using problem-solving and planning opportunities may help extend short-term activity changes into long-term behaviors [32, 34]. However, long-term usage and effects may be hard to estimate. In one study, about 45% of the subjects had stopped using health apps for various reasons including loss of interest and cost concerns [35]. All apps and websites should be explored before recommending them to patients. For instance, a 2015 review of 147 asthma apps found that 45 out of the 46 apps offering inhaler instructions omitted or misstated at least one step [36]. Of note, most, but not all, mobile apps or devices for self-management do not fall under the Federal Drug Administration regulatory approval process (https://www.fda.gov/medicaldevices/digitalhealth/mobilemedicalapplications; Accessed 3 Sept 2019).

available. They have been effectively used to promote medication compliance among patients with diabetes, hypertension, and heart disease [28], and also inform cancer patients

Are There Any Other Tools or Resources to Consider?

The American College of Lifestyle Medicine (www.lifestylemedicine.org; Accessed 2 Aug 2019) provides a variety of resources to help HCPs in their efforts to support lifestyle changes on the topics of diet, smoking, exercise, alcohol abuse, heart disease, arthritis, and more.

Is There a Need to Develop New Materials?

With the variety of resources available, why develop new ones? It may be necessary if existing content is too general or not specific enough for the target population. It may also be necessary if the content is not in accord with the practice needs or goals, not positive or engaging enough, or not "patient friendly" (i.e., written more for HCPs, uses complex terminology, or has other features making it difficult for the general public to understand). Also, existing educational materials not easily accessible to learners will need to be re-developed. Naturally, any educational materials that are outdated, inaccurate, or incomplete will need to be refreshed.

Should a Needs Assessment Be Conducted?

In some cases, assessing the need for new materials may be desirable if there is doubt about what resources are needed or the usefulness of existing resources. A needs assessment can help determine the target audience, messaging, or preferred delivery systems. One may also be required to apply for funding, either for resource development or for the needs assessment itself.

In developing a needs assessment, formulate the goals, the information desired, the amount of time required, and staff support to develop, conduct, and/or collate the data. Create questions that align specifically with goals and realistic options. Determine who will be asked to participate, ensuring an adequate number and representation to yield useful data. Finally, analyze the data and determine the action plan and type of materials to be developed [40]. There are 3 formats of needs assessments:

- *Key informant interviews*. Detailed information may be acquired through in-depth discussions with key stakeholders who have the knowledge or experience needed to address the topics. Pre-scripted questions provide a framework to help guide the interview process.
- *Surveys or questionnaires*. Questions should be written simply and clearly in a format easily understood by the general public. Test the survey on a sample group composed of a population similar to the survey recipients to determine if instructions and questions are clear enough to ensure accurate responses.
- *Focus groups*. These are pre-selected groups that engage in a focused discussion by a facilitator. The groups include representative samples of the target patient population, in order to understand the culture, needs, and resource development priorities. Focus groups are useful when information is needed that cannot be easily acquired through other means.

What Resources May Be Needed to Develop New Materials [38, 41, 42]?

- *Content experts*. These include dietitians, physiotherapists, mental health experts, or other HCPs, and depending on specific needs, any one or subset may be critical to ensure content meets current standards.
- *Writers*. Selecting people well experienced in developing patient education materials may be desirable depending on the quantity of materials to be developed and amount of time estimated to develop them. Scripting will be needed for any audiovisual (AV) materials. For special visuals, a designer, photographer, or videographer may be employed.
- *Budget and time allotments*. These are vital to the development and implementation of new materials and may require administrative support. Costs related to staffing and the purchase of supplies and equipment needed to produce materials must be determined and are strongly affected by the type of materials desired and the delivery method. For example, if iPods or computers will be used to share AV materials with patients in the office, additional hardware and software costs as well as viewing/storage space and security may be concerns. For print materials, the nature of use will affect cost. For example, a handy pocket-sized reference guide or a bound booklet may cost more than a tracking log or food guide.
- *Size*. For printed materials, page size should fit the intended use. Note that this will also affect writing and formatting, as well as the purchase of non-standard sized paper.
- *Printed cover or visual designs*. Users should find the cover appealing with an intent that is easy to grasp. Other graphics or illustrations should be easily understood, and this may involve additional design work.
- *Binding and paper type*. This can involve the use of heavy paper or laminated plastic.
- *Print on demand versus bulk ordering*. This will affect ongoing costs and storage needs.

- *AV materials*. If planning to develop AV materials such as videos, consider the cost, personnel, and environmental aspects. For a professional look, hiring a videographer to film a video may furnish a professional look and be desirable, but this can be quite costly. Various questions need to be posed. Who will be in the video? Patients? Healthcare staff? Will there be a narrator? The videographer should not be an actor or narrator (unless audio is to be added after filming). Having a director is useful to guide the filming, for example, to repeat an action, zoom in for close-ups, or stop if a correction is needed. Consider who will be filmed and what their roles will be. Their availability will need to be coordinated. In general, it is recommended to acquire a signed written consent by the actors permitting use of their images in an AV to be shared on a public website. One must also consider cost and acquisition of supplies or materials needed, such as products used for demonstrations or a good quality microphone or video recorder. For video filming, adequate space, good lighting, and availability are needed. If recording audio at the same time, privacy is needed to avoid extraneous noise. The filming background should be a neutral environment and devoid of potential distractions that may appear in the final footage. Investing in a video editing tool such as Microsoft Windows Movie Maker should be considered if within the budget. Other tool options include: Go! Animate (for cartoons), Google Story Builder (for video stories), or Stupeflix (to animate pictures or transform videos into a slide show).
- *Institutional design requirements*. Departments within one's institution may impose specific editorial, formatting, or design requirements for online or mobile device accessible materials, whether print or audiovisual.
- *Translators or a translation service*. This will be needed if materials need to be translated into another language. It is best to determine the values, health beliefs, and cultural perspectives of the target population before educational material development. This can be done as part of a needs assessment that also incorporates potential variations among subgroups of minority populations. Plan to use a translator that is qualified (preferably certified) and familiar with the cultural and linguistic nuances of the intended learners. A translated document should reflect the intended message; it should never be translated literally. If the source document is not written in simple, plain language, this will carry over to the translated document. Back translations (i.e., translation back to English) help ensure the material conveys an accurate message and tone and is best done by someone other than the original translator. Word processing or publishing software may be needed to ensure correct language characters or diacritical marks are used to ensure proper meaning if a professional translation service is not used [41, 42].

What Kinds of Materials Are Desired?

There are a number of options available to meet the needs and preferences of different cultures and ages.

Written or Print Materials

Brochures or handouts are most commonly used to educate patients and families. They are generally easier to produce or acquire than other types of materials. Effective learning depends on having the required reading skills to understand the content, whether in English or one's native tongue.

Fotonovelas have been studied in the Latino/Hispanic population as a culturally engaging way to communicate health information and desired health behaviors. Stories whose characters have relatable medical conditions help motivate patients in taking a greater interest in managing their own health [43]. Fotonovelas have been used to promote healthy eating [44] and address human immunodeficiency virus (HIV) precautions [43], depression, and mental health stigma [45, 46]. In one story, characters served as role models to target the stigma of depression, concerns about treatment, how they overcame barriers to seeking help, and the supportive role of family and friends. Examples of successful treatment served to reinforce positive health messaging as did the counter-examples of those failing to seek help resulting in negative consequences [46]. Another story of how a patient with diabetes can role model healthy lifestyle behavior is provided at https://www.cdc.gov/diabetes/ndep/toolkits/do-it-for-them.html (Accessed 3 Sept 2019). The key to creating a Fotonovela is character and script development. The process used to develop a Fotonovela includes identifying key messages and stakeholders, and creating a conversational tone, but also creating a culturally meaningful story line, writing the script based on the purpose and key messages to be delivered, and assigning realistic roles to the characters before selecting or developing illustrations. Photos or comic/graphic art type illustrations can be used when creating Fotonovelas. Photos can also be transformed into comic art via apps such as Comic Life, Comic Strip It Pro, Comic and Meme Creator, or Strip Designer [47].

Graphic novels refer to comic book style materials and are similar to fotonovelas as a way to model healthy behaviors. Although used primarily for children or teenagers, one such novel showcases the breast cancer experience for women [48]. However, if planning to use this format for an adult population, care must be taken to ensure they will be taken seriously. Some adults dismiss these as a source of valuable information, believing they do not address serious topics [49].

Visual aids combine text with graphs, illustrations, and/or pictures to visualize the key message and achieve meaningful learning. This may be helpful even if the learner has cognitive or literacy limitations [50], although person-ally explaining images at the time they are presented to the patient may be needed to help prevent misunderstandings [51]. Pictograms are images designed to convey a specific concept, instruction, or warning. Among the most familiar are restroom, highway, and *No Smoking* signs. In healthcare, pictograms have been used to communicate the steps of med-ication and inhaler usage, especially among those with low literacy. In one integrative review examining 11 studies, 10 showed improved learning with the use of pictograms; how-ever, the greatest effects were seen among those that received additional written or verbal information [51]. Pictographs also use symbols or figures to convey data in a chart, graph, or as icon arrays. Icon arrays have been used as an effec-tive way to communicate risk data [52]. Human-type figures (e.g., restroom icons) are more conducive to understanding cardiac risk data than those using blocks or ovals, which had a lower recall rate [53]. However, subjects' numeracy and graph literacy abilities play a key role in comprehending risk data [54].

Infographics combine limited text with images to commu-nicate information in a colorful and concise way (Fig. 14.1). They convey risk data, show nutritional information, and lead to better recall, especially in younger patients [8]. Well-designed infographics support comprehension and motivate health-promoting behaviors [55]. Special consideration may be needed with the elderly or those with low literacy [56]. For example, using simple line drawings with low levels of detail offer fewer distracting elements, making it easier to grasp the messaging [50, 57]. One source for data is www.healthdata.gov (Accessed 3 Sept 2019). Software such as Microsoft® PowerPoint® may be used to create charts or graphs. Online design tools such as Canva.com, Venngage.com, or Piktochart.com offer a step-by-step guide to creating infographics.

Other tools that may help engage and motivate patients include the use of self-management forms, such as food dia-ries or logs to record weight, blood pressure, or pain.

Audiovisual Materials

Videos are a common medium for educating patients. They are an ideal way to demonstrate specific procedures for immediate learning and may also help promote retention, even among those with low literacy [58, 59]. How video content is presented is a significant determinant of behav-ior change and outcomes – didactic presentations being least effective [60]. Videos may be acquired through ven-dors specializing in health education videos or accessed on professional or commercial websites that illustrate product use, procedures, or other topics of interest. Podcasts are audio or video files that can be downloaded and played on a mobile device, I-Pad, or computer. To meet specific

Protect Your Heart!

Heart attacks cause over 600,000 deaths each year. Start with these tips to keep your heart healthy.

Eat Healthy

Follow a diet low in fat that includes:
- Lean meats
- Fresh fruits and vegetables
- Whole grain cereals and breads
- Low fat dairy products

Keep Active

Aim to include at least 20 to 30 minutes each day of moderate activity that is safe for you. Examples include:
- Walking or running
- Bicycling
- Swimming
- Dancing
Start out slow and gradually do more.
Joining a gym, health or fitness club can help you keep on track.

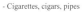

Avoid Tobacco

If you use any type of tobacco, quit!
If you've never used it, don't start!
This includes use of:
- Cigarettes, cigars, pipes
- Any type of smokeless tobacco
Ask your healthcare provider for help or go to www.smokefree.gov

Reduce Your Risk

Lower your chance of having a heart attack. Work with your healthcare provider to manage any health conditions or concerns, such as:
- High cholesterol
- High blood pressure
- Diabetes
- Weight control
- Stress

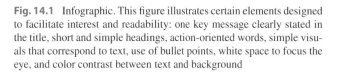

Source: Created by author for illustration purposes.

Fig. 14.1 Infographic. This figure illustrates certain elements designed to facilitate interest and readability: one key message clearly stated in the title, short and simple headings, action-oriented words, simple visu-als that correspond to text, use of bullet points, white space to focus the eye, and color contrast between text and background

needs, these may be self-developed. To create a video, podcast, audio file, or other AV, the following need to be considered once the topic and intended audience has been determined [61–63].

Video Length

The behavior or learning objective being targeted will affect the content and length of the AV and may need to be divided into several segments if too long to avoid information overload. In general, 5 to 8 minutes is ideal for a video. Longer than 9 minutes risks loss of attention, unless the time is needed to adequately demonstrate and teach a skill.

Script

Create a script following the conversational, Plain Language writing guidelines and also:

- Emphasize desired behaviors and benefits to achieve the learning goal.
- Incorporate interactive elements such as a quiz, decision-making options or problem-solving scenarios if feasible and appropriate to topic.
- Clearly indicate in the script what visuals correspond to the wording. This is helpful during filming if audio needs to be coordinated with visuals or if audio is added to the video after filming.
- Practice reading the script out loud. Get feedback on how it sounds to the listener. Speak slowly, especially if the AV is to be translated or dubbed. In Spanish, it may take 1½ times longer to speak the text.

Rehearse

Set up everything that will be needed for filming and do a dry run (or two) first. If the narrator is off camera, they can read during filming (but it shouldn't sound like reading). If on camera, they may wish to read from cue cards to ensure a smooth flow. Modulate voice to create a conversational tone.

Appearance

Those appearing in a video should wear comfortable clothing and appear appropriate to the situation. End users viewing the video should not be distracted by irrelevant details.

Filming

Allow plenty of time as several takes may be needed. Also, it is best to film everything at once to avoid changes in lighting, background, or appearance that would create a fragmented look and distraction in the final AV. This is especially true in regard to the actors' appearance. Depending on the topic, it may be desirable to film from different vantage points. It is more efficient to edit out footage after filming than to repeat the filming process. Upload final raw footage to the computer for editing. Save original footage separately from any edited version. During editing, key points may be posted into the AV to provide emphasis, but without distracting from the audio. For example, if discussing low-sodium foods, it may be hard to remember individual items. Showing a list of several foods on screen along with hearing and seeing them helps reinforce the information and aid in recall. Software such as PowerPoint may be used to embed written content into the AV.

Distribution

How will the AV be shared? If it will be embedded into an institution's website, the Internet Services (IS) or Information Technology (IT) department may impose criteria or limitations that may affect filming or posting. A readable transcript and an audio overview of the video should also be included.

Educational Video (Serious) Games

Educational video games are innovative patient education tools designed to entertain as they educate. As variables are manipulated in the game, users make behavior-based decisions. When game constructs help the user attain competence, become autonomous, and relate behavior to concepts in the game, the chance of success in achieving the desired behavior goals is increased [64, 65]. Serious games have been shown to increase knowledge and self-management in young patients with chronic conditions [66], cancer [67], and diabetes [64]. Interactive video games have also been used as decision-making aids in men with prostate cancer [68]. Gamesforchange.org (Accessed on 4 Sept 2019) is a nonprofit organization that supports concept development, strategic planning, vendor vetting, and consultation on all phases of patient education video game production and publishing. Another resource is seriousgamesforhealth.com (Accessed on 4 Sept 2019). Integrating the following guiding principles into game planning are believed to maximize game effectiveness [69–71].

Attention. Design elements such as graphics and sound should serve to motivate the user and keep their attention span. Characters, storyline, situations, and resolutions should be realistic and relatable. Avatars that are interesting help personalize and engage the user. Antagonists challenging the protagonist (representing the patient) depict issues of concern. Use different avatars for different roles. Ensure avatars enhance learning and not distract from the messaging.

Active learning. The user must interact with the game elements for learning to take place. Incorporate goal setting, goal monitoring, and problem-solving skills into any game designed to promote self-management. Avatars can guide users through the learning experience as surrogate instructors or as simulated learners.

Feedback. This is most effective when it is task oriented, allowing the user to immediately see the results of actions. Role modeling can embody coping, problem-solving, and decision-making scenarios. Choices should result in immediate feedback.

Consolidation. Learning and retention depend on game design that promotes concentration, integrates repetition, and allows pacing of new information to avoid information overload. Consider users' age, gender, and culture when writing the script.

For more information, Graafland et al. [72] cite specific criteria related to game description, rationale, functionality, validity, and data protection in great detail. Animations can be used in videos and interactive video games, and are of interest in developing materials for those with limited literacy or English skills. They are widely used to depict medical procedures and anatomical functions, such as blood flow, but can also be used to demonstrate self-care procedures. However, subjects who are cognitively limited were found to need extra time to process animation frames [50]. Use caution if using animated graphs to convey risk data, especially if patients are not skilled in understanding these depictions. In one study, Zikmund-Fisher et al. [73] found that animated graphs were not only unhelpful, but sometimes detrimental when subjects selected riskier treatments based on incorrect interpretations of the animations.

How Will Materials Be Delivered?

In addition to physically handing them to the patient, there are different ways to deliver educational materials to patients, especially as computer and interactive technologies become more advanced, available, and routine in day-to-day life. One advantage to using internet distribution methods is the ease and low cost of updates. Still, there are segments of the population not technologically savvy. Low computer or internet literacy skills could impede accessing electronic resources, which creates an additional training need. Before developing materials, consider which delivery methods would best suit the target population. In fact, multiple delivery modes may be considered to accommodate those who may have access or usage limitations or preferences.

The *"Cloud"* may be a convenient and relatively inexpensive way to house and distribute materials, which are maintained by a computing or data storage provider, such as Amazon, Google Drive, Dropbox, Backblaze, or Box.com. One may wish to consider whether a private, community, public, or hybrid infrastructure is best, once database storage needs are ascertained. Content would be easily retrieved or viewed by anyone with access and is not dependent on institutional affiliations.

Patient portals to electronic health records allow patients to access personalized health information via computer or mobile device. Healthcare professionals will need to collaborate with their institution's IS/IT departments in order to determine feasibility of installing desired materials for effi-cient opening, downloading, and/or printing by end users. Policy or licensing restrictions may exist that limit adding brochures, videos, or graphic files. As with any internet distribution method, usage depends on the patient's ability and willingness to access materials. One study tracking the use of sleep-related videos (insomnia, sleep apnea, and treatments) showed that only 20% of videos prescribed by physicians via portals were accessed by patients [74].

Computers based/I-Pads can facilitate viewing educational materials at home or in the healthcare setting, either by downloading files from the internet, loading discs, or installing permanent software applications [8]. One study effectively delivered low literacy, culturally appropriate materials to an underserved population even though training to use the computers was required [75].

Mobile devices (Smartphones) and apps can facilitate internet access by the patient. However, certain formatting and design elements need to be considered when developing these types of educational materials.

Getting Started with the Development Process

Once a decision is made to develop new materials, then the focus or goal of each new tool should be determined. Will it be to increase knowledge? Change attitudes? Acquire new skills? Learn problem-solving techniques? Or enhance decision-making? Decisions need to be made regarding the key messages and what specific behavior changes are being targeted.

Experts suggest that patient education materials be written at or below an eighth grade reading level as most people with a high school education (or higher) are comfortable reading at this level [38, 76]. Using Plain Language writing guidelines are usually adequate to achieve this. However, if the materials need to reach a patient population that is likely to read at a low reading level, consider writing to a fourth to sixth grade level.

Readability Assessment

As materials are being developed, a readability assessment tool can guide the writer to reassess writing style and vocabulary in order to improve readability. The Flesch-Kincaid Reading Grade Level and the Flesch Reading Ease tools are options found in some word processing programs such as Microsoft® Word. Reading ease is rated between 0 and 100. The higher the score, the easier the text is to read. A score greater than 60 is desirable. For accuracy in using a reading assessment tool, use paragraphs of at least 100 words that consist of full sentences. Do not include bulleted lists, headings, phrases, or abbreviations as these will result in inaccurate scores. Multisyllabic words and long sentences will result in a higher grade level and lower reading ease score, even if the words are considered common and easily understood (such as "family," "important," or "information"). This does not mean they need to be changed. Conversely, a low reading grade level does not necessarily mean that content is well written or easy to read and understand. Readabilityformulas. com (Accessed on 3 Aug 2019) provides more detail and access to readability formulas.

The Patient Education Materials Assessment Tools (PEMAT) can also guide production. Developed by the Agency for Healthcare Research and Quality (AHRQ), PEMAT is based on Plain Language writing principles and focuses on understandability and actionability of the content (https://www.ahrq.gov/; Accessed on 22 Aug 2019). PEMAT consists of a 26-item tool to assess printable materials, and a 25-item tool for AV materials that rate content, organization, wording, layout and design, and use of visual aids. These can be used to evaluate self-developed materials, as well as materials acquired elsewhere.

Plain Language Writing Guidelines

Plain Language is a communication style designed to provide information that is easy to read and understand for readers of nearly all literacy levels, thus making it easier to remember and use. Verbiage, syntax, formatting, and design elements all play a role in readability and engaging one's interest. The following Plain Language Writing Guidelines are recommended by the Centers for Medicare and Medicaid Services (CMS) and the Centers for Disease Control and Prevention (CDC), and may be applied not only to print materials, but also website content, scripting for videos, and other types of materials [38, 41, 42].

Writing Style

Use familiar, commonly used words instead of medical, scientific, technical terms or jargon, for example, "high blood pressure" instead of "hypertension." Explain or define any medical terms if they are needed. In general, short words (1 to 2 syllables) are easier to understand since longer words (and sentences) are associated with higher reading levels. However, there are some exceptions, for example, "information" is more readily understood by most people than "data." It is also important to "Keep it simple!" Use clear, focused messaging limited to what patients need to know. This is especially important when materials are one pagers such as Infographics. A casual, conversational style, especially for audible materials, creates a more natural, friendly tone that is more inviting and easier to read or listen to. Active voice is easier to read than passive voice. For example, use "Your doctor can explain..." instead of "This will be explained by your doctor." Action oriented verbs, such as "Take," "Lift,"

"Walk," and so on help ensure clarity. Words that require a judgment call should be clarified, such as "good," "normal," "adequate," "excessive," "small," "more," and so on. For example, stating "Take long walks (at least 15 minutes or more)" is acceptable. One should also keep lists down to 3 to 7 items and use bullets instead of listing items within a paragraph. Consider using subheadings to organize longer lists into manageable sections. If acronyms and abbreviations are likely to be familiar to the reader in patient education materials, use the initials first, and then write it out, for example, "HIV (Human Immunodeficiency Virus)." On the other hand, if the acronym or abbreviation is less familiar, or if there could be more than one meaning, then write it out first and then provide the initials, for example, "Abdominal Aortic Aneurysm (AAA)." Lastly, for medications, use both generic and brand names.

Numeracy

The simplest way to convey statistics or risk data is to use general words, such as most, many, or few, with percentages in parentheses; for example, "The chance of getting cancer from a CT scan is very slight (less than 1%)." Also, the word "chance" is deemed more easily understood than "risk of." Use numerals instead of writing out the numbers, "7" instead of "seven", as numbers are easier to process. If unsure about the reader's preference, use both imperial and metric labels, for example, 1 cup (240 ml), 2 teaspoons (10 ml), or 10 lbs. (4.5 kg).

Organization

Begin with the purpose of the material, for example, "This handout will explain how to limit the amount of salt in your diet." There should be one main message for a short handout (1–2 pages) or video (5–6 minutes) and no more than 4 main messages for longer materials. For example, a short handout might focus on stress management; a longer one on diabetes diet management with key points that address food shopping, reading labels, counting carbohydrates, and eating out. If relevant, order content chronologically. It is critical to prioritize. Place the most important topics near the beginning of each section, and very important points in a box or insert for emphasis. Key points can also be summarized at the end to reinforce important messages. This is a good way to introduce repetition without seeming redundant. Headings and subheadings can be incorporated to separate information into meaningful chunks to facilitate comprehension, but with care to avoid distraction with the added detail. Use advance organizers to introduce new information and provide context. For example, "To add fiber in your diet, eat fresh fruits and vegetables" instead of "Eat fresh fruits and vegetables to add fiber to your diet."

Text Design

Font sizes of 12 to 14 should be used, with no more than 1 to 2 simple font types per document. For clarity, heading font sizes should be at least 2 points larger than in the text. It is preferable to avoid *italic fonts* and ALL CAPS, which are more challenging to read. However, **bold** fonts can be used sparingly for emphasis, and are preferred over the use of underlined words. Contrast between font and page background color is also important and should be maximized. Black font on white background is best.

Lines and Spacing

Use left justification only. Including right justification causes uneven spacing and may confuse poor readers. Sentence lengths of 10 to 15 words are preferred, since sentences longer than 20 words may be harder for some readers to process. Shorter sentences are fine if used judiciously. However, long paragraphs of very short sentences may sound choppy yet may be necessary if writing for a fourth grade reading level or less. Line lengths of about 5 inches are easiest to read. For columns, use 40 to 50 characters per line. The effective use of white space improves reading ease. Use it to focus on key areas and avoid the appearance of text cluttering the page. Leave at least ½ to 1 inch margins around the page and between columns. In general, aim for a total of 10 to 35% of white space per page.

Writing for Health Literacy: Resources

The CDC offers several online courses at https://www.cdc.gov/healthliteracy/gettraining.html (Accessed 3 Sept 2019). These include using numbers and explaining risk, and creating easier to understand lists, charts, and graphs. In addition, The CMS Toolkit for Making Written Materials Clear and Effective is available at https://www.cms.gov/Outreach-and-Education/Outreach/writtenmaterialstoolkit/ (Accessed 3 Sept 2019).

Visual Elements

Visuals can be an effective aid to understanding and recall when used correctly to communicate a message. Visuals may consist of photographs, illustrations, or other types of artwork. They need to be culturally acceptable to readers and can be tested with a representative sample to confirm this [42].

General Concepts

Each visual should focus on one message or key point to help emphasize or explain the content. All visuals should contain a caption and placed near the respective text. Visuals should be numbered if used to convey sequential events, such as inhaler usage. High quality artwork and photographs make the message more credible. Therefore, images need to have sharp resolution and good color contrast and composition. They should show behavior or actions to be taken. If it is important to show an undesirable action, cross out the picture to denote a negative action (preferably in red), making sure the picture is clearly recognizable as an action to be avoided and captioned accordingly. If focusing on one important element within the image, use arrows or circles to draw attention. It is worth mentioning to avoid humor, which can be perceived as trivializing important information. Humor is subjective and may not be understood or appreciated by everyone, particularly from one ethnicity to another.

Drawings or Illustrations

Simple black-and-white line drawings are best. Color may be considered to emphasize or separate various elements (Fig. 14.2). An online site such as www.rapidresizer.com (Accessed on 22 Aug 2019) can convert images to line drawings.

Charts or Graphs

Simple bar charts or line graphs can be produced to convey information in an easily understood way. To do this, headings should be simple, data carefully presented, relationships clear, and explanations on interpretation provided. Furthermore, the relevance of these relationships to the reader and the specific health issue at hand should be described.

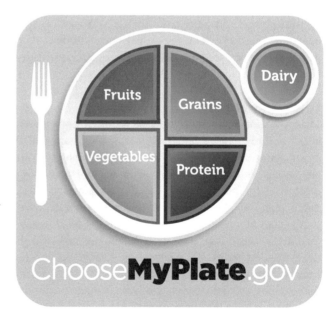

Fig. 14.2 Color illustration example on food portioning: Choose My Plate. (Source: United States Department of Agriculture)

Table 14.4 Internet image sources[a]

Site	Web address	Comments
CDC public health image library	https://phil.cdc.gov/	Free of charge; includes safe food handling, hygiene, and activity images; public domain
NIDDK	https://catalog.niddk. nih.gov/Catalog/ ImageLibrary/	Free of charge; includes anatomical, lifestyle, and activity images; public domain
Pixabay clipart	https://pixabay.com/ users/ openclipart-vectors-30363/	Free of charge, but one must join to use; wide variety of images (people, animals, food, activity, etc.); public domain, some images copy protected
Pexels	https://www.pexels. com/	Free of charge, but on must join to use; wide variety of images (ethnic people, exercise, food, etc.); public domain
Blausen medical on Wikiversity	https://en.wikiversity. org/wiki/WikiJournal of Medicine/Medical gallery of Blausen Medical 2014	Free of charge; anatomical pictures; public domain

[a]All websites accessed on August 22, 2019. Abbreviations: *CDC* Centers for Disease Control and Prevention, *NIDDK* National Institute of Diabetes and Digestive and Kidney Diseases

Photographs

Realistic images as photographs are particularly useful when context is needed to enhance comprehension. One must be careful to use photos of people that actually represent the target population. Photos can be bought online from commercial stock companies. Higher resolution photos work best for posters and other large formats. Lower resolution photos are fine for 8 × 11 inch or smaller-sized formats. Also, photos should be used without extraneous details, which can be distracting to readers.

Where to Get Images?

Images and/or photographs may be acquired from various sites. Be sure to check copyright or trademark status before downloading any materials, images or photographs, as using any visuals without permission may be a copyright infringement. Even for images in the public domain, elements within photographs may be copyright or trademark protected, such as a picture of a person standing in front of a McDonalds® sign. Check each image carefully before use and read the license and/or terms of agreement governing the site. For protected items, contact the source for permission to use. For photographs acquired privately, obtain written permission from the person in the photograph (Table 14.4).

Culture and Engagement

Culture

All educational materials should be reviewed and adapted for cultural competency and to avoid bias or any other potentially offensive messaging, especially in regard to gender, age, socioeconomic status, sexual orientation, disease, or disability. For instance, use person-first language ("patient with diabetes") instead of disease-first language ("diabetic person"). If creating materials for a specific culture, incorporate cultural elements that may appeal to them and promote engagement. Representative members can guide content developers to ensure acceptable terminology and images are used, as regional variations may exist. The use of strategies that are evidence-based for a particular ethno-cultural population is encouraged.

Engaging Patients

A positive and friendly tone is inviting and likely to engage readers. In other words, messaging should focus on desired behaviors ("do this/do that") instead of behaviors to avoid ("don't do this/don't do that"). Gain-framed messaging also helps engage patients by emphasizing the positive benefits of behavioral changes versus loss-framed messaging which focuses on the negative consequences of not following recommendations. Among 170 patients participating in a smoking cessation program, those who received gain-framed print and video materials showed a significantly higher abstinence rate after 6 months compared to those who received loss-framed information [77]. Gain-framed messaging is also used in *Benefits of Quitting Smoking*, found on smokefree.gov (Accessed on 4 Sept 2019).

Writing should also be personalized when addressing patients. Specifically, to write in the second person: "If you do this...." instead of "Patients who do this...." Using a question and answer format, such as with "Frequently Asked Questions" sections, helps to focus readers on topics of interest. Another example of interactive messaging is with thought-stimulating content or problem-solving scenarios, such as "List your asthma triggers: (1) _____ (2) _____ (3)_____," or "What might you do if...?" Video games, mobile apps, or wearable devices also promote engagement and interactivity by involving patients in their use.

Tips to Format Materials for Mobile Devices and Websites

Most internet readers scan the first few words or sentences, perusing headings and lists to seek useful information. If nothing quickly piques their interest, they leave the site. In addition to using Plain Language guidelines, a few useful formatting and design considerations to offset this are shown below [38].

Writing Style, Text, and Images

- Use at least a 12-point font. Smaller fonts create a crammed look and are harder to read.
- Limit use of numerical data in content.
- Use images that add value and load quickly for the end user.
- Line length should be about 50 characters for computer use; may use even less for mobile devices to accommodate 2- to 3-inch screen width and reduce scrolling.
- Keep sentences concise and paragraphs short (5 lines or less). Remove unneeded words, such as "this," "the," and "a," and use bullet points rather than whole sentences when possible.

Layout and Design

- Consider a table of contents with headings or page links at the top.
- Place primary menus in the left panel.
- Adjust page layout to avoid horizontal scrolling. Minimize down scrolling; hyperlink pages together instead of writing one long page.
- Be consistent in design and formatting for each page, especially regarding use of columns, buttons, text blocks, and alignment. This makes it easier to navigate.
- Provide visual cues to help the user know where they are, for example, color coding the pages and navigation menus or changing the color of a link that has already been clicked.
- Limit the number of clicks (2 or 3) needed to get to important information, keeping it as close to the home page as possible.
- Avoid using "click here" instructions (mobile users don't click).

American Disability Act Guidelines

The American Disability Act (ADA) offers certain guidelines to ensure web content is user friendly for all [39]. A few of these are as follows:

- Use HTML or RTF (rich text format), as they are more compatible with assistive technologies.
- Design site so users can select color and font sizes.

- Audio content needs to include written transcripts; videos should offer audio descriptions of the video's contents for the visually impaired.
- Include a "skip navigation" option that will let Screen Readers ignore navigation links.

Website Writing and Design Resources

- Complete ADA web design guidelines are at ada.gov/pca-toolkit/chap5toolkit.htm (Accessed 3 Sept 2019).
- Website content development, usability, and design guidelines by the US Department of Health and Human Services are at https://guidelines.usability.gov/ (Accessed 3 Sept 2019).
- The Guide to Writing and Designing Easy to Use Health Websites can be found at https://health.gov/healthliteracyonline/ (Accessed 3 Sept 2019).
- Making Website Content Senior Friendly is located at http://www.lgma.ca/assets/Programs~and~Events/Clerks~Forum/2013~Clerks~Forum/COMMUNICATIONS-Making-Your-Website-Senior-Friendly%2D%2DTip-Sheet.pdf (Accessed 3 Sept 2019).

Mobile App Development: An Application of Theory

To create ten Heart Failure mobile app modules, Athilingam et al. [37] used both the Cognitive Load Theory which suggests that working memory is enhanced if the cognitive load is maintained at a manageable level and Mayer's Theory of Multimedia Learning which supports the use of both audio and visual components to enhance learning. Each of the modules included formative feedback consisting of assessments that also reinforced content and consisted of 3 sections:

1. Information delivered via text and audio that used a conversational style
2. A HeartSmart section that used a quiz to evaluate knowledge
3. 3D-animated scenarios that enabled users to apply new knowledge

To ensure prompt and easy streaming, audio, images, and videos were compressed. At the time of publication, alpha and beta testing had been completed with plans to commence a clinical trial to evaluate outcomes. Among the testers, 70% reported learning new information, 95% felt very likely to use the app in the future, and 100% felt confident using it on a smartphone.

Final Evaluation of Materials

Before sharing newly developed materials and translations with patients, a series of diligent checks should be performed, primarily focusing on desired effects and user-friendliness. First, generate a prioritized list of items and concerns to be evaluated. Test to see how clearly content and visuals display on paper, a website, or a mobile device. For videos or podcasts, also check audio. Field test materials with a representative group of learners. For web and mobile devices, assess ease of navigation and search functions as well. Make corrections as needed and retest until satisfied that the product addresses all key points and is easy to use and understandable by learners. A feedback link to the website housing the materials may enhance performance through iterative improvements.

Hamilton Health Sciences (www.hamiltonhealthsciences. ca; Accessed on 7 Mar 2020) allows use or adaptation of the following patient evaluation questions with a 5-point rating scale (strongly agree to strongly disagree), but requests source acknowledgment:

- The words are easy to read.
- The information is easy to understand.
- Reading this helped me know ___ (or know how to ___).
- The information answered my questions.
- The [drawings, charts...] helped me understand the information.
- I would recommend this to other [patients, or persons with___] [38].

Conclusion

Plain Language guidelines for patient education material development can promote health literacy, a key factor in achieving positive health outcomes. Educational materials are a necessary part of the interactive process between patient and HCP. Providing quality materials allows for better choices in managing health. Creating and using materials that are engaging and personalized to meet learning needs brings patients one step closer to meeting their health management goals.

References

1. Kushner RF, Mechanick JI. Communication and behavioral change tools: a primer for lifestyle medicine counseling. In: Kushner RF, Mechanick JI, editors. Lifestyle medicine: a manual for clinical practice. 1st ed: Springer International Publishing; 2016. p. 17–28.
2. Medical Library Association. The librarian's role in the provision of consumer health information and patient education. Bull Med Libr Assoc. 1996;84:238–9.
3. Bastable SB. Overview of education in health care. In: The nurse as educator: principles of teaching and learning for nursing practice. 3rd ed. Sudbury: Jones and Bartlett; 2008.
4. Rankin SH, Stallings KD, London F. Patient education in health and illness. 5th ed. Philadelphia: Lippincott, Williams and Wilkins; 1996.
5. James J. Health policy brief: patient engagement. Health Affairs: Robert Wood Johnson Foundation, 2013 Feb 14; www.healthaffairs.org. Accessed on 2 May 2019.
6. Ng WI, Smith GD. Effects of a self-management education program on self-efficacy in patients with COPD: a mixed-methods sequential explanatory designed study. Int J Chron Obstruct Pulmon Dis. 2017;12:2129–39.
7. Wu SFV, Hsieh NC, Lin LJ. Prediction of self-care behavior on the basis of knowledge about chronic kidney disease using self-efficacy as a mediator. J Clin Nurs. 2016;25:2609–18.
8. Friedman AJ, Cosby R, Boyko S, et al. Effective teaching strategies and methods of delivery for patient education: a systematic review and practice recommendations. J Canc Educ. 2011;26:12–21.
9. Mechanick JI, Adams S, Davidson JA, et al. Transcultural diabetes care in the United States - a position statement by the American Association of Clinical Endocrinologists. Endocr Pract. 2019;25:729–65.
10. Shams L, Seitz AR. Benefits of multisensory learning. Trends Cogn Sci. 2008;12:411–7.
11. Grande SW, Faber MJ, Durand MA, et al. Classification model of patient engagement methods and assessment of feasibility in real-world settings. Patient Educ Couns. 2014;95:281–7.
12. McCarthy DM, Waite KR, Curtis LM, et al. What did the doctor say? Health literacy and recall of medical instructions. Med Care. 2012;50:277–82.
13. Waters EA, Biddle C, Kaphingst KA, et al. Examining the interrelations among objective and subjective health literacy and numeracy and their associations with health knowledge. J Gen Intern Med. 2018;33:1945–53.
14. Berkman N, Sheridan SL, Donahue KE, et al. Low health literacy and health outcomes: an updated systematic review. Ann Intern Med. 2011;155:97–107.
15. U.S. Dept of Health & Human Services, Washington DC. Plain Writing and Clear Communications. Available from: https://www.hhs.gov/open/plain-writing/index.html. Accessed on 5 April 2019.
16. Rosenfeld L, Rudd R, Emmons KM, et al. Beyond reading alone: the relationship between aural literacy and asthma management. Patient Educ Couns. 2011;82:110–6.
17. Nouri SS, Rudd RE. Health literacy in the "oral exchange": an important element of patient-provider communication. Patient Educ Couns. 2015;98:565–71.
18. National Network of Libraries of Medicine, Bethesda. Health Literacy. https://nnlm.gov/initiatives/topics/health-literacy. Accessed 7 May 2019.
19. Peters E, Hart S, Fraenkel L. Informing patients: the influence of numeracy, framing, and format of side effect information on risk perceptions. Med Decis Mak. 2011;31:432–6.
20. Golbeck A, Paschal A, Jones A, et al. Correlating reading comprehension and health numeracy among adults with low literacy. Patient Educ Couns. 2011;84:132–4.
21. Paige SR, Krieger JL, Stellefson M, et al. eHealth literacy in chronic disease patients: an item response theory analysis of the eHealth literacy scale (eHEALS). Patient Educ Couns. 2017;100:320–6.
22. Jacobs W, Amuta AO, Jeon KC. Health information seeking in the digital age: an analysis of health information seeking behavior among US adults. Cogent Soc Sci. 2017;3:1302785.

23. Cornett S. Assessing and addressing health literacy. Online J Issues Nurs. 2009;14:13. https://pdfs.semanticscholar.org/7e11/7e9d53f3 7a1e318ce7b85c0a5eb7d765aff4.pdf. Accessed 7 Mar 2020.

24. Ylitalo KR, Meyer MRU, Lanning BA, et al. Simple screening tools to identify limited health literacy in a low-income patient population. Medicine. 2018;97:e0110. https://www.ncbi.nlm.nih.gov/pmc/articles/PMC5882442/. Accessed 7 Mar 2020.

25. Parker RM, Baker DW, Williams MD, et al. The test of functional health literacy in adults: a new instrument for measuring patients' literacy skills. J Gen Intern Med. 1995;10:537–41.

26. Wallace L. Family medicine updates from the north American primary care research group. Ann Fam Med. 2006;4:85–6.

27. O'Hara J, Hawkins M, Batterham R, et al. Conceptualisation and development of the conversational health literacy assessment tool (CHAT). BMC Health Serv Res. 2018;18:199. https://www.ncbi.nlm.nih.gov/pmc/articles/PMC5863801/. Accessed 8 May 2019.

28. Yeung DL, Alvarez KS, Quinones ME, et al. Low-health literacy flashcards & mobile video reinforcement to improve medication adherence in patients on oral diabetes, heart failure, and hypertension medications. J Am Pharm Assoc. 2017;57:30–7.

29. Younus J, Kligman L. Mobile devices applications for patient education. Int J Cancer Res Mol Mech. 2016;2. https://sciforschenonline.org/journals/cancer-research/IJCRMM-2-128.php. Accessed 7 Mar 2020.

30. National Cancer Institute, Bethesda. Smokefree Apps. https://smokefree.gov/tools-tips/apps. Accessed 7 Mar 2020.

31. Zhao J, Freeman B, Li M. Can mobile phone apps influence people's health behavior change? An evidence review J Med Internet Res. 2016;18:e287. https://www.ncbi.nlm.nih.gov/pmc/articles/PMC5295827/. Accessed on 7 Mar 2020.

32. Ho K, Yao C, Lauscher HN. Health apps, wearables and sensors: the advancing frontier of digital health. BC Med J. 2017;59:503–6. https://www.bcmj.org/articles/part-2-health-apps-wearables-and-sensors-advancing-frontier-digital-health. Accessed 7 Mar 2020.

33. Appelboom G, Camacho E, Abraham ME, et al. Smart wearable body sensors for patient self-assessment and monitoring. Arch Pub Health. 2014;72. https://archpublichealth.biomedcentral.com/track/pdf/10.1186/2049-3258-72-28. Accessed on 7 Mar 2020.

34. Chiauzzi E, Rodarte C, DasMahapatra P. Patient-centered activity monitoring in the self-management of chronic health conditions. BMC Med. 2015;13:77. https://www.ncbi.nlm.nih.gov/pmc/articles/PMC4391303/. Accessed on 7 Mar 2020.

35. Krebs P, Duncan DT. Health app use among US mobile phone owners: a national survey. JMIR Mhealth Uhealth. 2015;3:e101. https://www.ncbi.nlm.nih.gov/pmc/articles/PMC4704953/. Accessed on 7 Mar 2020.

36. Huckvale K, Morrison C, Ouyang J, et al. The evolution of mobile apps for asthma: an updated systematic assessment of content and tools. BMC Med. 2015;13:58. https://www.ncbi.nlm.nih.gov/pmc/articles/PMC4391129/. Accessed on 7 Mar 2020.

37. Athilingam P, Osorio RE, Kaplan H, et al. Embedding patient education in mobile platform for patients with heart failure. Comput Inform Nurs. 2016;34:92–8.

38. Wizowski L, Harper T, Hutchings T. Writing health information for patients and families. 4th ed. Hamilton: Hamilton Health Sciences; 2014.

39. Information and Technical Assistance on the Americans with Disabilities Act, U.S. Department of Justice Civil Rights Division, Washington D.C. ADA best practices tool kit for state and local governments, Chapter 5, Website accessibility under Title II of the ADA, https://www.ada.gov/pcatoolkit/chap5toolkit.htm. Accessed on 7 Mar 2020.

40. Community toolbox. University of Kansas Center for Community Health and Development; c2018. Lawrence, KS. Chapter 3: Assessing community needs and resources (Sections 1,6,7), https://ctb.ku.edu/en/table-of-contents/assessment/assessing-community-needs-and-resources. Accessed on 7 Mar 2020.

41. Centers for Medicare and Medicaid Services (CMS). Baltimore, MD; Sept 2010. Toolkit for making written material clear and effective, https://www.cms.gov/Outreach-and-Education/Outreach/WrittenMaterialsToolkit/index.html. Accessed on 7 Mar 2020.

42. HHS, Centers for Disease Control and Prevention. Simply Put – A Guide for Creating Easy-To-Understand Materials, April 2009, 3rd Ed. https://stacks.cdc.gov/view/cdc/11938. Accessed on 7 Mar 2020.

43. Rural Women's Health Project (RWHP), Gainesville, 2018. The fotonovela. https://www.rwhp.org/fotonovela.html. Accessed on 7 Mar 2020.

44. Hinojosa MS, Nelson D, Hinojosa R, et al. Using fotonovelas to promote healthy eating in a Latino community. Am J Public Health. 2011;101:258–9.

45. Unger JB, Cabassa LJ, Molina GB, et al. Evaluation of a fotonovela to increase depression knowledge and reduce stigma among Hispanic adults. J Immigr Minor Health. 2013;15:398–406.

46. Cabassa LJ, Molina GB, Baron M. Depression fotonovela: development of a depression literacy tool for Latinos with limited English proficiency. Health Promot Pract. 2012;13:747–54.

47. Eaton K. Transforming your photos into comic strips. The New York Times 2014; May 14: Personal Technology: B13, https://www.nytimes.com/2014/05/15/technology/personaltech/transforming-your-photos-into-comics-strips.html. Accessed on 7 Mar 2020.

48. Lo-Fo-Wong DNN. Quality of care: distress, health care use and needs of women with breast cancer (Master's Thesis, University of Amsterdam, Amsterdam, NL) 2016; pp.1–232, https://pure.uva.nl/ws/files/2724276/178403_Lo_Fo_Wong_thesis_complete.pdf. Accessed on 7 Mar 2020.

49. Ashwal G, Thomas A. Are comic books appropriate health education formats to offer adult patients? AMA J Ethics. 2018;20:134–40.

50. Choi J. Literature review: using pictographs in discharge instructions for older adults with low-literacy skills. J Clin Nurs. 2011;20:2984–96.

51. Park J, Zuniga J. Effectiveness of using picture-based health education for people with low literacy: an integrative review. Cogent Med. 2016;3:1264679. https://cogentoa.com/article/10.1080/2331205X.2016.1264679. Accessed on 7 Mar 2020.

52. Galesic M, Garcia-Retamero R, Gigerenzer G. Using icon arrays to communicate medical risks: overcoming low numeracy. Health Psychol. 2009;28:210–6.

53. Zikmund-Fisher BJ, Witteman HO, Dickson M, et al. Blocks, ovals or people? Icon type affects risk perceptions and recall of pictographs. Med Decis Mak. 2014;34:443–53.

54. Damman OC, Vonk SI, van den Haak MJ, et al. The effects of infographics and several quantitative versus qualitative formats for cardiovascular disease risk, including heart age, on people's risk understanding. Patient Educ Couns. 2018;101:1410–8.

55. Arcia A, Suero-Tejeda N, Bales ME, et al. Sometimes more is more: iterative participatory design of infographics for engagement of community members with varying levels of health literacy. J Am Med Inform Assoc. 2016;23:174–83.

56. Berhenet M, Vaillancourt R, Pouliot A. Evaluation, modification, and validation of pictograms depicting medication instructions in the elderly. J Health Commun. 2016;21:27–33.

57. Van Beusekom M, Bos M, Wolterbeek R, et al. Patients' preferences for visuals: differences in the preferred level of detail, type of background and type of frame of icons depicting organs between literate and low-literate people. Patient Educ Couns. 2015;98:226–33.

58. Wilson EAH, Park DC, Curtis LM, et al. Media and memory: the efficacy of video and print materials for promoting patient education about asthma. Patient Educ Couns. 2010;80:393–8.

59. Wilson EAH, Makoul G, Bojarski EA, et al. Comparative analysis of print and multimedia health materials: a review of the literature. Patient Educ Couns. 2012;89:7–14.

60. Abed MA, Himmel W, Vormfelde S, et al. Video-assisted patient education to modify behavior: a systematic review. Patient Educ Couns. 2014;97:16–22.

61. WikiHow, Palo Alto, CA. How to make an educational video; 2019: Mar 19, https://www.wikihow.com/Make-an-Educational-Video. Accessed on 7 Mar 2020.

62. van Vliet LM, Hillen MA, van der Wall E, et al. How to create and administer scripted video-vignettes in an experimental study on disclosure of a palliative breast cancer diagnosis. Patient Educ Couns. 2013;91:56–64.

63. London F. The teaching toolbox. In: No time to teach. Philadelphia: Lippincott, Williams and Wilkins; 1999. p. 156–60.

64. Ricciardi F, DePaolis LT. A comprehensive review of serious games in health professions. Int J Comp Games Technol. 2014;787968. https://www.hindawi.com/journals/ijcgt/2014/787968/abs/. Accessed on 7 Mar 2020.

65. Thompson D, Baranowski T, Buday R. Conceptual model for the design of a serious video game promoting self-management among youth with type 1 diabetes. J Diabetes Sci Technol. 2010;4:744–9.

66. Charlier N, Zupancic N, Fieuws S, et al. Serious games for improving knowledge and self-management in young people with chronic conditions: a systematic review and meta-analysis. J Am Med Inform Assoc. 2016;23:230–9.

67. Kato PM, Cole SW, Bradlyn AS, et al. A video game improves behavioral outcomes in adolescents and young adults with cancer: a randomized trial. Pediatrics. 2008;122:e305–17.

68. Reichlin L, McArthur MN, Harris AM, et al. Assessing the acceptability and usability of an interactive serious game in aiding treatment decisions for patients with localized prostate cancer. J Med Internet Res. 2011;13:e4. https://www.ncbi.nlm.nih.gov/pmc/articles/PMC3221354/. Accessed on 7 Mar 2020.

69. Drummond D, Hadchouel A, Tesniere A. Serious games for health: three steps forward. Adv Simul. 2017;2:3. https://advancesinsimulation.biomedcentral.com/articles/10.1186/s41077-017-0036-3. Accessed on 7 Mar 2020.

70. Thompson D, Baranowski T, Buday R. Conceptual model for the design of a serious video game promoting self-management among youth with type 1 Diabetes. J Diabetes Sci Technol. 2010;4:744–9. https://journals.sagepub.com/doi/pdf/10.1177/193229681000400331. Accessed on 7 Mar 2020.

71. Pappas C. Top 10 tips on how to use avatars in e-learning. eLearning Industry. 2014. https://elearningindustry.com/top-10-tips-use-avatars-in-elearning. Accessed on 7 Mar 2020.

72. Graafland M, Dankbaar M, Mert A, et al. How to systematically assess serious games applied to health care. JMIR Serious Games. 2014;2:e11. https://www.ncbi.nlm.nih.gov/pmc/articles/PMC4307812/. Accessed on 7 Mar 2020.

73. Zikmund-Fisher BJ, Witteman HO, Fuhrel-Forbes A, et al. Animated graphics for comparing two risks: a cautionary tale. J Med Internet Res. 2012;14:e106. https://www.ncbi.nlm.nih.gov/pmc/articles/PMC3409597/?report=classic. Accessed on 7 Mar 2020.

74. Sampat A, Woo H, Aysola R, et al. Utilization of patient education videos prescribed through a patient portal. Sleep. 2018;41(Suppl 1):A391. https://academic.oup.com/sleep/article/41/suppl_1/A391/4988099. Accessed on 7 Mar 2020.

75. Zyskind A, Jones KC, Pomerantz KL, et al. Exploring the use of computer based patient education resources to enable diabetic patients from underserved populations to self-manage their disease. Inf Serv Use. 2009;29:29–43.

76. Safeer RS, Keenan J. Health literacy: the gap between physicians and patients. Am Fam Physician. 2005;72:463–8.

77. Toll BA, O'Malley SS, Katulak NA, et al. Comparing gain- and loss-framed messages for smoking cessation with sustained-release bupropion: a randomized controlled trial. Psychol Addict Behav. 2007;21:534–44.

Implementing Behavioral Medicine in a Lifestyle Medicine Practice

15

Sherri Sheinfeld Gorin and Catherine L. Davis

Abbreviations

AIDS	Acquired immunodeficiency syndrome
apps	Electronic applications
CBT	Cognitive behavioral therapy
DARNCAT	Desire, Ability, Reason, Need, Commitment, Activation, Taking steps
DPP	Diabetes Prevention Program
5 As	Ask/Assess, Advise, Assess/Agree, Assist, and Arrange
HCP	Healthcare professional
HIV	Human immunodeficiency virus
MET	Motivational enhancement therapy
MOHR	My Own Health Report
OARS	Open-ended questions, Affirmations, Reflections, and Summaries
SMART	Specific, Measurable, Attainable, Realistic, and Timely
T2D	Type 2 diabetes

Definition of Behavioral Medicine

Behavioral medicine relies on empirical evidence as well as conceptual models to explain behavior change at multiple levels (individual, family/group, practice, community, and policy). Behavioral medicine is inherently interdisciplinary, developing and integrating behavioral and biomedical knowledge, as well as incorporating techniques to apply to prevention, diagnosis, treatment, and rehabilitation [1]. These techniques are adapted to both the level of change as

S. S. Gorin (✉)
The University of Michigan, Department of Family Medicine, Ann Arbor, MI, USA

C. L. Davis
Georgia Prevention Institute, Department of Medicine, Medical College of Georgia at Augusta University, Augusta, GA, USA

well as the cultural context within which change occurs. Behavioral medicine addresses both physical and mental health and is closely related to fields such as health psychology, pediatric psychology, neuropsychology, geropsychology, rehabilitation psychology, and psychosomatic medicine [2]. The biopsychosocial model proposed by Engel presents similar concepts and serves as a critical reference [3, 4].

The Integrated Care Approach to Behavioral Medicine in Lifestyle Medicine

The integrated care approach configures a healthcare professional (HCP) with dedicated training and expertise in behavioral medicine as a core part of the medical team. Consequently, patients are routinely screened for behavioral concerns to promote patient engagement, including building trust and reducing barriers, such as stigma about mental health treatment. Referral to an off-site behavioral HCP can also be effective, particularly if the appointment can be made by the medical practice and followed up at subsequent visits. For example, in a recent study of integrated mental healthcare among patients diagnosed with diabetes, a behavioral HCP was introduced in the visit with another trusted HCP, thereby enhancing patient comfort while receiving behavioral treatment [5].

Brief, evidence-based treatments are most suitable to the primary care setting, with longer-term and more intensive treatments for those who are not responsive to the brief ones, or who have a more severe or urgent need (e.g., acute suicidality with intention and a plan, or serious mental illness such as psychotic disorders) [6]. Lifestyle behavior change requires a consistent approach with tapered maintenance and follow-up by the lifestyle medicine HCP to enhance adherence and address setbacks when they occur.

Diabetes education offers an example. Rather than a one-time course that patients undergo and thereby become permanently competent, diabetes self-management involves

© Springer Nature Switzerland AG 2020
J. I. Mechanick, R. F. Kushner (eds.), *Creating a Lifestyle Medicine Center*, https://doi.org/10.1007/978-3-030-48088-2_15

ongoing and recurring diabetes educator consultation to assist patients as they encounter challenging social, cultural, health, and other barriers to optimal self-care and also to learn how to handle setbacks. The diabetes educator also provides patients with new strategies as the available treatments progress. For instance, continuous glucose monitoring and partially automated insulin pump systems are a major advance over what was state of the art just a few years ago. As another example, new bariatric and metabolic procedures can improve diabetes and cardiovascular outcomes dramatically. Each of these modern treatments requires patient behavioral adherence to succeed.

Models of Change in Behavioral Medicine

Interventions at multiple levels help to overcome HCP barriers to implementing behavioral interventions, including limited HCP-patient encounter time and the need for specialized training. Behavior is multi-determined, affected by the culture, environment, clinical practice setting, family, and a range of individual patient factors. There are several widely used models of change that guide the delivery of behavioral medicine care. Many of these models offer explanations for behavior, and all offer levers for behavioral change. The Lifestyle Medicine Center can serve as the hub for behavioral counseling, while resources at other levels (e.g., policy, organizations, and community) can help patients to enact and sustain changes such as physical activity, smoking cessation, and healthy eating [7].

The Social Ecology Model

Ecology pertains to the relationships among organisms and their environments [8, 9]. The social ecology model, based on systems theory, and the early work of Bronfenbrenner [10], presume that the healthfulness of a situation and the well-being of participants are mutually influenced by aspects of the environment: physical (geography, architecture, and technology) and social (culture, economics, and politics) (Fig. 15.1).

Patient-environment interactions move through cycles of mutual influence, where each affects the other. The varied levels of human environments, such as worksites, are seen as complex systems in which each level is nested in more complex and distant levels. For example, the occupational health and safety of community work settings is directly influenced by state and local ordinances aimed at protecting public health and environmental quality [10–14].

The social ecology model recognizes the often-contradictory influences of environments and patients. For example, a socially supportive family or organization may

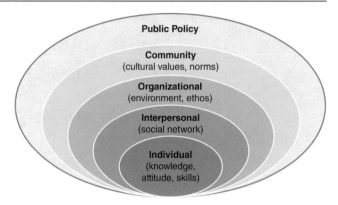

Fig. 15.1 The social ecology model. The social ecology framework posits that the healthfulness of a situation and the well-being of participants are mutually influenced by aspects of the environment: physical (geography, architecture, and technology) and social (culture, economics, and politics). Public policy, community, organizations, interpersonal networks, and individuals exert reciprocal influences on each other. (see Refs. [8, 9])

enable patients to cope more effectively with physical constraints (e.g., overcrowding and drab surroundings). A well-designed physical environment may not spur much health, however, if promotion of interpersonal or intergroup relations results in conflict and stress, or individuals are required to be socially isolated (as in the coronavirus disease 2019 pandemic).

A focus on the impact of the physical, human-made, or "built environment" on health has received renewed attention [15]. A "sense of place" is a widely discussed concept in fields as diverse as geography, environmental psychology, and art [16]. Place includes geography (e.g., sprawl), aggregated group properties (e.g., census-tract level income), as well as broader political, cultural, or institutional effects (e.g., county-level physician supply) [17].

Patients may live in geographic areas that encourage walking, biking, and social interaction [18, 19]. These environments can influence their likelihood to regularly engage in physical activity. Alternatively, harmful geographic settings can adversely affect health. For example, locales with increasing motor vehicle exhaust could exacerbate pulmonary disease [20]. The presence of neighborhood liquor stores could increase alcohol consumption with the associated adverse health consequences [21, 22]. Lack of grocery stores or places to purchase fresh fruits and vegetables (food deserts), coupled with the proximity of convenience stores and fast-food outlets, could promote unhealthy dietary consumption and eating patterns, especially for those with limited transportation options. Food deserts may also lead to food insecurity, defined by the U.S. Department of Agriculture as the household's limited or uncertain access to adequate food. Furthermore, food insecurity may result in individual hunger. The health impact of place (also including nature contact, buildings, public spaces, and urban form) may include physical, psychological, social, spiritual, and aesthetic outcomes [16], many of which have not yet been systematically examined.

The Chronic Care Model

The Chronic Care Model is among the most widely used health services intervention structures in the field, having directed innovation throughout major integrated healthcare systems (e.g., Group Health Cooperative and the Veterans Health Administration) as well as federal agencies (e.g., Centers for Medicare and Medicaid Services Innovation Center) [23]. The Chronic Care Model is based on the premise that improved chronic disease outcomes result from productive interactions among informed, activated patients and a prepared, proactive practice team [24].

Six components facilitate productive interchanges among lifestyle medicine HCPs, the larger clinical practice team, and patients in primary care [24]:

1. *Self-management support*, resulting from the HCP and patient working together via patient education and activation, various tools and resources, collaborative decision-making, and the use of clinical practice guidelines.
2. *Delivery system design*, involving the organization of the practice through clarifying care management roles, team-building, proactive patient follow-up, and implementing visit system changes to improve patient care.
3. *Decision support,* including guidance for HCP behavior and decision-making, with the institutionalization of clinical practice guidelines, protocols, prompts, and nudges; HCP education; and expert consultation support.

4. *Clinical information systems*, involving the gathering of information or improved use of information systems via a patient registry; the use of information for care management; and the provision of performance data.
5. *An organized health system*, resulting from the creation of a culture focused on quality through leadership support, HCP participation, and coherent system improvement.
6. *Community resources and policies,* arising from resources outside the center to facilitate linkages among patients and the community [25, 26].

All six components of the Chronic Care Model are considered necessary for improving healthcare in general, and apply widely across chronic illnesses, healthcare settings, and patient populations [27, 28] (Fig. 15.2).

Theoretical Models of Change: Family-, Group-, and Individual-Levels

Behavioral scientists have led the development and testing of models of change. There are several classic theories applicable to the Lifestyle Medicine Center that identify different health promotion strategies. Each of these theoretical models posits a trajectory for change in attitudes, beliefs, or behaviors.

Stimulus-Response Learning Theory

Stimulus-response theory includes classical conditioning (passive learning associating two stimuli) and operant conditioning (active learning associating action and consequence). This strict behaviorist approach relies on empirical observations to analyze behavior patterns, disregarding what was considered as the unmeasurable "black box" of cognition [29, 30]. Learning principles derived from this approach apply equally well to animals and people. In classical (Pavlovian) conditioning, the organism learns to associate a stimulus (e.g., buzz sound) with a biologi-

Fig. 15.2 The Chronic Care Model. The Chronic Care Model is based on the premise that improved chronic disease outcomes result from productive interactions among informed, activated patients and a prepared, proactive practice team. (See Refs. [24, 27, 28])

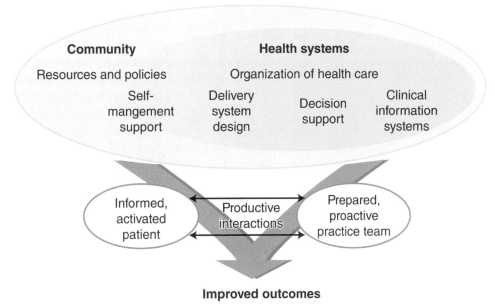

cally important event (e.g., food appearing), which results in an involuntary response to the first stimulus (e.g., salivation) even when no food is presented. In operant conditioning, the organism learns to respond to a stimulus (e.g., buzz sound) with a voluntary response (e.g., press lever) that results in a desired reward (e.g., food). Reinforcements (e.g., food reward and/or avoiding pain) increase the probability of a behavior, and punishments (e.g., pain and/or loss of food reward) decrease behaviors. Extinction (ceasing of a habitual behavior) is notoriously difficult to achieve with unpredictable reinforcements (e.g., child keeps misbehaving until parent gives in to demand). Given the slow progress of natural incentives for weight control and physical fitness (e.g., clothes fitting better, easier to climb stairs), more immediate incentives are a useful strategy to offset the intrinsically reinforcing value of energy-dense foods such as sweets, and sedentary activities such as screen time which may be required for work or school [31].

Stimulus control refers to behaviors which are triggered by a stimulus (i.e., cue), and are less likely to occur in the absence of that stimulus. Stimulus control strategies (placing cues to healthy behavior and removing cues to unhealthy behavior where the patient will encounter them) can enhance adherence to a particular lifestyle program [31]. As an example, for a person who finds donuts irresistible, avoiding visiting donut shops and bringing donuts home can help reduce eating donuts. Keeping walking shoes and a leash near the place where the patient sits down frequently and having a dog that wants to go for a walk (and will recognize the shoes as a cue) can help encourage physical activity. For a smoker, avoiding cues like spending time with friends who smoke, smelling tobacco smoke, or drinking alcohol if that was often paired with smoking, can help reduce the urge to smoke tobacco. Removing the television from the bedroom can help improve sleep habits. Making energy-dense, nutrient-poor foods (e.g., candy) less accessible, and putting an attractive bowl of fruit on the kitchen counter, or cut-up carrots and celery with an appealing dip in the front of the refrigerator or in a convenient to-go container, can encourage more nutritious food choices [31].

Social Learning Theory and Social Cognitive Theory

Social learning theory builds on stimulus-response theory by adding cognitive elements. It posits that learning novel behaviors (e.g., language and violence) can occur through social modeling (observation and imitation of others, such as parents) and without reinforcements [32]. Most learning occurs through modeling (i.e., social learning), such as watching others prepare and eat meals. Learning is affected by social influences, including reinforcements such as praise and inclusion in activities.

Bandura [33] built on social learning theory to develop social cognitive theory, where cognitive expectations, such as self-efficacy (e.g., feeling capable of stopping smoking), influence the behavior (e.g., smoking cessation). The cornerstone of the model is reciprocal determinism, or a dynamic interaction among the person, behavior, and the environment, within which the behavior is performed [34]. Individuals high in self-efficacy or more confident of their ability to maintain behavioral changes (e.g., smoking cessation or dietary changes) will execute them more readily with greater intensity and with greater perseverance in response to

initial failure than will individuals with comparatively lower self-efficacy [35, 36]. Rather than focusing on the training of behavior by environmental forces, social cognitive theory emphasizes the importance of knowledge, skill, and self-control. Self-regulatory processes, including self-generated inducements and expectations (e.g., telling oneself to exercise daily so that one can climb a flight of stairs more easily), are also highlighted in this theory.

Stages of Change

The stages of change model is based on the presumption that individuals move through a series of predictable behavioral stages:

1. *Precontemplation* (not ready) – considering the change
2. *Contemplation* (getting ready) – starting to think about initiating change
3. *Preparation* (ready) – seriously thinking about the change within a given time period (e.g., the next 6 months) or taking early steps to change
4. *Action* (making a change) – starting/stopping the target behavior within a 6-month period; individuals modify their behavior, experiences, or environment in order to overcome their problems; this requires a considerable commitment of time and energy
5. *Maintenance* (maintaining the change) – the target behavior change is maintained for more than 6 months; this includes preventing and recovering from relapse [37–40]

The name "transtheoretical" is often applied to the stages of change model as it includes elements from other theories, such as stimulus control from learning theories, a key strategy in the action and maintenance stages [31, 39]. Relapse occurs less often in the maintenance phase, once the healthy behavior change is more established, than in the action phase. Termination is sometimes included as the final stage of change, where the unhealthy behavior is no longer a temptation. However, this final stage may not be achievable for many people, particularly those with addictive behaviors. These stages are not necessarily linear. For example, the average smoker who quits reports at least several and often many relapses before achieving and maintaining abstinence [41]. Nevertheless, the stages of change model may suggest intervention points for different individuals at varied stages [40].

The mechanisms that drive movement through the stages of change are termed the processes of change [38]. These processes draw heavily on components of other models, such as the Health Belief Model described below [42], and describe decision-making regarding the adoption of a behavior. The decisional balance approach compares the strength of the target behavior's perceived pros with that of the perceived cons [43]. The relative weights that people assign to a behavior's pros and cons influence their decisions about behavioral change [43], such as continuing or ceasing to smoke.

Health Belief Model Theory

The goal of the Health Belief Model (as modified by Becker [42]) is to determine why some individuals who are illness-free take actions to avoid illness, whereas others fail to take protective actions. Another goal is to predict the conditions under which individuals would engage in simple preventive behaviors, such as immunizations. The model was based on the work of Kurt Lewin, who understood that the life space in which individuals live is composed of regions, some having a negative valence (one would seek to avoid), some a positive valence (one would seek to approach), and some a neutral valence [44].

The Health Belief Model suggests that before individuals take action, they must decide that the behavior, whether it is smoking, eating unhealthy foods, or engaging in unprotected sexual activity, creates a serious health problem. Moreover, they are personally susceptible to this health harm, and that moderating or stopping the behavior will be beneficial. The perceived barriers to undertaking a behavior are considered most important to health-promotive efforts [45]. An individual's perceived susceptibility to a disease and severity of harm are largely based on personal knowledge of the disease and potential outcomes. Although the combination of perceived susceptibility to, and severity of harm provides the force for action and the perception of high benefits and low barriers provides a course of action, it is the *cues to action* that start the process of change [46].

Cultural influences can have strong effects on health beliefs and practices, for example, in the use of complementary or alternative practices, differing disease causation beliefs, and perceptions of risk and personal agency [47]. Cultural beliefs and strong community ties can support health behaviors. Taboos and stigma (e.g., blood, sexually transmitted diseases, illness, and contagion) may hinder a patient from performing self-care in the presence of others or interfere with adherence to health behaviors (e.g., healthy eating, physical activity, taking medication, and vaccination), however. HCP understanding of cultural context can personalize treatment for patients in various communities [48].

Theory of Planned Behavior

This theory postulates that most volitional behavior can be predicted by beliefs, attitudes, and intentions. Therefore, efforts to change behavior should be directed at an individual's belief system. By altering the beliefs underlying attitudes or norms, changes in behavioral intentions, and subsequently in behavior, can also be induced [49, 50]. Individuals intend to do a behavior, such as brushing their teeth, when they evaluate it positively and believe that important others, such as parents, think they should do it [49].

Prospect Theory

This theory states that rather than being strictly rational, the degree to which a choice (or behavior) is seen as a gain or a loss can vary depending on how the consequences of the behavior are presented or framed [51]. When behavioral choices involve some risk, individuals will be more likely to accept these risks when information is framed in terms of relative disadvantages (i.e., losses or costs) of the outcomes. When behavioral choices involve little risk, individuals prefer options for which information is framed by relative advantages (i.e., gains or benefits). Choosing prevention behaviors (e.g., wearing a condom) is a risk-averse option for maintaining sexual health. These behaviors should be promoted with gain-framed messages, such as "using a condom during sexual intercourse can help to keep you healthy" [52]. Among asymptomatic or low risk patients, behaviors involving an uncertain, potentially negative outcome should be promoted with loss-framed messages (e.g., "failing to use a condom during sexual intercourse exposes you to various sexually transmitted diseases") [52]. As other examples, loss-framed messages could be shared with low risk or asymptomatic patients for human immunodeficiency virus (HIV) testing (where the patient may find out that they have HIV) or breast self-examination (where even benign lumps may raise concern about cancer). Message framing approaches, derived from prospect theory, have been applied to breast cancer screening, sunscreen use, HIV testing, condom use, human papillomavirus vaccination, and dental mouthwashes, as well as defining quality of life outcomes.

Behavioral Economics Theory

Behavioral economics, like prospect theory, recognizes that choices are not strictly rational [53]. A nudge is a cue (sometimes electronic) that influences choice, without removing options. Making the best choice, the default dramatically increases the proportion of people who choose it. Choice architecture refers to design decisions such as planning a cafeteria so that you have to go by the salad bar before you get to the grill, or offering a child a few healthy choices for a snack. Making the healthy option the easiest or most obvious choice (e.g., presenting fruit in an attractive bowl at the front of the display, with the less healthy items further back behind a latched lid) can increase the selection of fruit without removing the other options. Healthy lifestyle nudges include text message reminders to record dietary intake or an app that prompts physical activity breaks.

Stimulus control strategies, such as placing cues toward desired behaviors in one's routine (e.g., coming home to a dog that wants and might need to go for a walk; keeping ready-to-eat servings of vegetables with a healthy, tasty dip at the front of the refrigerator) and avoiding cues to unhealthy behavior (e.g., avoiding places where peers smoke, not bringing home large quantities of tempting unhealthy items), tend to increase healthful behaviors. Delay discounting refers to the degree to which people prefer smaller, more immediate rewards (immediate gratification) rather than larger, delayed rewards [54]. Episodic future thinking, projecting oneself into the future to pre-experience an event, is a promising strategy to offset delay discounting for behavior changes, including obesity treatment and reducing smoking [31, 32, 54, 55].

Effective Behavioral Interventions for Lifestyle Medicine

There is evidence for the influential role of behavioral interventions in cardiovascular disease, diabetes, cancer, HIV/AIDS, and chronic pain [56]. Behavioral risk factor modification (e.g., tobacco use, unhealthy eating, and physical inactivity) improves quality of life and reduces healthcare costs [57, 58]. Behavioral treatments for pain are underutilized and may be especially important given the current opioid epidemic [58]. Behavioral treatment is valuable for regimen adherence and reducing obesity [31, 59].

Obesity and diabetes are exemplary conditions for lifestyle medicine interventions. Reducing risks for type 2 diabetes (T2D) and other sequelae of obesity present common, daunting challenges for behavior change. According to a systematic review by the U.S. Preventive Services Task Force in 2018 [60], patients receiving behavior-based interventions had greater mean weight loss (−2.39 kg [95% CI, −2.86 to −1.93]; 67 studies [N = 22,065]) and less weight regain (−1.59 kg [95% CI, −2.38 to −0.79]; 8 studies [N = 1408]) at 12–18 months, compared with controls. In addition, 12 or more sessions per year of behavioral counseling delivered in-person, by phone, or electronically resulted in 4–7 kg weight loss, compared 1–2 kg weight loss with fewer sessions or counseling that did not include behavioral strategies such as motivational interviewing [61]. Furthermore, weight loss medication increased weight loss when added to behavioral treatment but also increased adverse events [60, 61].

The Diabetes Prevention Program (DPP) demonstrated that an intensive lifestyle intervention to lose weight through diet and physical activity was 58% effective in preventing or delaying onset of diabetes over 5 years, while metformin was only 31% effective [62]. The DPP was translated to the YMCA and has been adopted by the Centers for Disease Control and Prevention [63–66]. Lifestyle interventions based on the DPP are generally effective in community settings (~4% weight loss at 1 year) [63]. Very brief (<30 seconds) primary care physician advice with referral to a behavioral program (12 weekly sessions, 1 hour each) was also found effective in diabetes prevention (2.43 kg mean weight loss at 12 months; 1.04 kg mean weight loss at 12 months with just the very brief advice) in patients with obesity [64].

Specific behavioral interventions are useful in secondary prevention for patients with T2D. The Look AHEAD study reduced weight, cardiovascular risk factors, and medications in patients with T2D through an intensive lifestyle intervention [67]. The design and findings of this study have also been translated to group treatment at the YMCA. Such community settings offer durable and accessible support that is needed to maintain initial weight loss and lifestyle improvements [68].

Similarly, in chronic illnesses such as diabetes, diabetes self-management education should not be considered merely as a one-time treatment. Continuing support is needed to maintain the treatment regimen, especially when it is demanding for the patient, and to adjust for evolving treatment options [68, 69]. In addition, those with diabetes are prone to depression, which hampers adherence. In a small trial of distressed rural adults with T2D, a 12-session intervention tailored to severity, either cognitive behavioral therapy (CBT) with a psychologist for those with moderate to severe symptoms, or telephonic lifestyle coaching by a nurse for those with mild distress, have been shown to be feasible in a rural primary care clinic and effective in improving mood and adherence [5].

There is strong evidence for the effectiveness of brief clinician counseling in smoking cessation [70]. As described later in this chapter, brief motivational interviewing has demonstrated success in reducing drinking. The U.S. Preventive Services Task Force recommends offering adults with cardiovascular disease risk factors behavioral counseling interventions to promote a healthy diet and physical activity [71]. The overall magnitude of benefit related to these interventions is positive but small. Patients who are interested and ready to make behavioral changes may be most likely to benefit from behavioral counseling [70–75]. For example, the Patient-Centered Assessment and Counseling for Exercise approach has been successful [72].

Counseling of adults and children by HCPs can increase children's practices of safety behaviors (e.g., the use of seat belts, child safety seats, and bicycle helmets), although the prevalence of this counseling is low in the United States [73]. Brief counseling interventions aimed at high-risk individuals can increase condom use and prevent the spread of sexually transmitted diseases [74]. Recommendations by HCPs are central to adherence with cancer screening tests, such as those for the breast, colon, and cervix [75], particularly as the guidelines differ by patient characteristics, such as age. The HCP often serves as a motivator for guideline adherence by patients, through advice and referrals. Importantly, comprehensive, well-resourced follow-up, including referral to community resources, is essential to help patients gain the skills they need to change health habits, and to increase their preventive behaviors. These preventive behaviors, supported by the lifestyle medicine HCP, can result in improved health [76–78].

Evidence-Based Behavior Change Techniques

A number of techniques have been found to change behaviors toward health, across different types of patients, risk factors, and within varied contexts. The techniques that are most easily applied to Lifestyle Medicine Centers include goal setting and self-monitoring, shared decision-making, the five As, and motivational interviewing. CBT is a more comprehensive approach to encourage patient engagement for healthy change. CBT uses each of these techniques and is generally most effective when applied by specially trained and licensed mental health professionals.

Goal Setting and Self-Monitoring

After an assessment period, often using an automated or rapidly scored instrument, goal setting begins the change process. SMART (Specific, Measurable, Attainable, Realistic, and Timely) goals can begin the clinical collaboration for patient behavioral change, particularly when goals are reinforced by other team members (Table 15.1) [79]. Self-monitoring is essential to assess progress and identify challenges that call for a modified goal or behavioral strategy [31, 80, 81]. Technological solutions such as sensors and electronic applications (apps) can reduce the burden of self-monitoring.

Shared Decision-Making

Given the more recent view of healthcare decision-making as a partnership between patients and HCPs, there is growing interest in shared decision-making. In fact, the Patient Protection and Affordable Care Act of 2010 (H. R. 3590) [82] includes eight provisions to facilitate and encourage the use of the shared decision-making process. In shared decision-making, the patient and HCP participate in all phases of the decision-making process together, share treatment preferences, and reach an agreement on treatment choice. Shared decision-making engages both HCPs and patients, is informed by the best evidence available, and is weighted according to the specific characteristics and values of the patient [83]. Using formal shared decision-making processes can be especially useful in cases where more than

Table 15.1 SMART goals[a]

Smart item	Explanation	Example
Specific	Is the goal specific in units of increase or decrease?	I will increase my running mileage by 10% each week
Measurable	Is the goal measurable in observable units?	I will keep track of my running distance each day so that I can track my progress toward my goal
Attainable	Is the goal attainable for me?	Yes, given my current schedule and my desire to accomplish this goal, this is attainable
Realistic	Is the goal realistic for me?	Yes, I have everything I need to make this goal a reality. I have the support and resources in place
Timely	Is the goal attainable in a reasonable period of time?	I will sign up to run a 5K in 3 months and a 10K in 6 months

[a]Other examples of SMART goals are:

To increase adherence with medication and psychotherapy use for a depressed patient: I will take my fluoxetine (Prozac) each morning before I go to work and will go to Dr. Tappler's office every Tuesday at 4 pm, as scheduled, for the next month

To increase intake of fruits and vegetables: I will include at least one serving of vegetables for two meals each day and at least one serving of fruit per day over the next 4 weeks

To stop smoking: I will substitute a walk for my morning cigarette, and chew 4 mg of nicotine replacement gum every time that I feel like smoking. I will wear a nicotine patch on my left arm for the next 3 months

To increase physical activity: I will jog outside or use the elliptical machine at the gym at a moderate intensity for 30 minutes 4 times per week

See Refs. [143, 144, 146]

one treatment option is available and also when no treatment is considered best according to clinical evidence [84]. Shared decision-making is key to patient-centered care, defined as the extent to which discussions about care reflect the considered needs, values, and preferences of a well-informed patient [85].

One important prerequisite for shared decision-making is the mutual exchange of information between the patient and lifestyle medicine HCP, because the knowledge of both together is often greater than the knowledge of each separately, and can optimize the chances of successful management of an illness [86]. The patient discloses expectations, preferences, fears, attitudes toward risk, values, experience of illness, and social circumstances, whereas the HCP contributes expert medical knowledge on disease causes and mechanisms, symptoms, treatment options, and prognosis [87]. After an interactive process with a final agreement, the HCP and patient plan steps to put their shared decision into action. Often, these decisions are supported by tools for values clarification [88] and information about the benefits and harms of treatment choices [89].

5

168   S. S. Gorin and C. L. Davis

Shared decision-making is central to prostate cancer screening. Since the benefits are not clearer than the risks for prostate cancer screening using the Prostate-Specific Antigen test (PSA), major professional groups, such as the American Cancer Society, the American Urological Association, the American Academy of Family Practitioners, and the U.S. Preventive Services Task Force recommend informed or shared decision-making between age-eligible men and their primary care HCPs [90].

The Five As

The original five As framework (Ask, Advise, Assess, Assist, and Arrange, [91]) was developed for smoking-cessation counseling and has been adapted to other lifestyle changes, such as physical activity (Fig. 15.3) [7, 92]. The 5 As were first published alongside the 5 Rs to enhance moti-vation for tobacco cessation (Relevance, Risk, Rewards, Roadblocks, and Repetition) [93]. In 2002, The Counseling and Behavioral Interventions Work Group of the U.S. Preventive Services Task Force recommended adoption of the 5 As as a unifying framework for evaluating and describing health behavior counseling interventions in clinical settings [94].

A 2013 Cochrane review of randomized clinical trials on smoking cessation by physicians concluded that simple advice had a small effect on cessation rates [95]. Assuming an unassisted quit rate of 2–3%, a brief advice intervention can increase quitting by a further 1–3% at least 6 months post-counseling [95]. Additional components appear to have only a small effect, though there is a small additional benefit of more intensive interventions compared to very brief interventions [95]. Moreover, providing follow-up support after offering the advice may slightly increase the quit rates [96].

Fig. 15.3 The five As as applied to physical activity counseling. The five As framework (Ask, Advise, Assess, Assist, and Arrange) was first developed for smoking-cessation counseling and adapted to other lifestyle changes, such as physical activity [7, 91, 92] The updated five As substitute Assess for the first A, and Agree for the third A [94, 99, 100]

Assess	Physical activity level / Physical abilities / Beliefs and knowledge	**Individual** — "How much exercise do you currently get each day?" "What kinds of things make it hard to exercise?"
Advise	Health risks / Benefits of change / Appropriate "dose" of physical activity	**Health policy** — "The national guidelines recommend at least 150 minutes of moderate activity each week. I strongly recommend that you begin to move around more regularly. We always recommend starting from where you are and building up slowly."
Agree	Co-develop personalized action plan / Set specific physical activity goals based on interests and confidence level	**Social Support** — "I understand that you have a busy work and family schedule. How do you feel about starting with 20-minute walks for 3 days next week? Maybe you could also use that time to spend with your daughter?"
Assist	Identify barriers and create strategies to address them / Identify resources for physical activity and social support	**Community Resources** — "Do you have a gym, park, trail system, or other safe place to be active near your home or workplace?"
Arrange	Specify plan for follow-up (e.g. visits, phone calls, text messages) / Check on progress/maintenance of physical activity change	**Provider/Team** — "We would like to hear about how the walking is going for you. The nurse will call you in one week to check in and see if you have any questions or concerns."

Training programs have been designed to improve medical professionals' effectiveness, skills, and self-efficacy in this area [96, 97]. In the short term, they have been effective in improving HCPs' (particularly physicians') confidence and perceived effectiveness and increasing rates of asking, advising, and providing self-help materials for cessation [95, 97].

The U.S. Public Health Service clinical practice guideline summarized the effects of physicians' counseling on tobacco cessation, finding them more effective than any other professional group alone [98]. Various HCPs have been found to have critical influences on smoking cessation among their patients, yet they differ in their cessation efficacy [98]. Using a meta-analysis of 37 randomized clinical trials or quasi-experiments (with control groups) of HCP-delivered smoking cessation interventions, physicians (followed by multi-provider teams, dentists, and nurses) were found to be the most effective at inducing cessation [70]. These findings suggest that contact with an HCP will increase tobacco cessation; however, additional training in this area is warranted for nurses. Longer-term studies of smoking cessation, particularly among dentists and lifestyle medicine HCPs, are necessary [70].

Two Substitute As

The 5 As have been expanded to include elements of relationship formation (with the substitution of "Assess" for the first *A*, and "Agree" for the third *A*); these have been applied to other health behaviors to enhance patient self-management in chronic illness care [94, 99, 100]. This 5 As framework is closely linked to the principles of effective communication, as relationship skills (e.g., open-ended inquiry, reflective listening, and empathy) are essential elements of effective counseling interventions. However, unlike the 5 As for smoking cessation, these 5 As include a specific relationship-building component. Both 5 As frameworks have advantages as tools for learning and disseminating prevention behaviors [94, 101, 102].

Toward Routine Use of the 5 As in Clinical Practice

Given these findings, the lifestyle medicine HCP should ask about smoking at each visit, using a well-tested, brief model of the 5 As (Ask/Assess, Advise, Assess/Agree, Assist, and Arrange [91]). The Agency for Healthcare Research and Quality recommends that smoking be considered a "vital sign," like blood pressure and weight, and thus should be queried and recorded at each visit. A worksheet can integrate the 5 As in clinical practices (Fig. 15.4) [102], although proposed routine (and often automated) patient assessment and

Component	Who	What	When	Where	Resources needed	Notes
Assess						
Advise						
Agree						
Assist						
Arrange						

Fig. 15.4 Example office planning worksheet to integrate the five As into primary care practice. A worksheet can integrate the 5 As in clinical practice. These worksheets can be automated and integrated with the electronic medical record [102]

screening tools, and many electronic health records, also include cues for smoking cessation [103].

Motivational Interviewing

The widely disseminated clinical method of motivational interviewing arose through a convergence of behavioral science and clinical practice [104]. Motivational interviewing focuses on exploring and resolving ambivalence, and centers on motivational processes within the individual that facilitate change. Motivational interviewing supports change in a manner congruent with the person's own values and concerns, rather than coercing or imposing change. A definition of motivational interviewing is: "A collaborative, person-centered form of guiding to elicit and strengthen motivation for change" [104]. Components of motivational interviewing may be applied by the lifestyle medicine HCP, but it is best applied by a trained behavioral therapist.

The Motivational Interviewing Approach

Motivational interviewing focuses on building rapport in the initial stages of the counseling relationship. A central concept of motivational interviewing is the identification, examination, and resolution of ambivalence about changing behavior. With the client relationship central to the motivational interviewing process, the HCP expresses empathy, develops discrepancy, avoids argumentation, rolls with resistance, and supports self-efficacy [105].

Ambivalence – feeling two ways about behavior change – is seen as a natural part of the change process. By contrast, HCP exhortations or arguments for change tend to build resistance. Thus, when "change talk" is elicited or spontaneously expressed by the patient, the HCP provides positive affirmation and support to help build and deepen commit- ment [106, 107]. *Rolling with resistance* involves backing off when the patient expresses it, by acknowledging that change is difficult, while also inviting the patient to consider new information or perspectives [108, 109]. The HCP supports self-efficacy by helping the patient build on past successes, take achievable small steps toward change, and solve prob- lems to overcome barriers [110].

Motivation for change occurs when people perceive a mismatch between where they are and where they want to be; a lifestyle medicine HCP practicing MI works to develop this by helping patients examine the discrepancies between their current circumstances or behaviors and their values and future goals. To address client ambivalence and "roll with resistance," the HCP thoughtfully uses techniques and strate- gies that are responsive to the patient. These motivational interviewing strategies are built on three components of the counseling interchange: collaboration, evocation, and autonomy [108, 109, 111]. In short, the HCP employing motivational interviewing will seek to abide by four prin- ciples throughout treatment: express empathy, support self- efficacy, roll with resistance, and develop discrepancy [108, 109, 111].

Motivational Interviewing Strategies

The practice of motivational interviewing involves the skill- ful use of certain counseling techniques, including non- verbal communication, to establish a therapeutic alliance (or as it is originally termed, a "beneficial client-therapist attach- ment" [108]) and to capitalize on the patient's potential for change. These are known by the acronym OARS, which describes Open-ended questions, Affirmations, Reflections, and Summaries [109, 111].

Open-ended questions are those that are not easily answered by yes/no, or by a short, specific, limited response. Open-ended questions invite elaboration and thinking more deeply about an issue. On the other hand, closed-ended ques- tions (answerable by a simple yes/no) can be used for assessment.

Affirmations are statements that recognize patient strengths and support patient self-efficacy. They also assist in building rapport and in helping the patient see that change is possible. Affirmations include reframing behaviors or con- cerns as evidence of positive patient qualities.

Reflections, or reflective listening, are perhaps the most crucial skills in motivational interviewing. Reflections con- sist of repeating or rephrasing what the patient has said, para- phrasing the patient, or reflecting the patient's feelings. Through the use of these skills, the patient comes to feel that the HCP understands the issues from his or her perspective and is empathic. The HCP guides the patient toward resolv- ing ambivalence by focusing on the negative aspects of the *status quo* and the positive aspects of making change.

Summaries are a special type of reflection in which the clinician recaps what has occurred in all or part of a counsel- ing session. Summaries communicate interest and under- standing and call attention to important elements of the discussion. They may be used to shift attention or direction and to prepare the patient to move on. Summaries can high- light both sides of a patient's ambivalence about change and can promote the development of discrepancy by strategically selecting what information should be included and what can be minimized or excluded.

Change Talk

The HCP implements OARS alongside the patient's change talk. Change talk contains statements revealing the patient's motivation for, or commitment to, change. This is also con- ceptualized as DARNCAT:

- Desire (I want to change)
- Ability (I can change)
- Reason (It's important to change)
- Need (I should change)
- Commitment (I will make changes)
- Activation (I am ready, prepared, and willing to change)
- Taking steps (I am taking specific actions to change) [109, 111]

Example: Diabetes

A brief, scripted example of the use of motivational inter- viewing with a patient who has T2D to encourage eating less sugary foods follows:

- *Lifestyle Medicine HCP*: "You know, we've discussed this many times before; perhaps eating sugary foods is so important to you that you won't give it up, no matter what the cost." (*Come alongside*)
- *Patient response*: "I really should change; my health and staying around for my family is more important than eat- ing Krispy Kreme donuts®." (*Change talk*)
- *Lifestyle Medicine HCP*: "That's great to hear you say; in what (specific) ways could you reduce the sugary foods in your diet?" (*Ask for elaboration, examples*)

Practical Motivational Interviewing for Lifestyle Medicine

Brief versions of MI have been developed for use by HCPs in primary care and other healthcare settings [106, 109]. These brief versions, including Motivational Enhancement Therapy (MET), still include motivational interviewing strategies, but with emphasis on two specific dimensions of motivation: conviction about the need for change and confidence (self- efficacy) about taking action [108, 112]. Assessment is followed by tailoring of counseling to address the patient's level of conviction and confidence, agreeing on a realistic and achievable goal, and assisting the patient in developing a behavior change plan.

As a general rule, if both conviction and confidence are low, it is best to first focus on enhancing conviction. For patients with low conviction levels, effective counseling strategies include providing information and feedback (after asking the patient's permission), exploring ambivalence, and providing a menu of options for treatment and follow-up. Patients not ready to commit to action may agree to simply think about the possibilities for change or to seek assistance when they are ready to take action. For patients with low confidence, strategies include reviewing past experience, especially successes; teaching problem-solving and coping skills; and encouraging small steps that are likely to lead to an initial success. For all patients, a follow-up plan is essential as an important evidence-based ingredient of counseling interventions and successful health behavior change [93, 102, 111, 113].

Evaluation of Motivational Interviewing

Motivational interviewing has been found effective in decreasing substance abuse in a number of multisite clinical trials [112, 114]. Outcomes through 3 years of follow-up were similar for a 4-session MET (Motivational Enhancement Therapy, a specific motivational interviewing intervention) and the two 12-session treatment methods with which it was compared, yielding a cost-effectiveness advantage for MET [112, 115–117]. Similar positive findings emerged from the 3-site United Kingdom Alcohol Treatment Trial comparing MET with an 8-session family-involved behavior therapy [104, 118, 119].

The Clinical Trials Network of the U.S. National Institute on Drug Abuse has undertaken six multisite trials of motivational interviewing and MET as compared with treatment-as-usual for drug problems and dependence [120]. Motivational interviewing-based interventions promoted sustained reductions in alcohol use [121] and increased treatment retention [122]. It is important to note that MET exerted a significant beneficial effect at some sites, but not others [104, 121, 123].

In fact, not all clinical trials with motivational interviewing have been positive. For example, null findings have been reported among those with eating disorders [124], drug abuse and dependence [123, 125], tobacco use [126, 127], and problem drinking [128]. It is apparent that some HCPs are significantly more effective than others in delivering the same motivational interviewing-based treatment [116]; even in positive trials, a certain proportion of patients do not respond to MI [104].

The efficacy of MI also can vary across populations. A meta-analysis found that the effect size of motivational interviewing was doubled when the recipients were predomi-nantly from minority populations, as compared with white non-Hispanic Americans [129]. A retrospective analysis of Project MATCH data found that Native Americans responded better to MET, as compared with other treatments [130]. Similarly, the Clinical Trials Network studies found some evidence for differential benefit from MET among pregnant drug users from minority backgrounds relative to other women [104, 123]. Motivational interviewing appears to enhance diabetes education, even in non-Western cultures [131]. Given habits, preferences, and community factors including food availability, focusing on reducing portion sizes of calorie-dense and/or highly processed usual foods (such as sugar-sweetened beverages), and increasing fiber- and nutrient-dense fresh or minimally processed food intake may be helpful across cultures [132, 133].

Cognitive Behavioral Therapy (CBT)

CBT is the form of psychotherapy with the most extensive evidence base supporting its effectiveness [134]. On a base of essential trust and rapport, the therapist learns about the patient's concerns, coping strategies, and strengths. The trained therapist, using the following techniques, supports patients to change their behaviors:

- *Reframing* – showing someone another perspective on how to understand a situation
- *Self-talk* – attending to the things a person says to themselves, about themselves
- *Cognitive distortions* – identifying and challenging unhelpful self-talk, such as catastrophization, to replace it with more realistic and kind self-talk
- *Building skills* – such as self-monitoring, goal-setting, and relaxation
- *Behavioral activation* – increasing enjoyable activities in varied settings, with other people, to improve mood, over time [135]

Relaxation methods are also widely used in CBT and include slow deep breathing, imagery, mindfulness, meditation, and progressive muscle relaxation [135]. CBT addresses current challenges that the patient is experiencing, and typically includes behavioral homework assignments: self-monitoring of behavior, thoughts, and mood to identify patterns and assess progress, and practice at identifying and challenging unhelpful self-talk [135]. CBT was developed for treating depression in adults and has been applied successfully for treatment of a wide variety of problems including stress management, insomnia, anxiety disorders such as post-traumatic stress disorder, and adaptation to chronic health conditions, such as diabetes [135–138].

Assessing Practice Effectiveness for Patients: The "My Own Health Report" Tool

Lifestyle medicine is enhanced by a set of tools to assess health behavior and mental health. These tools allow the HCP to tailor the intervention, as well as begin to examine the effectiveness of the practice on patient outcomes. The "My Own Health Report" (MOHR) patient evaluation tool is evidence-based and assesses health behavior and mental health among patients in a primary care setting [77, 139, 140]. The MOHR tool is paired with a feedback system to promote patient counseling and collaborative goal setting between patients and HCPs in the Lifestyle Medicine Center.

The MOHR tool assesses 17 health behavior and psychosocial risk screening questions and 6 demographic questions [77, 139, 140]. Each of the screening items assessed by the MOHR tool is recommended by the U.S. Preventive Services Task Force (with the exception of sleep, quality of life, and anxiety) [77, 139, 140]. For those patients who initially screen positive for symptoms, additional follow-up services are provided. The electronic version of the MOHR tool [141] provides a score and categorizes patients' responses as being of "no concern," "some concern," or "high concern" [77, 139, 140]. For responses with some or high concern, patients are asked if they are ready to change and/or discuss the topic with their HCP [94, 99, 102, 142]. The MOHR tool provides patients with a summary containing motivational feedback, initial improvement steps, and space to create three SMART goals [143, 144]. An HCP summary is automatically shared with the practice via uploading to the electronic health record (sample SMART goals and feedback reports for patients and the practice team are found in Glasgow et al. [145] and Gorin and Krist [146]). The implementation of the MOHR tool was systematically evaluated within a practice-level, cluster-randomized, pragmatic implementation study using mixed methods [147].

Compared to patients from control practices, practices using the MOHR tool reported greater screening rates for each of the eight behaviors and mental health risks that were measured (range of differences, 5.3–15.8%, $p < 0.001$) [148]. Compared to controls, patients using the MOHR tool believed that their clinicians cared more for them and showed more interest in their concerns. Overall, the MOHR tool improved screening and goal setting.

Healthcare professionals who implemented the MOHR tool found that the patient and HCP reports helped to identify problem behaviors and streamlined the goal-setting process [149]. For example, one clinic "tie[d] the MOHR project into the clinic's patient-centered medical home initiative…[by] providing patients with support in self-management, self-efficacy, and behavior change [with] self-management tools" [149]. The MOHR tool provided access to information technology and human resources of health systems (such as nurses in call centers) to foster implementation and reach (e.g., for a weight-loss project) [149]. The MOHR tool offers considerable promise for assessing patient risk factors and encouraging shared goal setting between patients and HCPs.

Information Technology and the Lifestyle Medicine Center

Electronic and personal health records track and coordinate patient care. Many practices also use e-mail to communicate with patients, as well as mobile health (mHealth) approaches, such as telehealth, sensors, and text messages. Security and privacy remain key concerns throughout their use.

Mobile Health

Mobile health interventions are one of the fastest growing areas of activity in lifestyle medicine information technology. mHealth uses mobile devices, including any wireless device carried by a person that transmits or accepts health information. The growth in popularity of cell phones, now carried by a majority of the US adult population, with their rapidly increasing capabilities, screen resolutions, add-ons such as sensors, video chat, and increased storage, has resulted in an explosion in new ways to foster health management and preventive services.

Telehealth, a growing HCP tool, may rely on mHealth approaches. Telehealth is defined as the use of electronic information and telecommunications technologies to support and promote long-distance clinical healthcare, patient and professional health-related education, public health and health administration (according to the Health Resources and Services Administration). Telehealth has increased due to the availability of billing codes for reimbursement and, most recently, with the rapid alterations in healthcare delivery models due to the coronavirus disease 2019 pandemic. In addition to mHealth approaches, telehealth technologies include: live (synchronous) videoconferencing between a patient and HCP; and store-and-forward (asynchronous) videoconferencing to transmit the patient's health history to the HCP, usually a specialist. Other forms of remote electronic patient assessment and evaluation are discussed further in this chapter.

In 2017, 325,000 health-related apps were available for download on smartphones and tablets, with Android platforms the most popular [150]. Unfortunately, most digital health tools do not use behavior change theory [151]. Testing of these apps is rare, with resultant fraud, abuse, or even patient harm [152–154]. For example, in a case-control study, the performance of smartphone applications in assessing melanoma risk from photographs of skin lesions was evaluated; diagnostic accuracy of the apps varied considerably

[154]. Three of four smartphone applications incorrectly classified 30% or more of melanomas as not of concern. Reliance on these applications (which are not subject to regulatory oversight) in lieu of medical consultation, can delay the diagnosis of melanoma (and other diseases) and harm users [155]. Social media platforms have also been used to deliver lifestyle interventions, with modest effectiveness; however, social media is also rife with misinformation [152, 156].

> Nonetheless, online-delivered interventions are more accessible and scalable than in-person treatments. Evidence-based mHealth weight loss interventions include an 18-month smartphone-based behavioral obesity treatment with monthly weigh-ins that were comparable to gold standard group sessions [153]. Of note, a pragmatic trial of Rx Weight Loss, a physician-referred online weight loss program that was effective for initial weight loss (half of participants achieved 5% weight loss) [154], is underway in 60 primary care clinics to evaluate weight loss maintenance and utility of clinician supports [157].

A promising use of the cell phone is ecological momentary assessment, or repeated sampling of an individual's current behaviors and experiences in real time [158], to monitor smoking cessation or food choices. Unlike patient-reported behavior to the HCP, that can be biased and intermittent, the phone – which is carried throughout each day – can monitor behavior using sensors and/or diary entries. This monitoring can be timed appropriately (e.g., near lunch to query food choices) and can ask the patient specific questions in an easy-to-respond format. Data can be uploaded to centralized databases with online or mobile tracking tools. Visualizations can be viewed by the healthcare team and the patient, decisions made, and programs of treatment adjusted. Monitoring between visits is also possible with mobile health technologies. For example, sleep disorders or a smoking lapse may be recorded in real time by monitoring breathing patterns or movements.

Mobile health applications have the advantage of potential scalability to a large population, as devices are cheap and often already owned by the patient. These devices can be attached to specialized sensors, contain accelerometers and geographic location detection functions, collect, store, and transmit massive amounts of rich data in real time (allowing continuous data collection at many geographic locations), and therefore accommodate applications that provide real-time feedback.

Sensors

A number of sites and apps provide small wearable sensors capable of monitoring blood pressure, glucose, physical activity, and sleep (e.g., Apple Watch™, Omron HeartGuide™, Dexcom G6™, Freestyle Libre™, Medtronic Guardian™, Bodymedia™, Fit Armband BW 2™, Philips DirectLife™, FitBit™, Gruve™, and Zeo Personal Sleep Coach™). Recent developments in glucose monitoring and partially automated insulin dosing (i.e., hybrid closed-loop artificial pancreas) have dramatically improved the available treatments for patients with diabetes, especially those with type 1 diabetes [159, 160]. Also, new sensor technology (Sweatronics™) is capable of measuring cortisol levels from sweat, which may reflect the stress response.

Sensor data can allow rapid reactions to events or environments and provide interfaces for HCPs and patients or their families to facilitate comprehension. These approaches, called sensor-enhanced health information systems, have already been used for cardiac monitoring [161]. Continuous monitoring, for example, of gait abnormalities [161] can assist with the diagnosis and treatment of musculoskeletal conditions such as knee arthritis, using data from the patient's experiences with the activities of daily living. With the aging of the population, sensors may become more useful for at-home continuous monitoring and decision support to allow patients to remain at home with remote HCP support.

As one example of the promise of sensor-enhanced health information systems, the KNOWME Network, which is designed to reduce obesity among minority youth, is a suite of wearable, wireless sensors (a wireless body area network) that sends streaming data to a mobile phone for non-intrusive monitoring of metabolic health, vital signs such as heart rate and stress levels, and physical activity and other obesity-related behaviors [162]. The mobile phone collects, stores, and transmits data to a secure web server where data are analyzed and translated in real time. A record of behavior and health data that is time-stamped, synchronized, and geographically localized could be made available via secure Internet connections to a lifestyle medicine HCP. The phone allows for immediate, real-time feedback through the phone display and through text messaging, image, and voice tags. Some data will be immediately visualized on the phone for participants (for instance, a running tally of minutes of moderate to vigorous physical activity per day). In the future, networks such as KNOWME may yield a new generation of adaptive, personalized interventions for real-time monitoring, immediate data delivery, and rapid adaptive intervention response [162].

Short Message Service Text Reminders

Reminders are effective in engaging patients and prompting desired behaviors in a just-in-time manner. Two-way text messages can provide reminders, psychological support, triage, and verification of reported behaviors. For example, Text4baby is a widely disseminated application that provides advising prompts on healthy behaviors for pregnant women and mothers, such as prenatal care, safe sleep, immunizations, breastfeeding, and oral health [163]. Other applications include text message reminders for AIDS medication adherence, both in the United States and abroad.

A recent comprehensive meta-analysis of mobile health interventions found modest but significant effectiveness of text messages for improving appointment adherence relative to no reminders [164]. A study conducted after the meta-analysis found that text message reminders improved adherence to malaria treatment guidelines by 23% [165]. A systematic review by Militello et al. [166] showed that text messages may be more effective as reminders supporting disease management behavior change in children and teens than in adults [166]. However, the authors note that many studies were not of high quality, and more rigorous studies are needed to establish the benefits of mobile intervention for various modalities. This is particularly true as cell phone capabilities and new innovations have expanded rapidly to include video and photo transmission.

Cultural Sensitivity in Behavioral Change

Adapting the HCP's approach to the cultural contexts experienced by ethnic and racial minority and immigrant groups, in particular, is key to behavioral change. For example, upon immigration to the United States, Latino/a immigrant adolescents and their parents can experience cultural stressors that result from navigating multiple cultural contexts, hostile attitudes, and discrimination in their new communities. These cultural stressors can negatively influence family functioning, emotional well-being, and health-risk behaviors (such as cigarette smoking and binge drinking) among adolescents and parents [167]. A recent longitudinal study of 302 adolescent-caregiver pairs who were new immigrants to the United States found that preventive interventions, targeting families with poor functioning, might be most influential in the early years following immigration. Equally important to improving behavioral health among both new immigrant parents and adolescents are systematic community- and policy-focused strategies that combat discrimination against Latino/a families and improve the attitudes of community members about immigrants [167].

Multilevel (3 or more) interventions have positive effects on several health behavior outcomes among racial/ethnic minority groups; these outcomes include cancer prevention and screening, as well improving the quality of HCP and healthcare system processes such as patient navigation, according to a recent descriptive review (N = 26 studies) [168]. Further, culturally leveraging multilevel interventions, by adapting appropriate cultural meaning and context into the intervention materials, messages, and delivery systems, may improve their effectiveness [168–170].

Some Ethical Considerations on the Use of Online Technology in Lifestyle Medicine

The narrative encounter between patient and HCP, which is at the heart of the practice of medicine and which is central to online communication, cannot serve the needs of patients if they are unable to communicate their symptoms, unable to understand how to take their medications, or are too intimidated by the medical hierarchy and medical jargon to speak up [171]. Patients with low health literacy, those who are deaf or of limited English facility, those facing a stigma of substance abuse, and those otherwise disadvantaged face unique ethical challenges. The lifestyle medicine HCP should be guided by extant and emerging professional ethical guidelines and legal regulations, particularly to guard patients' privacy and the confidentiality of online and remote communications [171, 172].

Identifying Behavioral Change Experts

A number of trained HCPs may support patients' behavioral changes in the Lifestyle Medicine Center, alongside other clinicians. Clinical health psychologists are trained in behavioral theory and evidence-based practice in the context of health (disease prevention, medical treatment, and management of illnesses). Clinical health psychologists hold a doctoral degree in psychology (e.g., PhD or PsyD) that requires post-baccalaureate clinical training in health settings. The PhD degree requires research training and a dissertation, while the PsyD is clinically focused. Clinical health psychologists conduct research, provide clinical treatment, consult with other HCPs, and advise organizations and policy makers [173]. The American Board of Professional Psychology credential indicates the successful completion of training and experience requirements for a specialty in psychology, plus an examination demonstrating competency in that specialty. Only around 4% of licensed psychologists hold this credential. Dietitians, nurses, social workers, exercise scientists, physical therapists, diabetes care and education specialists (formerly called certified diabetes educators) [158], applied behavior analysts, and epidemiologists are examples of other experts who are skilled in assessing and supporting patients' behavior change.

Conclusion

Behavioral medicine provides an essential evidence base and personnel resource for lifestyle medicine. Resources are available to optimize a behavioral medicine program in a Lifestyle Medicine Center or Clinical Service Line (Table 15.2). Behavioral medicine HCPs play essential roles

Table 15.2 Professional and training resources in behavioral medicine for the lifestyle medicine healthcare professional[a]

Academy of Nutrition and Dietetics, https://www.eatright.org/

American Association of Diabetes Educators, https://www.diabeteseducator.org/

American College of Sports Medicine, https://www.acsm.org/

American Diabetes Association Mental Health Provider Directory Listing, https://professional.diabetes.org/mhp_listing

American Heart Association, https://www.heart.org/

American Psychological Association, https://www.apa.org

American Society for Metabolic and Bariatric Surgery, https://asmbs.org/about

Association for Behavioral and Cognitive Therapies, http://www.abct.org

Behavioral Research Program, National Cancer Institute, https://cancercontrol.cancer.gov/brp/

Exercise is Medicine, https://www.exerciseismedicine.org/

Find a Cognitive Behavioral Therapist, http://www.findcbt.org/FAT/

The "5 As," https://www.ahrq.gov/prevention/guidelines/tobacco/5steps.html

Jenny Craig, www.jennycraig.com

Motivational Interviewing Network of Trainers, https://motivationalinterviewing.org/

MyOwnHealthReport, https://MyOwnHealthReport.org

National Diabetes Education Program, https://www.cdc.gov/diabetes/ndep/

National Obesity Care Week, https://www.obesitycareweek.org/

Nutri/System, www.nutrisystem.com/

Obesity Action Coalition, https://www.obesityaction.org/

Obesity Medicine Association, https://obesitymedicine.org/

Obesity Medicine Education Collaborative, https://obesitymedicine.org/omec/

Overeaters Anonymous, www.oa.org/

Prevention Practice in Primary Care. Sheinfeld Gorin S, editor. New York: Oxford University Press; 2014. https://global.oup.com/academic/product/prevention-practice-in-primary-care-9780195373011?cc=us&lang=en&

SHAPE America (Society of Health and Physical Educators), https://www.shapeamerica.org/

Shared Decision Making, https://www.healthit.gov/sites/default/files/nlc_shared_decision_making_fact_sheet.pdf, http://informedmedicaldecisions.org/

Society for Health Psychology (American Psychological Association Division 38), https://societyforhealthpsychology.org/

Society of Behavioral Medicine, www.sbm.org

Society of Pediatric Psychology (American Psychological Association Division 54), https://societyofpediatricpsychology.org/

Strategies to Overcome and Prevent (STOP) Obesity Alliance, http://stop.publichealth.gwu.edu/

Text4baby, text4baby.org

TOPS (Take Off Pounds Sensibly) Club, Inc., www.tops.org/

TOPS Health Care Professionals, https://www.tops.org/tops/TOPS/Healthcare.aspx

Weight Watchers, www.weightwatchers.com

YMCA's Diabetes Prevention Program, https://www.ymca.net/diabetes-prevention

[a]All websites Accessed on March 7, 2020

in implementing lifestyle medicine interventions, as well as evaluating the effectiveness of Lifestyle Medicine Centers. The ideal lifestyle medicine practice team includes HCPs with behavioral expertise supplemented by specialized behavioral experts, such as health psychologists, diabetes educators, exercise scientists, and dieticians, to support their patients' healthy lifestyle changes.

References

1. Schwartz GE, Weiss SM. Behavioral medicine revisited: an amended definition. J Behav Med. 1978;1:249–51.
2. Dekker J, Stauder A, Penedo FJ. Proposal for an update of the definition and scope of behavioral medicine. Int J Behav Med. 2017;24:1–4.
3. Engel GL. The need for a new medical model: a challenge for biomedicine. Science. 1977;196:129–36.
4. Engel GL. The clinical application of the biopsychosocial model. Am J Psychiat. 1980;137:535–44.
5. Cummings DM, Lutes LD, Littlewood K, et al. Randomized trial of a tailored cognitive behavioral intervention in type 2 diabetes with comorbid depressive and/or regimen-related distress symptoms: 12-month outcomes from COMRADE. Diabetes Care. 2019;42:841–8.
6. Phelps R, Bray JH, Kearney LK. A quarter century of psychological practice in mental health and health care: 1990–2016. Am Psychol. 2017;72:822–36.
7. AuYoung M, Linke SE, Pagoto S, et al. Integrating physical activity in primary care practice. Am J Med. 2016;129:1022–9.
8. Moos RH. Social ecological perspectives on health. In: Stone GC, Cohen F, Adler NE, editors. Health psychology: a handbook. San Francisco: Jossey-Bass; 1979. p. 523–47.
9. Hawley AH. Human ecology; a theory of community structure. New York: The Ronald Press Company; 1950.
10. Emery FE, Trist EL. Towards a social ecology: contextual appreciations of the future in the present. New York: Plenum; 1972.

11. Cannon WB. The wisdom of the body. New York: W W Norton & Co.; 1939.

12. Katz D, Kahn RL. The social psychology of organizations. New York: Wiley; 1966.

13. Maruyama M. The second cybernetics: deviation-amplifying mutual causal processes. Am Sci. 1963;51:164–79.

14. Stokols D. Establishing and maintaining healthy environments: toward a social ecology of health promotion. Am Psychol. 1992;47:6–20.

15. Jackson RJ, Dannenberg AL, Frumkin H. Health and the built environment: 10 years after. Am J Public Health. 2013;103:1542–4.

16. Frumkin H. Healthy places: exploring the evidence. Am J Public Health. 2003;93:1451–6.

17. Sheinfeld Gorin S. Models for prevention. In: Sheinfeld Gorin S, editor. Prevention practice in primary care. New York: Oxford University Press; 2014. p. 57–92.

18. Putnam RD. Bowling alone: the collapse and revival of American community: Simon and Schuster; 2000.

19. Saelens BE, Sallis JF, Frank LD. Environmental correlates of walking and cycling: findings from the transportation, urban design, and planning literatures. Ann Behav Med. 2003;25:80–91.

20. Friedman MS, Powell KE, Hutwagner L, et al. Impact of changes in transportation and commuting behaviors during the 1996 Summer Olympic Games in Atlanta on air quality and childhood asthma. JAMA. 2001;285:897–905.

21. Jackson RJ. The impact of the built environment on health: an emerging field. Am J Public Health. 2003;93:1382–4.

22. Rabow J, Watts RK. The role of alcohol availability in alcohol consumption and alcohol problems. In: Galanter, M., editor. Recent developments in alcoholism: Genetics, behavioral treatment, social mediators and prevention, current concepts in diagnosis, Vol. 1. New York: Plenum Press; 1983. p. 285–302.

23. The CMS Innovation Center. https://innovation.cms.gov/. Accessed on 26 Oct 2019.

24. Rothman AA, Wagner EH. Chronic illness management: what is the role of primary care? Ann Int Med. 2003;138:256–61.

25. Grossman E, Keegan T, Lessler AL, et al. Inside the health disparities collaboratives: a detailed exploration of quality improvement at community health centers. Med Care. 2008;46:489–96.

26. Pearson ML, Wu S, Schaefer J, et al. Assessing the implementation of the chronic care model in quality improvement collaboratives. Health Serv Res. 2005;40:978–96.

27. Glasgow RE, Tracy Orleans C, Wagner EH, et al. Does the chronic care model serve also as a template for improving prevention? Milbank Q. 2001;79:579–612.

28. Tsai AC, Morton SC, Mangione CM, et al. A meta-analysis of interventions to improve care for chronic illnesses. Am J Manag Care. 2005;11:478–88.

29. Holland PC. Cognitive versus stimulus-response theories of learning. Learn Behav. 2008;36:227–41.

30. Skinner BF. Are theories of learning necessary? Psychol Rev. 1950;57:193–216.

31. Wilfley DE, Hayes JF, Balantekin KN, et al. Behavioral interventions for obesity in children and adults: evidence base, novel approaches, and translation into practice. Am Psychol. 2018;73:981–93.

32. Bandura A. Social learning theory. Oxford, UK: Prentice-Hall; 1977.

33. Bandura A. Health promotion by social cognitive means. Health Educ Behav. 2004;31:143–64.

34. Bandura A. Social foundations of thought and action. Prentice Hall: Englewood Cliffs, NJ; 1986.

35. Baer JS, Lichtenstein E. Cognitive assessment. In: Donovan DM, Marlatt GA, editors. Assessment of addictive behaviors. New York: Guilford Press; 1988. p. 189–213.

36. Devins GM. Social cognitive analysis of recovery from a lapse after smoking cessation: comment on Haaga and Stewart. J Consult Clin Psychol. 1992;60:29–31.

37. DiClemente CC. Motivational interviewing and the stages of change. In: Miller W, Rollnick R, editors. Motivational interviewing. New York: Guilford Press; 1991. p. 191–203.

38. Prochaska JO, DiClemente CC. Stages and processes of self-change of smoking: toward an integrative model of change. J Consult Clin Psychol. 1983;51:390–5.

39. Prochaska JO, Velicer WF. The transtheoretical model of health behavior change. Am J Health Prom. 1997;12:38–48.

40. Prochaska JO, Velicer WF, Guadagnoli E, et al. Patterns of change: dynamic typology applied to smoking cessation. Multivariate Behav Res. 1991;26:83–107.

41. Fisher E Jr, Bishop DB, Goldmuntz J, et al. Implications for the practicing physician of the psychosocial dimensions of smoking. Chest. 1988;93:69S–78S.

42. Becker MH. The tyranny of health promotion. Public Health Rev. 1986;14:15–23.

43. Janis IL, Mann L. Decision making: a psychological analysis of conflict, choice, and commitment. New York: Free Press; 1977.

44. Lewin K, Dembo T, Festinger L, et al. Level of aspiration. In: Hunt JM, editor. Personality and the behavioral disorders: a handbook based on experimental and clinical research. New York: Ronald Press; 1944. p. 333–78.

45. Janz NK, Becker MH. The health belief model: a decade later. Health Educ Q. 1984;11:1–47.

46. Rosenstock IM. The health belief model and preventive health behavior. Health Educ Monographs. 1974;2:354–86.

47. Andrews TJ, Ybarra V, Matthews LL. For the sake of our children: Hispanic immigrant and migrant families' use of folk healing and biomedicine. Med Anthropol Q. 2013;27:385–413.

48. Downs LS Jr, Scarinci I, Einstein MH, et al. Overcoming the barriers to HPV vaccination in high-risk populations in the US. Gynecol Oncol. 2010;117:486–90.

49. Ajzen I, Fishbein M. Understanding attitudes and predicting social behavior. New Jersey: Prentice Hall; 1980.

50. Ajzen I. Perceived behavioral control, self-efficacy, locus of control, and the theory of planned behavior. J Appl Soc Psychol. 2002;32:665–83.

51. Curry SJ, Emmons KM. Theoretical models for predicting and improving compliance with breast cancer screening. Ann Behav Med. 1994;16:302–16.

52. Salovey P, Williams-Piehota P. Field experiments in social psychology: message framing and the promotion of health protective behaviors. Am Behav Sci. 2004;47:488–505.

53. Royal Swedish Academy of Sciences. Press release: the prize in economic sciences 2017. https://www.nobelprize.org/uploads/2018/06/press-43.pdf. Accessed on 8 Mar 2020.

54. Weller RE, Cook EW 3rd, Avsar KB, et al. Obese women show greater delay discounting than healthy-weight women. Appetite. 2008;51:563–9.

55. Hollis-Hansen K, Seidman J, O'Donnell S, et al. Episodic future thinking and grocery shopping online. Appetite. 2019;133:1–9.

56. Sheinfeld Gorin S, Krebs P, Badr H, et al. Meta-analysis of psychosocial interventions to reduce pain in patients with cancer. J Clin Oncol 2012;30:539–47.

57. Fisher EB, Fitzgibbon ML, Glasgow RE, et al. Behavior matters. Am J Prev Med. 2011;40:e15–30.

58. Gatchel RJ, McGeary DD, McGeary CA, et al. Interdisciplinary chronic pain management: past, present, and future. Am Psychol. 2014;69:119–30.

59. Wu YP, Herbert LJ, Walker-Harding LR, et al. Introduction to the special issue on child and family health: the role of behavioral medicine in understanding and optimizing child health. Translat Behav Med. 2019;9:399–403.

60. Tronieri JS, Wadden TA, Chao AM, et al. Primary care interventions for obesity: review of the evidence. Curr Obes Rep. 2019;8:128–36.

61. LeBlanc ES, Patnode CD, Webber EM, et al. Behavioral and pharmacotherapy weight loss interventions to prevent obesity-related morbidity and mortality in adults: updated evidence report and systematic review for the US Preventive Services Task Force. JAMA. 2018;320:1172–91.

62. Knowler WC, Barrett-Connor E, Fowler SE, et al. Reduction in the incidence of type 2 diabetes with lifestyle intervention or metformin. New Engl J Med. 2002;346:393–403.

63. Ali MK, Echouffo-Tcheugui J, Williamson DF. How effective were lifestyle interventions in real-world settings that were modeled on the Diabetes Prevention Program? Health Aff (Millwood). 2012;31:67–75.

64. Aveyard P, Lewis A, Tearne S, et al. Screening and brief intervention for obesity in primary care: a parallel, two-arm, randomised trial. Lancet. 2016;388:2492–500.

65. Ackermann RT, Finch EA, Brizendine E, et al. Translating the Diabetes Prevention Program into the community. The DEPLOY Pilot Study. Am J Prev Med. 2008;35:357–63.

66. Ackermann RT, Liss DT, Finch EA, et al. A randomized comparative effectiveness trial for preventing type 2 diabetes. Am J Public Health. 2015;105:2328–34.

67. Pi-Sunyer X, Blackburn G, Brancati FL, et al. Reduction in weight and cardiovascular disease risk factors in individuals with type 2 diabetes: one-year results of the Look AHEAD trial. Diabetes Care. 2007;30:1374–83.

68. Marrero DG, Ackermann RT. Providing long-term support for lifestyle changes: a key to success in diabetes prevention. Diabetes Spectrum. 2007;20:205–9.

69. Powers MA, Bardsley J, Cypress M, et al. Diabetes self-management education and support in type 2 diabetes. Diabetes Educ. 2017;43:40–53.

70. Sheinfeld Gorin S, Heck JE. Meta-analysis of the efficacy of tobacco counseling by health care providers. Cancer Epidemiol Prev Biomarkers. 2004;13:2012–22.

71. U.S. Preventive Services Task Force. Draft Recommendation Statement Healthy Diet and Physical Activity to Prevent Cardiovascular Disease in Adults With Risk Factors: Behavioral Counseling Interventions. https://www.uspreventiveservicestaskforce.org/uspstf/draft-recommendation/diet-and-physical-activity-to-prevent-cardiovascular-disease-in-adults-with-risk-factors-counseling. Accessed May 29, 2020.

72. Calfas KJ, Hagler AS. Physical activity. In: Sheinfeld Gorin S, Arnold J, editors. Health promotion in practice. San Francisco, CA: Jossey-Bass; 2006. p. 192–221.

73. Chen J, Kresnow MJ, Simon TR, et al. Injury-prevention counseling and behavior among US children: results from the second Injury Control and Risk Survey. Pediatrics. 2007;119:e958–65.

74. Noar SM. Behavioral interventions to reduce HIV-related sexual risk behavior: review and synthesis of meta-analytic evidence. AIDS Behav. 2008;12:335–53.

75. Mandelblatt JS, Yabroff KR. Effectiveness of interventions designed to increase mammography use: a meta-analysis of provider-targeted strategies. Cancer Epidemiol Prev Biomarkers. 1999;8:759–67.

76. Goetzel RZ, Staley P, Ogden L, et al. A framework for patient-centered health risk assessments: providing health promotion and disease prevention services to Medicare beneficiaries. US Department of Health and Human Services, Centers for Disease Control and Prevention, Atlanta, GA; 2011. Available at: http://www.cdc.gov/policy/opth/hra/. Accessed on 29 May 2020.

77. Krist AH, Phillips SM, Sabo RT, et al. Adoption, reach, implementation, and maintenance of a behavioral and mental health assessment in primary care. Ann Fam Med. 2014;12:525–33.

78. Shekelle PG, Tucker JS, Maglione MA, et al. Health risk appraisals and Medicare. Santa Monica: RAND Corporation; 2003.

79. Glasgow RE. Medical office-based interventions. In: Snoek F, Skinner TC, editors. Psychology in diabetes care. 2nd ed. Hoboken, NJ: Wiley; 2005. p. 109–33.

80. Michie S, Abraham C, Whittington C, et al. Effective techniques in healthy eating and physical activity interventions: a meta-regression. Health Psychol. 2009;28:690–701.

81. Carver CS, Scheier MF. Control theory: a useful conceptual framework for personality-social, clinical, and health psychology. Psychol Bull. 1982;92:111–35.

82. An act entitled The Patient Protection and Affordable Care Act, 42 U.S.C., §18001 et seq. 2010.

83. Healthwise. http://informedmedicaldecisions.org/. Accessed on 1 Aug 2019.

84. Health IT.gov National Learning Consortium. Shared Decision Making. [Fact sheet]. 2013, https://www.healthit.gov/sites/default/files/nlc_shared_decision_making_fact_sheet.pdf. Accessed on 8 Mar 2020.

85. Sepucha KR, Fowler FJ Jr, Mulley AG Jr. Policy support for patient-centered care: the need for measurable improvements in decision quality. Health Aff. 2004;23(Suppl Variation):VAR54–62.

86. Charles C, Gafni A, Whelan T. Shared decision-making in the medical encounter: what does it mean? (or it takes at least two to tango). Social Sci Med. 1997;44:681–92.

87. Coulter A. Paternalism or partnership?: patients have grown up—and there's no going back. BMJ. 1999;319:719–20.

88. Llewellyn-Thomas HA. Patients' health-care decision making: a framework for descriptive and experimental investigations. Med Decis Making. 1995;15:101–6.

89. Greenfield S, Kaplan S, Ware JE. Expanding patient involvement in care. Ann Intern Med. 1985;102:520–8.

90. Smith RA, von Eschenbach AC, Wender R, et al. American Cancer Society guidelines for the early detection of cancer: update of early detection guidelines for prostate, colorectal, and endometrial cancers. CA Cancer J Clin. 2001;51:38–75.

91. Agency for Healthcare Research and Quality. Five Major Steps to Intervention (The "5 A's"). https://www.ahrq.gov/prevention/guidelines/tobacco/5steps.html. Accessed 29 May 2020.

92. Glynn TJ, Manley MW. How to help your patients stop smoking: a National Cancer Institute manual for physicians. Bethesda, MD: Smoking, Tobacco, and Cancer Program, Division of Cancer Prevention and Control, National Cancer Institute, U.S. Dept. of Health and Human Services, Public Health Service, National Institutes of Health; 1989.

93. Fiore M. United States tobacco use and dependence guideline panel. Treating tobacco use and dependence. Respir Care. 2000;45:1200–62.

94. Whitlock EP, Orleans CT, Pender N, et al. Evaluating primary care behavioral counseling interventions: an evidence-based approach. Am J Prev Med. 2002;22:267–84.

95. Stead LF, Buitrago D, Preciado N, Sanchez G, Hartmann-Boyce J, Lancaster T. Physician advice for smoking cessation. Cochrane Database Systemat Rev. 2013:CD000165.

96. Kawakami M, Nakamura S, Fumimoto H, et al. Relation between smoking status of physicians and their enthusiasm to offer smoking cessation advice. Int Med. 1997;36:162–5.

97. Cornuz J, Zellweger J-P, Mounoud C, et al. Smoking cessation counseling by residents in an outpatient clinic. Prev Med. 1997;26:292–6.

98. Fiore MC, Jaén CR, Baker TB, et al. Treating tobacco use and dependence: 2008 update U.S. Public Health Service Clinical Practice Guideline executive summary. Respir Care. 2008;53:1217–22.

99. Glasgow RE, Davis CL, Funnell MM, et al. Implementing practical interventions to support chronic illness self-management. Joint Comm J Qual Safety. 2003;29:563–74.

100. Glasgow RE, Funnell MM, Bonomi AE, et al. Self-management aspects of the improving chronic illness care breakthrough series: implementation with diabetes and heart failure teams. Ann Behav Med. 2002;24:80–7.

101. Fligor BJ, Neault MW, Mullen CH, et al. Factors associated with sensorineural hearing loss among survivors of extracorporeal membrane oxygenation therapy. Pediatrics. 2005;115:1519–28.

102. Glasgow RE, Goldstein MG. Introduction to the principles of health behavior change. In: Woolf S, editor. Health promotion and disease prevention in clinical practice. 2nd ed. Philadelphia: Williams and Wilkins; 2007. p. 129–47.

103. My Own Health Report project: A nationwide preventive health effort. http://healthpolicy.ucla.edu/programs/health-economics/projects/mohr/Pages/default.aspx. Accessed 29 May 2020.

104. Miller WR, Rose GS. Toward a theory of motivational interviewing. Am Psychol. 2009;64:527–37.

105. Miller WR. Motivational enhancement therapy with drug abusers. Albuquerque, NM: Department of Psychology and Center on Alcoholism, Substance Abuse, and Addictions, University of New Mexico; 1995.

106. Rollnick S, Mason P, Butler C. Health behavior change: a guide for practitioners. London: Churchill Livingstone; 1999.

107. Miller WR, Rollnick S, Moyers TB. Motivational interviewing (7 videotape series). Albuquerque, NM: University of New Mexico; 1998.

108. Horvath AO, Luborsky L. The role of the therapeutic alliance in psychotherapy. J Consult Clin Psychol. 1993;61:561–73.

109. Rollnick S, Butler CC, McCambridge J, et al. Consultations about changing behaviour. BMJ. 2005;331:961–3.

110. Miller W, Rollnick S. Motivational interviewing: preparing people for change. 2nd ed. New York: The Guilford Press; 2002.

111. Goldstein MC, Whitlock EP, DePue J. Multiple health risk behavior interventions in primary care: summary of research evidence. Am J Prev Med. 2004;27(2 Suppl):61–79.

112. Project MATCH Research Group. Matching alcoholism treatments to client heterogeneity: project MATCH posttreatment drinking outcomes. J Stud Alcohol. 1997;58:7–29.

113. Norris SL, Nichols PJ, Caspersen CJ, et al. The effectiveness of disease and case management for people with diabetes: a systematic review. Am J Prev Med. 2002;22:15–38.

114. Miller WR, Zweben A, DiClemente CC, et al. Motivational enhancement therapy manual: a clinical research guide for therapists treating individuals with alcohol abuse and dependence. Project MATCH Monograph Series v.2. DHHS Publication No. (ADM) 92–1894. Rockville MD: National Institute on Alcohol Abuse and Alcoholism; 1992.

115. Babor TF, Del Boca FK, editors. Treatment matching in alcoholism. Cambridge, UK: Cambridge University Press; 2003.

116. Project MATCH Research Group. Matching alcoholism treatments to client heterogeneity: project MATCH three-year drinking outcomes. Alcoholism Clin Exp Res. 1998;22:1300–11.

117. Holder HD, Cisler RA, Longabaugh R, et al. Alcoholism treatment and medical care costs from Project MATCH. Addiction. 2000;95:999–1013.

118. UKATT Research Team. United Kingdom alcohol treatment trial (UKATT): hypotheses, design and methods. Alcohol Alcoholism. 2001;36:11–21.

119. UKATT Research Team. Effectiveness of treatment for alcohol problems: findings of the randomised UK alcohol treatment trial (UKATT). BMJ. 2005;331:541.

120. Carroll KM, Farentinos C, Ball SA, et al. MET meets the real world: design issues and clinical strategies in the Clinical Trials Network. J Subst Abuse Treat. 2002;23:73–80.

121. Ball SA, Martino S, Nich C, et al. Site matters: multisite randomized trial of motivational enhancement therapy in community drug abuse clinics. J Consult Clin Psychol. 2007;75:556–67.

122. Carroll KM, Ball SA, Nich C, et al. Motivational interviewing to improve treatment engagement and outcome in individuals seeking treatment for substance abuse: a multisite effectiveness study. Drug Alcohol Depend. 2006;81:301–12.

123. Winhusen T, Kropp F, Babcock D, et al. Motivational enhancement therapy to improve treatment utilization and outcome in pregnant substance users. J Subst Abuse Treat. 2008;35:161–73.

124. Treasure JL, Katzman M, Schmidt U, et al. Engagement and outcome in the treatment of bulimia nervosa: first phase of a sequential design comparing motivation enhancement therapy and cognitive behavioural therapy. Behav Res Ther. 1999;37:405–18.

125. Miller WR, Yahne CE, Tonigan JS. Motivational interviewing in drug abuse services: a randomized trial. J Consult Clin Psychol. 2003;71:754–63.

126. Baker A, Richmond R, Haile M, et al. A randomized controlled trial of a smoking cessation intervention among people with a psychotic disorder. Am J Psychiat. 2006;163:1934–42.

127. Colby SM, Monti PM, Barnett NP, et al. Brief motivational interviewing in a hospital setting for adolescent smoking: a preliminary study. J Consult Clin Psychol. 1998;66:574–8.

128. Kuchipudi V, Hobein K, Flickinger A, et al. Failure of a 2-hour motivational intervention to alter recurrent drinking behavior in alcoholics with gastrointestinal disease. J Stud Alcohol. 1990;51:356–60.

129. Hettema J, Steele J, Miller WR. Motivational interviewing. Annu Rev Clin Psychol. 2005;1:91–111.

130. Villanueva M, Tonigan JS, Miller WR. Response of Native American clients to three treatment methods for alcohol dependence. J Ethn Subst Abuse. 2007;6:41–8.

131. Chee WSS, Gilcharan Singh HK, Hamdy O, et al. Structured lifestyle intervention based on a trans-cultural diabetes-specific nutrition algorithm (tDNA) in individuals with type 2 diabetes: a randomized controlled trial. BMJ Open Diabetes Res Care. 2017;5:e000384.

132. Via MA, Mechanick JI. Nutrition in type 2 diabetes and the metabolic syndrome. Med Clin North Am. 2016;100:1285–302.

133. Hill JO, Galloway JM, Goley A, et al. Scientific statement: socioecological determinants of prediabetes and type 2 diabetes. Diabetes Care. 2013;36:2430–9.

134. Beck JS. Cognitive behavior therapy: basics and beyond. 2nd ed. New York, NY: Guilford Press; 2011.

135. Murphy R, Straebler S, Cooper Z, et al. Cognitive behavioral therapy for eating disorders. Psychiatr Clin North Am. 2010;33:611–27.

136. van Straten A, van der Zweerde T, Kleiboer A, et al. Cognitive and behavioral therapies in the treatment of insomnia: a meta-analysis. Sleep Med Rev. 2018;38:3–16.

137. Kaczkurkin AN, Foa EB. Cognitive-behavioral therapy for anxiety disorders: an update on the empirical evidence. Dialogues Clin Neurosci. 2015;17:337–46.

138. Li C, Xu D, Hu M, et al. A systematic review and meta-analysis of randomized controlled trials of cognitive behavior therapy for patients with diabetes and depression. J Psychosom Res. 2017;95:44–54.

139. Estabrooks PA, Boyle M, Emmons KM, et al. Harmonized patient-reported data elements in the electronic health record: supporting meaningful use by primary care action on health behaviors and key psychosocial factors. J Am Med Informat Assoc. 2012;19:575–82.

140. Lindblad R, Gore-Langton R. Identifying core behavioral and psychosocial data elements for the electronic health record. Bethesda, MD: National Institutes of Health and Society of Behavioral Medicine; 2011.

141. MyOwnHealthReport. https://myownhealthreport.org/. Accessed on 25 Oct 2019.

142. Krist AH, Woolf SH, Frazier CO, et al. An electronic linkage system for health behavior counseling: effect on delivery of the 5A's. Am J Prev Med. 2008;35:S350–8.

143. Croteau J, Ryan D. Achieving your SMART health goals. https://bewell.stanford.edu/achieving-your-smart-health-goal/. Accessed on 29 Oct 2019.

144. O'Neill J. SMART goals, SMART schools. Educ Leadership. 2000;57:46–50.

145. Glasgow RE, Kessler RS, Ory MG, et al. Conducting rapid, relevant research: lessons learned from the My Own Health Report project. Am J Prev Med. 2014;47:212–9.

146. Gorin SS, Krist AH. Using MOHR for behavior change: a webinar for providers, 2013. http://connectpro72759986.adobeconnect.com/p8rvj6lrauv/; http://healthpolicy.ucla.edu/programs/health-economics/projects/mohr/Documents/MOHRwebinar3-6-13.pdf. Accessed on 8 Mar 2020.

147. Krist AH, Glenn BA, Glasgow RE, et al. Designing a valid randomized pragmatic primary care implementation trial: the my own health report (MOHR) project. Implement Sci. 2013;8:73. https://doi.org/10.1186/1748-5908-8-73.

148. Krist AH, Glasgow RE, Heurtin-Roberts S, et al. The impact of behavioral and mental health risk assessments on goal setting in primary care. Transl Behav Med. 2016;6:212–9.

149. Balasubramanian BA, Heurtin-Roberts S, Krasny S, et al. Factors related to implementation and reach of a pragmatic multisite trial: the my own health report (MOHR) study. J Am Board Fam Med. 2017;30:337–49.

150. Pohl M. 325,000 mobile health apps available in 2017 – Android now the leading mHealth platform. 2017. https://research-2guidance.com/325000-mobile-health-apps-available-in-2017. Accessed on 29 Oct 2019.

151. Klonoff DC. Behavioral theory: the missing ingredient for digital health tools to change behavior and increase adherence. J Diabetes Sci Technol. 2019;13:276–81.

152. Waring ME, Jake-Schoffman DE, Holovatska MM, et al. Social media and obesity in adults: a review of recent research and future directions. Curr Diab Rep. 2018;18:34.

153. Thomas JG, Bond DS, Raynor HA, et al. Comparison of smartphone-based behavioral obesity treatment with gold standard group treatment and control: a randomized trial. Obesity. 2019;27:572–80.

154. Thomas JG, Leahey TM, Wing RR. An automated Internet behavioral weight-loss program by physician referral: a randomized controlled trial. Diabetes Care. 2015;38:9–15.

155. Wolf JA, Moreau JF, Akilov O, et al. Diagnostic inaccuracy of smartphone applications for melanoma detection. JAMA Dermatol. 2013;149:422–6.

156. An R, Ji M, Zhang S. Effectiveness of social media-based interventions on weight-related behaviors and body weight status: review and meta-analysis. Am J Health Behav. 2017;41:670–82.

157. Espel-Huynh HM, Wing RR, Goldstein CM, et al. Rationale and design for a pragmatic effectiveness-implementation trial of online behavioral obesity treatment in primary care. Contemp Clin Trials. 2019;82:9–16.

158. American Association of Diabetes Educators. Press release: a new title for the specialty. Am Assoc Diab Educ. 2019. https://www.diabeteseducator.org/about-adces/media-center/press-releases/press-releases/2019/08/20/a-statement-from-the-american-association-of-diabetes-educators%2D%2D-a-new-title-for-the-specialty. Accessed on 13 Mar 2020.

159. American Diabetes Association. 7. Diabetes technology: standards of medical care in diabetes – 2020. Diabetes Care. 2020;43(Suppl 1):S77–88.

160. Shan R, Sarkar S, Martin SS. Digital health technology and mobile devices for the management of diabetes mellitus: state of the art. Diabetologia. 2019;62:877–87.

161. Marschollek M, Gietzelt M, Schulze M, et al. Wearable sensors in healthcare and sensor-enhanced health information systems: all our tomorrows? Healthcare Informat Res. 2012;18:97–104.

162. Emken BA, Li M, Thatte G, et al. Recognition of physical activities in overweight Hispanic youth using KNOWME Networks. J Phys Act Health. 2012;9:432–41.

163. Wellpass. Text4baby 2017, text4baby.org. Accessed on 11 Aug 2019.

164. Free C, Phillips G, Watson L, et al. The effectiveness of mobile-health technologies to improve health care service delivery processes: a systematic review and meta-analysis. PLoS Med. 2013;10:e1001363.

165. Zurovac D, Sudoi RK, Akhwale WS, et al. The effect of mobile phone text-message reminders on Kenyan health workers' adherence to malaria treatment guidelines: a cluster randomised trial. Lancet. 2011;378:795–803.

166. Militello LK, Kelly SA, Melnyk BM. Systematic review of text-messaging interventions to promote healthy behaviors in pediatric and adolescent populations: implications for clinical practice and research. Worldviews Evid-Based Nurs. 2012;9:66–77.

167. Lorenzo-Blanco EI, Meca A, Pina-Watson B, et al. Longitudinal trajectories of family functioning among recent immigrant adolescents and parents: links with adolescent and parent cultural stress, emotional well-being, and behavioral health. Child Dev. 2019;90:506–23.

168. Gorin SS, Badr H, Krebs P, et al. Multilevel interventions and racial/ethnic health disparities. J Natl Cancer Inst Monogr. 2012;2012:100–11.

169. Fisher TL, Burnet DL, Huang ES, et al. Cultural leverage: interventions using culture to narrow racial disparities in health care. Med Care Res Rev. 2007;64(5 Suppl):243S–82S.

170. Resnicow K, Baranowski T, Ahluwalia JS, et al. Cultural sensitivity in public health: defined and demystified. Ethnicity Dis. 1999;9:10–21.

171. Tauqeer Z. To understand and be understood: the ethics of language, literacy, and hierarchy in medicine. AMA J Ethics. 2017;19:234–7.

172. Beauchamp TL, Childress JF. Principles of biomedical ethics. 7th ed. New York: Oxford University Press; 2013.

173. American Psychological Association. Clinical Health Psychology 2019. https://www.apa.org/ed/graduate/specialize/health. Accessed on 29 Sept 2019.

The Role of the Registered Dietitian Nutritionist in a Lifestyle Medicine Program

Holly R. Herrington, Patricia P. Araujo, and Bethany Doerfler

Abbreviations

ACEND	Accreditation Council for Education in Nutrition and Dietetics
AMA	American Medical Association
AND	Academy of Nutrition and Dietetics (formerly known as Academy of Dietetics and Nutrition)
CBNS	Board for Certification of Nutrition Specialists
CNS	Certified Nutrition Specialist
DASH	Dietary Approaches to Stop Hypertension
HCPs	Healthcare professionals
HER	Electronic health record
HTN	Hypertension
MNT	Medical nutrition therapy
NCD	Non-communicable diseases
NCPM	Nutrition Care Process and Model
NE	Nutrition education
NHANES	National Health and Nutrition Examination Survey
PHI	Protected health information
RD	Registered dietitian
RDN	Registered dietitian nutritionist
T2D	Type 2 diabetes

H. R. Herrington (✉)
Northwestern Memorial Hospital, Center for Lifestyle Medicine, Chicago, IL, USA
e-mail: hherring@nm.org

P. P. Araujo
Northwestern Medicine, Center for Lifestyle Medicine, Chicago, IL, USA
e-mail: patricia.araujo@nm.org

B. Doerfler
Northwestern Medicine, Digestive Health Center, Chicago, IL, USA
e-mail: Bethany-doerfler@northwestern.edu

Introduction to Nutritional Care

Diet and nutrition are fundamental aspects of lifestyle medicine and the care of patients with noncommunicable diseases (NCDs). The registered dietitian (RD) and the registered dietitian nutritionist (RDN) credential have identical meanings and legal definitions. However, the RDN credential is often used by RDs who want to emphasize the nutrition aspect of their credential to the public and to other healthcare professionals (HCPs) [1]. Throughout this chapter, the term RDN will be used for consistency. The RDN is an integral member of the interdisciplinary team and there is strong evidence that medical nutritional therapy (MNT) is an effective intervention for the prevention and treatment of multiple medical conditions, including obesity, diabetes, renal disease, cardiovascular disease, gastrointestinal disorders, and hyperlipidemia, among others [2]. Table 16.1 displays the specialty areas that a RDN may provide MNT for the prevention and treatment of NCDs, as well as outcomes measured in the outpatient setting [3–5].

As an active team member, the RDN is expected to work closely with individual patients to support informed decision-making, self-care behaviors, problem solving, and active collaboration with the healthcare team to improve clinical outcomes, health status, and quality of life in a cost-effective manner [6]. In addition, when guiding patients toward more healthy diets, the RDN should consider the patient's confidence and self-efficacy for diet and lifestyle change, as well as the presence or absence of social support.

Medical Nutrition Therapy

Healthy eating patterns and regular physical activity can help patients achieve and maintain good health and reduce the risk of chronic disease. The role of the RDN is to provide MNT by using multiple diet nutrition therapies, technology, and evidence-based research to provide effective dietary treatments to a

© Springer Nature Switzerland AG 2020
J. I. Mechanick, R. F. Kushner (eds.), *Creating a Lifestyle Medicine Center*, https://doi.org/10.1007/978-3-030-48088-2_16

Table 16.1 Specialty areas for medical nutrition therapy provided by a registered dietitian nutritionist[a]

	Assessment	Associated conditions	Interventions	Monitoring	Evaluation	Insurance coverage
Obesity/ weight loss	Current weight, height, BMI, associated medical issues, past diet attempts, weight loss goals, weight history graph	Weight gain, overweight, obesity, severe obesity	Weight loss goal of 10% over 6 months, 1–2 lbs. of weight loss per week Increased physical exercise with a goal of 150–300 minutes per week	Initial visit (30–60 minutes), follow-up every 2 weeks until weight loss goal is achieved; Follow-up can be conducted in person or via telemedicine	Weight loss of 1–2 lbs. per week, 5–10% weight loss over 6 months	Not covered or limited visits per year or needs qualifying condition
Diabetes	Current weight, height, BMI, fasting glucose labs, A1C, current medications, secondary medical diagnosis (e.g., obesity, cardiac, and hypertension)	Clarify type: Type 1 type 2, gestational, or prediabetes	Weight loss, monitoring of macronutrient intake, specifically carbohydrates and saturated fats	Initial visit (30–60 minutes); follow-up every 2 weeks until goal is achieved conducted in person or via telemedicine	Weight loss, reduction in A1C, and improvement in fasting glucose levels	Covered by insurance, number of visits per year varies by insurance provider
General wellness and healthy eating	Current weight, BMI, overall health status, patients stated goals for seeking out MNT (following a specific diet, learning how to prepare foods, basic questions regarding nutrition, etc.)	May have no associated medical diagnosis	MNT for general nutritional concerns	Initial visit (30–60 minutes); follow-up as needed for patient to feel confident	Patient's ability to change diet, overcoming barriers to achieving dietary goals	Not typically covered by insurance unless associated with a medical diagnosis
Bariatric procedure	Current weight, height, BMI, dietary history, current dietary intake, past history of eating disorder	BMI criteria with/without obesity associated complication (e.g., diabetes, HTN, sleep apnea)	Education on post-procedure dietary guidelines Pre-procedure guidelines may vary among centers (e.g., weight loss and dietary change prior to procedure) MNT for glycemic control	Candidacy for procedure must be evaluated at least one time by a RDN; Follow-up visits and monitoring prior to procedure may vary among centers	Initially, weight loss of 10% excess body weight per month following procedure Total weight loss following procedure will vary by procedure	Covered by most insurance companies
NAFLD/ NASH Other liver conditions	Current weight, height, BMI, laboratory values (e.g., ALT/ AST), FibroScan, current dietary intake	Overweight, obesity	Weight loss goal of 5–10% current weight over the next 6 months Dietary reduction of carbohydrates, specifically refined carbohydrates and sugar intake Increased physical activity with a goal of 150–300 minutes per week	Initial dietary evaluation for weight loss and MNT for NAFLD/ NASH; Follow-up every 2 weeks until weight loss goal achieved. Follow-up visits may be conducted in person or via telemedicine	Labs drawn every 6–12 months	Not typically covered for weight loss or fatty liver. Insurance plans will vary for coverage depending on the carrier or plan
Renal conditions	Dietary history, nutritional/herbal supplements, scored sodium questionnaire, glycemic control, protein/ inflammatory markers, kidney function, anemia, blood lipids, electrolytes, body weight/composition, weight changes, fluid status, waist circumference, social history	CKD all stages, CKD s/p transplant, ARF, altered renal function	Appropriate energy intake (23–25 kcal/kg), high protein/protein controlled diet, may need to adjust intake of potassium, sodium, phosphorus	Every 1–3 months, more frequently if needed to maintain adequate nutrition	Weight changes, fluid shifts, renal function, electrolytes, knowledge regarding dietary approaches, changes in nutrient supplementation	2 or 3 hours per year as covered under Medicare Additional hours might be needed based on nutritional status or change in condition

Table 16.1 (continued)

	Assessment	Associated conditions	Interventions	Monitoring	Evaluation	Insurance coverage
Oncology	Nutritional assessment tool (i.e., PG-SGA), diet history (food and nutrient intake, FFQ, 24 hour typical day recall), nutritional/herbal supplements, nutrition support intake, food avoidances/ intolerances, dietary pattern changes, difficulty chewing or swallowing, glucose, immunity/inflammatory markers, anemia, body weight/composition, weight changes, fluid status, nutrition-focused physical exam, signs of vitamin/mineral deficiencies, grip strength	All types of cancers, inpatient oncology units, transplant recipients, survivorship	High calorie/high protein diets, calorie restriction for weight loss, food safety education, nutrition support, supplementation if needed (fish oil, medical food supplements, glutamine), education on symptom management for cancer treatment	Initial visits and subsequent visits to be determined by the patient/ HCP based on nutritional status, presence of cachexia, malnutrition, obesity, coverage/ ability to pay, and ability to access clinic	Changes in weight, appetite, taste/smell, ability to chew/ swallow, supplementation, and blood counts	Not typically covered by insurance. Many cancer centers provide nutritional services free of charge to patients
Vegetarian eating pattern	Diet history (food and nutrient intake, FFQ, 24 hour typical day recall), protein intake (amino acid profile), micronutrient intake (e.g., B12, iron, zinc, folate, and calcium), fatty acid intake (EPA/DHA), nutritional /herbal supplements, CBC, anemia, iron, ferritin, B12, zinc, vitamin D, MMA, lipid profile, body weight, weight changes, bone density, reasons for following vegetarian diet, and signs of disordered eating.	May have no associated medical diagnosis	Adequate calories/ protein, complementary mixtures of amino acids from plant foods, supplementations if needed (vitamin D, zinc, iron, B12, calcium, fish oil/ EFA, folate)	Initial and subsequent visits to be determined by the patient/ HCP based on nutritional status	Adherence to plan/ supplementation, increased knowledge regarding dietary approaches	Not typically covered by insurance

ªAbbreviations: *A1C* hemoglobin A1c, *ALT* Aspartate transaminase, *AST* Alanine transaminase, *ARF* Acute renal failure, *BMI* Body mass index, *CBC* Complete blood count, *CKD* Chronic kidney disease, *DHA* Docosahexaenoic acid, *EAL* Evidence analysis library, *EFA* Essential fatty acids, *EPA* Eicosapentaenoic acid, *FFQ* Food Frequency Questionnaire, *HCP* Healthcare professional, *HTN* Hypertension, *MMA* Methylmalonic acid, *MNT* Medical nutrition therapy, *NAFLD* Nonalcoholic fatty liver disease, *NASH* Nonalcohol steatohepatitis, *PG-SGA* Patient-Generated Subjective Global Assessment, *RDN* Registered dietitian nutritionist. Adapted from Refs [3–5]

wide variety of patients (Table 16.2). Current research, including observational population studies and interventional studies that investigate specific eating patterns, have provided therapeutic dietary guidance and guidelines for risk factor reduction and improved health outcomes over a range of chronic diseases [7–11]. The 2015–2020 Dietary Guidelines for Americans provide dietary recommendations based on the current body of nutrition science and are used to assist HCPs and policymakers to guide Americans in making healthy food and beverage choices (Table 16.3) [12]. These guidelines are updated every 5 years.

Healthy eating patterns can be tailored to an individual's personal preferences, thus enabling patients to choose the diet that is right for them. Recognizing that individuals will need to make shifts in food and beverages choices in order to achieve a healthy eating pattern, the 2015–2020 Dietary Guidelines for Americans embody the idea that healthy eating patterns are not strict prescriptions, but an adaptable framework to allow individuals to enjoy foods that meet their personal, financial, cultural, and traditional preferences [12].

Table 16.2 Goals of medical nutrition therapy in lifestyle therapies

Achieve and maintain healthy body weight, improve comorbid conditions or decrease health risk reduction through a variety of healthy eating patterns, promote and support weight loss or maintenance, while emphasizing a variety of nutrient-dense foods
Assess and evaluate patients' nutritional needs based on personal preferences, health literacy, access to healthy foods, willingness and ability to make lifestyle or behavioral changes, barriers to change, ease of adherence, practicality, sustainability, and effectiveness at promoting long-term lifestyle changes
Maintain and foster good patient relationships by providing nonjudgmental messages about food choices and by using judgment free language
Provide patients with practical tools for developing healthy eating patterns through a variety of dietary strategies

Table 16.3 2015–2020 US Dietary Guidelines key recommendations[a]

Consume a healthy eating pattern that accounts for all foods and beverages within an appropriate calorie level	
A healthy eating pattern includes:	A healthy eating pattern limits:
A variety of vegetables from all of the subgroups—dark green, red, and orange, legumes (beans and peas), starchy, and other	Saturated fats and trans fats, added sugars, and sodium
Fruits, especially whole fruits	Consume less than 10% of calories per day from added sugars
Grains, at least half of which are whole grains	
Fat-free or low-fat dairy, including milk, yogurt, cheese, and/or fortified soy beverages	Consume less than 10% of calories per day from saturated fats
A variety of protein foods, including seafood, lean meats and poultry, eggs, legumes (beans and peas), nuts, seeds, and soy products	Consume less than 2300 mg per day of sodium
	If alcohol is consumed, it should be consumed in moderation—up to 1 drink per day for women and up to 2 drinks per day for men (but less is better)
Healthy oils (e.g., canola and extra virgin olive)	

[a]Based on data from the US Department of Agriculture, Agricultural Research Service and US Department of Health and Human Services, Centers for Disease Control and Prevention. See https://health.gov/our-work/food-nutrition/2015–2020-dietary-guidelines (Accessed on 23 Mar 2020)

Use of Dietary Plans and Patterns

Scientific evidence supporting dietary guidance has grown and evolved over the decades. Although the evidence continues to be substantial that there are relationships among individual nutrients, foods, food groups, and health outcomes, individual nutrients are not consumed in isolation. Therefore, more recent emphasis has been focused on consuming nutrients in various combinations over time (an eating pattern), which may be more predictive of overall health status and disease risk than individual foods or nutrients. Therefore, MNT and dietary guidelines, in the context of chronic disease prevention and management, have become more focused on overall eating patterns and various health outcomes [12].

Associations Between Eating Patterns and Health

There is currently strong evidence that shows healthy eating patterns, especially those that are higher in fruit and vegetable intake, are associated with a reduced risk of cardiovascular disease (CVD), type 2 diabetes (T2D), certain types of cancers (such as colorectal and postmenopausal breast cancers), overweight, and obesity [7–11, 13]. Emerging evidence also suggests that relationships may exist between eating patterns and some neurocognitive disorders and congenital anomalies [13].

Within this body of evidence, recurring characteristics of healthy eating patterns have been identified as higher intakes of vegetables and fruits, whole grains, fat-free or low-fat dairy, seafood, legumes, and nuts. Additionally, reduced intake of meats (including processed meats), processed poultry, sugar-sweetened foods and beverages, and refined grains are also identified as characteristics of healthy eating patterns. These characteristics of a healthy eating pattern can be realistically achieved by a wide variety of dietary strategies and approaches. The 2015–2020 Dietary Guidelines for Americans also recommend that a healthy weight be achieved or maintained to reduce overall risk for disease [12].

Specific Dietary Plans for Promoting a Healthy Eating Pattern

Utilizing any of the variety of diet plans that encompass healthy eating patterns may be useful for HCPs making dietary recommendations. Three evidence-based dietary approaches are reviewed below, with a comprehensive list shown in Table 16.4 [13].

The Mediterranean Diet

Based on the eating patterns of populations that live on the shores of the Mediterranean Sea, this plant-based eating pattern does not prescribe specific amounts of any one food group. Instead, it offers a guide in which to base food groups, those to choose most often to least often in an overall diet. Vegetables, fruits, nuts, whole grains, and unsaturated fatty oils are chosen to be the largest component of the diet. Seafood and fish are the second largest component with at least two servings weekly suggested. Poultry and dairy are advised in moderation while red meat and sweets are to be consumed "less often." In the 2015–2020 Dietary Guidelines for Americans, the Mediterranean diet approach is one of the three model diets highlighted for healthy eating patterns based on research from the past 5 years. The Mediterranean diet has also been shown to help decrease risk of T2D and cardiovascular disease [14].

Table 16.4 Dietary approaches associated with healthy eating patterns (energy deficit used to promote weight loss)

Higher-protein diet (25% of total calories from protein, 30% of total calories from fat, and 45% of total calories from carbohydrate), with provision of foods that create an energy deficit

Higher-protein Zone™-type diet (5 meals/d, each with 40% of total calories from carbohydrate, 30% of total calories from protein, and 30% of total calories from fat) without formal prescribed energy restriction, but with an overall energy deficit

Lacto-ovo-vegetarian-style diet with prescribed energy deficit

Low-calorie diet with prescribed energy deficit

Low-carbohydrate diet (initially <20 g/d carbohydrate) without formal prescribed energy restriction, but with a realized energy deficit

Low-fat vegan-style diet (10–25% of total calories from fat) without formal prescribed energy restriction, but with a realized energy deficit

Low-fat diet (20% of total calories from fat) without formal prescribed energy restriction, but with a realized energy deficit

Low-glycemic-load diet, either with formal prescribed energy restriction or without formal prescribed energy restriction, but with realized energy deficit

Lower-fat (<30% fat), high-dairy (four servings/day) diets, with or without increased fiber and/or low-glycemic-index (low-glycemic-load) foods, with prescribed energy deficit

Macronutrient-targeted diets (15% or 25% of total calories from protein; 20% or 40% of total calories from fat; 35%, 45%, 55%, or 65% of total calories from carbohydrate) with prescribed energy deficit

Mediterranean-style diet with prescribed energy deficit

Moderate-protein diet (12% of total calories from protein, 58% of total calories from carbohydrate, and 30% of total calories from fat) with provision of foods that realize an energy deficit

Provision of high-glycemic-load or low-glycemic-load meals with prescribed energy deficit

The AHA-style step 1 diet (prescribed energy restriction of 1500–1800 kcal/d, <30% of total calories from fat, <10% of total calories from saturated fat)

Adapted from Ref. [13]

Under the care of the RDN, this diet can be applied to individuals with minimal nutritional risk. However, there is concern for potential weight gain if patients are adding more calorie dense foods (such as healthy fats) without adjusting for total calorie intake. Emphasis should be placed on following the eating pattern in its entirety as opposed to adding individual foods in a patient's current eating pattern.

The DASH Diet

The Dietary Approaches to Stop Hypertension (DASH) diet is another specific healthy eating pattern that encourages food choices that are low in total fat, saturated fat, and cholesterol while also choosing higher amounts of fruits, vegetables, and whole grains. Protein is supplied by low-fat dairy, fish, poultry, and nuts, while red meat, sweets, and sugary beverages are limited. The DASH diet is high in fiber, potassium, calcium, and magnesium and low in sodium. This approach combines all the attributes of a diet that promotes overall health, but has been specifically noted for its effect on lowering blood pressure in those patients who have hypertension (HTN). The DASH diet has also been shown to reduce blood pressure in patients who may not have been diagnosed with HTN and are looking to avoid this diagnosis [15]. While this dietary pattern has many benefits, adherence can be difficult. Those patients who are unable to plan meals or prepare meals at home may find this more challenging. Foods are generally categorized and are not easy to decipher or follow without the guidance of the RDN. Those patients with lactose intolerance or food allergies (such as nuts) may also need assistance finding alternative choices [15, 16].

Healthy Vegetarian Eating Pattern

The Healthy Vegetarian Eating Pattern was developed considering food choices of self-identified vegetarians in the National Health and Nutrition Examination Survey (NHANES) and provides recommendations to meet the 2015–2020 Dietary Guidelines for Americans [12] for those who follow a vegetarian diet. The Healthy Vegetarian Eating Pattern includes protein and fiber sources from legumes (beans and peas), soy products, nuts and seeds, and whole grains. It contains no meats, poultry, or seafood. This eating pattern is high in calcium and dietary fiber.

Numerous professional medical organizations, including the American Heart Association, The National Lipid Institute, and the American College of Cardiology, have identified vegetarian or vegan eating patterns to be effective in improving cardiovascular disease outcomes. Eating a vegetarian or vegan-style food pattern has been shown to decrease total and LDL cholesterol due to the lower intake of saturated fats. Recent studies have shown that individuals who follow a vegetarian eating pattern have an overall lower risk for heart disease, T2D, HTN, obesity, and some types of cancer [17–20].

When planned for and executed under the guidance of the RDN, a vegetarian eating pattern can be nutritionally adequate for both adults and children, and may lower the risk of developing chronic diseases. However, there are areas of concern for potential deficiencies. Patients following a vegetarian or vegan eating pattern are at risk for under-consuming protein. The RDA for protein intake for adults is 0.8 grams of protein for every kilogram of body weight. It is important to note that a person following a vegetarian diet may be able to achieve this goal by including dairy products, fish, eggs, legumes, nuts, soy, and vegetarian-based protein supplements. However, those wishing to avoid animal products altogether need more careful planning to reach adequate protein intake. Additionally, patients following a vegetarian or vegan diet pattern may become deficient in some vitamins or minerals, such as vitamin D, vitamin B12, calcium, and omega-3 fatty acids [21].

Individual Choices Within Healthy Eating Patterns

When addressing healthy eating patterns with patients, it is imperative to be knowledgeable about specific individual preferences of how or when food may be consumed. Lifestyle modifications that incorporate healthy eating and exercise patterns continue to be the foundation of overall MNT, but the standard model of lifestyle modification is not effective or sustainable for many patients. This often leads them to seek alternative or "quicker" approaches. Over the past decade, many diet patterns have arisen, both healthy and unhealthy, which have led to consumer and HCP confusion. Despite the growing popularity of fad diets to facilitate weight loss and reduce chronic disease risk, there are limited studies that suggest these popular regimens are beneficial. Fad diets, including but not limited to juicing, detoxing, fasting, or high fat/low carbohydrate intake, are attractive to many patients as results are seen quickly. However, these diets are typically short-lived. Nonetheless, a review of the literature does suggest that some fad diets and exercise plans do lead to health improvements and/or weight loss. These studies are limited and are all based on the concept of caloric restriction. Overall, the long-term sustainability of many of these fad diets has been widely questioned in the current literature [22].

A characteristic trait of individuals who follow fad diets is dichotomous thinking, the belief that foods are "good" or "bad" and perceived failure is likely to come to those who cannot adhere to the strict regimen of the fad diet. When a single food is emphasized, confusion and controversy can hinder, rather than facilitate, adoption of healthy dietary patterns. Following an overall healthy eating pattern, as opposed to emphasizing "good" or "bad" food lists, may better help patients adhere to longer term lifestyle changes which may, in turn, lead to sustainable dietary and healthy improvements.

The RDN in a Lifestyle Medicine Center should be able to discuss healthy eating patterns as a whole, but also specific topics including short-term fad diets, timing of meals, meal skipping, use of meal replacements, and snacking. A skilled RDN would reduce the probability of relapse into unhealthy food patterns and behaviors by increasing knowledge and self-efficacy, teaching coping skills, and incorporating personal choices in individualized eating patterns. An RDN will also assist individuals with making choices that fit into their budget, as well as cultural boundaries. This individualized education is more comprehensive and involves context-based judgment that is likely more sustainable than dichotomous approaches over time [23].

Timing of Meals

A wide source of confusion among HCPs as well as patients involves the timing of meals and snacks. Scientific evidence for the optimal number, timing, and size of meals is lacking.

It has been hypothesized that eating small, frequent meals enhances fat loss and helps to achieve better weight maintenance. Several observational studies have supported this, indicating that feeding frequency is positively associated with reductions in fat mass and body fat percentage as well as an increase in fat-free mass [24–28].

The evidence surrounding consumption of breakfast or increased feeding frequency has also supported disease risk reduction and prevention of chronic disease. Although limited, evidence suggests that skipping breakfast is associated with atherosclerosis and cardiovascular disease. A prospective cohort review of data from the National Health and Nutrition Examination Survey III 1988 to 1994 showed that skipping breakfast was associated with a significantly increased risk of mortality from cardiovascular disease [29]. Additionally, regular breakfast consumption is important for the prevention of T2D. A recent systematic review of eight studies involving 106,935 participants revealed that breakfast skipping is associated with a significantly increased risk of T2D [30].

Recent studies on snack timing, obesity, and related eating behaviors have shown that greater morning snacking was associated with increased fruit and vegetable consumption, while greater evening snacking was associated with higher BMI, higher intake of fast food, French fries, and soft drinks, and higher percentage of time eating while distracted. Evening snacking may be more detrimental to healthy eating patterns and healthy weight compared to snacking at other times of day. Therefore, the RDN should suggest that reducing evening snacks or discussing healthier food options at nighttime may be an important and simple message for changing healthy eating patterns [31, 32]. Potential strategies to decrease nighttime eating might include increased consumption of high fiber foods, increased intake of fruits and vegetables, and planned snacks earlier in the day.

Meal or Snack Replacements

For patients who feel overwhelmed with too many food options, have difficulty controlling portions or demonstrate difficulty with meal preparation or shopping, the use of meal replacements (e.g., liquid meals, meal bars, and calorie-controlled packaged meals) may be used as part of the diet component of a comprehensive weight management program. Substituting 1–2 daily meals or snacks with meal replacements is a successful weight loss and weight maintenance strategy [33, 34].

More evidence for implementing the use of meal replacements for weight and disease risk management is demonstrated in the Action for Health in Diabetes (Look AHEAD) trial. Look AHEAD is a 16-center, randomized controlled trial, with the purpose to investigate the influence of weight loss achieved via an intensive lifestyle intervention (ILI) on long-term cardiovascular health in adults with overweight or obesity and T2D. Participants were prescribed a low-energy (1200–1800 kcal/day) low-fat (< 30% kcal from fat, with <10% from saturated fat) diet. The diet also included a meal replacement (MR) plan, in which for the first 4 months, MRs (beverages and food bars) were recommended to be consumed to replace two meals per day and one to two snacks per day. This study was the first investigation to assess diet quality and food group consumption for individuals with T2D who were prescribed a reduced energy, low-fat plan using MR.

At 12 months, a significantly greater percentage of participants met recommendations for energy from fat and saturated fat; cholesterol; and daily servings from the fruit, vegetable, milk, yogurt and cheese, fats, oils, and sweets food groups than the control group. Additionally, the greatest percentage of participants meeting dietary recommendations were those consuming ≥2 MR/day, followed by those consuming 1 to <2 MR/day and < 1 MR/day, respectively. The findings that consuming a reduced-energy, low-fat MR plan is associated with improved diet quality is similar to what has been found in other investigations that have examined changes in diet quality with an MR plan in healthy patients with overweight and obesity [35].

Reducing Nutrition Confusion

Regardless of how patients may choose to implement healthy eating patterns, guided directives are more likely to result in healthy dietary and lifestyle changes when they have a consistent emphasis on a balanced and moderate total dietary pattern. To reduce confusion from the volume and inconsistencies of nutrition advice, the RDN or other HCPs should consider tailoring dietary advice when designing nutrition education messages or programs for patients [34].

The RDN or HCP should:

- Promote variety, proportionality, moderation, and gradual improvement in dietary habits. Patients can make small changes and improvements to diet and lifestyle each day which may be less overwhelming than making too many changes at once.
- Emphasize food patterns, rather than changes in specific nutrients or foods.
- Be aware of social, cultural, economic, and emotional meanings that might be attached to some foods and allow for flexibility whenever possible. Social and cultural aspects of food consumption are essential for planning educational programs to help correct nutritional problems.
- Provide guidance on appropriate ways to include foods that have physiological benefits (e.g., containing fiber and other phytonutrients) beyond simple macronutrient content as part of a healthy diet [36].

All food and beverage choices are part of an eating pattern. Medical professionals in a Lifestyle Medicine Center can work with patients in a variety of methods to adapt their personal choices when developing a healthy eating pattern. Tailored eating patterns should accommodate physical health, cultural, ethnic, traditional, and personal preferences, as well as personal food budgets, food insecurity or accessibility. Eating patterns that are tailored to individual choices and preferences are more likely to be motivating, accepted, and maintained over time, which may lead to significant shifts in dietary intake and improved health. Individual factors that are unique to the individual include age, sex, socioeconomic status, food accessibility, cultural restrictions, the presence of a disability, physical health, knowledge and skills, and personal preferences. These must all must be considered when helping a patient devise a healthy eating pattern. Providing education with specific goals, such as improving individual food choices, is most effective when delivered by a wide variety of nutrition and physical activity professionals working alone or in multidisciplinary teams (Table 16.4) [13].

Differentiating Registered Dietitian Nutritionist from Other Healthcare Professionals

RDNs are nutrition content experts who are nationally and locally licensed to deliver MNT to individuals. As mentioned earlier, RDN is an optional credential that dietitians can use to incorporate the term "nutritionist" in their title [1]. By way of training, RDNs complete a minimum of a bachelor's degree at an accredited university or college and course work approved by the Accreditation Council for Education in Nutrition and Dietetics (ACEND) of the Academy of Nutrition and Dietetics [37] and beginning in 2024, RDNs will be required to complete a graduate degree [38]. Completed ACEND-accredited supervised practice typically takes place at a healthcare facility, community agency, as well as food service corporations. Often this process takes place over 12 months and candidates accumulate 1200 hours before eligibility is granted to sit for the registration exam. This national board exam is administered by the Commission on Dietetic Registration [38]. Once credentials for RDN have been met, the RDN must maintain 75 hours of continuing medical education every 5 years [39]. Additional advanced areas of practice and certification for RDNs are unique to this field, including advanced practice certifications for renal disease, adult and pediatric obesity, sports nutrition, oncology, and gerontology nutrition. Currently in many states, RDNs are the only nutrition professional that is licensed to provide nutrition care plans. RDNs can play vital role in integrating key concepts of nutrition, health, and lifestyle into either healthcare, academia, or business.

Health Coach

Health coaching is a relatively new position created to help patients implement healthy lifestyle changes. In contrast to RDNs, health coaches are not content experts in health or disease; they do not diagnose or prescribe, unless a health coach has expertise through another profession that allows expert advice to be given [40]. Health and wellness coaches can partner with patients seeking assistance with implementation of either medically directed or self-directed behavior change. Standard behavioral strategies include active listening, motivational interviewing, and development of behavior change plans. Health and wellness coaches are trained in core areas of chronic disease, evidence-based treatments, and the delivery of behavioral change plans [41]. Core training and certification often focuses on recommendations provided by public health groups such as the Center for Disease Control or National Institutes of Health. Training consists of ≥15 hours in health promotion, disease prevention, and the associated lifestyle recommendations for optimal treatment [42]. Coaches can also act as a liaison between the medical team and the patient, but do not provide prescriptive MNT [41, 43].

Nutritionist

Where there are legal standards for RDNs, the term "nutritionist" is less standardized and less regulated. A nutritionist can have nutrition training or no nutrition training. The Board for Certification of Nutrition Specialists (CBNS) offers nutritionists the opportunity to earn the certified nutrition specialist (CNS) credential. To become a CNS, nutritionists must complete a master's or doctoral degree in a field-related discipline; complete 1000 hours of supervised practical experience; successfully pass the CBNS certification examination; and complete continuing professional education needed to maintain certification [44]. Medical healthcare institutions need to integrate credentialed nutrition professionals into their healthcare team. For example, the RDN can work with a health coach to provide both a nutrition care plan and the behavioral aspects of nutrition change. Nutritionists may be able to provide sound nutrition advice, but limitations exist on uniform standards of training and other barriers to integration [41].

Integrating the RDN into Clinical Nutrition Research

The RDN applies clinical research into nutrition care plans. Oftentimes, appropriate nutrition assessment methods can be

Table 16.5 Academic and clinical domains for registered dietitian nutritionists

Research interest and program initiatives	Role of Registered Dietitian Nutritionist
Medical school and medical staff training	Development of nutritional competencies and training materials for undergraduate and graduate medical education along with continuing medical education. Creation of assessment screening tools to guide medical care
Clinical settings: outpatient	Designing research protocols with appropriate nutrition assessment techniques and study related materials to evaluate role of nutrition on disease activity and outcomes
Clinical settings: in-patient and healthcare economy	Evaluation of critical quality assurance standards, including length of stay, healthcare utilization, health-related quality of life, and minimizing nutritional risk in hospitalized patients
Innovations	Integration of emerging nutrition science and technology to evaluate the feasibility and acceptability of nutrition interventions for patients in a particular clinical setting

lacking in medical studies. Integrating the RDN in study design, assessment, and execution can improve the likelihood that nutritional assessment methods and related confounders are appropriately controlled. There are several academic and clinical domains that benefit when an RDN is involved in research activities (Table 16.5) [45–47].

Delivery of Services

Traditionally, nutritional therapy and education are provided face-to-face. However, with the emergence of new technology, more innovative approaches are being employed [47].

In-Person Service Delivery

In-person nutritional interventions can be provided individually or in a group setting. The AHA/ACC/TOS Guideline for the management of overweight and obesity in adults recommends both individual and group weight loss interventions, but recommends high frequency (14 or more sessions in 6 months) encounters and delivery by a trained interventionist in both [13].

Individual

In-person, face-to-face dietary counseling in a private setting, or a medical office, is the most traditional approach. In this method, the patient meets the RDN for a dedicated individual session. In-person visits can include the provision of nutrition education by HCPs, or MNT by the RDN or other nutrition professional. The main difference between nutrition education and MNT is that the former reinforces nutritional knowledge, while the latter is individualized and includes nutritional diagnosis and interventions, such as counseling, focused on the management of disease [41].

In one-to-one in-person counseling, RDNs and other nutritional professionals follow standards in the Nutrition Care Process, a systematic process to provide a framework for MNT, which includes a nutritional assessment, diagnosis, interventions, monitoring, and evaluation [48]. The Nutrition Care Process and Model (NCPM), accepted by the American Dietetic Association, now known as the Academy of Nutrition and Dietetics, set the ground for a standard approach to nutritional care interventions for RDNs and dietetic practitioners globally [47]. The development of NCPM shifted the old practice of dietitians providing only diet instructions into a new practice integrating behavioral sciences and biological sciences as components of nutrition care [47].

Dietetic consultations delivered by RDNs in primary care offices positively influence markers for diet quality, diabetes control, weight loss, gestational weight gain [49], and slowing the progression to dialysis [50]. It is anticipated that RDNs will provide similar positive outcomes in Lifestyle Medicine Centers.

From the lifestyle medicine physician's perspective, potential challenges for offering face-to-face nutrition interactions are the need for dedicated staff, physical space, proper equipment, and supplies (such as food models, software for diet analysis/drafting, equipment for measuring anthropometrics, body composition, and energy expenditure) all of which increase costs. From a patient's perspective, face-to-face interaction requires increased time and the burden of commuting, along with associated costs. These barriers make it even more difficult to provide face-to-face care in locations with less access to resources, such as rural settings [51].

Group

Group nutritional interventions are sessions for ≥2 patients at a time but typically composed of 8–12 patients [52]. Group counseling can be as effective as individual counseling, or sometimes more, in delivering nutritional and lifestyle-focused interventions (i.e., for the management of prediabetes, diabetes and obesity) [52–55]. Group therapy that is family-based has been shown to be an effective lifestyle intervention in childhood obesity [56]. A randomized controlled trial also indicated that group therapy delivery by a multidisciplinary team can reduce early signs of cardiovascular disease in children with obesity [57]. New findings indicate that group cognitive behavioral therapy for obesity may be a useful treatment approach though more research in this area is needed [58].

For a Lifestyle Medicine Center, potential advantages of group interventions are optimizing physical space and the HCP's time. However, the practice needs to have a large room to accommodate a group setting. Another potential benefit to group intervention is that group therapy for weight loss has lower dropout rates when compared to individual nutritional counseling [59]. In addition, group settings can provide patients with a communal atmosphere with peer support reinforcing that they are "not alone" in facing an NCD. Group settings can also be a good avenue for facilitating other nontraditional methods of education, such as cooking demonstrations, supermarket tours, hands-on workshops (such as label reading), and family-based group education. To optimize the ambiance and dynamics of group therapy, it is helpful to set ground rules and enlist an experienced and trained HCP.

Remote Service Delivery

The possibilities for long-distance nutritional interventions are numerous and continue to grow as new technologies emerge. These technologies can be both exciting and intimidating for HCPs in the field of lifestyle medicine.

Telehealth

The administration of healthcare and education remotely using electronic technologies for communication is known as telehealth [60]. Telehealth pertains to any aspect of healthcare and can be administered through different mediums, including the internet, with video-conferencing or e-mail, text messages, smartphone apps, or other types of remote communications [60, 61]. In contrast, telenutrition refers to the specific area of nutrition care using technologies employed by an RDN for a remote patient [60]. Telenutrition is poised for expanded use by RDNs due to growing accessibility of technology, improvements in data transmission, and lower cost than in-person encounters [62].

Potential advantages to telehealth from a practice and practitioner's perspective are access to a wider range of potential patients and more possibilities for the delivery of care [63]. Telehealth is particularly promising in the field of obesity since many interventions require high frequency follow-up visits, and not surprisingly, most telehealth nutritional interventions are in obesity [61].

Even as telehealth becomes more accepted in the treatment of chronic diseases, HCPs should keep in mind that not all patients will be suitable candidates for this type of intervention. The HCP should consider the patient's current medical condition technology skills, and the accessibility of hardware and communications equipment [64]. Considerations for the delivery of education using technology are the target audience and method of information delivery [62, 65]. It is important to consider the target audience's financial stability, educational level, and age, since those characteristics appear to influence whether people seek health information online or offline; with those who seek information online often being younger, more educated, and more affluent [65]. There is a wide variability in the delivery of web-based education and the individual results [66].

An important concern for web-based education is the safety and privacy of protected health information (PHI). Specifically, this technology raises concern regarding the protection of patient's health data and inappropriate use [67]. Consumers are concerned with their PHI used in health apps being shared with unauthorized third parties [67]. All aspects of telehealth and telenutrition that involve the transfer of patient data should comply with the Health Insurance Portability and Accountability Act, as well as institutional, state, and federal regulations [64]. Practitioners should also be aware of any additional state and licensure regulations that might compromise the delivery of telenutrition. In the case where the practitioner holds licensure in a different state than the one they are providing services through telehealth, it is important to verify regulations in both states.

A final potential barrier to adopting web-based and mobile-based interventions is limited reimbursement for services rendered [67]. Medicare covers face-to-face MNT for individual initial assessments and reassessments for specific diseases (such as diabetes and kidney disease) [68]. However, telenutrition coverage by public payers is usually limited [63, 68]. Specifically, there is only limited coverage under Medicare for telehealth delivered MNT, Diabetes Self-Management Training, and intensive behavioral therapy for obesity care to patients who reside in approved rural areas, and in a few states Medicaid also covers telenutrition interventions for other patient populations [63]. Lifestyle Medicine Centers should verify public and private coverage within states relevant to the telehealth practice.

Mobile

The wide accessibility of mobile phones makes mobile health a promising method for the delivery of nutrition education. However, despite being labeled promising and possibly effective, there is insufficient evidence supporting mobile health interventions for healthy eating [69]. A systematic review reported that only one fourth of studies showed a statistically significant improvement in lifestyle (including weight management, healthy diet, exercise), using a mobile app [70]. Other reviews previously showed some modest improvement in lifestyle using app-based interventions; however, studies had limitations and most concluded that more research was needed [71–73]. Some evidence suggests that telehealth could improve metrics for patients with

T2D, but the magnitude is unknown and more research is also needed in this area [74].

Nevertheless, a potential benefit of mobile-based intervention is that it may allow patients to have a more active participation in their heath than usually allowed by more standard medical practices, potentially encouraging adherence through engagement [67]. In addition, it is argued that mobile-based interventions can have lower costs, though the initial cost for technology development can be considerable.

Telephone

Telephone care is a promising way of delivering lifestyle interventions. Telephone consultations of 10–15 minutes can prevent weight regain when compared to self-directed or interactive technology interventions [75] and telephone care exhibits comparable results with face-to-face interactions minimizing weight regain [76–78]. Studies analyzing the effect of telehealth on hemoglobin A1c for patients with T2D indicate that the best outcome was derived with telephone-based interventions [74]. Some benefit of telephone counseling for lifestyle behaviors has also been seen with oncology patients [77, 79, 80].

The advantages of telephone-based interventions are that it is less costly than standard face-to-face interventions [51, 78] and decreases the need for dedicated clinic space, supplies, and ancillary staff. Telephone-based interventions also increase access to patients who reside in secluded areas. From a patient's perspective, telephone consultations can save time, cost, and burden associated with commuting. However, individual phone counseling still requires HCP time [51]. Telephone delivered group-based educational intervention may decrease the amount of HCP time required, however, there is insufficient evidence regarding effectiveness [51].

Coding and Billing

Offering nutrition interventions by a trained nutritional professional in a Lifestyle Medicine Center creates a cost for both the lifestyle practice and for the patient. Being able to provide the patient with different payment options and being able to collect for these services can improve value for all parties leading to a sustainable healthcare activity. However, it is important to be knowledgeable of billing nuances as well as regulatory issues that might impede payment arrangements.

Costs to the Patient

The provision of nutrition education and MNT is not always covered by insurances and can be cost prohibitive to some patients. Therefore, different models can be employed when charging patients for these services [81].

Self-Pay

The patient is responsible for covering 100% of the cost of the nutrition consultation with payment typically expected at the time of service. These can be promoted as individual consultations or as "bundle" deals, where discounted prices are offered when more than one service is purchased together [81]. If possible, and preferably part of an initial business plan for the Lifestyle Medicine Center, price points for nutritional services can be fixed to be competitive in the local market (e.g., establishing prices that are a fraction of prevailing charges in the community, but still manageable with a profit margin).

Health-Saving Accounts or Flexible Spending Accounts

Patients are allowed to use flexible spending accounts offered by their employer for nutritional sessions [81]. Although, this can help them cover the cost of the sessions, there still needs to be a perceived value by the patient in having the nutritional sessions.

Billing Insurance

Services rendered are billed to the patient's primary, and if applicable, secondary insurance. The patient might be ultimately responsible for copays, deductibles, or services not covered by their insurance. Coverage for MNT is still limited, and patients should receive fair warning of any potential bills prior to accepting services.

Medicare

Since 2002, MNT services delivered by nutritional professionals are covered by Medicare Part B under the "National Coverage Determination for Medical Nutrition Therapy" when the treating physician refers the patient [68]. Under Medicare Part B, MNT is covered for diagnosis of diabetes, kidney disease, and post-kidney transplantation (within 3 years of transplant), and it includes 3 hours within the first year of the initial referral and 2 hours in subsequent years, unless additional hours are ordered by a treating physician based on a change in condition [68, 82]. Appropriate codes (Table 16.6) and associated diagnosing codes (Table 16.7) should be used when billing Medicare for MNT [68, 83].

Table 16.6 MNT coding for Medicare

CPT code	Initial/reassessment	Individual/group	Time increments
97802	Initial	Individual	15 minutes
97803	Reassessment	Individual	15 minutes
97804	N/A	Group	30 minutes

[a]Abbreviation: *CPT* Current procedural terminology; Adapted from Ref. [68]

Table 16.7 Diagnosis codes that could be used for Medicare Part B medical nutrition therapy services[a]

Diabetes mellitus	Chronic kidney disease	Kidney transplant
"E10.2—Type 1 diabetes mellitus with kidney complications	N18.5—Chronic kidney disease, stage 5 (excludes chronic kidney disease, stage 5, requiring chronic dialysis)	Z94.0—Kidney transplant status"
E10.5—Type 1 diabetes mellitus with circulatory complications	N18.4—Chronic kidney disease, stage 4	
E10.65—Type 1 diabetes mellitus with hyperglycemia	N18.3—Chronic kidney disease, stage 3	
E10.9—Type 1 diabetes mellitus without complications		
E11.4—Type 2 diabetes mellitus with neurological complications		
E11.64—Type 2 diabetes mellitus with hypoglycemia		
E11.8—Type 2 diabetes mellitus with unspecified complications		

[a]International Classification of Diseases (ICD)-10 codes provided. Adapted from Ref. [83]

Table 16.8 Intensive behavioral therapy for obesity coding for Medicare[a]

Code	Individual/group	Time increments
G0447	Individual	15 minutes
G0473	Group	30 minutes

[a]Adapted from Ref. [68]. https://www.cms.gov/Outreach-and-Education/Medicare-Learning-Network-MLN/MLNMattersArticles/downloads/MM7641.pdf

In addition, dietary intervention provided as part of intensive behavioral therapy for patients with obesity (defined by a BMI >30 kg/m^2) can be covered by Medicare when provided by a primary care physician/advance care provider or nutritional professional supervised by a primary care physician [68]. Intensive behavioral therapy is covered weekly for the first month, every other week from month 2 to 6, and then monthly for months 7 to 12 if the recipient has achieved at least 3 kilograms weight loss throughout the first 6 months [68]. Table 16.8 discusses IBT coding for Medicare [68].

Medicaid

Medicaid coverage is determined by the state based on a set of standard national guidelines, so it is important for the facility to verify coverage in their specific State of practice [84]. MNT could be covered as an optional benefit under "Other diagnostic, screening, preventive and rehabilitative services," and if covered, the State will determine the frequency, duration, and other specifics [84].

Commercial Carriers

Commercial insurances can have different policies for non-physician services, and these should be reviewed individually with individual insurances [85]. Patients may also be given the option to pay for services up front but be provided with visit documentation so they can apply for insurance reimbursement on their own [81].

Costs to the Lifestyle Medicine Center

Different options are available for the lifestyle medical center to offer nutritional services, such as having a nutrition professional on-site or offering referrals to nutrition professionals off-site. To determine the best option for offering these services, the lifestyle medical center should analyze the volume of patients, demand and capacity to pay for nutritional services, market value, and possible revenue. These considerations are best evaluated when the Lifestyle Medicine Center business plan is being created.

On-Site Nutrition Professional

In this case, the Lifestyle Medicine Center employs the nutrition professional who works full- or part-time on-site. The salary of the nutrition professional is paid by the Lifestyle Medicine Center and can be calculated hourly or on an annual basis. This model might work well for centers that have a high volume of patients and want a dedicated nutrition professional onsite. The facility must be aware of the nutrition professional's and their HCP's billing policy regarding non-physician services, as well as any State regulations which can impede payment arrangements [85]. For example, "Fee splitting" laws can forbid, in some states, to share the fees that a HCP receives from providing services with another professional not involved in the service delivered [85]. However, in most states, if the physician bills for the services of an RDN or nutritional professional that are employed by them, this would (likely) not be fee splitting [85].

Off-Site Nutrition Professional

In this model, the nutrition professional and the HCPs work together by sharing the same patients through an established referral process. In general, the nutrition professional would be off-site, but exceptions occur where the nutrition professional sees patients on-site but is not employed by the Lifestyle Medicine Center. These options might work well for facilities that do not have a large volume of patients or that do not want to have a dedicated nutrition professional on-site, or when the cost of having a dedicated nutrition professional does not outweigh the anticipated benefits or prof-its. Potential drawbacks to this process are poor communication among HCPs and less cohesion with this multidisciplinary approach, thus it is important that parties establish an effective way of communicating for this model. Fee splitting issues also apply for this off-site model [85]. Moreover, the AMA code of medical ethics considers receiving financial incentive for referring a patient for a service unethical [86]. Whether electronic or written, referral should explicitly state the medical necessity and rationale for MNT.

Patient Educational and Counseling Resources

Written

Written materials can be a helpful and informative resource for patients to highlight and further explain important counseling points, and also for the patient to refer to after the consultation. Materials can be personalized to the patient, such as an after-visit summary, or take the form of generic pre-written handouts.

After-Visit Summaries

These summaries are notes written by the HCP to the patient at the time of the consultation, which reflect important points addressed during the counseling session, such as diagnosis, treatment plan, and follow-up appointment [87]. In the Lifestyle Medicine Center, the after-visit summary can be used to outline patient-oriented lifestyle goals. Although the after-visit summary is individualized, it can often be time-consuming to complete. If these summaries are based on a prepopulated template in the electronic health record (EHR), self-populated, and not carefully reviewed by the HCP and staff, there can be significant error and confusion [87].

Pre-written Materials

Pre-written materials are routinely used in medical offices. They are often based on a specific topic and can be brief or extensive. The advantage of using pre-written materials is that they are practical, though may not be specific to the patient's care plan. Pre-written educational resources can be provided by a third party commercial entity or created by the lifestyle medicine program.

Public/Commercial Handouts

When using pre-written materials, it is important to verify any copyrights before distributing to patients (government educational material and materials from not-for-profit agencies can often be reproduced for patient education free of charge, but some require a payment). Table 16.9 lists credible resources that lifestyle practices can refer to for patient education. This is a partial list and many other resources are available. Another tool not mentioned below is "UpToDate,"

Table 16.9 Resources[a]

General nutrition	*The Academy of Dietetics and Nutrition*
	  https://www.eatright.org/
	Harvard T.H. Chan School of Public Health- The Nutrition Source
	  https://www.hsph.harvard.edu/nutritionsource/
	USDA Food and Nutrition Service
	  https://www.fns.usda.gov/tn/nutrition-education-materials
	USDA
	  https://www.nutrition.gov/basic-nutrition/printable-materials-and-handouts

Obesity/weight loss	*The Obesity Action Coalition*
	  https://www.obesityaction.org/get-educated/public-resources/brochures-guides/
	Centers for Disease Control and Prevention
	  https://www.cdc.gov/obesity/resources/factsheets.html
	NIH National Heart, Lung and Blood Institute
	  https://www.nhlbi.nih.gov/health/educational/wecan/tools-resources/parent-tip-sheets.htm
	Rethink Obesity (registered trademark of Novo Nordisk):
	  https://www.rethinkobesity.com/resources/educational-materials.html

Physical activity	*NIH National Heart, Lung, and Blood Institute*
	  https://www.nhlbi.nih.gov/health/educational/wecan/tools-resources/physical-activity.htm
	NIH National Institute on Aging
	  https://www.nia.nih.gov/health/exercise-physical-activity
	CDC Centers for Disease Control and Prevention
	  https://www.cdc.gov/physicalactivity/resources/index.htm
	American Heart Association
	  https://www.heart.org/en/healthy-living/fitness

Diabetes	*The Academy of Dietetics and Nutrition*
	  https://www.dce.org/publications/education-handouts
	NIH National Institute of Diabetes and Digestive and Kidney Diseases
	  https://www.niddk.nih.gov/health-information/diabetes/overview
	Lilly Diabetes
	  https://www.lillydiabetes.com/resources
	American Diabetes Association
	  https://professional.diabetes.org/content/diabetes-educator-resources
	MedlinePlus
	  https://medlineplus.gov/diabetes.html
	American Association of Diabetes Educators
	  https://www.diabeteseducator.org/living-with-diabetes/Tools-and-Resources

Kidney disease	*NIH National Institute of Diabetes and Digestive and Kidney Diseases*
	  https://www.niddk.nih.gov/health-information/communication-programs/nkdep
	National Kidney Foundation
	  https://www.kidney.org/kidneydisease

Cardiovascular disease/ hypertension	*American Heart Association*
	  https://www.heart.org/en/health-topics/consumer-healthcare/patient-education-resources-for-healthcare-providers
	Medline Plus
	  https://medlineplus.gov/heartdiseases.html

Cancer	*NIH National Cancer Institute*
	  https://www.cancer.gov/publications/patient-education
	American Institute for Cancer Research
	  https://www.aicr.org/resources/media-library/
	American Cancer Society
	  https://www.cancer.org/treatment/survivorship-during-and-after-treatment/staying-active/nutrition.html?sitearea=ETO
	American Society of Clinical Oncology
	  https://www.cancer.net/about-us/asco-answers-patient-education-materials

[a]All websites accessed on 23 Mar 2020

available for many HCPs, which has patient educational materials in a variety of topics. In some EHR (e.g., Epic), educational materials for each patient are suggested automatically and can be selected and printed in the after-visit summary.

Self-Developed Handouts

Providing self-developed handouts is a personalized approach for the Lifestyle Medicine Center to cater to its populations' specific needs; however, it is labor intensive and the handouts need to be periodically updated. When writing materials, the content should be clear, accurate, up-to-date, organized, cohesive, engaging, motivating, and written in a conversational style at a level that the reader can understand [88]. Readability tools are often used to generate a grade level for educational materials, but there is limited usefulness to applying a readability level to a general patient population [88]. Instead, readability might be better suited for generating a range of difficulty levels for the material catering to a specific patient population [88]. Topics to consider when developing written materials for patients include available medical interventions (e.g., tests/exams, referrals, pharmacotherapy, and surgical options), community-based programs and resources, commercial services or products (e.g., commercial weight loss programs, meal delivery programs, and food/supplement recommendations). Useful center materials may also include meal replacement recommendations, online resources, helpful websites, smartphone applications, and behavior modification tools (e.g., self-monitoring tools such as food diaries, online/electronic food trackers, exercise logs, and electronic devices, such as pedometers). Materials should also help the patient focus on making goals for physical activity, diet plans including portion sizes, calorie recommendations, menu examples, relevant pictures, and infographics.

Virtual Resources

In lieu of or in combination with written educational materials, patients can also be referred to electronic resources such as websites, smartphone applications, and DVDs. Prior to making recommendations to specific third-party resources, the Lifestyle Medicine Center should verify that the resource is providing safe and credible information. Resources could be provided from professional organizations, universities, large medical institutions, government agencies, and from individuals. Virtual resources of interest should be informational (e.g., focused on diseases, diet/nutrition, lifestyle, physical activity, and psychology) and interactive (e.g., focused on behavior changes and self-monitoring). Examples of smartphone applications that exist in different categories are listed in Table 16.10. An important consideration for virtual resources is that many specific products, i.e. specific smartphone applications, have not undergone rigorous/formal testing.

Table 16.10 Websites and phone applications[a]

	Smartphone applications
Obesity and weight loss	Bariatric Surgery: Baritastic - Bariatric Tracker® Bariatric IQ® BariatricPal® Food Tracking: MyFitnessPal® CalorieKing Food Search® Lose It!- Calorie Counter® Noom® Bitesnap:® Photo Food Journal WW Weight Watchers Reimagined® Behavior Change: Way of Life - Habit Tracker Chains.cc® Coach.me - Goals & Habits®
General nutrition	General Nutrition: FoodSwitch® Eat This Much - Meal Planner® Fooducate - eat better coach® Sugar Rush - Discover Added Sugars in Your Food® Menu/Cooking Planner: Meal Planner Pal® Paprika Recipe Manager3® Healthy Recipes - SparkRecipes® Epicurious® Tasty® Food Network Kitchen® NYT Cooking® Yummly Recipes + Shopping List® Allrecipes Dinner Spinner® Healthy Crockpot Recipes®

Table 16.10 (continued)

	Smartphone applications
Physical activity	P.A./Training Apps: Nike Training Club®
	J&J Official 7 Minute Workout®
	7 Minute Workout: Fitness App®
	JEFIT Workout Planner Gym Log®
	FitStar Yoga®
	12 Minute Athlete®
	Aaptiv: #1 Audio Fitness App®
	Daily Yoga: Workout and Fitness®
	Simply Yoga - Home Instructor®
	LOTUS Yoga and Meditation®
	Yoga for Begginers Mind+Body®
	Map My Walk® or Map My Run® (by Under Armour)
	Fitness Buddy: Train at Home®
	Endomondo®
Diabetes	DM general:
	DiabetesPal®
	One Drop for Diabetes Health®
	Diabetes: M®
	Blood sugar management/diary:
	Glucose Buddy Diabetes Tracker®
	Glucose-Blood Sugar Tracker®
	MySugr Diabetes Tracker Log®
	BG Monitor Diabetes®
	Health2Sync®
	Sugarmate®
	Carbohydrate counting:
	Carb Manager: Keto Diet App®
	Recipes:
	Diabetes Recipe App®
Cardiovascular disease/hypertension	Heart rate monitoring: Instant Heart Rate: HR Monitor®
	Blood pressure monitoring:
	SmartBP: Smart Blood Pressure®
	Qardio Heart Health®
	Blood Pressure Companion®
	Blood Pressure Monitor®
Cancer	Support/network:
	BELONG Beating Cancer Together®
	My Cancer Coach®
	LivingWith™: Cancer Support®
	Symptom tracker:
	chemoWave: cancer health app®
	Care management: Cancer.Net Mobile®
	Supplements:
	AboutHerbs®

ᵃAll websites accessed on 23 Mar 2020

Selling of Point-of-Service Products

Selling health-related products might sound appealing to a lifestyle medical center that routinely recommends nutritional supplements and meal substitutes. Selling these products might also be a source of revenue for the practice, while offering patients easy access to obtain recommended products. However, in addition to considering potential financial incentives, the Lifestyle Medicine Center must consider professional ethics, conflicts of interest, and patient safety.

Ethical and Legal Considerations

Ethical considerations regarding the sale of health products in physician's offices are addressed in the American Medical Association (AMA) Code of Medical Ethics' Opinions on Physicians' Financial Interests Opinion 8.063. The AMA says that the selling of health-related products can take away from the primary responsibility of the physician, which is to care for the patient's interests, even before the physician's own interest [89]. In addition, the practice of selling health-related products may place pressure on the patient and potentially affect patient's trust [89]. According to the AMA code of ethics, physicians should take the following steps to minimize negatives when selling health-related products in their offices or in websites: (1) only sell products that have sound scientific validity, (2) lessen conflicts of interest by selling only products that fulfills an immediate need of the patient or by offering products free or at cost, (3) fully disclose any financial relationships with manufactures/distributors of the products, and (4) avoid products that are sold exclusively in physician's offices [89].

In addition, Lifestyle Medicine Centers should be informed of any State laws that might dictate the extent that selling products at a medical office is permitted. For example, Illinois 225 ILCS 60/22 reads that the department (Illinois General Assembly) may take action against "Promotion of the sale of drugs, devices, appliances or goods provided for a patient in such manner as to exploit the patient for financial gain of the physician" [90].

Safety Considerations

When dispensing health products, the Lifestyle Medicine Center should also take caution to assure the safety of the patient. Products should be kept as per manufacturers' recommendation in order to preserve the quality and shelf life. Products that are expired should be discarded, and a first in first out methodology should be considered to help optimize the dispensing of these products. For nutritional supplements, offices should work with manufacturers and distributors to make sure that products are free of contaminants and that nutritional labels and health claims are accurate and not misleading. In addition, it is prudent that HCPs who are recommending products to a specific patient ensure that these products are safe for that patient to take, that there are no contraindications, allergies, food and drug interactions, or other potential harms.

Clinic Environment and Physical Layout of Clinic Space

The physical environment of the office and clinic space plays a critical role in the patient pathway of care. The physical requirements of the center can influence the relationship between the HCP and the patient and may greatly improve the healthcare experience for patients. Simple design steps can enhance workflow efficiency and patient safety, as well as patient and team interactions and satisfaction, making it more likely that patients may seek help and to be receptive to counseling [91].

Providing adequate space, having comfortable furniture, and supplying appropriate equipment are basic necessities to improving quality of care and promoting active participation during the counseling session [91–93]. The specific requirements will depend on the patient population being served in the Lifestyle Medicine Center. To improve the patient experience and increase the likelihood of seeking medical care, close attention should be paid toward assuring proper furniture, stocking the clinic room, making available appropriate teaching tools, and training and educating the clinic staff.

Nutrition knowledge is an integral component of health literacy, where low health literacy is associated with poor health outcomes. Having food models readily available in the clinic helps to further facilitate understanding of the nutrition education provided. To help increase nutrition literacy, there are numerous tools available for HCPs that are geared toward increasing nutrition knowledge and comprehension. Food models are an effective learning strategy across all ages and literacy levels. The use of food models can be instrumental in changing patients' knowledge about nutrition guidelines and portion sizes [94]. Food models can also increase confidence in reading and understanding nutrition food labels and facilitate intentional changes toward a healthy eating pattern [94].

In addition to using food models to help enrich nutrition literacy, the center should consider space for storing teaching models, additional equipment for instruction, as well as adequate spaces for large groups (Table 16.11).

Table 16.11 Considerations for equipping the Lifestyle Medicine Center

Food models
Portion control models:
MyPlate portion control plate
Measuring cups
Measuring spoons
Anatomical model set:
1–5 lbs. fat and muscle replicas
Food scale
Body weight scale (kg/lbs)
Body fat analyzer (e.g., bioelectrical impedance)
Tape measure for waist circumference
Storage space for meal analysis tools:
Food frequency questionnaire
Food diaries
Handouts
Office space for counseling:
Can be shared or individual office space
Classroom or conference room:
Nutrition classes
Community programs
Meetings
Kitchen space:
Cooking classes
Culinary medicine

Multidisciplinary Team

Patients and HCPs need to collaborate on how to optimize lifestyle management from the time of the initial comprehensive medical evaluation through all subsequent evaluations and follow-up visits. To enhance care, patients and HCPs should work together when assessing complications and management of comorbid conditions. Having a shared philosophy of treatment within a multidisciplinary team in the clinic can help increase the likelihood patients may reach their health goals.

The healthcare team at a Lifestyle Medicine Center should include medical care (MDs or DOs, and advance practice providers [nurse practitioners and/or physician assistants]), dietary care (RDN), and emotional/psychological care (PhD or licensed clinical social worker [LCSW]). Employment of other HCPs who can extend this care includes a health coach and/or behavioral counselor. Additionally, integrating community resources (e.g., social media, houses of worship, community centers, and support groups) can significantly extend the reach and impact of HCPs with respect to lifestyle counseling (Table 16.12) [95].

Using both interdisciplinary and multidisciplinary strategies, each HCP has their own role to help the patient reach positive outcomes. The interdisciplinary strategies allow the common or shared philosophy of treatment and healthcare goals to be more specifically targeted through individual

expertise of the multidisciplinary team. By using the HCPs own expertise to develop individual care goals, multidisciplinary teams can integrate specific intervention goals into a comprehensive care plan. In other words, if each HCP focuses on a single, shared goal with each team member, then applying strategies to achieve those goals through multiple areas of expertise (e.g., medical approach, dietary approach, and psychological approach) will promote clinical success.

Interdisciplinary and multidisciplinary care must occur to bring about improved patient outcomes [91]. Shared philosophies in treatment of the patient should also include shared treatment practices, such as using "people first" language, making the patient feel supported and empowered, and increasing motivation to reach his or her goals. Multidisciplinary team members should consider the impact that language has on building therapeutic relationships and to choose positive words and phrases that place people first [96]. The words used to describe excess weight can be embarrassing and reinforce stigma for many patients. Negativity is demotivating in reaching weight loss goals. The use of people-first language ("patient with obesity" or "having obesity"), as opposed to condition/disease-first language ("obese patient"), is recommended terminology for both academic and clinical settings [96, 97].

Another strategy that should be implemented across the multidisciplinary team is the use of motivational interviewing techniques. Motivational interviewing is a client-centered

Table 16.12 Roles and responsibilities of a multidisciplinary team[a]

Team member	Role	Responsibility
Physician, advanced practice provider	Interpretation of routine anthropometrics (e.g., weight, BMI, WC, BP), laboratory and other tests Assessment of biological and social determinants of health Prescriptions and other interventions	- Counseling/coaching/behavioral interventions on diet/lifestyle change to achieve a healthy weight or reduced risk of disease development or progression - Assist patients in controlling health outcomes: e.g., reaching lower blood pressure or lowering glucose levels, and improving lipid levels - Managing medications
Registered dietitian nutritionist, certified diabetes educator	Provide dietary and nutrition counseling to help reach patient focused goals	- Counseling/coaching/behavioral interventions on diet/lifestyle change to achieve improved health and develop healthy eating patterns - Utilize numerous dietary interventions to help a patient incorporate healthy foods appropriate for the medical condition being managed
Clinical psychologist, licensed social worker	Assessment of psychosocial, behavioral, environmental, and attributes that may improve or interfere with reaching healthy goals, healthy eating patterns, and/ or weight loss	- Implementing behavioral and psychological techniques to help patients reach health goals - Many patients may also be counseled for depression, anxiety, eating disorders, or other psychological conditions that interfere with reaching health centered goals
Exercise therapist, physical therapist	Instruction on exercise to increase patient's activity, reduce physical injury risks, and improve disease risk outcomes	- Create individualized plans and instruction on exercise and activity - Assist patients in reaching recommended exercise goals
Medical assistants, customer service representative, office staff	Greet and register patients in the waiting room or check-in areas Collect patient anthropometrics Assist patients with insurance and billing	- Provide patients with respect and care - Participate in high-touch environment - Encourage patients to return to the Lifestyle Medicine Center

[a]Includes healthcare professionals and staff. Abbreviations: *BMI* Body mass index, *BP* Blood pressure, *WC* Waist circumference. Adapted from Ref. [95]

counseling style for eliciting behavior change by helping patients explore and resolve ambivalence and or resistance towards behavior change. Training in counseling techniques, such as motivational interviewing can be challenging for healthcare providers.

To help ensure the most up-to-date, effective methods of working with patients, clinic staff, and team members should be required to receive continuing education and training in lifestyle counseling, including counseling on nutrition and physical activity, motivational interviewing skills, exercise therapies, and pharmacotherapy when indicated.

Summary

Helping individuals select the dietary approach that is most likely to achieve long-term and sustainable health outcomes may be the most important contribution that the lifestyle medicine HCP can make. MNT, provided by an RDN, or through the use of a multidisciplinary team, should be focused on healthy eating patterns instead of targeting one or more specific food groups. Achieving a healthy eating pattern can be accomplished through a variety of dietary approaches including the DASH diet, the Mediterranean diet, or a vegetarian lifestyle. It is most important that HCPs work with patients to help develop a plan that is individually tailored, is easy to implement, and sustainable over the long term. Considerations that may impact a patient's food choices include socioeconomic factors, cultural preferences, and taste preference.

There are multiple methods for providing interventions, and the choice will depend on the patient population as well as the Lifestyle Medicine Center's capabilities and objectives. In-person practice is the most conventional, but long-distance service, such as telehealth, has the potential of providing new and existing benefits for both patients and HCPs.

References

1. Commission on Dietetic Registration. RDN credential - frequently asked questions, 2020. https://www.cdrnet.org/news/rdncredential-faq. Accessed on 23 Mar 2020.
2. Academy of Nutrition and Dietetics Evidence Analysis Library. Medical nutrition therapy, 2019. https://www.andeal.org/topic.cfm?menu=5284. Accessed on 23 Mar 2020.
3. Academy of Nutrition and Dietetics Evidence Analysis Library. Chronic kidney disease, 2018. https://www.andeal.org/topic.cfm?menu=5303. Accessed on 23 Mar 2020.
4. Academy of Nutrition and Dietetics Evidence Analysis Library. Oncology, 2013. https://www.andeal.org/topic.cfm?menu=5291. Accessed on 23 Mar 2020.
5. Academy of Nutrition and Dietetics Evidence Analysis Library. Vegetarian nutrition, 2011. https://www.andeal.org/topic.cfm?menu=5271. Accessed on 23 Mar 2020.
6. American Diabetes Association. Lifestyle management: standards of medical care in diabetes—2019. Diabetes Care. 2019;42(Suppl 1):S46–60.
7. Cespedes EM, Hu FB. Dietary patterns: from nutritional epidemiologic analysis to national guidelines. Am J Clin Nutr. 2015;101:899–900.
8. Romero-Gomez M, Zelber-Sagi S, Trenell M. Treatment of NAFLD with diet, physical activity and exercise. J Hepatol. 2017;67:829–46.
9. Van Horn L, McCoin M, Kris-Etherton PM, et al. The evidence for dietary prevention and treatment of cardiovascular disease. J Am Diet Assoc. 2008;108:287–331.
10. American Diabetes Association. Obesity management for the treatment of type 2 diabetes: standards of medical care in diabetes-2019. Diabetes Care. 2019;42(Suppl 1):S81–90.
11. Isakova T, Nickolas TL, Denburg M, et al. KDOQI US Commentary on the 2017 KDIGO Clinical Practice Guideline update for the diagnosis, evaluation, prevention, and treatment of chronic kidney disease-mineral and bone disorder (CKD-MBD). Am J Kidney Dis. 2017;70:737–51.
12. U.S. Department of Health and Human Services and U.S. Department of Agriculture. 2015–2020 Dietary guidelines for Americans, 2015. http://health.gov/dietaryguidelines/2015/guidelines/. Accessed on 23 Mar 2020.
13. Jensen MD, Ryan DH, Apovian CM, et al. AHA/ACC/TOS guideline for the management of overweight and obesity in adults: a report of the American College of Cardiology/American Heart Association Task Force on Practice Guidelines and The Obesity Society. J Am Coll Cardiol. 2014;63(25 Pt B):2985–3023.
14. Penalvo JL, Oliva B, Sotos-Prieto M, et al. Greater adherence to a Mediterranean dietary pattern is associated with improved plasma lipid profile: the Aragon health workers study cohort. Rev Esp Cardiol. 2015;68:290–7.
15. Steinberg D, Bennett GG, Svetkey L. The DASH diet, 20 years later. JAMA. 2017;317:1529–30.
16. The President and Fellows of Harvard College-The Nutrition Source. DASH, 2020. https://www.hsph.harvard.edu/nutrition-source/healthy-weight/diet-reviews/dash-diet/. Accessed on 23 Mar 2020.
17. Abbasi J. Cardiovascular corner: low lipids, metformin, and plant-based diets. JAMA. 2019;322:15–6.
18. Dinu M, Abbate R, Gensini GF, et al. Vegetarian, vegan diets and multiple health outcomes: a systematic review with meta-analysis of observational studies. Crit Rev Food Sci Nutr. 2017;57:3640–9.
19. Chuang SY, Chiu TH, Lee CY, et al. Vegetarian diet reduces the risk of hypertension independent of abdominal obesity and inflammation: a prospective study. J Hypertens. 2016;34:2164–71.
20. Huang RY, Huang CC, Hu FB, et al. Vegetarian diets and weight reduction: a meta-analysis of randomized controlled trials. J Gen Intern Med. 2016;31:109–16.
21. Craig WJ. Nutrition concerns and health effects of vegetarian diets. Nutr Clin Pract. 2010;25:613–20.
22. Obert J, Pearlman M, Obert L, et al. Popular weight loss strategies: a review of four weight loss techniques. Curr Gastroenterol Rep. 2017;19:61.
23. Quagliani D, Hermann M. Practice paper of the academy of nutrition and dietetics abstract: communicating accurate food and nutrition information. J Acad Nut Diet. 2012;112:759.
24. Kahleova H, Lloren JI, Mashchak A, et al. Meal frequency and timing are associated with changes in body mass index in Adventist Health Study 2. J Nutr. 2017;147:1722–8.
25. Canuto R, da Silva GA, Kac G, et al. Eating frequency and weight and body composition: a systematic review of observational studies. Public Health Nutr. 2017;20:2079–95.
26. Georgiopoulos G, Karatzi K, Yannakoulia M, et al. Eating frequency predicts changes in regional body fat distribution in healthy adults. Q J Med. 2017;110:729–34.

27. Tamez M, Rodriguez-Orengo JF, Mattei J. Higher eating frequency, but not skipping breakfast, is associated with higher odds of abdominal obesity in adults living in Puerto Rico. Nutr Res. 2020;73:75–8.

28. House BT, Shearrer GE, Boisseau JB, et al. Decreased eating frequency linked to increased visceral adipose tissue, body fat, and BMI in Hispanic college freshmen. BMC Nutr. 2018;4:10.

29. Rong S, Snetselaar LG, Xu G, et al. Association of skipping breakfast with cardiovascular and all-cause mortality. J Am Coll Cardiol. 2019;73:2025–32.

30. Bi H, Gan Y, Yang C, et al. Breakfast skipping and the risk of type 2 diabetes: a meta-analysis of observational studies. Public Health Nutr. 2015;18:3013–9.

31. Njike VY, Smith TM, Shuval O, et al. Snack food, satiety, and weight. Adv Nutr. 2016;7:866–78.

32. Barrington WE, Beresford SAA. Eating occasions, obesity and related behaviors in working adults: does it matter when you snack? Nutrients. 2019;11(10):E2320. https://doi.org/10.3390/nu11102320.

33. Tovar AR, Caamano Mdel C, Garcia-Padilla S, et al. The inclusion of a partial meal replacement with or without inulin to a calorie restricted diet contributes to reach recommended intakes of micronutrients and decrease plasma triglycerides: a randomized clinical trial in obese Mexican women. Nutr J. 2012;11:44.

34. Freeland-Graves JH, Nitzke S. Position of the academy of nutrition and dietetics: total diet approach to healthy eating. J Acad Nutr Diet. 2013;113:307–17.

35. Raynor HA, Anderson AM, Miller GD, et al. Partial meal replacement plan and quality of the diet at 1 year: action for health in diabetes (Look AHEAD) Trial. J Acad Nutr Diet. 2015;115:731–42.

36. Freeland-Graves J, Nitzke S. Position of the American Dietetic Association: total diet approach to communicating food and nutrition information. J Am Diet Assoc. 2002;102:100–8.

37. Academy of Nutrition and Dietetics. Qualifications of a registered dietitian nutritionist, 2020. https://www.eatright.org/food/resources/learn-more-about-rdns/qualifications-of-a-registered-dietitian-nutritionist. Accessed on 23 Mar 2020.

38. Commission on Dietetic Registration. RD examination—eligibility requirements, 2020. https://www.cdrnet.org/rd-eligibility. Accessed on 23 Mar 2020.

39. Commission on Dietetic Registration. Maintaining your credential—at a glance, 2020. https://www.cdrnet.org/maintain. Accessed on 23 Mar 2020.

40. National Board for Health & Wellness Coaching. Welcome. https://nbhwc.org/. Accessed on 23 Mar 2020.

41. Academy of Nutrition and Dietetics. MNT versus nutrition education, 2020. https://www.eatrightpro.org/payment/coding-and-billing/mnt-vs-nutrition-education. Accessed on 23 Mar 2020.

42. National Society of Health Coaches. NSHC health coach program details, 2020. https://www.nshcoa.com/health-coach-program-details. Accessed on 23 Mar 2020.

43. Academy of Nutrition and Dietetics. Scope of practice, 2020. https://www.eatrightpro.org/practice/quality-management/scope-of-practice. Accessed on 23 Mar 2020.

44. American Nutrition Association. Current CNS. https://theana.org/certify/currentCNS. Accessed on 23 Mar 2020.

45. Kris-Etherton PM, Akabas SR, Bales CW, et al. The need to advance nutrition education in the training of health care professionals and recommended research to evaluate implementation and effectiveness. Am J Clin Nutr. 2014;99(5 Suppl):1153s–66s.

46. Bruemmer B, Harris J, Gleason P, et al. Publishing nutrition research: a review of epidemiologic methods. J Am Diet Assoc. 2009;109:1728–37.

47. Hammond MI, Myers EF, Trostler N. Nutrition care process and model: an academic and practice odyssey. J Acad Nutr Diet. 2014;114:1879–94.

48. Thompson KL, Davidson P, Swan WI, et al. Nutrition care process chains: the "missing link" between research and evidence-based practice. J Acad Nutr Diet. 2015;115:1491–8.

49. Mitchell LJ, Ball LE, Ross LJ, et al. Effectiveness of dietetic consultations in primary health care: a systematic review of randomized controlled trials. J Acad Nutr Diet. 2017;117:1941–62.

50. de Waal D, Heaslip E, Callas P. Medical nutrition therapy for chronic kidney disease improves biomarkers and slows time to dialysis. J Ren Nutr. 2016;26:1–9.

51. Perri MG, Ariel-Donges AH, Shankar MN, et al. Design of the rural LEAP randomized trial: an evaluation of extended-care programs for weight management delivered via group or individual telephone counseling. Contemp Clin Trials. 2019;76:55–63.

52. Renjilian DA, Perri MG, Nezu AM, et al. Individual versus group therapy for obesity: effects of matching participants to their treatment preferences. J Consult Clin Psychol. 2001;69:717–21.

53. Academy of Nutrition and Dietetics Evidence Analysis Library. NC: group vs. individual counseling, 2008. https://www.andeal.org/topic.cfm?menu=3151&cat=3549. Accessed on 23 Mar 2020).

54. Rickheim PL, Weaver TW, Flader JL, et al. Assessment of group versus individual diabetes education: a randomized study. Diabetes Care. 2002;25:269–74.

55. Endevelt R, Peled R, Azrad A, et al. Diabetes prevention program in a Mediterranean environment: individual or group therapy? An effectiveness evaluation. Prim Care Diabetes. 2015;9:89–95.

56. Kalavainen MP, Korppi MO, Nuutinen OM. Clinical efficacy of group-based treatment for childhood obesity compared with routinely given individual counseling. Int J Obes. 2007;31:1500–8.

57. Farpour-Lambert NJ, Martin XE, Bucher Della Torre S, et al. Effectiveness of individual and group programmes to treat obesity and reduce cardiovascular disease risk factors in pre-pubertal children. Clin Obes. 2019;9:e12335.

58. Dalle Grave R, Calugi S, Bosco G, et al. Personalized group cognitive behavioural therapy for obesity: a longitudinal study in a real-world clinical setting. Eat Weight Disord. 2018;25:337–46.

59. Minniti A, Bissoli L, Di Francesco V, et al. Individual versus group therapy for obesity: comparison of dropout rate and treatment outcome. Eat Weight Disord. 2007;12:161–7.

60. Academy of Nutrition and Dietetics. Practicing telehealth, 2020. https://www.eatrightpro.org/practice/practice-resources/telehealth/practicing-telehealth. Accessed on 23 Mar 2020.

61. Knotowicz H, Haas A, Coe S, et al. Opportunities for innovation and improved care using telehealth for nutritional interventions. Gastroenterology. 2019;157:594–7.

62. Harris J, Felix L, Miners A, et al. Adaptive e-learning to improve dietary behaviour: a systematic review and cost-effectiveness analysis. Health Technol Assess. 2011;15:1–160.

63. Stein K. Remote Nutrition Counseling: considerations in a new channel for client communication. J Acad Nutr Diet. 2015;115:1561–76.

64. Rollo ME, Hutchesson MJ, Burrows TL, et al. Video consultations and virtual nutrition care for weight management. J Acad Nutr Diet. 2015;115:1213–25.

65. Heetebry I, Hatcher M, Tabriziani H. Web based health education, E-learning, for weight management. J Med Syst. 2005;29:611–7.

66. Cook DA, Garside S, Levinson AJ, et al. What do we mean by web-based learning? A systematic review of the variability of interventions. Med Educ. 2010;44:765–74.

67. European Commission. GREEN PAPER on mobile health ("mHealth"). Belgium;Brussels. 2014. p. 1–20. https://ec.europa.eu/transparency/regdoc/rep/1/2014/EN/1-2014-219-EN-F1-1.Pdf.

68. Schaum KD. Medical nutrition therapy, obesity behavioral therapy, and smoking cessation counseling reimbursement Q & A's. Adv Skin Wound Care. 2017;30:250–5.

69. McCarroll R, Eyles H, Ni MC. Effectiveness of mobile health (mHealth) interventions for promoting healthy eating in adults: a systematic review. Prev Med. 2017;105:156–68.

70. Covolo L, Ceretti E, Moneda M, et al. Does evidence support the use of mobile phone apps as a driver for promoting healthy lifestyles from a public health perspective? A systematic review of randomized control trials. Patient Educ Couns. 2017;100:2231–43.

71. Schoeppe S, Alley S, Van Lippevelde W, et al. Efficacy of interventions that use apps to improve diet, physical activity and sedentary behaviour: a systematic review. Int J Behav Nutr Phys Act. 2016;13:127.

72. Payne HE, Lister C, West JH, et al. Behavioral functionality of mobile apps in health interventions: a systematic review of the literature. JMIR Mhealth Uhealth. 2015;3:e20.

73. Zhao J, Freeman B, Li M. Can mobile phone apps influence people's health behavior change? An evidence review. J Med Internet Res. 2016;18:e287.

74. Lee PA, Greenfield G, Pappas Y. The impact of telehealth remote patient monitoring on glycemic control in type 2 diabetes: a systematic review and meta-analysis of systematic reviews of randomised controlled trials. BMC Health Serv Res. 2018;18:495.

75. Svetkey LP, Stevens VJ, Brantley PJ, et al. Comparison of strategies for sustaining weight loss: the weight loss maintenance randomized controlled trial. JAMA. 2008;299:1139–48.

76. Perri MG, Limacher MC, Durning PE, et al. Extended-care programs for weight management in rural communities: the treatment of obesity in underserved rural settings (TOURS) randomized trial. Arch Intern Med. 2008;168:2347–54.

77. Harrigan M, Cartmel B, Loftfield E, et al. Randomized trial comparing telephone versus in-person weight loss counseling on body composition and circulating biomarkers in women treated for breast cancer: the Lifestyle, Exercise, and Nutrition (LEAN) Study. J Clin Oncol. 2016;34:669–76.

78. Radcliff TA, Bobroff LB, Lutes LD, et al. Comparing costs of telephone vsfFace-to-face extended-care programs for the management of obesity in rural settings. J Acad Nutr Diet. 2012;112:1363–73.

79. Moug SJ, Bryce A, Mutrie N, et al. Lifestyle interventions are feasible in patients with colorectal cancer with potential short-term health benefits: a systematic review. Int J Color Dis. 2017;32:765–75.

80. Spencer JC, Wheeler SB. A systematic review of Motivational Interviewing interventions in cancer patients and survivors. Patient Educ Couns. 2016;99:1099–105.

81. Ulatowski K. Guide to insurance and reimbursement. Today's Dietitian. 2017;19:40.

82. Academy of Nutrition and Dietetics. Medicare MNT, 2020. https://www.eatrightpro.org/payment/medicare/mnt. Accessed on 23 Mar 2020.

83. Academy of Nutrition and Dietetics. Diagnosis codes for medicare MNT, 2020. https://www.eatrightpro.org/payment/coding-and-billing/diagnosis-and-procedure-codes/diagnosis-codes-for-medicaremnt. Accessed on 23 Mar 2020.

84. Academy of Nutrition and Dietetics. Medicaid medical nutrition therapy, 2020. https://www.eatrightpro.org/payment/nutrition-services/medicaid/medicaid-medical-nutrition-therapy. Accessed on 23 Mar 2020.

85. Academy of Nutrition and Dietetics. Items to consider when establishing an RDN/MD partnership, 2020. https://www.eatrightpro.org/payment/business-practice-management/services-fees-and-management-resources/items-to-consider-when-establishing-an-rdnmd-partnership. Accessed on 23 Mar 2020.

86. American Medical Association. Fee splitting, 2020. https://www.ama-assn.org/delivering-care/ethics/fee-splitting. Accessed on 23 Mar 2020.

87. William Ventres. After-visit confusion. Agency for healthcare research and quality - cases & commentaries Rockville, MD, 2014.

88. Jeanne McGee for U.S. Department of Health & Human Services Centers for Medicare & Medicaid Services. TOOLKIT for making written material clear and effective, 2010. https://www.cms.gov/Outreach-and-Education/Outreach/WrittenMaterialsToolkit/. Accessed on 23 Mar 2020.

89. AMA Council on Ethical and Judicial Affairs. AMA code of medical ethics' opinions on physicians' financial interests. AMA J Ethics. 2015;17:739–43.

90. Illinois General Assembly. Illinois compiled statutes. Springfield, IL. http://www.ilga.gov/legislation/ilcs/ilcs3.asp?ActID=1309. Accessed on 23 Mar 2020.

91. Forhan M, Risdon C, Solomon P. Contributors to patient engagement in primary health care: perceptions of patients with obesity. Prim Health Care Res Dev. 2013;14:367–72.

92. Gunn R, Davis MM, Hall J, et al. Designing clinical space for the delivery of integrated behavioral health and primary care. J Am Board Fam Med. 2015;28(Suppl 1):S52–62.

93. Kirkpatrick MK, Esterhuizen P, Drake D. An optimal caring/healing environment for obese clients. Bariatric Nurs Surg Patient Care. 2009;4 https://doi.org/10.1089/bar.2009.9978.

94. Santalo MI, Gibbons S, Naylor PJ. Using food models to enhance sugar literacy among older adolescents: evaluation of a brief experiential nutrition education intervention. Nutrients. 2019;11:E1763. https://doi.org/10.3390/nu11081763.

95. Dietz WH, Solomon LS, Pronk N, et al. An integrated framework for the prevention and treatment of obesity and its related chronic diseases. Health Aff (Millwood). 2015;34:1456–63.

96. Dickinson JK, Maryniuk MD. Building therapeutic relationships: choosing words that put people first. Clin Diabetes. 2017;35:51–4.

97. Kyle TK, Puhl RM. Putting people first in obesity. Obesity (Silver Spring). 2014;22:1211.

Mary Ann McLaughlin and Frank Vera

Abbreviations

AACVPR	American Association of Cardiovascular Pulmonary Rehabilitation
ACSM	American College of Sports Medicine
AHA	American Heart Association
ASCVD	Atherosclerotic Cardiovascular Disease
ASEP	American Society of Exercise Physiology
CVD	Cardiovascular disease
ECG	Electrocardiogram
EP	Exercise physiologist
HCP	Healthcare professional
MET	Metabolic equivalent of task
PA	Physical activity
RPE	Rating of perceived exertion

Introduction

The US healthcare system has evolved and now assigns greater value to early and sustainable lifestyle and behavioral changes that are associated with better health for the individual and society as a whole. Strategies are being employed to change healthcare systems to focus on primary prevention – a philosophy that is not only cost-effective but also, more importantly, decreases the burden of disease, increases the quality of life, and saves lives [1]. This paradigm shift, from an overwhelming dependence on tertiary prevention that essentially waits for disease to become symptomatic to primordial, primary, and secondary prevention that is oriented to averting disease development and progression, has fomented a culture of interdisciplinary collaboration and patient care. To support this trajectory and fruition of healthcare, the discipline of exercise science figures as an essential and fundamental component in comprehensive care and lifestyle medicine.

The origin of exercise science dates back to ancient cultures. Hippocrates (460–370 BC) advocated for moderate exercise to maintain and improve health status [2]. This concept was later promoted by Galen (129–200 AD), who believed that trained individuals had superior health, respiration, metabolism, muscle tone, and strength [3]. One of the first books on exercise was written by Cristobal Mendez (1500–1561 AD), which contained information regarding the benefits and specific descriptions of exercise, as well as their relative levels of importance [4]. These and other works recognized by the early twentieth-century European scientists can be considered as the genesis of the framework around which one understands "exercise physiology." The first physiology research laboratories were established in the USA in the 1920s. Notably, the Harvard Fatigue Laboratory, which operated from 1927 to 1947, attracted many prominent scientists who were interested in exploring exercise physiology research topics such as cardiovascular and hemodynamic responses to exercise, work capacity, and fatigue. The scientists who trained there ultimately established exercise physiology laboratories in other medical schools and science departments. Subsequently, the dissemination of peer-reviewed research studies raised the public's awareness of the benefits of exercise [5]. Moreover, progress toward understanding human physiology under exercise and stress created pathways for certain individuals to become experts in the field. As a result, exercise scientists or exercise physiologists (EPs) became more prominent and valued as healthcare professionals (HCPs). Most recently, the 2019 American College of Cardiology (ACC) and American Heart

M. A. McLaughlin (✉)
Icahn School of Medicine at Mount Sinai, New York, NY, USA

Marie-Josee and Henry R. Kravis Center for Cardiovascular Health at Mount Sinai Heart, New York, NY, USA
e-mail: maryann.mclaughlin@mountsinai.org

F. Vera
Marie-Josee and Henry R. Kravis Center for Cardiovascular Health at Mount Sinai Heart, New York, NY, USA

© Springer Nature Switzerland AG 2020
J. I. Mechanick, R. F. Kushner (eds.), *Creating a Lifestyle Medicine Center*, https://doi.org/10.1007/978-3-030-48088-2_17

Association (AHA) reviewed scientific evidence and established "Guidelines on the Primary Prevention of Cardiovascular Disease," which included recommendations on exercise [6]. Although clinicians support the guidelines and recommend exercise, many patients fail to engage in exercise due to lack of experience or training. By providing education, instruction, and monitoring to those at risk for atherosclerotic cardiovascular disease (ASCVD), as well as those with complex cardiac conditions, EPs play an integral role in improving cardiovascular health.

The Exercise Physiologist: Roles and Responsibilities

As HCPs become more aware of the profound implications of lifestyle medicine, attention should also be focused on the important roles and team dynamics involved in delivering this healthcare model. Exercise science is based on fundamentals of biology and human physiology. Utilizing EPs provides a durable method to optimize clinical outcomes and enrich clinical practice. An EP is an HCP that works with other HCPs to assist in programing and implementing safe exercise for individuals across the spectrum of wellness to illness. Over the past 20 years, the depth and scope of exercise science have shown increasing applications to medicine. The exercise physiology discipline has adopted the initiative "Exercise Is Medicine," founded by the American College of Sports Medicine, which was endorsed by other professional bodies and practicing clinicians [7]. Exercise physiology interventions prevent and manage chronic disease or injury, as well as target the restoration of optimal physical function and wellness. The scope of EP responsibilities includes diagnostic and functional testing, exercise prescription, exercise supervision, patient counseling, education, and analysis of outcomes.

The curriculum for exercise physiologists includes rigorous academic coursework and clinical training. Many universities and colleges have departments that offer courses on kinesiology and sports sciences and also both undergraduate and graduate degrees. The EP typically receives a bachelor's degree in exercise physiology, exercise science, or kinesiology and health. Educational programs include coursework in biology, chemistry, anatomy, kinesiology, nutrition, exercise psychology, and statistics, in addition to clinical work. Some programs require students to conduct laboratory research (e.g., in an exercise physiology or biometric laboratory) with formal data collection and analysis. Postgraduate degrees are available in exercise physiology, exercise science and nutrition, and strength and conditioning/fitness entrepreneurship. Master of science level coursework may include areas of emphasis, including biomechanics, exercise physiology, motor development/control, strength conditioning, and sport and exercise psychology. Certification exams are administered by the American Society of Exercise Physiologists (ASEP), which require continuing education for recertification every 5 years. Additional certifying organizations include the American Association of Cardiovascular and Pulmonary Rehabilitation (AACVPR) and the American College of Sports Medicine (ACSM). The ACSM offers the following credentialing activity for clinical applications: clinical certifying organizations such as these require strict guidelines and prerequisites in order to sit for an exam. For example, all three national organizations require a minimum of either a bachelor's or a master's degree in the related field, as well as more than 1200 h of clinical hands-on experience. Furthermore, ASEP requires demonstration of competence in certain academic courses. In comparison, the requirements of non-clinical certifications, such as personal trainers or fitness instructors, are far less stringent. The National Academy of Sports Medicine (NASM) and National Strength and Conditioning Organization (NASC) are among the most well-known and recognized organizations for personal training and fitness. The only requirements necessary to test for NASM and NASC certifications are age of 18 years or older, high school diploma, and current CPR/AED certification. In addition to the coursework and clinical education, an EP requires certain humanistic skills to effectively perform in a healthcare environment:

1. Strong communication skills
2. Proficiency in detailed-oriented tasks
3. Empathy for patients with acute and chronic medical conditions

More specifically, in order to determine optimal exercise and fitness regimens, an EP must be able to demonstrate the following competencies:

1. Assessment of medical history to predict risk during exercise
2. Performance and interpretation of data from exercise treadmill stress tests
3. Measurement of blood pressure, oxygen level, blood glucose, heart rhythm on electrocardiogram (ECG), and determination of optimal exercise fitness regimens

According to the Bureau of Labor statistics, approximately 50% of EPs are self-employed, 26% work in hospitals, and fewer than 5% work in physician offices or other ancillary health offices (e.g., occupational medicine) [8]. It is anticipated that the demand for EPs will continue to rise with the expansion of medical fitness and Lifestyle Medicine Centers. For instance, in patients who are diagnosed with chronic diseases, EPs can promote positive physical, physiological, and behavioral changes in response to physical stress that are necessary to optimize health.

Lifestyle Medicine Centers and Clinical Service Lines: Physical Performance Programs

Evidence

Implementation of clinical service lines that include physical performance programs can improve health and provide sustainable high-quality outcomes. Exercise physiologists are pivotal examples of non-physician HCPs that support the continuum of care for various models of

wellness and rehabilitation. According to the World Health Organization, physical inactivity ranks as the fourth leading risk factor for global mortality and has major implications on the prevalence of non-communicable diseases [9]. Physical inactivity is a primary contributor to more than 20 chronic diseases [10]. In other words, exercise can modulate the course of illness for a significant number of chronic diseases. The EP assists physicians in managing chronic diseases, such as cardiovascular, pulmonary, musculoskeletal, and metabolic disorders, as part of an interdisciplinary, comprehensive care approach. In addition, evidence for improvement in outcomes for cancer treatment, digestive disorders, and neurologic disorders lends credence to increased involvement by EPs (Table 17.1) [11–33].

Table 17.1 Medical conditions with evidence of benefit from exercise

Condition	Description	Reference
Cardiovascular		
Congestive heart failure	Improves functional capacity, quality of life, and prognosis	[11]
Coronary artery disease	Decreases CVD risk, all-cause mortality risk, and CVD mortality risk	[12]
Ehlers-Danlos syndrome	Cornerstone treatment	[13]
Hypertension	Reduces cardiovascular risk; prevents, treats, and controls hypertension	[14]
Peripheral arterial disease	Although there is limited data to identify clinical characteristics that can consistently predict responsiveness to exercise programs, experts agree that all patients with PAD should have access to exercise programs to improve walking performance	[15]
Postural orthostatic tachycardia syndrome	Improves with physical reconditioning in most patients: short-term progressive exercise training program	[16]
Gastrointestinal		
Diverticulosis	Frequent low-intensity exercise periods have protective effects on the gastrointestinal tract and may reduce the risk of diverticulosis. An increase in colonic motor activity via hormonal, vascular, and mechanical aspects, leading to reduced colonic transit time, has been suggested as an underlying mechanism	[17, 18]
Gallbladder disease	Benefits to ectopic fat distribution in the liver and decreases risk for gallbladder disease	[19, 20]
Non-alcoholic fatty liver disease	Benefits in NAFLD due to weight loss and other pathways	[20]
Metabolic		
Metabolic syndrome/insulin resistance	Mitigates metabolic syndrome risk factors	[10]
Obesity	Studies have demonstrated that exercise has a positive effect on body weight in patients who are overweight or obese	[21]
Musculoskeletal		
Arthritis	Decreases pain, improves reported energy levels and function, and helps maintain bone and cartilage tissue health	[22]
Osteoporosis	Participation in a structured exercise program demonstrates improved balance and lower extremity strength in women	[23]
Neurologic/psychiatric		
Cognitive dysfunction	There is a positive association between physical activity and cognition	[24]
Anxiety	Reduces symptoms of anxiety among sedentary patients with chronic illness	[25]
Multiple sclerosis	Improves well-being via cardiovascular improvement, other systemic changes, and better central nervous system function	[26]
Parkinson's disease	Lowers risk for development and decreases motor symptoms	[27]
Stroke	There are many public health guidelines on the recommended volume and intensity of physical for optimal health. Although separate guidelines for stroke prevention do not exist, the recommendations for primary stroke prevention are consistent with the current US guidelines: at least 40 min per day of moderate to vigorous intensity aerobic PA 3–4 days/week	[28]

(continued)

Table 17.1 (continued)

Condition	Description	Reference
Oncologic		
Breast cancer	Improves longevity among survivors	[29]
Colon cancer	Protects against proximal and distal colon cancers with a significant reduction of 27% for active individuals	[30]
Endometrial cancer	Affords modest protection	[31]
Pulmonary		
Asthma	Improves control	[32]
Obstructive sleep apnea	Meta-analysis has shown effect of exercise in reducing severity in patients with minimal changes in body weight	[33]

Abbreviations: *CVD* cardiovascular disease, *NAFLD* non-alcoholic fatty liver disease, *OSA* obstructive sleep apnea, *PA* physical activity, *PAD* peripheral arterial disease, *POTS* postural orthostatic tachycardia syndrome

Organizational Structure

An effective framework for providing lifestyle modification and collaborative interdisciplinary care in primary health settings is largely lacking in the USA. Typically, there is a gap in the delivery, maintenance, and follow-up of patients in whom lifestyle modification has been prescribed. The evidence of the benefit of physical activity for optimal health underpins support for integration of an EP into medical practice. The use of interdisciplinary teams in primary health care settings has been shown to improve utilization of resources, cost-effectiveness, and health outcomes.

Within a sponsoring health system is the Lifestyle Medicine Center or Clinical Service Line. Within this service line, specific programs are built that utilize EPs, such as cardiac rehabilitation (typically for secondary prevention in patients who have had a cardiovascular event) and medical fitness (typically for primary prevention of cardiovascular disease, or primary or secondary prevention in those with other chronic diseases). In their fundamental core, these programs are systematically designed to follow specific elements of care and performance measures created by national government organizations. Utilizing guidelines set by the Center for Medicare and Medicaid Services (CMS), as well as other national health organizations, Lifestyle Medicine Centers operate in an intricate process that includes everything from equipment and technology to logistics and regulations. For example, according to the most recent decision memo from CMS, cardiac rehabilitation programs must include, but are not limited to, a comprehensive approach to therapy (medical evaluation, a program to modify cardiac risk factors, exercise prescription, education, and counseling), be medically supervised by a physician, and immediate availability to cardio-pulmonary, emergency, diagnostic, and therapeutic life-saving equipment [34].

Another requirement by CMS for cardiac rehabilitation is a physician's signature every 30 days on patient treatment plans. This requirement is to ensure that the individualized treatment plan (ITP) created for each patient is cleared, acknowledged, and deemed appropriate by the medical director of the program. Although this is a CMS requirement and national standard, most programs function within the confinement of hospitals or medical office buildings and follow further regulations and policies beyond CMS requirements; it is up to the discretion of the sponsoring institution to go beyond these CMS guidelines when operating Lifestyle Medicine Centers according to their hospital standards.

Cardiac rehabilitation programs are also required to implement emergency and untoward event training for all staff members who have direct care with their patients. Creating an annual emergency training calendar provides for up-to-date life-saving skills and practice methods to sustain a safe, medically supervised environment. In addition to monthly periodic trainings for staff members, programs utilize day-to-day diagnostic tools and software programs to ensure that safe exercise parameters are met for their patients. One example of this is the use of direct telemetry that wirelessly monitors ECG activity during exercise. The benefit of providing this element of care is to enhance the supervision and identification of certain cardiac rhythms that ultimately improves the efficacy of patient care and clinical outcomes. In some cases, cardiac rehabilitation programs utilize the integrated function of third-party software programs that communicate with electronic medical record (EMR) databases. This allows seamless interaction and continuity of care between the patient and physician.

By using an effective organizational structure for these programs, the EP provides supervision that ensures safe exercise and intensity progression to higher levels of fitness. The EP's duty is to deliver substantial and accurate clinical guidance that adheres to evidence-based clinical guidelines and strategies set by the physician, while also following national institutional recommendations (such as from the ACSM, the AACVPR, and the AHA).

To illustrate, patients recovering from cardiac-related events or procedures are recommended to participate in secondary prevention programs, such as cardiac rehabilitation or pulmonary rehabilitation. Here, patients receive individualized treatment plans prescribed by EPs as a strategy to reduce the risk of having recurring events. The AACVPR has developed "Guidelines for Cardiac Rehabilitation and Secondary Prevention Programs" [35], and EPs working in cardiac rehabilitation programs must remain up-to-date in cardiopulmonary resuscitation/advanced cardiovascular life support training and ECG evaluation. As EPs join various programs within the Lifestyle Medicine Clinical Service Line, different organizational structures can be explored, developed, and evaluated. The EP may be salaried or work on a per diem basis. Typically, the EP manager reports to the medical director (MD) of the program and works closely with other HCP and staff, including a nutritionist and nurse. The EP manager provides direct oversight of staff EPs and is responsible for assessing skill level and providing education of current medical and exercise guidelines. Weekly educational seminars may be given by MDs in related areas (endocrinology, cardiology, pulmonology, orthopedics, psychiatry, physical medicine and rehabilitation, gastroenterology, and nutrition), which provide important knowledge to remain current in delivering the most up-to-date treatment.

Role of the Exercise Physiologist

Once a patient has been referred to the Lifestyle Medicine Center for intensive lifestyle change, which may involve the cardiac rehabilitation or medical fitness programs, the care team begins a comprehensive review and implementation of interventions. Although organizational structures vary among institutions, the EP is generally involved in conducting the assessment, identifying risk factors, developing protocols, and implementing lifestyle management solutions as they pertain to physical activity. For example, in cardiac rehabilitation, this evaluation begins with an in-depth review of their past medical history, assessment of their current functional status, screening of significant psychosocial factors, and prescription of an exercise regimen that is tailored to specific needs and personal goals (Table 17.2). A comprehensive portfolio of individualized treatment plans and education includes the following domains: exercise, nutrition, weight management, tobacco use, and psychosocial (Tables 17.3a, 17.3b, 17.3c, 17.3d, and 17.3e). Each domain incorporates certain processes, such as clinical assessment and goals, intervention, reassessment, and discharge from the program.

Clinical Assessment and Goals

Prior to developing an individualized treatment plan, the EP evaluates the individual's medical conditions and physician orders for therapy. The EP reviews current and past medical history, surgical history, cardiac risk factor assessment, social history (including social support), risk of alcohol or substance use, and medication use. A clinical assessment includes evaluation of baseline physical measures: height,

Table 17.2 Key recommendations for integrating the assessment and promotion of physical activity into clinical practice

Physical activity assessment is a priority during all patient visits, particularly those at high risk for or diagnosed with one or more chronic disease. The two central questions include:
  "On average, how many days per week do you engage in moderate or greater intensity physical activity (such as a brisk walk)?"
  "On average, how many minutes do you engage in this physical activity on those days?"
If responses to the questions above indicate the individual is below the recommended U.S. PA guideline recommendation of 150 min/ week, individuals should be advised of the health benefits of regular PA and encouraged to gradually increase either their frequency or duration of activity.
Wearable devices or smartphones can objectively assess physical activity levels. Self-tracking is helpful to some individuals to increase their physical activity levels in the short term. A more structured promotion/referral/behavior change plan is needed for the maintenance of effects.
As recommended by the US guidelines for Americans, a comprehensive assessment of physical activity should include engaging in muscle-strengthening, resistance, and flexibility exercises for major muscle groups at least twice a week. The following question can be used:
  "How many days a week do you perform muscle-strengthening exercises, such as body weight exercises or resistance training?"
Behavior change is a dynamic phenomenon; attempting to change unhealthy behaviors often entails a series of states. Identifying behavioral readiness should tailor the PA counseling.
In addition to behavioral readiness, assessment of physical readiness for exercise constitutes an important step for physical activity promotion. The deleterious health effects of inactivity far outweigh the risks of adverse events triggered by exercise. Following a pre-exercise screening protocol can reduce these risks and build trust between the healthcare professional and the patient.

See Ref. [39]

weight, body mass index, blood pressure, heart rate, oxygen saturation, and heart rhythm (via ECG). Nutrition, weight, and body composition are also evaluated and the EP then develops a multifaceted plan for improvement. All members of the lifestyle medicine team have had formal education in nutrition and attend appropriate lectures regarding current clinical guidelines. Nutrition assessment and education may be augmented by an intervention with a registered dietitian nutritionist.

Psychological Assessment

"Activation for change" is vital for patient engagement and success. The concept of "readiness to learn" involves three main features: emotional status, cognition, and motivation level. The EP is trained in motivational interviewing to understand and assist patients in reaching maximal health outcomes. The EP also provides ongoing education and counseling on topics, such as nutrition, smoking cessation, risk factor modification, and psychosocial counseling to help lower perceived levels of anxiety and stress.

Psychosocial assessment and intervention is an integral part of the lifestyle medicine plan. All HCPs participating in

Table 17.3a Individualized treatment plan for exercise for a medical fitness program

<table>
<tr>
<th colspan="3">Assessment/Plan
Date: ____________ Time:________ Initi.____________</th>
<th>Re-Assessment
Date:______ Time:____
Initial:______________</th>
<th>Re-Assessment
Date:______ Time:____
Initial:______________</th>
</tr>
<tr>
<td rowspan="3">EXERCISE (Required)</td>
<td rowspan="3">□ Sedentary Lifestyle as a Risk Factor
□ Not a Risk Factor at This Time – engages in regular exercise
□ Low activity tolerance
□ ADL difficulty
□ Sedentary or <150 min/week
□ Angina with Exercise
□ O2 Support ________L/min
□ unfamiliar w/ exercise equip.
<u>Initial Exercise Level</u>
DASI Calculated METs: _____
1st Ex MET Range: _________
Recommended Initial Exercise Prescription
<u>Frequency:</u>
Attend CR _____ days/week
For _______ weeks
<u>Intensity</u>
RPE 11-14
□ 40-80% DASI
□ THR based on Karvonen formula or Duke Activity Status Index
<u>OR</u>
□ RHR +20-30 bpm
□ RHR +10-20 bpm
<u>Mode:</u>
□ Treadmill (TM)
□ Upright Bike
□ Recumbent Bike
□ Rec. Elliptical
□ Upright Elliptical
□ Recumbent Stepper
□ Arm Ergometer
□ Hand Weights
□ Cybex Weight Machines
□ Stability/Flexibility/Balance Exercise
<u>Duration:</u>
• 5-10 min warm-up
• 5-10 min aerobic conditioning or as tolerated on 2-3 different pieces of equip
• 5-10 min cool-down
<u>Progression:</u>
Exercise workloads will be progressed gradually within the limits of the patients ability. In the absence of clinical symptoms and problems the following guidelines will be used: <u>Increase intensity at 0.2-2.0 METs every 1-3 weeks dependent on RPE/HR response to a goal of __________ Mets, as tolerated.</u></td>
<td>Plan
Goals/Intervention/Edu
□ Attend Cardiac Rehab 2-3days/week
□ Increase aerobic duration 2-5 min per session as tolerated to goal of 30-40 minutes total
□ Increase METs: 0.2-2.0 METs every 1-3 weeks until MET goal achieved
□ Orient to exercise equip
□ Resistance train 2-3 days/week
□ Core/Balance Training
□ Return to work/lifestyle
□ Exercise Coaching/educ
□ Review home exercise guidelines
□ Initiate home exercise
□ Continue w/home Exercise
□ Self-monitoring (HR, RPE, progression)</td>
<td><u>Current Exercise Prescription</u>
Mode:____________________
Attendance: ________ times/wk
Time: _________ mins.
Current MET Level: _________
RPE 11-14
□ Weight Training : ________ lbs
□ Core/Balance Training
<u>Progression over next 30 days:</u>
(Complete @ least 2 of Following)
Increase of : ________ minutes
______MPH ______ % Grade
______RPMS _____WATTS
______Resistance Level on…
____
To achieve/maintain THR, RPE of 11-14 and MET goal _________
Home exercise: Y N
Mode: __________________
Freq: _______ times/week
Time: _______ minutes
Notes: ________________</td>
<td><u>Current Exercise Prescription</u>
Mode:____________________
Attendance: ________ times/wk
Time: _________ mins.
Current MET Level: _________
RPE 11-14
□ Weight Training : ________ lbs
□ Core/Balance Training
<u>Progression over next 30 days:</u>
(Complete @ least 2 of Following)
Increase of : ________ minutes
______MPH ______ % Grade
______RPMS _____WATTS
______Resistance Level on…
____
To achieve/maintain THR, RPE of 11-14 and MET goal _________
Home exercise: Y N
Mode: __________________
Freq: _______ times/week
Time: _______ minutes
Notes: ________________</td>
</tr>
<tr>
<td>Re-Assessment
Date:______Time:____
Initial:______________</td>
<td colspan="2">Discharge Assessment
And Long-term Goals (LTG)
Date:_________ Time:_________ Init:_________</td>
</tr>
<tr>
<td><u>Current Exercise Prescription</u>
Mode:____________________
Attendance: ________ times/wk
Time: _________ mins.
Current METLevel: _________
RPE 11-14
□ Weight Training : ________ lbs
□ Core/Balance Training
<u>Progression over next 30 days:</u>
(Complete @ least 2 of Following)
Increase of : ________ minutes
______MPH ______ % Grade
______RPMS _____WATTS
______Resistance Level on…
____
To achieve/maintain THR, RPE of 11-14 and MET goal _________
Home exercise: Y N
Mode: __________________
Freq: _______ times/week
Time: _______ minutes
Notes: ________________</td>
<td colspan="2"><u>LTG:</u> >150 minutes moderate exercise/week, MET level >6.0 (or as appropriate for patient), resistance training 2-3 days/week, return to work and/or lifestyle activities
Entry DASI METs: ______ Exit DASI METs: ______
Entry/Exit DASI MET% Change: _______
Peak <u>Exercise Session</u> METs on DC_________
Peak <u>Exercise Session</u> METs % Change _________
Min of Exercise: ______________
□ Resistance training 2-3 days/week
□ Returned to work
□ Returned to Lifestyle/Activities
□ Exercise >150 minutes/week
□ Self-Monitoring Exercise
□ Enrolled in maintenance program or local gym
□ Progress
□ No Progress
□ Met Goals
Discharge Exercise Plan: ______________
Mode: ________________________
Fre:_______times/week Time: ______ min</td>
</tr>
</table>

Example of individualized exercise treatment plan adapted for Cardiac Rehab and Medical Fitness Program sources: Ascension Seton Hospital Medical Center Cardiac Rehabilitation Program, Salim B. Street and Catherine Spranger, Kyle, Texas and Marie-Josee and Henry Kravis Center for Cardiovascular Health at Mount Sinai, New York, NY

Table 17.3b Individualized treatment plan for nutrition for a medical fitness program

	Assessment/Plan		Re-Assessment	Re-Assessment
	Date: _____ **Time:** _____ **Initi.** _____		**Date:** _____ **Time:** ____ **Initial:** _____	**Date:** _____ **Time:** ____ **Initial:** _____

<table>
<tr>
<td rowspan="4">NUTRITION (Required)</td>
<td>

☐Nutrition as a Risk Factor
☐Not a Risk Factor at This Time – *maintenance of heart healthy diet encouraged*

☐ Rate Your Plate Score
   < 54 Score: _____
      Diet high in sodium?
        ☐ Yes ☐ No
     Eats out routinely/freq'ly?
        ☐ Yes ☐ No
☐ Caffeine Consumption
   Yes / No
   Amount: _____
☐ Alcohol Consumption
   Yes / No
   Amount: _____

</td>
<td>

Plan Goals/Intervention/Edu
☐ Maintain current diet habits
☐ Heart Healthy Diet
☐ ↓ Portion size (wt mgmt)
☐ Diabetic Diet
☐ Decrease Sodium Intake
☐ Practice heart healthy restaurant eating
☐ Decrease/eliminate caffeien
☐ Decrease/eliminate alcohol
☐ Recommend 1:1 dietary consult
☐ Participate in Nutrition coaching/educ classes
☐ Patient specific nutrition goals

(See Patient Specific "SMART" Goals)

</td>
<td>

Pt follows diet recommendations

☐ Heart Healthy ☐ Diabetic

☐ ↓ Portion Size ☐ ↓Salt/fluid

☐ ↓ Caffeine   ☐ ↓ Alcohol

Current
Dietician Consult Completed
☐Yes ☐ No ☐ N/A

Staff/Patient Coaching
☐Yes ☐ No

☐ **Progressing**
☐ **Not Progressing**
☐ **Meeting Goals**
Notes: _____
_____
_____
_____

</td>
<td>

Pt follows diet recommendations

☐ Heart Healthy ☐ Diabetic

☐ ↓ Portion Size ☐ ↓Salt/fluid

☐ ↓ Caffeine   ☐ ↓ Alcohol

Current
Dietician Consult Completed
☐Yes ☐ No ☐ N/A

Staff/Patient Coaching
☐Yes ☐ No

☐ **Progressing**
☐ **Not Progressing**
☐ **Meeting Goals**
Notes: _____
_____
_____
_____

</td>
</tr>
<tr>
<td colspan="2">

Re-Assessment
Date: _____ **Time:** ____
Initial: _____

</td>
<td colspan="2">

Discharge Assessment
And Long-term Goals (LTG)
Date: _____ **Time:** _____ **Init:** _____

</td>
</tr>
<tr>
<td colspan="2">

Pt follows diet recommendations

☐ Heart Healthy ☐ Diabetic

☐ ↓ Portion Size ☐ ↓Salt/fluid

☐ ↓ Caffeine   ☐ ↓ Alcohol

Current
Dietician Consult Completed
☐ Yes ☐ No ☐ N/A

Staff/Patient Coaching
☐ Yes ☐ No

☐ **Progressing**
☐ **Not Progressing**
☐ **Meeting Goals**
Notes: _____
_____
_____
_____

</td>
<td colspan="2">

LTG: Rate your plate score >55. **Patient able to verbalize understanding of life-long adherence to Heart Healthy Diet and/or Diabetic, low sodium/fluid restriction diet as appropriate for individual patient.** Decrease/eliminate caffeine and/or alcohol from diet.

Discharge

Rate Your Plate score: _____ (>55)
☐ **Progress**
☐ **No Progress**
☐ **Met Goals**

Notes: _____
_____
_____
_____
_____

</td>
</tr>
</table>

Example of individualized exercise treatment plan adapted for Cardiac Rehab and Medical Fitness Program sources: Ascension Seton Hospital Medical Center Cardiac Rehabilitation Program, Salim B. Street and Catherine Spranger, Kyle, Texas and Marie-Josee and Henry Kravis Center for Cardiovascular Health at Mount Sinai, New York, NY

Table 17.3c Individualized treatment plan for weight management for a medical fitness program

Assessment/Plan Date:_____ Time:_____ Initi._____		Re-Assessment Date:_____ Time:____ Initial:_____	Re-Assessment Date:_____ Time:____ Initial:_____
□ **Weight Management Risk Factor** □ **Not a Risk Factor at This Time** □ BMI >30 (Obesity) □ Waist Circumference **Men** >40 inches **Women** >35 inches □ Sedentary or <150 min/week □ Angina with Exercise □ O2 Supp. _____ L/min □ Unfamiliar w/ex. Equip. **Initial** Height: _____ in Weight: _____ lbs BMI: _____ Waist: _____ in *Healthy Weight Range per BMI table:* _____	**Plan Goals/Intervention/Edu** □ Heart Healthy Diet □ Weight Loss 0.5-2lb/wk □ Understanding Your Healthy weight range and BMI □ Recommend 1:1 dietary consult □ Participate in Weight Management/ Nutrition coaching □ Set Goal Weight of _____ lbs by end of program □ Exercise >300 min/wk □ Weight Gain (as appropriate for individual patient)	Pt follows diet recommendations □ Heart Healthy □ Diabetic □ ↓ Portion Size □ ↓Salt/fluid **Current** Weight: _____ BMI: _____ Dietician Consult Completed □ Yes □ No □ N/A Staff/Patient Coaching □ Yes □ No □ **Progressing** □ **Not Progressing** □ **Meeting Goals** Notes: _____	Pt follows diet recommendations □ Heart Healthy □ Diabetic □ ↓ Portion Size □ ↓Salt/fluid **Current** Weight: _____ BMI: _____ Dietician Consult Completed □ Yes □ No □ N/A Staff/Patient Coaching □ Yes □ No □ **Progressing** □ **Not Progressing** □ **Meeting Goals** Notes: _____

CORE COMPONENTS- WEIGHT MANAGEMENT

Re-Assessment Date:_____ Time:____ Initial:_____	Discharge Assessment And Long-term Goals (LTG) Date:_____ Time:_____ Init:_____
Pt follows diet recommendations □ Heart Healthy □ Diabetic □ ↓ Portion Size □ ↓Salt/fluid **Current** Weight: _____ BMI: _____ Dietician Consult Completed □ Yes □ No □ N/A Staff/Patient Coaching □ Yes □ No □ **Progressing** □ **Not Progressing** □ **Meeting Goals** Notes: _____	**LTG:** BMI <25, waist circumference <35 inches for women or <40 inches for men, 0.5-2lbs/week weight loss until targeted optimal body weight achieved, following heart healthy diet, exercising >300 minutes/week. **Discharge** Weight: _____ BMI: _____ Waist: _____ in Total Weight Loss: _____ Minutes of exercise/week: _____ □ **Progress** □ **No Progress** □ **Met Goals** □ Referred to weight control support group **Notes:** _____

Example of individualized exercise treatment plan adapted for Cardiac Rehab and Medical Fitness Program sources: Ascension Seton Hospital Medical Center Cardiac Rehabilitation Program, Salim B. Street and Catherine Spranger, Kyle, Texas and Marie-Josee and Henry Kravis Center for Cardiovascular Health at Mount Sinai, New York, NY

Table 17.3d Individualized treatment plan for tobacco cessation for a medical fitness program

CORE COMPONENTS – TOBACCO USE	Assessment/Plan Date: _____ Time: _____ Initi. _____		Re-Assessment Date: _____ Time: ____ Initial: _____	Re-Assessment Date: _____ Time: ____ Initial: _____

	□Tobacco Use Risk Factor
	□Not a Risk Factor at This Time – (as evidenced by…)
	
	□ Current Smoker
	  • Cigarettes
	  • E-cigarettes
	  • Cigar/Pipe
	  • Hookah
	□ Smoked within the previous 6 mo.
	□ Exposed to second-hand smoke
	□ Recreational Drug Use
	
	Quit Date: _____
	
	Pack(s)/Day: _____
	
	Years Smoking: _____
		Plan
		Goals/Intervention/Edu
		□ Effects of tobacco/smoking-risks of continued behavior
		□ Attend Smoking cessation counseling
		□ Set Quit Date
		_____
		□ Eliminate/Reduce tobacco to _____/day
		□ Refer to MD for medical management
		□ Avoid second-hand smoke
		□ Reduce/eliminate recreational drug use
			Tobacco Use: □ Yes □ No
			
			Amount of tobacco per day:
			_____
			
			□ New Quit Date:
			_____
			
			Staff/Patient Coaching
			□ Yes □ No
			
			□ **Progressing**
			□ **Not Progressing**
			□ **Meeting Goals**
			
			Notes: _____
			_____
			_____
			_____
			_____
				Tobacco Use: □ Yes □ No
				
				Amount of tobacco per day:
				_____
				
				□ New Quit Date:
				_____
				
				Staff/Patient Coaching
				□ Yes □ No
				
				□ **Progressing**
				□ **Not Progressing**
				□ **Meeting Goals**
				
				Notes: _____
				_____
				_____
				_____
				_____

	□ Has someone to help them quit □ Using medication to quit □ 3rd hand smoke □ Smokeless tobacco	**Re-Assessment** Date: _____ Time: ____ Initial: _____ **Tobacco Use:** □ Yes □ No Amount of tobacco per day: _____ □ New Quit Date: _____ Staff/Patient Coaching □ Yes □ No □ **Progressing** □ **Not Progressing** □ **Meeting Goals** Notes: _____ _____ _____ _____ _____	**Discharge Assessment** **And Long-term Goals (LTG)** Date: _____ Time: _____ Init: _____ **LTG:** Complete Smoking Cessation and Avoidance of 2nd hand smoke □ Completely Smoke-Free □ On Smoking Cessation Medication □ Smoking Cessation Resources Given/attended counseling/classes Tobacco use reduced to: _____ pack(s)/day □ **Progress** □ **No Progress** □ **Met Goals** Notes: _____ _____ _____ _____ _____ _____	

Example of individualized exercise treatment plan adapted for Cardiac Rehab and Medical Fitness Program sources: Ascension Seton Hospital Medical Center Cardiac Rehabilitation Program, Salim B. Street and Catherine Spranger, Kyle, Texas and Marie-Josee and Henry Kravis Center for Cardiovascular Health at Mount Sinai, New York, NY

Table 17.3e Individualized treatment plan for psychosocial factors for a medical fitness program

		Assessment/Plan Date: _____ Time: _____ Initi. _____	**Plan**	**Re-Assessment** Date: _____ Time: ____ Initial: _____	**Re-Assessment** Date: _____ Time: ____ Initial: _____
PSYCHOSOCIAL *(Required)*		☐ Psychosocial Risk Factor ☐ Not a Risk Factor at This Time – maintenance of healthy psychosocial wellbeing encouraged ☐ Poor Coping skills ☐ Stress/Anxiety per pt. repor Low / Med / High ☐ Abnormal sleep patterns ☐ Currently seeing counselor/physician ☐ On Psychotropic Medication ☐ S/Sx of depression ☐ Ferrans & Powers QOL Score _____ Ferrans & Powers <u>Total QOL Reference Mean Score 23</u> (SD 4.04)	**Plan** **Goals/Intervention/Edu** ☐ Maintain current psych/social wellbeing ☐ Discuss Psychosocial impacts on health ☐ Participate in Psychosocial Coaching ☐ Mental Health referral as needed ☐ Teach & support self-help strategies ☐ Increase/Resume social functioning ☐ Return to work ☐ Improve Ferrans & Powers Score ☐ Importance of adequate sleep ☐ Sleep study referral	***Improved Quality of Life*** Demonstrates responsibility for health-related behavior change/maintenance ☐ Yes ☐ No Stress /Anxiety per pt. report improving? ☐ Yes ☐ No ☐ N/A Depression Symptoms Improving? ☐ Yes ☐ No ☐ N/A Ferrans & Powers score: _____ Sleep Issues improving? ☐ Yes ☐ No ☐ N/A Staff / Patient Coaching ☐ Yes ☐ No ☐ N/A ☐ Progressing ☐ Not Progressing ☐ Meeting Goals Notes: _____ _____ _____	***Improved Quality of Life*** Demonstrates responsibility for health-related behavior change/maintenance ☐ Yes ☐ No Stress /Anxiety per pt. report improving? ☐ Yes ☐ No ☐ N/A Depression Symptoms Improving? ☐ Yes ☐ No ☐ N/A Ferrans & Powers score: _____ Sleep Issues improving? ☐ Yes ☐ No ☐ N/A Staff / Patient Coaching ☐ Yes ☐ No ☐ N/A ☐ Progressing ☐ Not Progressing ☐ Meeting Goals Notes: _____ _____ _____
		Ferrans & Powers <u>Subscales</u> **Health/Function** _____ *(Avg sc 23.10)* (SD 4.47) **Social & Economic** _____ *(Avg sc 21.83)* (SD 4.11) **Psychological/Spiritual** _____ *(Avg sc 22.95)* (SD 5.21) **Family** _____ *(Avg sc 25.60)* (SD 4.49) *Lowest of scores to be focus of Plan- goals/interventions/educ*	**Re-Assessment** Date: _____ Time: ____ Initial: _____ ***Improved Quality of Life*** Demonstrates responsibility for health-related behavior change/maintenance ☐ Yes ☐ No Stress /Anxiety per pt. report improving? ☐ Yes ☐ No ☐ N/A Depression Symptoms Improving? ☐ Yes ☐ No ☐ N/A Ferrans & Powers score: _____ Sleep Issues improving? ☐ Yes ☐ No ☐ N/A Staff / Patient Coaching ☐ Yes ☐ No ☐ N/A ☐ Progressing ☐ Not Progressing ☐ Meeting Goals Notes: _____ _____ _____	**Discharge Assessment** **And Long-term Goals (LTG)** Date: _____ Time: _____ Init: _____ **LTG:** Use relaxation techniques when stressors identified, verbalized resources available for depressions and/or stress, and maximize coping skills. Decrease vulnerability to stress. Improved QOL scores. Maintains healthy psychosocial wellbeing. **Final Ferrans & Powers Score:** Health/Function: _____ Social & Economic: _____ Psychological/Spiritual : _____ Family: _____ ☐ **Health-Related Behavior Change** ☐ **Improved Stress Management Skills** ☐ **Mental Health Referral Completed (if needed)** ☐ **Sleep Study Referral Completed (if needed)** ☐ **Progress** ☐ **No Progress** ☐ **Met Goals** Notes: _____ _____ _____ _____ _____ _____	

Example of individualized exercise treatment plan adapted for Cardiac Rehab and Medical Fitness Program sources: Ascension Seton Hospital Medical Center Cardiac Rehabilitation Program, Salim B. Street and Catherine Spranger, Kyle, Texas and Marie-Josee and Henry Kravis Center for Cardiovascular Health at Mount Sinai, New York, NY

an outpatient Lifestyle Medicine Center are trained in motivational interviewing as well as in the administration and scoring of specific inventories to assess depression, including the Beck Depression Inventory and the Patient Health Questionnaire [36, 37]. By using tools such as the Ferrans and Powers Quality of Life Index [38], the EP can identify areas in a patient's life that require closer attention. In some cases, patients can be referred to other specialists that provide cognitive-behavioral therapy.

Exercise Assessment

Although exercise is considered an important component of a healthy lifestyle, the US adults spend >7 h per day in sedentary activities (Fig. 17.1). National guidelines on health promotion recommend that adults should be counseled to optimize a physically active lifestyle (Tables 17.4 and 17.5). In addition to recommendations for aerobic exercise, components of exercise prescriptions include recommendations for muscular strength and flexibility (Tables 17.6a and 17.6b). Exercise prescriptions are developed using protocols set by ACSM and AACVPR guidelines. During a patient's exercise therapy session, EPs follow strict guidelines to precisely titrate the patient's intensities. For instance, EPs are constantly adjusting and monitoring the metabolic equivalent of task (MET) with exercise in the context of a patient's impaired cardiovascular system. Cycle ergometer wattage is adjusted, as well as treadmill speeds and inclines. This is done to ensure that the patient stays within safe exercising parameters. Similarly, in cardiac rehabilitation programs, EKG telemetry monitoring

Table 17.4 Recommendations for exercise and physical activity

COR	LOE	Recommendations
I	B-R	1. Adults should be routinely counseled in healthcare visits to optimize a physically active lifestyle [40, 41]
I	B-NR	2. Adults should engage in at least 150 min per week of accumulated moderate-intensity or 75 min per week of vigorous-intensity aerobic physical activity (or an equivalent combination of moderate and vigorous activity) to reduce ASCVD [42–47]
IIa	B-NR	3. For adults unable to meet the minimum physical activity recommendations (at least 150 min per week of accumulated moderate-intensity or 75 min per week of vigorous-intensity aerobic physical activity), engaging in some moderate- or vigorous-intensity physical activity, even if less than this recommended amount, can be beneficial to reduce ASCVD risk [44, 45]
IIb	C-LD	4. Decreasing sedentary behavior in adults may be reasonable to reduce ASCVD risk [42, 48–50]

See Ref. [6]

Abbreviations: *ASCVD* atherosclerotic cardiovascular disease, *COR* class of recommendation, *LOE* level of evidence, *NR* non-randomized, *LD* limited data

Table 17.5 Definitions and examples of different intensities of physical activity[a]

Intensity	METs	Examples
Sedentary behavior	1–1.5	Sitting, reclining, or lying; e.g., watching television
Light	1.6–2.9	Walking slowly, cooking, or light housework
Moderate	3.0–5.9	Brisk walking (2.4–4 mph), biking (5–9 mph), or recreational swimming
Vigorous	≥6	Jogging/running, biking (≥10 mph), singles tennis, or swimming laps

See Ref. [6]

Abbreviations: *MET* metabolic equivalents, *mph* miles per hour
[a]Sedentary behavior is defined as any waking behavior characterized by an energy expenditure ≥1.5 METs while in a sitting, reclining, or lying posture. Standing is a sedentary activity in that it involves ≤1.5 METs, but it is not considered a component of sedentary behavior

Hours Per Day Spent in Various States of Activity

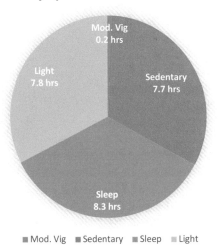

■ Mod. Vig ■ Sedentary ■ Sleep ■ Light

Fig. 17.1 Intensities of physical activity. The US adults spend >7 h/day on average in sedentary activities. Replacing sedentary time with other physical activity involves increasing either moderate- to vigorous-intensity physical activity or light-intensity physical activity. (Data modified from Young et al. [53])

allows the EP to view the patient's rhythm during exercise. This allows the EP to keep the patient's heart rate within their exercising ranges. Moreover, EPs are specifically trained in ECG interpretation to identify any abnormal rhythms that may be present during strenuous activities. In addition, EPs also use patients' subjective assessments, such as the Borg Rate of Perceived Exertion (RPE), that gauge effort levels (Table 17.7). Using objective and subjective data guarantees that patients are working within sustainable levels for the best possible outcomes. In some situations, the EP adjusts treatment plans using clinical judgment to change the course or plan of care that provides the best opportunities for optimal outcomes. Individualized exercise prescriptions follow the FITT principle – Frequency, Intensity, Time, and Type – and include the following components:

Table 17.6a Components of an exercise prescription for muscular strength and endurance for cardiac patients

Component	Recommendation
Intensity	Resistance that allows ~10–15 repetitions without significant fatigue RPE of 11–13 on Borg 6–20 scale Complete movement through as full a range of motion as possible, avoiding breath holding and straining (Valsalva maneuver) by exhaling during the exertion phase of the motion and inhaling during the recovery phase Maintain a secure but not overly tight grip on the weight handles or bar to prevent an excessive BP response RPP should not exceed that identified as threshold for CRE exercise
Volume	Minimum of one set per exercise May increase to two or three sets once accustomed to the regimen and, if greater gains are desired, ~8–10 different exercises using all major muscle groups of the upper and lower body: chest press, shoulder press, triceps extension, bicep curls, lat (latissimus dorsi) pull-down, lower back extension, abdominal crunch or curl-up, quadriceps extension, leg curls (hamstrings), and calf raise
Frequency	2 or 3 nonconsecutive days/week
Type	Variable: free weights, weight machines, resistance bands, pulley weights, dumbbells, and light wrist or ankle weights Select equipment that is safe, effective, and accessible
Progression	Training loads may be increased by ~5% when the patient can comfortably achieve the upper limit of the prescribed repetition range

See Ref. [51]

Abbreviations: *RPE* rating of perceived exertion, *BP* blood pressure, *RPP* rate pressure product = Heart *rate* × systolic blood *pressure*, *CRE* cardiorespiratory endurance

Table 17.6b Components of an exercise prescription for musculoskeletal flexibility

Component	Recommendation
Intensity	Hold to a position of mild discomfort (not pain) Exercises should be performed in a slow, controlled manner, with a gradual progression to greater ranges of motion
Duration	Gradually increase to 30 s, then as tolerable to 90 s for each stretch; breathing normally 3–5 repetitions for each exercise
Frequency	2 or 3 nonconsecutive days/week
Type	Static, with a major emphasis on the lower back and thigh regions

See Ref. [51]

1. Type of exercise activity (walking, rowing, and cycling)
2. Specific workloads (walking speed and watts)
3. Duration and frequency of activity
4. Intensity guidelines based on target hemodynamics (heart rate and blood pressure), as well as estimated Borg RPE
5. Precautions due to other comorbid conditions (balance, orthopedic limitations, etc.)

Table 17.7 Rating of perceived exertion

Borg's scale	Modified Borg scale
6 –	0 – At rest
7 – Very, very light	
8 –	1 – Very easy
9 – Very light	2 – Somewhat easy
10 –	
11 – Fairly light	3 – Moderate
12 –	4 – Somewhat hard
13 – Somewhat hard	5 – Hard
15 – Hard	6 –
16 –	7 – Very hard
17 – Very hard	8 –
18 –	
19 –Very, very hard	9 –
20 –	10 – Very, very hard

See Ref. [52]

In addition to exercise prescriptions, a comprehensive medical fitness program ideally models the individualized treatment plan used in AACVPR programs. The plan includes diagnosis, type, frequency, duration of services to be rendered, and goals set for individual patients. Relative determinants for progression of activity incorporate information from initial assessment, physical assessment, and response to previous activity. Symptoms such as dyspnea, chest pain, lightheadedness, and diaphoresis are important variables to determine the need for termination of activity. Examples of symptom assessments according to the AACVPR include the Borg RPE. In addition, scores targeting different systems include the following:

- Dyspnea assessment utilizes a 5-point scale (0: no dyspnea, 1: mild/noticeable, 2: mild/some difficulty, 3: moderate difficulty, 4: severe/cannot continue).
- Angina assessment utilizes 5-point scale (0: no angina, 1: light, 2: moderate/bothersome, 3: severe, 4: worse pain ever experienced).
- Claudication pain scale utilizes 5-point scale (0: no pain, 1: minimal pain, 2 moderate pain, 3 intense pain, 4: maximal pain).

Impact of the Exercise Physiologist

The EP demonstrates an understanding of anatomy and physiology, giving them the conceptual basis for applying biomechanics and the human kinetic chain (the action and response of overlapping segmental joints throughout the human body during muscle activation). The EP is able to provide corrective exercise programs for patients with impaired movement patterns and/or chronic muscular dysfunctions. The EP communicates periodic updates on patients' progress through clinical outcomes reports and multi-session reviews. Under the supervision and guidance of practicing physicians, EPs coordinate and manage patient care throughout their therapeutic journey. Wellness programs that specialize in treating multiple physical disabilities utilize the expertise of the EP to reduce the impact of chronic pain and debilitation. Currently, EPs are not required to obtain a license to participate in patient care. However, EPs are encouraged to become certified through national governing bodies and are therefore highly valued participants in the lifestyle medicine care team.

Conclusion

The collaborative effort of multidisciplinary teams in lifestyle management programs drives practical and sustainable solutions to improve health for our society. One cannot fathom such impact created by a single person or entity, but rather by a cohesive team. Specifically, the impact of the EP within this care model can be viewed as a structural component that brings all aspects of care related to physical activity to the hands of the patient. By extension, a culture of active participation in healthcare results, empowering and motivating patients to tackle any health adversity that faces them. Above all, the communication between physician and EP is integral to the success of this team, particularly within a Lifestyle Medicine Center and Clinical Service Line. The EP is a great resource for physicians in tracking patients' health status with preventive care strategies. Exercise physiologists are HCPs who promote life-long optimum health and fitness and promote effective rehabilitative services. In addition to providing clinical interventions, EPs may advance the field of exercise physiology through critical thinking and research. There is a promising future for EPs as they ultimately impact the general public in providing and developing preventive exercise training strategies to reduce the burden of chronic disease. Indeed, EPs bridge the gap between scientific research and implementation of healthy lifestyles.

References

1. Benjamin RM. The national prevention strategy: shifting the nation's health care system. Public Health Rep. 2011;126:774–6.
2. Berryman JW. Exercise and the medical tradition from Hippocrates through antebellum America: a review essay. In: Berryman JW, Park RJ, editors. Sport and exercise sciences: essays in the history of sport medicine. Urbana: University of Illinois; 1992. p. 1–57.
3. Tipton CM. The history of "Exercise Is Medicine" in ancient civilizations. Adv Physiol Educ. 2014;38:109–17.
4. Tipton CM, editor. History of exercise physiology. Champaign: Human Kinetics; 2014.
5. Tipton CM. Contemporary exercise physiology: fifty years after the closure of Harvard fatigue laboratory. Exerc Sport Sci Rev. 1998;26:315–39.
6. Arnett DK, Blumenthal RS, Albert MA, et al. 2019 ACC/AHA guidelines on the primary prevention of cardiovascular disease: executive summary. J Am Coll Cardiol. 2019;74:1376–414.
7. Jonas S, Phillips EM. ACSM's exercise is medicine: a Clinician's guide to exercise prescription. Philadelphia: Lippincott, Williams & Wilkins; 2009.
8. U.S. Bureau of Labor Statistics Office of Occupational Statistics and Employment Projections. Exercise physiologists. https://www.bls.gov/ooh/healthcare/mobile/exercise-physiologists.htm. Accessed on 17 Mar 2020.
9. World Health Organization. Global recommendations on physical activity for health. Geneva: WHO; 2010.
10. Booth FW, Roberts CK, Laye MJ. Lack of exercise is a major cause of chronic diseases. Compr Physiol. 2012;2:1143–21.
11. Zores F, Iliou MC, Gellen B, et al. Physical activity for patients with heart failure: position paper from the heart failure (GICC) and cardiac rehabilitation (GERS-P) Working Groups of the French Society of Cardiology. Arch Cardiovasc Dis. 2019;112:723–31.
12. Moholdt T, Lavie CJ, Nauman J. Sustained physical activity, not weight loss, associated with improved survival in coronary heart disease. J Am Coll Cardiol. 2018;71:1094–101.
13. Simmonds JV, Herbland A, Hakim A, et al. Exercise beliefs and behaviours of individuals with Joint Hypermobility Syndrome/Ehlers-Danlos Syndrome – hypermobility type. Disabil Rehabil. 2019;41:445–55.
14. Sharman JE, La Gerche A, Coombes JS. Exercise and cardiovascular risk in patient with hypertension. Am J Hypertens. 2015;28:147–58.
15. Treat-Jacobson D, McDermott MM, Bronas UG, et al. Optimal exercise programs for patients with peripheral artery disease: a scientific statement from the American Heart Association. Circulation. 2019:e10–33. https://doi.org/10.1161/CIR.0000000000000623.
16. Fu Q, VanGundy TB, Galbreath MM, et al. Cardiac origins of the postural orthostatic tachycardia syndrome. J Am Coll Cardiol. 2010;55:2858–68.
17. Peters HP, De Vries WR, Vanberge-Henegouwen GP, et al. Potential benefits and hazards of physical activity and exercise on the gastrointestinal tract. Gut. 2001;48:435–9.
18. Aldoori WH, Giovannucci EL, Rimm EB, et al. Prospective study of physical activity and the risk of symptomatic diverticular disease in men. Gut. 1995;36:276–82.
19. Wilund KR, Feeney LA, Tomayk EJ, et al. Endurance exercise training reduces gallstone development in mice. J Appl Physiol. 2008;104:761–5.
20. Molina-Molina E, Lunardi Baccetto R, Wang DG, et al. Exercising the hepatobiliary-gut axis. The impact of physical activity performance. Eur J Clin Invest. 2018;48:e12958.
21. Shaw KA, Gennat HC, O'Rourke P, et al. Exercise for overweight or obesity. Cochrane Database Syst Rev. 2006:CD003817. https://doi.org/10.1002/14651858.CD003817.pub3.
22. Nelson AE, Allen KD, Golightly YM, et al. A systematic review of recommendations and guidelines for the management of osteoarthritis: the chronic osteoarthritis management initiative of the U.S. bone and joint initiative. Semin Arthritis Rheum. 2014;43:701–12.
23. Sahni P, Nieves JW. Determining the effects of a 4-week structured strength and flexibility exercise program on functional status of subjects with osteoporosis. HSS J. 2019;15:241–6.
24. Erickson KI, Hillman C, Stillman CM, et al. Physical activity, cognition, and brain outcomes: a review of the 2019 physical activity guidelines. Med Sci Sports Exerc. 2019;51:1242–51.
25. Herring MP, O'Connor PJ, Dishman RK. The effects of exercise training on anxiety symptoms among patients: a systematic review. Arch Inter Med. 2010;170:321–31.
26. Guo LY, Lozinsky B, Yong VW. Exercise in multiple sclerosis and its models: focus on the central nervous system outcomes. J Neurosci Res. 2019;98:509–23.

27. Xu X, Fu Z, Le W. Exercise and Parkinson's disease. Int Rev Neurobiol. 2019;147:45–74.

28. Howard VJ, McDonnell MN. Physical activity in primary stroke prevention: just do it! Stroke. 2015;46:1735–9.

29. Patel AV, Friedenreich CM, Moore SC, et al. American College of Sports Medicine roundtable report on physical activity, sedentary behavior, and cancer prevention and control. Med Sci Sports Exerc. 2019;51:2391–402.

30. Boyle T, Keegel T, Bull F, et al. Physical activity and risks of proximal and distal colon cancers: a systematic review and meta-analysis. J Natl Cancer Inst. 2012;104:1548–61.

31. Kushi LH, Doyle C, McCullough M, et al. American Cancer Society guidelines on nutrition and physical activity for cancer prevention: reducing the risk of cancer with healthy food choices and physical activity. CA Cancer J Clin. 2012;62:30–67.

32. Lang JE. The impact of exercise on asthma. Curr Opin Allergy Clin Immunol. 2019;19:118–25.

33. Ifftikhar IH, Kline CE, Youngstedt SD. Effects of exercise training on sleep apnea: a meta-analysis. Lung. 2014;192:175–84.

34. Decision Memo for Cardiac Rehabilitation Programs (CAG-00089R). https://www.cms.gov/medicare-coverage-database/details/nca-decision-memo.aspx?NCAId=164&NcaName=Cardiac+Rehabilitation+Programs&DocID=CAG-00089R. Accessed on 17 Jan 2020.

35. Williams MA, Roitman JL. Guidelines for cardiac rehabilitation and secondary prevention programs. 5th ed: American Association of Cardiovascular and Pulmonary Rehabilitation. Champaign, IL: Human Kinetics; 2013.

36. Beck AT, Ward CH, Mendelson M, et al. An inventory for measuring depression. Arch Gen Psychiatry. 1961;4:561–71.

37. Kroenke K, Spitzer RL, Williams JB. The PHQ-9 validity of a brief depression severity measure. J Gen Intern Med. 2001;16:606–13.

38. Ferrans and Powers. Quality of life index: cardiac version. https://qli.org.uic.edu/questionaires/questionnairehome.htm. Accessed on 30 July 2019.

39. Lobelo F, Rohm Young D, Sallis R, et al. Routine assessment and promotion of physical activity in healthcare settings: a scientific statement from the American Heart Association. Circulation. 2018;137:e495–522.

40. Orrow G, Kinmonth AL, Sanderson S, et al. Effectiveness of physical activity promotion based in primary care: systematic review and meta-analysis of randomised controlled trials. BMJ. 2012;344:e1389.

41. Sanchez A, Bully P, Martinez C, et al. Effectiveness of physical activity promotion interventions in primary care: a review of reviews. Prev Med. 2015;76(suppl):S56–67.

42. Ekelund U, Steene-Johannessen J, Brown WJ, et al. Does physical activity attenuate, or even eliminate, the detrimental association of sitting time with mortality? A harmonised meta-analysis of data from more than 1 million men and women. Lancet. 2016;388:1302–10.

43. Hamer M, Chida Y. Walking and primary prevention: a meta-analysis of prospective cohort studies. Br J Sports Med. 2008;42:238–43.

44. Kyu HH, Bachman VF, Alexander LT, et al. Physical activity and risk of breast cancer, colon cancer, diabetes, ischemic heart disease, and ischemic stroke events: systematic review and dose-response meta-analysis for the Global Burden of Disease Study, 2013. BMJ. 2016;354:i3857.

45. Sattelmair J, Pertman J, Ding EL, et al. Dose response between physical activity and risk of coronary heart disease: a meta-analysis. Circulation. 2011;124:789–95.

46. Zheng H, Orsini N, Amin J, et al. Quantifying the dose-response of walking in reducing coronary heart disease risk: meta-analysis. Eur J Epidemiol. 2009;24:181–92.

47. Wahid A, Manek N, Nichols M, et al. Quantifying the association between physical activity and cardiovascular disease and diabetes: a systematic re-view and meta-analysis. J Am Heart Assoc. 2016;5:e002495.

48. Biswas A, Oh PI, Faulkner GE, et al. Sedentary time and its association with risk for disease incidence, mortality, and hospitalization in adults: a systematic review and meta-analysis. Ann Intern Med. 2015;162:123–32.

49. Chomistek AK, Manson JE, Stefanick ML, et al. Relationship of sedentary behavior and physical activity to incident cardiovascular disease: results from the Women's Health Initiative. J Am Coll Cardiol. 2013;61:2346–54.

50. Patterson R, McNamara E, Tainio M, et al. Sedentary behaviour and risk of all-cause, cardiovascular and cancer mortality, and incident type 2diabetes: a systematic review and dose response meta-analysis. Eur J Epidemiol. 2018;33:811–29.

51. Williams MA, Haskell WL, Ades PA, et al. Resistance exercise in individuals with and without cardiovascular disease: 2007update. A scientific statement from the American Heart Association Council on Clinical Cardiology and Council on Nutrition, Physical Activity, and Metabolism. Circulation. 2007;116:572–84.

52. Borg GA. Psychophysical bases of perceived exertion. Med Sci Sports Exerc. 1982;14:377–81.

53. Young DR, Hivert MF, Alhassan S, et al. Sedentary behavior and cardiovascular morbidity and mortality: a science advisory from the American Heart Association. Circulation. 2016;134:e262–79.

The Inpatient Lifestyle Medicine Consultation Service

18

Jeffrey I. Mechanick

Abbreviations

ABCD	Adiposity-based chronic disease
CMBCD	Cardiometabolic-based chronic disease
CR	Cardiac rehabilitation
CVD	Cardiovascular disease
DBCD	Dysglycemia-based chronic disease
HCP	Healthcare professional
RVU	Relative value unit

Introduction

Lifestyle medicine is the nonpharmacologic and nonprocedural management of chronic disease. Implicit in this definition, though not obvious, is the notion that individuals can have multiple chronic diseases, highlighting the need for concurrent prevention of chronic disease risk, progression, and complications. Lifestyle medicine is commonly regarded as an outpatient endeavor that focuses on primordial, primary, secondary, and tertiary prevention exclusively in non-acute settings. However, there is an emerging role for lifestyle medicine in the acute setting, with specific reference to inpatients who are a captive audience for interventions that can not only help treat the immediate problem but also prevent that problem from recurring, while also managing other chronic diseases (Table 18.1). Perhaps the first reference of this concept is by Turner et al. [1] in 1972, focusing attention on primary prevention of risk factors for heart disease to avert admissions to the coronary care unit. This concept was extended by a study by Thornley and Turner [2], where patients in the coro-

Table 18.1 Examples of concurrent prevention types for an inpatient lifestyle medicine consult[a]

Clinical target	Prevention type	Lifestyle intervention
Hyperosmolar hyperglycemia	Tertiary	Consistent carbohydrate diet for better glycemic control in the hospital
Acute hypertensive emergency	Tertiary	Stress reduction techniques, low-sodium diet
Type 2 diabetes	Secondary	Medical nutrition therapy; behaviors to improve medication adherence to prevent another episode related to diabetes complications
Postoperative, post-ICU CABG	Secondary	Dietary counseling by RDN, phase I cardiac rehabilitation[b], additional counseling by lifestyle medicine HCP on stress reduction, physical activity, sleep, alcohol moderation, tobacco cessation, etc.
Cardiovascular disease	Primary	In all patients, regardless of active inpatient problem list, to provide counseling on healthy eating to lose weight and improve glycemic status; physical activity ; behaviors to avoid tobacco product use; and other cardiometabolic risk factors
Cancer	Primary	In all patients, regardless of active inpatient problem list, to review routine cancer screening and risk factors, and then counsel regarding healthy eating, physical activity, tobacco cessation, stress reduction, etc.

Abbreviations: *CABG* coronary artery bypass grafting, *HCP* healthcare professional, *ICU* intensive care unit, *RDN* registered dietitian nutritionist

[a]Primordial prevention strategies can also be discussed and facilitated with the patient by providing a list of community and public services (e.g., walking paths in the park, nutrition facts label postings in restaurants, and educational lectures on health). Quaternary prevention strategies are exercised at all encounters to limit interventions to only those that are ethical, evidence-based, with net anticipated benefit, and within the patients established inpatient care plan

[b]Cardiac rehabilitation phase I is inpatient, whereas phases II and III are outpatient

J. I. Mechanick (✉)
The Marie-Josée and Henry R. Kravis Center for Cardiovascular Health at Mount Sinai Heart, and the Division of Endocrinology, Diabetes and Bone Disease, Icahn School of Medicine at Mount Sinai, New York, NY, USA
e-mail: jeffrey.mechanick@mountsinai.org

© Springer Nature Switzerland AG 2020
J. I. Mechanick, R. F. Kushner (eds.), *Creating a Lifestyle Medicine Center*, https://doi.org/10.1007/978-3-030-48088-2_18

nary care unit who have had a myocardial infarction had an earlier hospital discharge when there was rapid mobilization (by 2–4 days), compared with mobilization at 5 days or later, representing a form of secondary prevention.

This new imperative to integrate lifestyle medicine within standards of inpatient care is substantiated by the findings of Haynes [3]. Based on a questionnaire completed by recently discharged adult hospital patients (N = 190), over 80% agreed with screening for all chronic disease risk factors, with the majority of those with various risks wanting to change their behaviors [3]. However, only a third received health education, primarily on admission, though the majority wanted it upon discharge [3]. Overall, over 80% agreed that the hospital was an appropriate place to receive health education and that details of how this can be continued in the community should also be provided [3]. This paradigm of inpatient lifestyle medicine care can be viewed as a comprehensive approach and fits squarely in a strategy that optimizes population health in a cost-effective manner.

There are many challenges to building an inpatient lifestyle medicine program. For virtually all inpatient settings, this type of program is nascent and will therefore need to leverage many resources – both easy and hard to find – and then successfully integrate in a hospital environment with

demonstrable and durable clinical successes and fiscal responsibility. From a pragmatic standpoint, a series of discrete action steps in the development process can be followed. These action steps are designed to address specific and anticipated challenges derived from the experiences of others who have succeeded in creating inpatient lifestyle medicine programs (Table 18.2). Since the necessary resources vary based on objectives and unique hospital settings, human resources need to be considered at an early developmental stage (Table 18.3). In general, relatively long (weeks to months) dedicated inpatient lifestyle medicine programs, e.g., those that target weight loss, diabetes control, behavioral modification, or metabolic syndrome risk factor reduction, are not officially part of a hospital-based consultative service, though over time, they could be incorporated into a more mature, robust program.

As an example, there is a Lifestyle Medicine Inpatient Consultation Service currently operational and functioning as a clinical service line for a neurology rehabilitation stroke team, within a sponsoring organization (Loma Linda University Health System) [4]. Initiation of this inpatient lifestyle medicine service line required 2 years to plan, test, and develop and now operates half a day per week with a preventive medicine attending, two preventive medicine resi-

Table 18.2 Challenges and action steps to creating an inpatient lifestyle program∗

Program component	What is the challenge?	Action steps
Healthcare culture	Recalcitrant	1- Environmental scan: to collect data on chronic disease, readmission rates, epidemiology, urban infrastructure, and then develop needs assessment
		2- To formulate proposal and present to institutional stakeholders
		3- To include a formal strategic plan
		4- Once approved, to leverage implementation science to build a program and recruit human, physical, and technological resources
Education	Inadequate	5- To organize educational sessions for program leaders, healthcare professionals and staff, administration, and patients/families
Hospital infrastructure	Incomplete	6- To identify gaps in the existing infrastructure and present plans to close the gaps for the program to operate at acceptable levels
Economics	Necessity	7- Necessary for durability of the enterprise, notwithstanding startup and subsequent financial support from the sponsoring healthcare system, grants, and private donations
		8- Requires dedicated financial competency, accountability
		9- Requires a formal business plan incorporating all aspects of operations and strategy
Evidence	Limited	10- Additional environmental scanning, initially of external scientific data, and then internal (via registry, clinical trials, etc.) scientific data, for adaptation and sustainability
		11- Curate data and concepts for educational use and future interrogation/mining for program optimization, clinical trial design, research, and publications
Metrics	Ill-defined	12- Based on the scientific evidence, to generate a core set of clinical metrics individually for each patient and aggregated for the program's patient population over a specified time period
		13- Based on the scientific evidence, to generate an ancillary set of clinical metrics, many may be aspirational, that can be implemented *ad hoc* for individual patients, or over time for aggregated markers of performance
		14- To generate a set of economic endpoints to establish value designations, as well as indices of financial performance to guide strategic growth, marketing, and adaptation/optimization
Operations	Need for innovation	15- To develop a plan for location, human resources, equipment, and process based on the strategic and business plans
Resources	Variability	16- To generate a list based on strategic and business plans to generate a list of human and other resources that subserve the strategic, business, and operational plans of the program

Table 18.3 Human resources for development of an inpatient Lifestyle Medicine Clinical Service Line[a]

Development stage	Position	Description
Initial	Physician (MD or DO)	Team leader with a relevant specialization (e.g., preventive care, primary care, general internal medicine, nutrition, obesity, endocrinology); has training and experience in lifestyle medicine
Initial	Administrator	New or already working with the team leader; manages logistics, billing, and other support functions
Initial/subsequent	RN or APP	Works directly with the team leader and directly supervises other team members; has training and experience in various aspects of lifestyle medicine (e.g., nutrition, physical activity, and mind-body)
Subsequent	Dietitian (RN, RDN)	Focuses on nutritional and dietary components of care; coordinates with other team members to provide comprehensive lifestyle medicine care
Subsequent	Exercise physiologist or physical therapist	Focuses on physical activity; coordinates with other team members to provide comprehensive lifestyle medicine care
Subsequent	Behavioralist (MD, PhD, or MS/MA)	Focuses on promoting healthy behaviors in a wide range of areas; coordinates with other team members to provide comprehensive lifestyle medicine care
Subsequent	Research coordinator	Focuses on clinical studies with experience in aspects of lifestyle medicine, clinical trials, epidemiology, statistics, and/or primary writing for publication
Subsequent	Trainees	Medical students, residents, fellows, and visiting students, trainees, staff, and faculty

Abbreviations: *APP* Advanced Practice Provider (e.g., nurse practitioner or physician's assistant), *DO* Doctor of Osteopathic medicine, *MA* Masters of Arts, *MD* Medical Doctor (allopathic), *MS* Masters of Science, *PhD* Doctor of Philosophy, *RD* Registered Dietitian, *RDN* Registered Dietitian Nutritionist, *RN* Registered Nurse

[a]Subsequent additions to the clinical service line depend on the mission set by the team leader, specific needs of the hospital and sponsoring health system, and funding/resource constraints

dents, other visiting residents, and medical students [4]. The inpatient service coordinates with the outpatient clinic, which has five physicians and operates 5 days a week [5]. Salary lines for physicians in this inpatient service line are based on the resource-based relative value scale. This scale refers to three relative value unit (RVU) databases (work product, practice expense, and malpractice expense) that determine a reimbursement formula for Medicare. As of 2018, the inpatient service line generates RVUs that approximate a breakeven point; however, the main challenges that remain are building the referral base [4].

Services

Nutrition

Inpatient nutrition is a "teachable moment" that can be leveraged through education to improve clinical outcomes, both short- and long terms [6]. This applies to food options presented not only at the bedside but also in the cafeteria and various formats of food merchandising, such as kiosks, gift and snack shops, and vending machines [6]. Incorporating farmers' market models both inside and outside the hospital facility can accentuate the healthy eating messaging to patients, families, employees, and host of other people navigating around the premises.

As a rule, every hospitalized patient receives a routine nutritional assessment on admission with mandated regular follow-up typically performed by a dietitian (registered dietitian or registered dietitian nutritionist). In patients that are identified to be at high risk, a nutrition support team may be consulted, especially if enteral and/or parenteral nutrition support is required. However, there is a practice gap that an inpatient lifestyle medicine service can fill that addresses patients with chronic diseases not requiring nutrition support, but for whom comprehensive secondary prevention strategies are needed. Additionally, there is a need to identify patients with risk factors for chronic disease, for which primary prevention tactics need to be implemented.

The strategy for individualized nutritional management, as part of an inpatient lifestyle medicine program, is to take inventory of the patient's chronic diseases that may or may not be related to the admitting diagnosis. Then, to classify management tactics based on the presence or absence of pre-disease (risk factors) and disease states. Primary prevention recommendations are fashioned for the pre-disease states and secondary prevention recommendations for the disease states. Tertiary preventive nutritional interventions would be applied to the acute presenting problem, corresponding to complication(s) from the disease state. Since dietary interventions may vary for each of these levels of prevention, the healthcare team will need to prioritize which elements to emphasize in the inpatient setting. Nonetheless, all patients should be provided healthy diets in the hospital regardless of their risk factors (a form of primordial prevention). For example, depressive symptoms, which often complicate an inpatient admission, can be reduced in patients with chronic diseases (e.g., cardiovascular disease [CVD] and metabolic syndrome) with the consumption of healthy diets[7–9].

Physical Activity

Sufficient physical activity is not only associated with improved clinical outcomes and impact of chronic diseases, but also lower expenditures for acute admissions [10]. Heart failure is a challenging clinical scenario in the hospital, particularly when there is acute decompensation with consequent worsening of other organ systems (e.g., chronic kidney disease) [11]. Physiological mechanisms of action for physical activity in this setting are mainly derived from animal studies and include vasodilation (e.g., via increased nitric oxide synthase and nitric oxide, decreased angiotensin II) [12, 13], decreased chemoreflex-mediated reduction in renal blood flow [14], decreased renin-angiotensin-aldosterone system hyperactivity (e.g., via reduced catecholamines and prostaglandins) [15, 16], and decreased oxidative stress [17], inflammation [18], renal fibrosis [19], and renal apoptosis [20]. Exercise training for inpatients with acute decompensated heart failure, with or without renal dysfunction, generally exhibits demonstrable beneficial effects on cardiac and renal status in clinical trials [21–31].

In a Norwegian study of a psychodynamic approach to 244 inpatients with eating disorders, a comprehensive approach to exercise oriented to the entire body was implemented [32]. This consisted of five components: an initial assessment; psychoeducation (focusing on the relationship between physical activity and health); connections among body, emotion, and social situations; exercise groups; and supervision by educated personnel [32]. Specific activities include rest, relaxation, outdoor activities (e.g., walks and hiking), body awareness, and weekend excursions, with coordinated outpatient care after discharge [32].

It is important to establish continuity of care with respect to physical activity during and after hospitalization. In a questionnaire study of hospital-based outpatient services for patients with musculoskeletal disorders, various communication formats facilitated inpatient/outpatient coordinated care: printed materials mailed out, e-mail and telephone contact, text messaging, and private internet-based social network messages [33]. For patients treated in the hospital with obesity-related complications, counseling should be provided about the benefits and implementation of regular exercise and physical activity after discharge [34].

One particular form of physical activity that can be introduced during a hospital stay is physical therapy, an allied health profession that addresses disability and functional impairment due to a variety of organ system disorders, and primarily, but not exclusively, focused on movement and the musculoskeletal system. This modality is generally recommended for inpatients with the intent of continuing after discharge. In a retrospective study ($N = 1003$) by Hartley et al. [35] of patients admitted to a medicine service, early physical therapy assessment (<24 h) was associated with reduced length of stay and odds of needing care on discharge. Though causality was not demonstrable, this beneficial effect was thought to be due to prevention of hospital-related deconditioning among frail, older adults [35].

Behavioral

Behavioral medicine is based on the biological, social, and psychological drivers of health and disease, and agents of behavioral change include healthcare professionals (HCP; nurses, social workers, psychologists, and physicians [also including medical students and residents]). Behavioral medicine consultation services are typically rendered in the outpatient setting, but recently inpatient behavioral medicine consultation services have been developed. Although these inpatient behavioral medicine services most commonly concentrate on improving adherence to medical interventions, they can be expanded to address various aspects of preventive care. This ranges from population-based (all admissions) primordial prevention and health promotion to decrease chronic disease risk factors, to primary prevention for patients at risk to avert frank disease, to secondary prevention to avert subsequent episodes, complications, and readmissions, to tertiary prevention with lifestyle and pharmacotherapy interventions to address primary complaints and the admission diagnosis, in order to minimize suffering and decrease mortality.

There are various dimensions to the problem of how unhealthy behaviors translate into chronic disease management, particularly within a hospital-based community. As it turns out, and certainly not surprisingly, unhealthy behaviors and poor health status are not only manifested by patients but also by hospital staff and HCPs. Moreover, unhealthy behaviors tend to cluster and interact among patients, HCP, and staff, in the hospital setting, resulting in a direct or indirect influence on patient care [36]. Mechanisms for this influence include adverse effects on adaptive learning, implementation of evidence-based policy and practice, and knowledge mobilization [37]. The main features of knowledge mobilization in hospital care include effective governance, influential leadership, supportive architecture, appropriate resourcing and rewards, active conflict management, leveraged pre-collaboration assets, stakeholder ownership and trust, shared vision and goals, knowledge sharing, strategic communication, continuous learning, and capacity building as a core activity [37]. In addition, the clustering of unhealthy behaviors in the hospital also affects vulnerable populations, such as the economically disadvantaged. If a network of behaviors among all those involved in hospital care can be centered on positive health, then better outcomes can be expected.

Gate et al. [38] designed an inpatient behavioral intervention based on the COM-B system (*C*apability, *O*pportunity, *M*otivation, and *B*ehavioral change) and Behavioral Change Wheel, delivered by a health psychologist. The intervention was a 4-week behavioral change program, consisting of a detailed baseline assessment, personalized goal setting, psychological skills development, motivational support, and referral to a community resource [38]. The intervention was feasible, acceptable to the patient, and resulted in improved self-efficacy, health and well-being scores, achievement of lifestyle and health management goals, and successful referrals to community services [38]. Cramer et al. [39] evaluated a 14-day integrative medicine inpatient program ($N = 2486$), consisting of aerobic exercise (e.g., walking, running, cycling, and swimming), meditative movement therapies (e.g., Yoga, Tai Chi, and Qigong), and relaxation techniques (e.g., progressive relaxation, mindfulness meditation, breathing exercises, and guided imagery). Practice frequency for each of these activities was predicted by self-efficacy (ranging from not-confident to absolutely confident), stage of change (ranging from pre-contemplation to preparation stages), and health locus of control (ranging from internal [health controlled by oneself] to external-social [health controlled by others] to external-fatalistic [health controlled by chance/destiny]) behavioral changes, and if successful can lead to improved adherence with health-promoting and lifestyle modification recommendations [39].

In a small ($N = 8$) pilot study of patients with severe mental illness (where cardiovascular risk factors such as obesity and metabolic syndrome have increased prevalence [40, 41]), brief nutritional and psychoeducation interventions (two 50-min within a single week) were associated with greater awareness (comparing pre- and post-assessment questionnaires) of healthy eating and physical activity habits [42]. Inpatient stress management programs can also be initiated to improve responses to stressors through daily activity structuring (balancing work, plan, and leisure), identification and expressions of emotions more constructively, greater sense of self-worth, and better ability to function comfortably in groups [43].

Among oncology patients, the elucidation of psychological stress factors affecting behaviors can improve care. This is especially relevant in the management of chronic pain, substance abuse, and malingering, by improving communication skills with the patient [44]. Integrated behavioral medicine programs have been proposed for inpatient and outpatient oncological care, with innovative models that incur little expense to patients and sponsoring health systems (via complementary services provided by volunteers [medical residents and behavioral medicine externs] and minimal billable time by state-mandated clinical psychologist supervision) [45].

Motivational tools are important to improve development of healthy lifestyle behaviors. In a sample of 17 patients with chronic heart failure, recruited from hospital and outpatient settings, motivations for improvement were interrogated using the Temporal Self-Regulation Theory framework [46]. Five motivational themes were found: two self-care motivators (consideration of family's future and one's own past), one demotivator (fatalistic consideration of one's own future), and two barriers for behavioral change (difficulty with physical activity and deviating from dietary habits and norms) [46]. In a pediatric inpatient population, lifestyle behavior change can be facilitated through discussions of personal experience of effectiveness, constraints associated with hospitalization, appropriateness of advice within specific care plans, job role priorities, and perceived benefits [47].

No doubt, the greatest challenge in establishing an inpatient behavioral medicine consultation service is training candidate HCPs, particularly physicians. Three teaching models have been presented by Kertesz et al. [48], which can be implemented by new or established inpatient lifestyle medicine programs: the New Hanover Regional Medical Center model (affiliated with the University of North Carolina at Chapel Hill), the Indiana University – Methodist family medicine residency model, and the University of Nebraska Medical Center model.

Specialized Programs

Many hospitals have incorporated various innovative programs to improve patients' experiences. However, the value of these programs has only recently been analyzed, quantified, and placed in the context of clinical outcomes. Since these inpatient programs do not involve medications or procedures, and they can be incorporated after a hospitalization, in the outpatient setting, as part of daily living experiences. Spirituality is also a component of inpatient lifestyle medicine and is covered in Chapter 20 by Costello et al. Wearable technologies can be useful for coordinating the inpatient and outpatient experiences; these devices are discussed in Chapter 13 by Mechanick and Zhao.

Art-Based Programs
Art therapy is a form of psychological therapy and therefore falls into the behavioral sciences. The visual arts can be particularly therapeutic in patients who have difficultly expressing feelings and emotions verbally, such as those with schizophrenia [49], dementia [50], traumatic brain injury

[51], seizure disorder [51], acute stress disorder [51], history of sexual abuse [51], or in a palliative care setting [52]. Sculpting is a form of art therapy that can improve emotional expression in patients with seizure disorder [53]. Art therapy can also improve symptoms of distress in cancer inpatients [54]. Art therapy may be conducted individually where relationships are forged between the patient and therapist, or in groups where an added benefit can be connecting with other group members. Innovations, such as augmented reality (e.g., a paint interaction system), hold great promise in helping inpatients begin to overcome mental and physical barriers [55].

Music therapy is a form of art-based therapy. In a cohort of 46 inpatients in a palliative care program, live music was associated with reported benefits of expression of spirituality, comfort, relaxation, escape, and reflection [56]. Songwriting is another modality in music therapy and can allow for exploration of "self-concept" (beliefs about oneself providing a sense of who they are in the world) in patients with neurological injury [57]. In one study, the calmness related to music therapy in hospitalized patients with Alzheimer's disease was associated with increased melatonin levels [58]. The Louis Armstrong Department of Music that is associated with several medical institutions consists of music therapists and other clinicians that receive training in music psychotherapy and provides services to adult and pediatric inpatients with chronic obstructive pulmonary disease, cardiovascular disease, neurodegenerative disease and stroke, cancer, intellectual disabilities, and other musicians with performance-related issues [59].

Imagery

Motor imagery is a technique that is characterized by mental rehearsals of voluntary motor acts without any actual motor activity and is based on simulation theory. The quality of this process exhibits a circadian variation with best results in the late morning, as demonstrated in older adults in a rehabilitation program [60]. Guided imagery is a technique that is characterized by mental engagement of all the senses to create a perception of stimulus with the intention of activating a beneficial psychological or physiological response [61]. In a pilot study by Jallo et al. [62], guided imagery in hospitalized pregnant women ($N = 19$) was associated with decreased stress and systolic blood pressure measurements, which are postulated to confer better health postpartum. In a 3-month study by Patricolo et al. [63], guided imagery (30-min session offered daily) in patients transferred from the intensive care unit to a progressive care unit was associated with decreased pain and anxiety and was qualitatively comparable to the effects of massage (15-min session offered daily). Additional implementation studies for guided imagery in the hospital have focused on the role of oncology nurses and pain control [64]. Studies are also underway investigating computerized positive mental imagery training in inpatient mental health settings [65].

Massage Therapy

Hospital-based massage therapy can be a useful adjunct to a Lifestyle Medicine Clinical Service Line, though a list of specific competencies and a mechanism for standardized training are still needed [66]. In a specialist palliative care unit, the majority of patients surveyed ($N = 179$) wanted a complementary therapy, of which massage and reflexology were the most popular [67]. In a single-arm feasibility study ($N = 109$), massage therapy was associated with reduction in anxiety, distress, fatigue, pain, and tension in patients with hematologic malignancies admitted to the bone marrow transplant service [68]. Mechanisms of action for massage therapy are still unclear. It is thought that the relief of muscle spasms and improvement in blood flow and metabolite excretion can ameliorate neurogenic symptoms and decrease analgesic medication requirements [69, 70]. However, adverse effects have also been described, including hematoma and abdominal symptoms (pain, vomiting, and constipation) [70]. In a meta-analysis of seven randomized trials ($N = 479$) involving patients with essential hypertension, Chinese massage ("Tuina") increased the therapeutic benefit of anti-hypertensive medications, though when used alone, it was not better than the medications [71]. These results could be viewed as positive, but more likely as non-informative since the results are of limited interpretive value due to clinical heterogeneity and low methodological quality of the included studies [71]. In short, hospital-based massage therapy needs to be studied scientifically and practitioners diligently trained. Prior to implementation, patients should be queried in terms of anticoagulant use, insertion of medical appliances or devices, and presence of wounds or hematomas, with work limited to just lymphatic drainage when in doubt [70].

Meditation and Movement Therapies

Meditation, mindfulness, and movement therapies are often performed concurrently and are therefore considered together here. Several meta-analyses have demonstrated the benefits of meditation and mindfulness on stress, substance abuse disorder (including tobacco and alcohol), and negative emotional states [72–75]. Transcendental meditation is a popular technique based on the repetition of a meaningless sound ("mantra") for an inward calming of the mind. This technique is practiced for 20 minutes twice a day, taught by certified instructors, and associated with positive effects on stress, anxiety, cardiovascular health, and alcohol use disorder, among others [76–80].

Mindfulness is a technique of approaching a situation objectively in the current moment, in a nonjudgmental way with openness, patience, compassion, and acceptance [81].

Mindfulness can be viewed as naturally occurring dispositional traits that are developed over time through meditation and other interventions and can be assessed with self-reported questionnaires. Trait mindfulness correlates more strongly with substance-abuse disorder in the inpatient setting, compared with the outpatient setting [82]. Mindfulness can be applied to patients' attitudes and HCPs' approaches to clinical problems [83]. In a small ($N = 30$) randomized controlled study by Parswani et al. [84], mindfulness based on the methods of Kabat-Zinn [85] and Segal [86] was taught and practiced for 1–1.5 h in weekly sessions for 8–10 weeks, started about 3 months after a cardiac event, and associated with decreased symptoms in anxiety, depression, and stress, compared with controls. In this study, mindfulness incorporated meditation, walking, pleasure activities, and cognitive restructuring, while also addressing eating habits and breathing [84]. Mindfulness instruction can also be delivered through internet-based applications [85]. Other clinical hospital settings in which mindfulness training and practice have resulted in beneficial effects include decreased postoperative pain following gynecological surgery [87], acute pain in a medical service [88], mood in adolescents in a psychiatric ward [89, 90], and stress reduction for caregivers of bone marrow transplant patients [91].

Tai chi is a low-intensity aerobic exercise, characterized by controlled breathing and graceful movements, that is well suited for inpatients with chronic disease, disability, and frailty. Qigong is a similar physical activity but involves simpler and repetitive movements. Together, as inpatient interventions, these exercises can reduce pain, depression, and falls and can improve balance, cognition, and cardiovascular conditioning [92–95]. In a medical-surgical unit, small-group, video-guided, beginner-level Tai chi and Qigong classes, supervised by physical therapists, 3 times a week, were feasible and associated with greater patient mobility [96]. In a small ($N = 22$) randomized study of patients who had a stroke, Tai chi was associated with improvements in balance, gait, physical function, pain, vitality, general health, and mental health [97]. Qigong was also associated with improved quality of life scores in patients with stroke ($N = 68$) on inpatient medical and rehabilitation wards [98]. In another small study of inpatients with diabetes ($N = 10$), Qigong walking was associated with lower blood sugars [99]. In patients with anorexia nervosa in a young adult psychiatric inpatient service, the response to Qigong was explored by analyzing interview data and classifying barriers and incentives to interventions; the authors found that Qigong may be able to enhance the anorexia nervosa recovery process [100]. However, in a Cochrane review of active mind-body movement therapies in patients with chronic obstructive pulmonary disease, of which the majority of studies used Tai chi or Qigong in the treatment group, and many of the studies examined inpa-

tient programs, there was no benefit, with an exception when considering only the low-quality evidence, in which quality of life scores was improved [101].

Yoga combines meditation, breathing, physical postures, and movements, and has been found to be therapeutic for sleep, muscle strength, inflammation, pain, fatigue, nausea, and other quality of life metrics over a wide range of clinical settings [102–109]. In a prospective cohort study of 486 inpatients with a hematological malignancy, Mascaro et al. [110] found that 40-min individualized yoga sessions were associated with decreased fatigue and anxiety. Inpatients on the psychiatric service can realize sustained benefits in reductions of anxiety after a yoga session for up to a full day [111]. Kupershmidt and Barnable [112] presented a yoga breathing protocol (Pranayama) that improves peak expiratory flow rate and forced expiratory volume and can be applied to the inpatient setting. Adherence with Yoga as an anti-hypertensive lifestyle intervention can be facilitated with six motivational telephone counseling sessions at months 1, 2, 3, 6, 9, and 12 after discharge from inpatient rehabilitation [113]. In a rehabilitation and complex continuing care hospital, patients receiving a Yoga class, 50–60 min weekly for 8 weeks, had improved pain-related factors and psychological experiences [114]. The ramifications of symptom improvement with Yoga are not confined to these clinical metrics alone. For instance, in the Urban Zen Initiative on an inpatient oncology unit at Beth Israel Hospital in New York, economic benefits and cost-savings were also established with an immersive healing environment that included Yoga and other integrative medicine approaches [115].

Pet- and Animal-Assisted Therapy

Within the theoretical framework of human caring [116], and the nursing professional practice model of relationship-based care [117], lies animal therapy and family pet visitation programs [118]. Pet therapy can utilize service or therapy animals, as well as home pets, and should involve grooming/bathing of animals within 24 h of patient exposure [118]. Beneficial effects reported in the literature are based on relatively weak data, including case reports, but affirm the ability to implement animal-assisted therapies in the hospital setting. These benefits include improvements in hemodynamics in those with CVD; behavioral changes, including decreased anxiety [119]; improved clinical course after stroke in acute rehabilitation units [119, 120]; higher satisfaction scores among trauma patients [121]; decreased psychological symptoms in critical illness [122]; and decreased pain perception in pediatric patients, with [123, 124] or without cancer [125]. Potential mechanisms that can mediate these effects include increased phenylethylamine (an amphetamine-like neurotransmitter; [126]), lower adrenal axis activation [127], and blunting of autonomic responses [128].

Scenarios

The new field of inpatient lifestyle medicine requires grounding in scientific evidence. The different skills and services that comprise an inpatient lifestyle medicine consultative service can be applied to specific clinical settings. Two of these settings are presented below: cardiometabolic risk mitigation and cancer. As with outpatient care, the phenotypic expression of chronic disease results from the contextualization of genetic and genomic factors by the physical (human-made ["built"] and natural) and nonphysical (cultural) environment. Therefore, the first step in the inpatient evaluation is, notwithstanding the admission diagnosis and primary acute illness, to identify relevant drivers that configure one or

more chronic disease states. It is these contributory chronic disease states that are the target of an inpatient lifestyle medicine management plan, implemented within a preventive care paradigm (Fig. 18.1).

Cardiometabolic Risk Mitigation

Cardiovascular disease, particularly coronary heart disease and stroke, accounts for most deaths, both domestically in the USA [129] and globally [130]. Key mechanistic drivers for CVD are metabolic in nature, namely adiposity-based chronic disease (ABCD; [131]) and dysglycemia-based chronic disease (DBCD; [132]), giving risk to the "cardiometabolic" terminology used to describe risk, syndrome, and

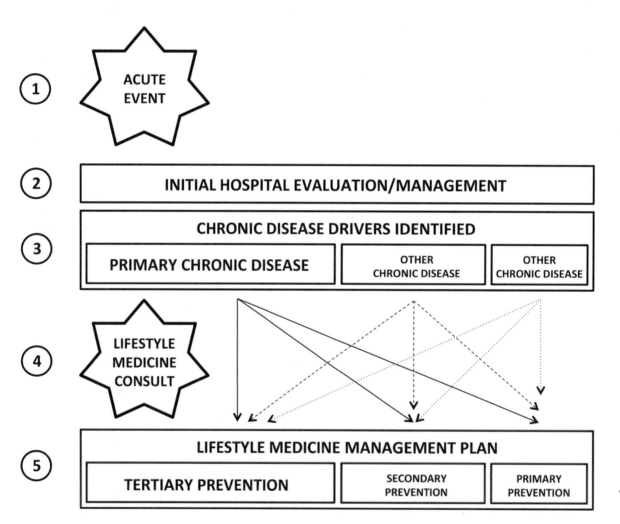

Fig. 18.1 Strategic plan and implementation tactics for an inpatient lifestyle medicine consult. Events in numerical order are provided on left. Event 1 – the patient presents to the primary inpatient care team with an acute illness or episode. Event 2 – routine evaluation and management are performed oriented to the acute clinical problem. Event 3 – the primary team thinks about pathogenesis and identifies the primary drivers and chronic diseases that led to the acute problem, and also identifies other chronic diseases that are relevant to the patient's

recovery. Event 4 – a lifestyle medicine consult is ordered to address relevant drivers and chronic disease states that can optimize clinical outcomes and minimize the need for pharmacotherapy and procedures. Event 5 – the lifestyle medicine plan is formulated and implemented using appropriate and available services (nutritional, physical activity based, behavioral, etc.) prioritizing the primary chronic disease and concurrently incorporating different prevention modalities

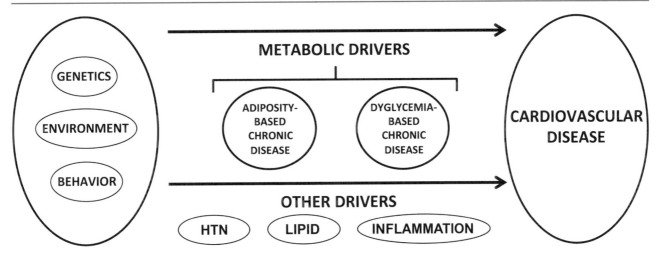

Fig. 18.2 Cardiometabolic-based chronic disease. "Cardiometabolic" = cardiovascular disease with metabolic drivers or causes. Primary drivers are genetics, environment, and behavior. Metabolic drivers are derived from primary drivers, lead to cardiovascular disease, and are interrelated: abnormal adiposity (amount, distribution, and/or function) is associated with dysglycemia (insulin resistance, pre-diabetes, type 2 diabetes, and vascular complications). Other drivers are also metabolic syndrome traits. Each of these mechanistic events can be viewed as targets for sustainable preventive care, which should be initiated as early as possible. Abbreviation: HTN hypertension

disease. When integrated, a new pathophysiological model of cardiometabolic-based chronic disease (CMBCD; [133, 134]) provides a structure for early and sustainable preventive care to reduce morbidity and mortality for individual patients and populations (Fig. 18.2). In fact, Kontis et al. [135] used global data and projections from 2015 to 2040 to find that just three lifestyle medicine interventions could save about 94 million lives within 25 years: [a] scaling up access to blood pressure treatment to 70%, [b] reducing sodium intake to 30%, and [c] eliminating *trans*-fat intake. It is within this context that hospitalized patients provide an exceptional opportunity to not just casually mention, or allude to the need for CMBCD risk mitigation, but to formally design a preventive care plan that centers on lifestyle medicine, utilizing many of the inpatient services outlined above.

Cardiovascular Disease

Hospitalized patients with an acute CVD event or presentation are typically managed with actions that are part of tertiary prevention (e.g., to reduce symptoms, suffering, or mortality with pharmacology, percutaneous coronary intervention, and/or surgical procedure). However, sequential secondary prevention strategies are indicated to prevent subsequent events and progression of disease, which consist not only of various medications (e.g., anticoagulants, statins, and sodium glucose transport protein 2 inhibitors) but also of formal cardiac rehabilitation (CR) and structured lifestyle change. In addition, concurrent primary and secondary prevention strategies for other chronic disease/pre-disease states (e.g., malignancy and degenerative conditions) can also be implemented in patients with established CVD. In contrast,

Table 18.4 Cardiometabolic-based chronic disease prevention strategies for hospitalized patients[a]

Presentation	Prevention type	Strategy
CMBCD	Primary	To mitigate non-CMBCD risk factors in patients at risk for other chronic diseases
	Secondary	To prevent disease progression in patients with other chronic diseases
		To prevent disease progression in patients with early CMBCD
	Tertiary	To prevent suffering and mortality in patients with advanced CMBCD or events
Non-CMBCD	Primary	To mitigate CMBCD risk factors
	Secondary	To prevent disease progression in patients with early CMBCD

Abbreviations: *CMBCD* Cardiometabolic-based chronic disease
[a]Many of these prevention strategies can be conducted sequentially or concurrently. The key modifiable CMBCD risk factors are unhealthy eating patterns, physical inactivity, tobacco use, abnormal adiposity, dysglycemia, hypertension, dyslipidemia, stress, and poor sleep hygiene

in hospitalized patients admitted for non-CVD oriented problems, primary prevention strategies for CVD should be evaluated and implemented (Table 18.4).

In the secondary prevention scenario, patients have already experienced a CVD event or procedure. Secondary prevention of CMBCD progression incorporates lifestyle change and judicious pharmacotherapy. Lifestyle interventions focus on modifiable risk factors (e.g., "Life's Simple 7[®]" by the American Heart Association, https://www.heart.org/en/professional/workplace-health/lifes-simple-7 [Accessed December 14, 2019], consisting of "Stop

Smoking," "Eat Better," "Get Active," "Lose Weight," "Manage Blood Pressure," "Control Blood Pressure," and "Reduce Blood Sugar").

In a study of 113,971 patients using registry data from 193 different hospitals, Kumbhani et al. [136] found that adherence to secondary prevention strategies was highest in those patients having a percutaneous coronary intervention, compared with coronary artery bypass graft surgery or no intervention groups. In an Australian/New Zealand study of 2299 inpatient acute coronary syndrome survivors, only about one-quarter received optimal secondary prevention, with the others generally having unstable angina, age over 70 years, or admission to a private (compared with public) hospital [137]. Unfortunately, the occurrence of major acute cardiovascular events after secondary prevention efforts correlates with psychosocial factors, particularly in men [138].

Cardiac rehabilitation programs are frequently initiated in the hospital and then continued in the outpatient setting. Inpatient CR interdisciplinary teams are oriented toward environmental drivers, clinical dimensions, complexity, and competencies, consisting of nurses, physiotherapists, dietitians, and psychologists, and resulting in "minimal care" pathways [139]. The lifestyle medicine specialist would be ideal for overseeing inpatient CR programs. In a randomized, controlled study of patients with chronic heart failure ($N = 475$), a self-management patient education program (five patient-centered interactive 60–75 min sessions focusing on behavior), as part of inpatient CR, was superior to the use of usual care [140]. Inpatient CR consists of chest physiotherapy with early ambulation and active physical exercise and can improve disabilities associated with acute decompensated heart failure [141], following cardiac surgery [142, 143], and with a left ventricular assist device [144]. Long-term outpatient secondary prevention programs following inpatient CR mitigate CVD risk factors and subsequent events, including those patients with lower education levels [145].

There are many challenges to addressing CVD prevention through lifestyle medicine in the hospital, not the least of which is gaining acceptance and traction as a valuable component of the care team. However, one critical aspect is the high prevalence of stress-related disorders accompanied by unhealthy lifestyles and the presence of CMBCD risk factors among hospital team members themselves [146, 147]. Hence, the lifestyle medicine consultant should exhibit and relate healthy personal behaviors, while attending to the health of hospital patients and possibly even the health of colleagues.

Diabetes

Any chronic state of significant hyperglycemia, including both type 2 diabetes (T2D) and type 1 diabetes, poses a risk for CVD, organ dysfunction, and other diabetes-related complica-

tions. However, insulin resistance (which is normoglycemic), pre-diabetes (a milder form of hyperglycemia), and T2D (a more severe form of hyperglycemia) each contributes to the risk of CVD, as represented in the DBCD [132] and CMBCD models [133, 134]. It is for this reason that any inpatient with DBCD (that is, with or at risk for T2D) merits an evaluation, discussion, and implementation of a formal program for structured lifestyle change, regardless of the admitting diagnosis. Unfortunately, among those patients with DBCD who are in lower socioeconomic strata, patient engagement with the healthcare system is limited [148]. This is generally due to the prevailing emphasis on acute care and not chronic disease management or prevention. Moreover, younger patients with DBCD are more dependent on family and community guidance, and not receptive to hospital care that is hamstrung by staff shortages, ineffective communication, and general lack of patient-empowerment interventions [148].

A lifestyle medicine consultant and inpatient team can potentially fill these gaps: self-management education, patient empowerment, and lifestyle modification [149]. For instance, Sullivan et al. [150] found that health coaching in the hospital setting that emphasizes diabetes self-management, motivation, self-efficacy, and empowerment was associated with reduced 30-day readmission rates. Since the use of inpatient specialized diabetes teams, compared with a primary service team, is associated with improved cost-effectiveness (lower 30-day readmission rates to medical services, better transition of care and adherence with outpatient follow-up, and reduced inpatient diabetes costs) [151], an inpatient lifestyle medicine team would benefit from specialized diabetes training. From a pragmatic standpoint, a hospital's structured glucose management program can take the form of any of four care models, led by an endocrinologist, advanced practice provider, pharmacist, or virtual glucose management team [152]. Therefore, any inpatient lifestyle medicine consultation service would need to be adapted and configured according to the preferred hospital model.

One of the most important components to lifestyle modification in inpatient DBCD care involves nutrition, being a centerpiece for educational programs for HCPs [153] and small-group interactive education for patients [154]. Behavioral methods are also important, and in a study by Schumann et al. [155], the incorporation of a psychologist in the rehabilitation setting facilitated instruction regarding self-management, nutrition, physical activity, and glycemic control. Pictorial dietary assessment tools can also be valuable and their use has been associated with more accurate estimates of protein/calorie intakes and reduced time to complete food intake records [156]. Inpatient nutritional care for patients with DBCD is basically oriented along the following lines and should be included in formal discussions and team collaborations:

- Optimization of glycemic control according to specific targets
- Provision of medical nutrition therapy and synchronization of carbohydrate with insulin or insulin secretagogues
- Counseling and management of overweight/obesity, or ABCD
- Promotion of healthy eating patterns that take into account comorbidities
- Primary and secondary prevention of diabetes complications, especially CVD
- Nutritional risk screening, case finding, and assessment in the context of malnutrition and optimal nutrition support

Other aspects of lifestyle medicine applicable to DBCD in the inpatient setting are also included in educational materials and formal discussions. These include physical activity (both aerobic and strength training), sleep hygiene, stress reduction, and evidence-based, judicious use of dietary supplements.

Obesity

Adiposity-based chronic disease encompasses patients with increased adipose tissue mass ("overweight" or "obese" by body mass index thresholds), abnormal adipose tissue distribution (e.g., ectopic fat or increased waist circumference), and/or abnormal adipocyte function [131]. Various clinical scenarios in the hospital would benefit from a lifestyle medicine consult for patients with ABCD in general, and obesity in particular (Table 18.5). Specifically, patients with more severe forms of ABCD undergoing surgery, particularly bariatric surgery, should receive lifestyle medicine counseling pre- and postoperatively [157]. In addition to consultative services that address the special needs and risks of patients

with ABCD, inpatient weight loss programs for adults and children can be incorporated into a burgeoning lifestyle medicine service. Obesity medicine overlaps with lifestyle medicine – both include expertise and knowledge about other modalities of treatment, such as pharmacotherapy and bariatric procedures.

Cancer

There are three broad and clear indications for an inpatient lifestyle medicine consultation in patients with cancer. Implementation of primary prevention serves to mitigate any risk factors and molecular mechanisms for chronic disease, including other malignancies (especially with tobacco cessation [158–161], alcohol moderation [162–164], healthy eating patterns [165, 166], weight loss if overweight/obese [167–173], and more physical activity [166, 174, 175]). Secondary prevention optimizes lifestyle in an evidence-based way that has been associated with improved responses to therapy (e.g., reducing the adverse effects of tobacco [176], alcohol [177, 178], unhealthy eating patterns [], overweight/obese [183–187], and physical inactivity [188–191] on a variety of cancer outcomes). Lastly, tertiary prevention addresses the current hospital admission that may have been precipitated by nutritional issues, including prolonged undernutrition [192–195], or a stress-induced event or series of events [196–198]. In addition to these preventive care strategies, the inpatient lifestyle medicine team can facilitate many specific services that address adverse behaviors, create a more tranquil and relaxing setting, and provide ongoing education with smooth transition to the outpatient setting [199–201].

Conclusion

The high prevalence of chronic disease and changing care models that focus on preventive medicine necessitates the incorporation of a formal Lifestyle Medicine Clinical Service Line in routine inpatient care. There are many challenges to initializing inpatient lifestyle medicine consultative teams that include changing the hospital culture to address chronic disease and comprehensive health, coordinating inpatient and outpatient care, educating patients and hospital personnel, and funding. It is recommended that champions of lifestyle medicine first perform an environmental scan of the urban infrastructure, needs of the target patient population, and available services by their healthcare system to then assemble a team, create a viable strategic plan and budget, secure funding, and operationalize on a small scale. Over time, this endeavor can expand by scaling up (incorporating new services) and out (over a larger geography), and then

Table 18.5 Clinical scenarios for inpatient lifestyle medicine consultation for obesity

Scenario	Approach
Patient-driven	Risk assessment that includes genetic, environmental, and behavioral primary drivers, adiposity and dysglycemia metabolic drivers, and other CVD risk factors; provision of educational counseling and materials regarding healthy eating, physical activity, and healthy behaviors; and post-discharge care setup and assistance with wearable technologies, community engagement, gym facilities, etc.
Bariatric surgery	Preoperative or postoperative assessment as above with outpatient follow-up and coordination with bariatric surgery team
Cardiac surgery	Preoperative or postoperative assessment as above with focus on CMBCD risk factors, outpatient follow-up, and judicious pharmacotherapy with the possibility of bariatric procedures
Severe obesity	Assessment as above including discussions about pharmacotherapy and bariatric procedures

Abbreviation: *CMBCD* Cardiometabolic-based chronic disease

adapt to emerging problems and technologies. Sustainability of lifestyle interventions post-hospital discharge is critical to health and the mitigation of chronic disease risk. Blending inpatient lifestyle medicine with more conventional outpatient services can improve continuity of care, individual patient outcomes, and population health.

References

1. Turner R, Illingworth D, Burt A. Anti-coronary care: the case for primary and secondary prevention. Br Heart J. 1972;34:960–1.
2. Thornley PE, Turner RWD. Rapid mobilization after acute myocardial infarction. First step in rehabilitation and secondary prevention. Br Heart J. 1977;39:471–6.
3. Haynes CL. Health promotion services for lifestyle development within a UK hospital – patients' experiences and views. BMC Public Health. 2008;8:284. https://doi.org/10.1186/1471-2458-8-284.
4. Cramer T, Wilson A, Rea B. Lifestyle medicine inpatient consultation services at Loma Linda University Health: a novel approach in a tertiary care center. Am J Lifestyle Med. 2018;12:227–9.
5. Cramer T, Rea B. The lifestyle medicine outpatient clinic at Loma Linda University Health. Am J Lifestyle Med. 2018;12:425–7.
6. Aggawal M, Grady A, Desai D, et al. Successful implementation of healthful nutrition initiatives into hospitals. Am J Med. 2020;133:19–25.
7. Sanchez-Villegas A, Martínez-Gonzalez MA, Estruch R, Salas-Salvadó J, Corella D, Covas M-I, et al. Mediterranean dietary pattern and depression: the PREDIMED randomized trial. BMC Med. 2013;11:208. https://doi.org/10.1186/741-7015-11-208.
8. Perez-Cornago A, Lopez-Legarrea P, de la Iglesia R, Lahortiga F, Martinez JA, Zulet MA. Longitudinal relationship of diet and oxidative stress with depressive symptoms in patients with metabolic syndrome after following a weight loss treatment: the Resmena Project. Clin Nutr. 2014;33:1061–7.
9. Parletta N, Zarnowiecki D, Chol J, et al. A Mediterranean-style dietary intervention supplemented with fish oil improves diet quality and mental health in people with depression: A randomized controlled trial (HELFIMED). Nutr Neurosci. 2019;22(7):474–87. https://doi.org/10.1080/1028415X.2017.1411320.
10. Marashi A, Ghassem Pour S, Li V, et al. The association between physical activity and hospital payments for acute admissions in the Australian population aged 45 and over. PLoS One. 2019;14:e0218394. https://doi.org/10.1371/journal.pone.0218394.
11. Cops J, Haesen S, De Moor B, et al. Exercise intervention in hospitalized heart failure patients, with evidence on congestion-related complications: a review. Heart Failure Rev. 2019. https://doi.org/10.1007/s10741-019-09833-x.
12. Van Craenenbroeck AH, Van Craenenbroeck EM, Kouidi E, et al. Vascular effects of exercise training in CKD: current evidence and pathophysiological mechanisms. Clin J Am Soc Nephrol. 2014;9:1305–18.
13. Zheng H, Li YF, Zucker IH, et al. Exercise training improves renal excretory responses to acute volume expansion in rats with heart failure. Am J Physiol Ren Physiol. 2006;291:F1148–56.
14. Marcus NJ, Pügge C, Mediratta J, et al. Exercise training attenuates chemoreflex mediated reductions of renal blood flow in heart failure. Am J Phys Heart Circ Phys. 2015;309:H259–66.
15. Ikeda T, Gomi T, Sasaki Y. Effects of swim training on blood pressure, catecholamines and prostaglandins in spontaneously hypertensive rats. Jpn Heart J. 1994;35:205–11.
16. Braith RW, Welsch MA, Feigenbaum MS, et al. Neuroendocrine activation in heart failure is modified by endurance exercise training. J Am Coll Cardiol. 1999;34:1170–5.
17. de Souza PS, da Rocha LG, Tromm CB, et al. Therapeutic action of physical exercise on markers of oxidative stress induced by chronic kidney disease. Life Sci. 2012;91:132–6.
18. Agarwal D, Elks CM, Reed SD, et al. Chronic exercise preserves renal structure and hemodynamics in spontaneously hypertensive rats. Antioxid Redox Signal. 2012;16:139–52.
19. Peng CC, Chen KC, Hsieh CL, et al. Swimming exercise prevents fibrogenesis in chronic kidney disease by inhibiting the myofibroblast transdifferentiation. PLoS One. 2012;7:e37388. https://doi.org/10.1371/journal.pone.0037388.
20. Chen KC, Peng CC, Hsieh CL, et al. Exercise ameliorates renal cell apoptosis in chronic kidney disease by intervening in the intrinsic and the extrinsic apoptotic pathways in a rat model. Evid Based Complement Alternat Med. 2013:368450–13.
21. Reeves GR, Whellan DJ, O'Connor CM, et al. A novel rehabilitation intervention for older patients with acute decompensated heart failure: the REHAB-HF pilot study. JACC Heart Fail. 2017;5:359–66.
22. Mudge AM, Denaro CP, Scott AC, et al. Addition of supervised exercise training to a post-hospital disease management program for patients recently hospitalized with acute heart failure: the EJECTION-HF randomized phase 4 trial. JACC Heart Fail. 2018;6:143–52.
23. Oliveira MF, Santos RC, Artz SA, et al. Safety and efficacy of aerobic exercise training associated to non-invasive ventilation in patients with acute heart failure. Arq Bras Cardiol. 2018;110:467–75.
24. Scrutinio D, Passantino A, Catanzaro R, et al. Inpatient cardiac rehabilitation soon after hospitalization for acute decompensated heart failure: a propensity score study. J Cardiopulm Rehabil Prev. 2012;32:71–7.
25. Tanaka S, Kamiya K, Matsue Y, et al. Effects of acute phase intensive electrical muscle stimulation in frail elderly patients with acute heart failure (ACTIVE-EMS): rationale and protocol for a multicenter randomized controlled trial. Clin Cardiol. 2017;40:1189–96.
26. Forestieri P, Bolzan DW, Santos VB, et al. Neuromuscular electrical stimulation improves exercise tolerance in patients with advanced heart failure on continuous intravenous inotropic support use-randomized controlled trial. Clin Rehabil. 2018;32:66–74.
27. Groehs RV, Antunes-Correa LM, Nobre TS, et al. Muscle electrical stimulation improves neurovascular control and exercise tolerance in hospitalised advanced heart failure patients. Eur J Prev Cardiol. 2016;23:1599–608.
28. Tanaka S, Masuda T, Kamiya K, et al. A single session of neuromuscular electrical stimulation enhances vascular endothelial function and peripheral blood circulation in patients with acute myocardial infarction. Int Heart J. 2016;57:676–81.
29. Ambrosy AP, Mulder H, Coles A, et al. Renal function and exercise training in ambulatory heart failure patients with a reduced ejection fraction. Am J Cardiol. 2018;122:999–1007.
30. Toyama K, Sugiyama S, Oka H, et al. Exercise therapy correlates with improving renal function through modifying lipid metabolism in patients with cardiovascular disease and chronic kidney disease. J Cardiol. 2010;56:142–6.
31. Hama T, Oikawa K, Ushijima A, et al. Effect of cardiac rehabilitation on the renal function in chronic kidney disease – analysis using serum cystatin-C based glomerular filtration rate. Int J Cardiol Heart Vasc. 2018;19:27–33.
32. Danielsen M, Rø Ø, Bjørnelv S. How to integrate physical activity and exercise approaches into inpatient treatment for eating disorders: fifteen years of clinical experience and research. J Eat Disord. 2018;6:34. https://doi.org/10.1186/s40337-018-0203-5.
33. McPhail SM, Schippers M, Maher CA, et al. Patient preferences for receiving remote communication support for lifestyle physical activity behavior change: the perspective of patients with musculoskeletal disorders from three hospital services. BioMed Res Int. 2015:8; Article ID 390352. https://doi.org/10.1155/2015/390352.

34. Akkary E, Cramer T, Chaar O, et al. Survey of the effective exercise habits of the formerly obese. J Soc Laparoendosc Surg. 2010;14:106–14.
35. Hartley PJ, Keevil VL, Alushi L, et al. Earlier physical therapy input is associated with a reduced length of hospital stay and reduced care needs on discharge in frail older inpatients: an observational study. J Geriatr Phys Ther. 2019;42:E7–E14.
36. Blake H, Mo PKH, Lee S, et al. Health in the HNS: lifestyle behaviours of hospital employees. Perspect Public Health. 2012;132:213–5.
37. Wutzke S, Rowbotham S, Haynes A, et al. Knowledge mobilization for chronic disease prevention: the case of the Australian Prevention Partnership Centre. Health Res Policy Sys. 2018;16:109. https://doi.org/10.1186/s12961-018-0379-9.
38. Gate L, Warren-Gash C, Clarke A, et al. Promoting lifestyle behaviour change and well-being in hospital patients: a pilot study of an evidence-based psychological intervention. J Public Health. 2015;38:e292–300.
39. Cramer H, Lauche R, Moebus S, et al. Predictors of health behavior change after an integrative medicine inpatient program. Int J Behav Med. 2014;21:775–83.
40. Gurusamy J, Gandhi S, Damodharan D, et al. Exercise, diet and educational interventions for metabolic syndrome in persons with schizophrenia: a systematic review. Asian J Psychiatr. 2018;36:73–85.
41. Fan X, Liu EY, Freudenreich O, et al. Higher white blood cell counts are associated with an increased risk for metabolic syndrome and more severe psychopathology in non-diabetic patients with schizophrenia. Schizophr Res. 2010;118:211–7.
42. Wu C, Chiang M, Natarajan R, et al. Pilot lifestyle education intervention for patients with severe mental illness during the inpatient stay. Asian J Psychiatr. 2019;40:15–7.
43. Courtney C, Escobedo B. A stress management program: inpatient-to-outpatient continuity. Am J Occup Ther. 1990;44:306–10.
44. Moore DA, Markman ES, McMahon CE, et al. Utilization of behavioral medicine services to refine medical diagnostic formulation in the face of uncertain symptom presentation. Case Rep Oncol. 2016;9:493–8.
45. Markman ES, Moore DA, McMahon CE. Integrated behavioral medicine in cancer care: utilizing a training program model to provide psychological services in an urban cancer center. Curr Oncol Rep. 2018;20:677. https://doi.org/10.1007/s11912-018-0677-y.
46. Chew HSJ, Sim KLD, Chair SY. Motivation, challenges and self-regulation in heart failure self-care: a theory-driven qualitative study. Int J Behav Med. 2019. https://doi.org/10.1007/s12529-019-09798-z.
47. Elwell L, Powell J, Wordsworth S, et al. Health professional perspectives on lifestyle behavior change in the paediatric hospital setting: a qualitative study. BMC Pediatr. 2014;14:71, http://www.biomedcentral.com/1471-2431/14/71.
48. Kertesz JW, Delbridge EJ, Felix DS. Models for integrating behavioral medicine on a family medicine in-patient teaching service. Int J Psychiatry Med. 2014;47:357–67.
49. Crawford MJ, Killaspy H, Kalaitzaki E, et al. The MATISSE study: a randomized trial of group art therapy for people with schizophrenia. BMC Psychiatry. 2010;10:65, http://www.biomedcentral.com/1471-244X/10/65.
50. Peisah C, Lawrence G, Reutens S. Creative solutions for severe dementia with BPSD: a case of art therapy used in an inpatient and residential care setting. Int Psychogeriatr. 2011;23(6):1011–3.
51. Rhondali W, Lasserre E, Filbet M. Art therapy among palliative care inpatients with advanced cancer. Palliat Med. 2012;27:571–2.
52. Bitonte RA, De Santo M. Art therapy: an underutilized, yet effective tool. Ment Illn. 2014;6:5354. https://doi.org/10.4081/mi.2014.5354.
53. Brown SE, Sheila T, Pestana-Knight E. Development and use of the art therapy seizure assessment sculpture on an inpatient epilepsy monitoring unit. Epilepsy Behav Case Rep. 2017;9:6–9.
54. Nainis N, Paice JA, Ratner J, et al. Relieving symptoms in cancer: innovative use of art therapy. J Pain Symptom Manag. 2006;31:162–9.
55. Donnari S, Canonico V, Fatuzzo G, et al. New technologies for art therapy interventions tailored to severe disabilities. Psychiatr Danub. 2019;31(suppl 3):462–6.
56. Peng CS, Baxter K, Lally KM. Music intervention as a tool in improving patient experience in palliative care. Am J Hosp Palliat Med. 2019;36:45–9.
57. Baker FA, Tamplin J, MacDonald RAR, et al. Exploring the self through songwriting: an analysis of songs composed by people with acquired neurodisability in an inpatient rehabilitation program. J Music Ther. 2017;54:35–54.
58. Kumar AM, Tims F, Cruess DG, et al. Music therapy increases serum melatonin levels in patients with Alzheimer's disease. Altern Ther Health Med. 1999;5:49–57.
59. The Louis Armstrong Department of Music Therapy. https://www.mountsinai.org/locations/music-therapy. Accessed 10 Nov 2019.
60. Rulleau T, Mauvieux B, Toussaint L. Influence of circadian rhthyms on the temporal features of motor imagery for older adult inpatients. Arch Phys Med Rehabil. 2015;96:1229–34.
61. Giedt JF. Guided imagery. A psychoneuroimmunological intervention in holistic nursing practice. J Holist Nurs. 1997;15(2):112–27.
62. Jallo N, Cozens R, Smith M, et al. Effects of a guided imagery intervention on stress in hospitalized pregnant women. Holist Nurs Pract. 2013;27:129–39.
63. Patricolol GE, LaVoie A, Slavin B, et al. Beneficial effects of guided imagery or clinical massage on the status of patients in a progressive care unit. Crit Care Nurse. 2017;37:62–9.
64. Burhenn P, Olausson J, Villegas G, et al. Guided imagery for pain control. Clin J Oncol Nurs. 2014;18:501–3.
65. Blackwell SE, Westermann K, Woud ML, et al. Computerized positive mental imagery training versus cognitive control training versus treatment as usual in inpatient mental health settings: study protocol for a randomized controlled feasibility trial. Pilot Feasibility Stud. 2018;4:133. https://doi.org/10.1186/s40814-018-0325-1.
66. Brennan MK, Healey D, Tague C, et al. Hospital based massage therapy specific competencies. J Bodyw Mov Ther. 2019;23:291–4.
67. Harte J, Leahy H, McCarthy J, et al. Exploring patients' interest in complementary therapies in a specialist palliative care unit. Int J Palliat Nurs. 2019;25:108–10.
68. Kuon C, Wannier R, Harrison J, et al. Massage for symptom management in adult inpatients with hematologic malignancies. Glob Adv Health Med. 2019;8:1–6. https://doi.org/10.1177/2164956119849390.
69. Hauschulz J, Clark S, Bauer B, et al. Resolution of postsurgical diplopia, paresthesia, and weakness following inpatient massage therapy: a case report. Glob Adv Health Med. 2019;8:1–4. https://doi.org/10.1177/2164956119852396.
70. Sharma I, Joseph D, Kirton O. Traumatic complications of inpatient massage therapy: case report and literature review. Trauma Case Rep. 2018;18:1–4. https://doi.org/10.1016/j.tcr.2018.11.003.
71. Yang X, Zhao H, Wang J. Chinese massage (Tuina) for the treatment of essential hypertension: a systematic review and meta-analysis. Complement Ther Med. 2014;22:541–8.
72. Sedlmeier P, Eberth J, Schwarz M, et al. The psychological effects of meditation: a meta-analysis. Psychol Bull. 2012;138:1139–71.
73. Goyal M, Singh S, Sibinga EM, et al. Meditation programs for psychological stress and wellbeing: a systematic review and meta-analysis. JAMA Int Med. 2014;174:357–68.

74. Brewer JA, Mallik S, Babuscio TA, et al. Mindfulness training for smoking cessation: results from a randomized controlled trial. Drug Alcohol Depend. 2011;119:72–80.

75. Bowen S, Witkiewitz K, Clifasefi SL, et al. Relative efficacy of mindfulness-based relapse prevention, standard relapse prevention, and treatment as usual for substance use disorders: a randomized clinical trial. JAMA Psychiatry. 2014;71:547–56.

76. Orme-Johnson DW, Barnes VA. Effects of the transcendental meditation technique on trait anxiety: a meta-analysis of randomized controlled trials. J Altern Complement Med. 2014;20:330–41.

77. Schneider RH, Carr T. Transcendental meditation in the prevention and treatment of cardiovascular disease and pathophysiological mechanisms: an evidence based review. Adv Integr Med. 2014;1:107–12.

78. Bai Z, Chang J, Chen C, Li P, Yang K, Chi I. Investigating the effect of transcendental meditation on blood pressure: a systematic review and meta-analysis. J Hum Hypertens. 2015;29(11):653–62.

79. Schneider RH, Grim CE, Rainforth MV, et al. Stress reduction in the secondary prevention of cardiovascular disease. Circ Cardiovasc Qual Outcomes. 2012;5:750–8.

80. Gryczynski J, Schwartz RP, Fishman MJ, et al. Integration of Transcendental Meditation® (TM) into alcohol use disorder (AUD) treatment. J Subst Abuse Treat. 2018;87:23–30.

81. Dobkin PL, Laliberte V. Being a mindful clinical teacher: can mindfulness enhance education in a clinical setting? Med Teach. 2014;36:347–52.

82. Karyadi KA, VanderVeen JD, Cyders MA. A meta-analysis of the relationship between trait mindfulness and substance use behaviors. Drug Alcohol Depend. 2014;143:1–10. https://doi.org/10.1016/j.drugalcdep.2014.07.014.

83. Gilmartin H, Goyal A, Hamati MC, et al. Brief mindfulness practices for healthcare providers – a systematic literature review. Am J Med. 2017;130:1219.e1–1219.e17.

84. Parswani MJ, Sharma MP, Iyengar SS. Mindfulness-based stress reduction program in coronary heart disease: a randomized control trial. Int J Yoga. 2013;6:111–7.

85. Kabat-Zinn J. Full catastrophic living: using the wisdom of your body and mind to face stress, pain and illness. New York: Delacourt; 1990.

86. Segal Z, Williams M, Teasdale J. Mindfulness-based cognitive therapy for depression: a new approach to preventing relapse. New York: Guilford Press; 2002.

87. Weston E, Raker C, Huang D, et al. The association between mindfulness and post-operative pain: a prospective cohort study of gynecologic oncology patients undergoing minimally invasive hysterectomy. J Minim Invasive Gynecol. 2019. https://doi.org/10.1016/j.jmig.2019.08.021.

88. Miller-Matero LR, Coleman JP, Smith-Mason CE, et al. A brief mindfulness intervention for medically hospitalized patients with acute pain: a pilot randomized clinical trial. Pain Med. 2019:1–6. https://doi.org/10.1093/pm/pnz082.

89. Sams DP, Handley ED, Alpert-Gillis LJ. Mindfulness-based group therapy: impact on psychiatrically hospitalized adolescents. Clin Child Psychol Psychiatry. 2018;23:582–91.

90. Blum H, Rutt H, Nash C, et al. Mindfulness meditation and anxiety in adolescents on an inpatient psychiatric unit. J Health Care Chaplain. 2019. https://doi.org/10.1080/08854726.2019.1603918.

91. Vinci C, Reblin M, Jim H, et al. Understanding preferences for a mindfulness-based stress management program among caregivers of hematopoietic cell transplant patients. Complement Ther Clin Pract. 2018;33:164–9.

92. Li F, Harmer P, Fitzgerald K, et al. Tai chi and postural stability in patients with Parkinson's disease. N Engl J Med. 2012;366:511–9.

93. Hwang H-F, Chen S-J, Lee-Hsieh J, et al. Effects of homebased Tai Chi and lower extremity training and self-practice on falls and functional outcomes in older fallers from the emergency department – a randomized controlled trial. J Am Geriatr Soc. 2016;64:518–25.

94. Wang X-Q, Pi Y-L, Chen P-J, et al. Traditional Chinese exercise for cardiovascular diseases: systematic review and meta-analysis of randomized controlled trials. J Am Heart Assoc. 2016;5:e002562.

95. Wayne PM, Walsh JN, Taylor-Piliae RE, et al. Effect of tai chi on cognitive performance in older adults: systematic review and meta-analysis. J Am Geriatr Soc. 2014;62:25–39.

96. Bao GC, Dillon J, Jannat-Khah D, et al. Tai chi for enhanced inpatient mobilization: a feasibility study. Complement Ther Med. 2019;46:109–15.

97. Kim HY, Kim YL, Lee SM. Effects of therapeutic Tai Chi on balance, gait, and quality of life in chronic stroke patients. Int J Rehabil Res. 2015;38:156–61.

98. Chen C-H, Hung K-S, Chung Y-C, et al. Mind-body interactive qigong improves physical and mental aspects of quality of life in inpatients with stroke: a randomized control study. Eur J Cardiovasc Nurs. 2019:1–9. https://doi.org/10.1177/1474515119860232.

99. Iwao M, Kajiyama S, Mori H, et al. Effects of qigong walking on diabetic patients: a pilot study. J Altern Complement Med. 1999;5:353–8.

100. Gueguen J, Piot M-A, Orri M, et al. Group Qigong for adolescent inpatients with anorexia nervosa: incentives and barriers. PLoS One. 2017;12:e0170885. https://doi.org/10.1371/journal.pone.0170885.

101. Gendron LM, Nyberg A, Saey D, et al. Active mind-body movement therapies as an adjunct to or in comparison with pulmonary rehabilitation for people with chronic obstructive pulmonary disease. Cochrane Database Syst Rev. 2018;10:CD012290. https://doi.org/10.1002/14651858.CD012290.pub2.

102. Feuerstein G. The yoga tradition. Prescott: Hohm Press; 1998.

103. Mustian KM, Sprod LK, Janelsins M, et al. Multicenter, randomized controlled trial of yoga for sleep quality among cancer survivors. J Clin Oncol. 2013;31:3233–41.

104. Vardar Yağlı N, Şener G, Arıkan H, et al. Do yoga and aerobic exercise training have impact on functional capacity, fatigue, peripheral muscle strength, and quality of life in breast cancer survivors? Integr Cancer Ther. 2015;14:125–32.

105. Chandwani KD, Perkins G, Nagendra HR, et al. Randomized, controlled trial of yoga in women with breast cancer undergoing radiotherapy. J Clin Oncol. 2014;32:1058–65.

106. Danhauer SC, Addington EL, Sohl SJ, et al. Review of yoga therapy during cancer treatment. Support Care Cancer. 2017;25:1357–72.

107. Carson JW, Carson KM, Porter LS, et al. Yoga of awareness program for menopausal symptoms in breast cancer survivors: results from a randomized trial. Support Care Cancer. 2009;17:1301–9.

108. Raghavendra RM, Nagarathna R, Nagendra HR, et al. Effects of an integrated yoga programme on chemotherapy-induced nausea and emesis in breast cancer patients. Eur J Cancer Care (Engl). 2007;16:462–74.

109. Bower JE, Greendale G, Crosswell AD, et al. Yoga reduces inflammatory signaling in fatigued breast cancer survivors: a randomized controlled trial. Psychoneuroendocrinology. 2014;43:20–9.

110. Mascaro J, Waller AV, Wright L, et al. Individualized, single session yoga therapy to reduce physical and emotional symptoms in hospitalized hematological cancer patients. Integr Cancer Ther. 2019;18:1–8. https://doi.org/10.1177/1534735419861692.

111. Bukar NK, Eberhardt LM, Davidson J. East meets west in psychiatry: yoga as an adjunct therapy for management of anxiety. Arch Psychiatr Nurs. 2019;33:371–6.

112. Kupershmidt S, Barnable T. Definition of a Yoga breathing (Pranayama) protocol that improves lung function. Holist Nurs Pract. 2019;33:197–203.

113. Schröer S, Mayer-Berger W, Pieper C. Effect of telerehabilitation on long-term adherence to yoga as an antihypertensive lifestyle intervention: results of a randomized controlled trial. Complement Ther Clin Pract. 2019;35:148–53.

114. Curtis K, Kuluski K, Bechsgaard G, et al. Evaluation of a specialized Yoga program for persons admitted to a complex continuing

care hospital: a pilot study. Evid Based Complement Alternat Med. 2016:6267879. https://doi.org/10.1155/2016/6267879.

115. Kligler B, Homel P, Harrison LB, et al. Cost savings in inpatient oncology through an integrative medicine approach. Am J Manag Care. 2011;17:779–84.

116. Watson J. Nursing: the philosophy and science of caring. Revised ed. Boulder: University Press of Colorado; 2008.

117. Koloroutis M, Manthey M, Felgen J, et al. Relationship-based care: a model for transforming practice. 1st ed. Minneapolis: Creative Health Care Management; 2004.

118. Sehr J, Eisele-Hlubocky L, Junker R, et al. Family pet visitation. Am J Nurs. 2013;113:54–9.

119. Cole KM, Gawlinski A, Steers N, et al. Animal-assisted therapy in patients hospitalized with heart failure. Am J Crit Care. 2007;16:575–85.

120. Burres S, Edwards NE, Beck AM, et al. Incorporating pets into acute inpatient rehabilitation: a case study. Assoc Rehabil Nurs. 2016;41:336–41.

121. Stevens P, Kepros JP, Mosher BD. Use of a dog visitation program to improve patient satisfaction in trauma patients. J Trauma Nurs. 2017;24:97–101.

122. Hetland B, Bailey T, Prince-Paul M. Animal assisted interactions to alleviate psychological symptoms in patients on mechanical ventilation. J Hosp Palliat Nurs. 2017;19:516–23.

123. Urbanski BL, Lazenby M. Distress among hospitalized pediatric cancer patients modified by pet-therapy intervention to improve quality of life. J Pediatr Oncol Nurs. 2012;29:272–82.

124. Chubak J, Hawkes R, Dudzik C, et al. Pilot study of therapy dog visits for inpatient youth with cancer. J Pediatr Oncol Nurs. 2017;34:331–41.

125. Sobo EJ, Eng B, Kassity-Krich N, et al. Canine visitation (pet) therapy: pilot data on decreases in child pain perception. J Holist Nurs. 2006;24:51–7.

126. Odendaal JS, Lehmann SM. The role of phenylethylamine during positive human-dog interaction. Acta Vet Brno. 2000;69:183–8.

127. Odendaal JS, Meintjes RA. Neurophysiological correlates of affiliative behaviour between humans and dogs. Vet J. 2003;165:296–301.

128. Virues-Ortega J, Buela-Casal G. Psychophysiological effects of human-animal interaction: theoretical issues and long-term interaction effects. J Nerv Ment Dis. 2006;194:52–7.

129. Centers for Disease Control and Prevention. Deaths and mortality. https://www.cdc.gov/nchs/fastats/deaths.htm. Accessed on 14 Dec 2019.

130. World Health Organization. The top 10 causes of death. https://www.who.int/news-room/fact-sheets/detail/the-top-10-causes. Accessed on 14 Dec 2019.

131. Mechanick JI, Hurley DL, Garvey WT. Adiposity-based chronic disease as a new diagnostic term: American Association of Clinical Endocrinologists and the American College of Endocrinology position statement. Endocr Pract. 2017;23:372–8.

132. Mechanick JI, Garber AJ, Grunberger G, et al. Dysglycemia-based chronic disease: an American Association of Clinical Endocrinologists position statement. Endocr Pract. 2018;24:995–1011.

133. Mechanick JI, Farkouh ME, Newman JD, et al. Cardiometabolic-based chronic disease: adiposity and dysglycemia drivers. J Am Coll Cardiol. 2020;75:525–538.

134. Mechanick JI, Farkouh ME, Newman JD, et al. Cardiometabolic-based chronic disease: addressing knowledge and clinical practice gaps in the preventive care plan. J Am Coll Cardiol. 2020;75:539–555.

135. Kontis V, Cobb LK, Mathers CD, et al. Three public health interventions could save 94 million lives in 25 years. Circulation. 2019;140:715–25.

136. Kumbhani DJ, Fonarow GC, Cannon CP, et al. Temporal trends for secondary prevention measures among patients hospitalized with coronary artery disease. Am J Med. 2015;128:426.e1–9.

137. Redfern J, Hyun K, Chew DP, et al. Prescription of secondary prevention medications, lifestyle advice, and referral to rehabilitation among acute coronary syndrome inpatients: results from a large prospective audit in Australia and New Zealand. Heart. 2014;100:1281–8.

138. Kure CE, Chan YK, Ski CF, et al. Gender-specific secondary prevention? Differential psychosocial risk factors for major cardiovascular events. Open Heart. 2016;3:e000356. https://doi.org/10.1136/openhrt-2015-000356.

139. Fattirolli F, Bettinardi O, Angelino E, et al. What constitutes the 'minimal care' interventions of the nurse, physiotherapist, dietician and psychologist in cardiovascular rehabilitation and secondary prevention: a position paper from the Italian Association for Cardiovascular Prevention, Rehabilitation and Epidemiology. Eur J Prev Cardiol. 2018;25:1799–810.

140. Meng K, Musekamp G, Schuler M, et al. The impact of a self-management patient education program for patients with chronic heart failure undergoing inpatient cardiac rehabilitation. Patient Educ Couns. 2016;99:1190–7.

141. Motoki H, Nishimura M, Kanai M, et al. Impact of inpatient cardiac rehabilitation on Barthel Index score and prognosis in patients with acute decompensated heart failure. Int J Cardiol. 2019. https://doi.org/10.1016/j.ijcard.2019.06.071.

142. Zanini M, Nery RM, de Lima JB, et al. Effects of different rehabilitation protocols in patient cardiac rehabilitation after coronary artery bypass graft surgery. J Cardiopulm Rehabil Prev. 2019;00:1–7. https://doi.org/10.1097/HCR.0000000000000431.

143. Marcassa C, Giordano A, Giannuzzi P. Five-year hospitalisations and survival in patients admitted to inpatient cardiac rehabilitation after cardiac surgery. Eur J Prev Cardiol. 2016;23:1609–17.

144. Reiss N, Schmidt T, Langheim E, et al. Inpatient cardiac rehabilitation of LVAD patients – updated recommendations from the Working Group of the German Society for Prevention and Rehabilitation of Cardiovascular Diseases. Thorac Cardiovasc Surg. 2019. https://doi.org/10.1055/s-0039-1691837.

145. Mayer-Berger W, Simic D, Mahmoodzad J, et al. Efficacy of a long-term secondary prevention programme following inpatient cardiovascular rehabilitation on risk and health-related quality of life in a low-education cohort: a randomized controlled study. Eur J Prev Cardiol. 2014;21:145–52.

146. Mittal TK, Cleghorn CL, Cade JE, et al. A cross-sectional survey of cardiovascular health and lifestyle habits of hospital staff in the UK: do we look after ourselves? Eur J Prev Cardiol. 2018;25:543–50.

147. Kurnat-Thoma E, El-Banna M, Oakcrum M, et al. Nurses' health promoting lifestyle behaviors in a community hospital. Appl Nurs Res. 2017;35:77–81.

148. Abrahams N, Gilson L, Levitt NS, et al. Factors that influence patient empowerment in inpatient chronic care: early thoughts on a diabetes care intervention in South Africa. BMC Endocr Disord. 2019;19:133. https://doi.org/10.1186/s12902-019-0465-1.

149. Lambrinou E, Hansen TB, Beulens JWJ. Lifestyle factors, self-management and patient empowerment in diabetes care. Eur J Prev Cardiol. 2019;26:55–63.

150. Sullivan VH, Hays MM, Alexander S. Health coaching for patients with type 2 diabetes mellitus to decrease 30-day hospital readmissions. Prof Case Manag. 2019;24:76–82.

151. Bansal V, Mottalib A, Pawar TK, et al. Inpatient diabetes management by specialized diabetes team versus primary service team in non-critical care units: impact on 30-day readmission rate and hospital cost. BMJ Open Diabetes Res Care. 2018;6:e000460. https://doi.org/10.1136/bmjdrc-2017-000460.

152. Drincic AT, Akkireddy P, Knezevich JT. Common models used for inpatient diabetes management. Curr Diab Rep. 2018;18:10. https://doi.org/10.1007/s11892-018-0972-x.

153. Mathioudakis N, Bashura H, Boyer L, et al. Development, implementation, and evaluation of a physician-targeted inpatient glycemic management curriculum. J Med Educ Curr Dev. 2019;6:1–10.

154. Reusch A, Strobl V, Ellgring H, et al. Effectiveness of small-group interactive education vs. lecture-based information-only programs on motivation to change and lifestyle behaviours. A prospective controlled trial of rehabilitation inpatients. Patient Educ Couns. 2011;82:186–92.

155. Schumann K, Touradji P, Hill-Briggs F. Inpatient rehabilitation diabetes consult service: a rehabilitation psychology approach to assessment and intervention. Rehabil Psychol. 2010;55:331–9.

156. Budiningsari D, Shahar S, Manaf ZA, et al. Evaluation of pictorial dietary assessment tool for hospitalized patients with diabetes: cost, accuracy, and user satisfaction analysis. Nutrients. 2018;10:27. https://doi.org/10.3390/nu10010027.

157. Mechanick JI, Apovian C, Brethauer S, et al. Clinical practice guidelines for the perioperative nutrition, metabolic, and nonsurgical support of patients undergoing bariatric procedures – 2019 update: cosponsored by American Association of Clinical Endocrinologists/American College of Endocrinology, The Obesity Society, American Society for Metabolic & Bariatric Surgery, Obesity Medicine Association, and American Society of Anesthesiologists. Endocr Pract. 2019;25:1–75.

158. Ni Y, Shi G, Qu J. Indoor PM$_{2.5}$, tobacco smoking and chronic lung diseases: a narrative review. Environ Res. 2019. https://doi.org/10.1016/j.envres.2019.108910.

159. Sarlak S, Lalou C, Amoedo ND, et al. Metabolic reprogramming by tobacco-specific nitrosamines (TSNAs) in cancer. Semin Cell Dev Biol. 2019. https://doi.org/10.1016/j.semcdb.2019.09.001.

160. Tomar SL, Hecht SS, Jaspers I, et al. Oral health effects of combusted and smokeless tobacco products. Adv Dent Res. 2019;30:4–10.

161. Zhang Y, He J, He B, et al. Effect of tobacco on periodontal disease and oral cancer. Tob Induc Dis. 2019;17:40. https://doi.org/10.18332/tid/106187.

162. Song BJ, Abdelmegeed MA, Cho YE, et al. Contributing roles of CYP2E1 and cytochrome P450 isoforms in alcohol-related tissue injury and carcinogenesis. Adv Exp Med Biol. 2019;1164:73–87.

163. Huang C, Zhang Y, Zhong S. Alcohol intake and abnormal expression of Brf1 in breast cancer. Oxidative Med Cell Longev. 2019;4818106. https://doi.org/10.1155/2019/4818106.

164. Mello FW, Melo G, Pasetto JJ, et al. The synergistic effect of tobacco and alcohol consumption on oral squamous cell carcinoma: a systematic review and meta-analysis. Clin Oral Investig. 2019;23:2849–59.

165. Panta P, Sarode SC, Sarode GS, et al. Can healthy diet intercept progression of oral potentially malignant disorders? Oral Oncol. 2018;85:106–7.

166. Allison RL. Back to basics: the effect of healthy diet and exercise on chronic disease management. S D Med. 2017;Spec No:10–18.

167. Paternoster S, Falasca M. The intricate relationship between diabetes, obesity and pancreatic cancer. BBA Rev Cancer. 2020;1873:188326. https://doi.org/10.1016/j.bbcan.2019.188326.

168. Wang K, Yu XH, Tang YJ, et al. Obesity: an emerging driver of head and neck cancer. Life Sci. 2019;233:116687. https://doi.org/10.1016/j.lfs.2019.116687.

169. Saitta C, Pollicino T, Raimondo G. Obesity and liver cancer. Ann Hepatol. 2019;18:810–5.

170. Zhou B, Wu D, Liu H, et al. Obesity and pancreatic cancer: an update of epidemiological evidence and molecular mechanisms. Pancreatology. 2019;19:941–50.

171. Nindrea RD, Aryandono T, Lazuardi L, et al. Association of overweight and obesity with breast cancer during premenopausal period in Asia: a meta-analysis. Int J Prev Med. 2019;10:192. https://doi.org/10.4103/ijpvm.IJPVM.372.18.

172. Donovan MG, Wren SN, Cenker M, et al. Dietary fat and obesity as modulators of BC risk: focus on DNA methylation. Br J Pharmacol. 2019. https://doi.org/10.1111/bph.14891.

173. Tumminia A, Vinciguerra F, Parisi M, et al. Adipose tissue, obesity and adiponectin: role in endocrine cancer risk. Int J Mol Sci. 2019;20:2863. https://doi.org/10.3390/ijms20122863.

174. Lugo D, Pulido AL, Mihos CG, et al. The effects of physical activity on cancer prevention, treatment and prognosis: a review of the literature. Complement Ther Med. 2019;44:9–13.

175. Chan DSM, Abar L, Cariolou M, et al. World cancer research fund international: continuous update project-systematic literature review and meta-analysis of observational cohort studies on physical activity, sedentary behavior, adiposity, and weight change and breast cancer risk. Cancer Causes Control. 2019;30:1183–200.

176. Jassem J. Tobacco smoking after diagnosis of cancer: clinical aspects. Transl Lung Cancer Res. 2019;8(Suppl 1):S50–8.

177. Marziliano A, Teckie S, Diefenbach MA. Alcohol-related head and neck cancer: summary of the literature. Head Neck. 2019. https://doi.org/10.1002/hed.26023.

178. Mujcic A, Blankers M, Bommele J, et al. The effectiveness of distance-based interventions for smoking cessation and alcohol moderation among cancer survivors: a meta-analysis. Psychooncology. 2019. https://doi.org/10.1002/pon.5261.

179. Lee MK, Park SY, Choi GS. Facilitators and barriers to adoption of a healthy diet in survivors of colorectal cancer. J Nurs Scholarsh. 2019;51:509–17.

180. Lawler S, Maher G, Brennan M, et al. Get healthy after breast cancer – examining the feasibility, acceptability and outcomes of referring breast cancer survivors to a general population telephone-delivered program targeting physical activity, healthy diet and weight loss. Support Care Center. 2017;25:1953–62.

181. Ryu SW, Son YG, Lee MK. Motivators and barriers to adoption of a healthy diet by survivors of stomach cancer: a cross-sectional study. Eur J Oncol Nurs. 2019;44:101703. https://doi.org/10.1016/j.ejon.2019.101703.

182. Cho D, Park CL. Barriers to physical activity and healthy diet among breast cancer survivors: a multilevel perspective. Eur J Cancer Care. 2018:27. https://doi.org/10.1111/ecc.12772.

183. Amin MN, Hussain S, Sarwar S, et al. How the association between obesity and inflammation may lead to insulin resistance and cancer. Diabetes Metab Syndr Clin Res Rev. 2019;13:1213–24.

184. Santoni M, Cimadamore A, Massari F, et al. Key role of obesity in genitourinary tumors with emphasis on urothelial and prostate cancers. Cancers. 2019;11:1225. https://doi.org/10.3390/cancers11091225.

185. Zimta AA, Tigu AB, Muntean M, et al. Molecular links between central obesity and breast cancer. Int J Mol Sci. 2019;20:5364. https://doi.org/10.3390/ijms20215364.

186. Aurilio G, Piva F, Santoni M, et al. The role of obesity in renal cell carcinoma patients: clinical-pathological implications. Int J Mol Sci. 2019;20:5683. https://doi.org/10.3390/ijms20225683.

187. Warner AB, McQuade JL. Modifiable host factors in melanoma: emerging evidence for obesity, diet, exercise, and the microbiome. Curr Oncol Rep. 2019;21:72. https://doi.org/10.1007/s11912-019-0814-2.

188. Balhareth A, Aldossary MY, McNamara D. Impact of physical activity and diet on colorectal cancer survivors' quality of life: a systematic review. World J Surg Oncol. 2019;17:153. https://doi.org/10.1186/s12957-019-1697-2.

189. Wang Y, Song H, Yin Y, et al. Cancer survivors could get survival benefits from postdiagnosis physical activity: a meta-analysis. Evid Based Complement Alternat Med. 2019:1940903. https://doi.org/10.1155/2019/1940903.

190. Coughlin SS, Caplan LS, Williams V. Home-based physical activity interventions for breast cancer patients receiving pri-

231

mary therapy: a systematic review. Breast Cancer Res Treat. 2019;178:513–22.
191. Avancini A, Sartori G, Gkountakos A, et al. Physical activity and exercise in lung cancer care: will promises be fulfilled? Oncologist. 2019. https://doi.org/10.1634/theoncologist.2019-0463.
192. Forslund M, Ottenblad A, Ginman C, et al. Effects of a nutrition intervention on acute and late bowel symptoms and health-related quality of life up to 24 months post radiotherapy in patients with prostate cancer: a multicenter randomized trial. Support Care Cancer. 2019. https://doi.org/10.1007/s00520-019-05182-5.
193. Crowder SL, Douglas KG, Yanina Pepino M, et al. Nutrition impact symptoms and associated outcomes in post-chemoradiotherapy head and neck cancer survivors: a systematic review. J Cancer Surviv. 2018;12:479–94.
194. Barr RD, Gomez-Almaguer D, Jaime-Perez JC, et al. Importance of nutrition in the treatment of leukemia in children and adolescents. Arch Med Res. 2016;47:585–92.
195. Kiss N, Gilliland S, Quinn P, et al. Evaluating the effectiveness of a nutrition assistant role in a head and neck cancer clinic. Nutr Diet. 2019;76:21–7.

196. PDQ Supportive and Palliative Care Editorial Board. Cancer-related post-traumatic stress (PDQ®): health professional version. PDQ Cancer Inform Summ 2002–2019, Oct 30. https://www-ncbi-nlm-nih-gov.eresources.mssm.edu/pubmed/26389172.
197. Kruk J, Aboul-Enein BH, Bernstein J, et al. Psychological stress and cellular aging in cancer: a meta-analysis. Oxidative Med Cell Longev. 2019:1270397. https://doi.org/10.1155/2019/1270397.
198. Marziliano A, Tuman M, Moyer A. The relationship between post-traumatic stress and post-traumatic growth in cancer patients and survivors: a systematic review and meta-analysis. Psychooncology. 2019. https://doi.org/10.1002/pon.5314.
199. Strauss-Blasche G, Gnad E, Ekmekcioglu C, et al. Combined inpatient rehabilitation and spa therapy for breast cancer patients. Cancer Nurs. 2005;28:390–8.
200. Gjerset GM, Loge JH, Gudbergsson SB, et al. Lifestyles of cancer survivors attending an inpatient educational program – a cross-sectional study. Support Care Cancer. 2016;24:1527–36.
201. Klocker J, Klocker-Kaiser U, Pipam W, et al. Long-term improvement of the bio-psycho-social state of cancer patients after 3 weeks of inpatient oncological rehabilitation. Wien Med Wochenschr. 2018;168:350–60.

Transcultural Lifestyle Medicine

Ramfis Nieto-Martínez and Juan P. González-Rivas

Abbreviations

BMI   Body Mass Index
DPP   Diabetes Prevention Program
EVM   Ecological Validity Model
FEV1   Forced Expiratory Volume first second
FINDRISC Finland Diabetes Risk Score
FVC   Forced Vital Capacity
HCP   Healthcare Professional
MNA   Mini Nutritional Assessment
NHANES National Health and Nutrition Examination Survey
SDOH Social Determinants of Health
T2D   Type 2 Diabetes
tDNA   transcultural Diabetes Nutrition Algorithm

The original version of this chapter was revised and updated. The correction to this chapter can be found at https://doi.org/10.1007/978-3-030-48088-2_32

R. Nieto-Martínez (✉)
LifeDoc Health, Memphis, TN, USA

Harvard TH Chan School of Public Health,
Harvard University, Boston, MA, USA

Foundation for Clinical, Public Health, and Epidemiological
Research of Venezuela (FISPEVEN), Caracas, Venezuela
e-mail: nietoramfis@hsph.harvard.edu

J. P. González-Rivas
International Clinical Research Center,
St Anne's University Hospital, Brno, Czech Republic

Harvard TH Chan School of Public Health,
Harvard University, Boston, MA, USA

Foundation for Clinical, Public Health, and Epidemiological
Research of Venezuela (FISPEVEN), Caracas, Venezuela

Introduction

An Arab patient, who barely speaks English, is evaluated by a Hispanic doctor in a healthcare center in Miami. The patient has increased adiposity and waist circumference on exam and a fasting blood glucose of 130 mg/dl. Lifestyle, foods, and traditions can vary greatly between Western and Arab peoples. These particularities need to be properly identified and managed to avoid disparities in healthcare delivery. Besides the language gap, what other ethno-cultural differences should be addressed to provide adequate lifestyle medicine recommendations for this patient with cardiometabolic risk factors?

Epidemiologically, populations from different ethnicities and cultures exhibit diverse phenotypes and burdens of disease. In the USA, in 2013, heart disease was the leading cause of death in Caucasian and African American women, but cancer was the leading cause among American Indian/Alaska Native, Asian/Pacific Islander, and Hispanic women [1]. In the USA, in 2017, racial-ethnic minorities represented 38.8% of the population: Hispanic 18.1%, Native American 13.4%, Asian 5.8%, Native American/Alaska Native 1.3%, Pacific Islander 0.2%, and mixed 2.7% [2]. However, minority groups constituted only 13.4% of the 147,815 primary care physicians in a cohort study [2].

Physiological determinants are contextualized by physical, cultural, and behavioral factors to create chronic disease phenotypes (Fig. 19.1). Inflammation is a common pathophysiological pathway in almost all chronic diseases [3]. For example, at comparable levels of overweight and insulin resistance, African American adolescents with obesity showed a higher inflammatory response and lower concentration of glucagon-like peptide 1 than Caucasian adolescents with obesity, which may act synergistically to foster the progression from obesity to type 2 diabetes (T2D) [4]. Social determinants of health (SDOH) are equally important. Lower rates of health services use in Hispanic and African Americans have been reported, which could be attributed to lower income, poorer education, and less private health insurance coverage, compared with

Fig. 19.1 The role of cultural factors in the lifestyle medicine management of chronic disease. Lifestyle medicine can exert beneficial effects on molecular drivers (genetics and epigenetics), context (environment, culture, and behavior), and phenotype of chronic disease

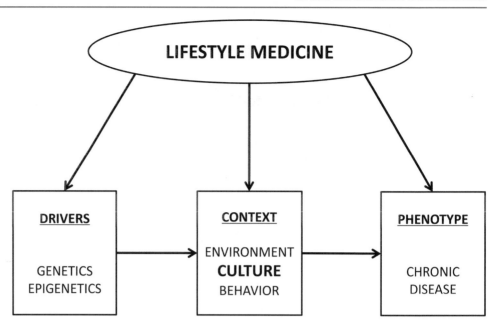

Caucasians [5]. However, some disparities can result from the interactions between patients and their healthcare professional (HCP) (e.g., racial bias, patient preferences, or poor communication) [5]. In this context, cultural competency – a set of consistent behaviors, attitudes, and policies that enable a system, agency, or individual to work within a cross-cultural context or situation effectively – must be applied [6].

In addition to differences among the racial-ethnic subgroups, cultural heterogeneity also occurs within each subgroup. An ever-expanding mosaic of ethno-cultural variety in the USA, among other nations, imposes a challenge to the individual healthcare system. Another global threat is population displacement [7]. Moving to another country can be part of the planned migration process, but forced displacement due to natural disasters, wars or social, politic, or economic conflicts can overburden the healthcare system of the asylum/receiving countries, imposing the need to consider ethno-cultural information to ensure the health of migrant populations [7, 8].

Data from National Health and Nutrition Examination Survey (NHANES) 2011–2016 in the USA reported that healthy lifestyle advice to adults with chronic conditions by HCPs is low, and lowest in those with overweight/obesity [9]. This shortcoming must be urgently addressed in order to implement early and sustainable strategies that can reduce the burden of chronic disease. Obviously, it is not possible for each patient to be evaluated by an HCP of the same ethno-cultural origin, but each HCP must know basic aspects of transcultural lifestyle medicine. Lifestyle medicine interventions ideally must be based on the best evidence available, and cultural differences and needs must be recognized and effectively incorporated in healthcare [6]. Certain cultural factors, such as language barriers, belief systems, availability of food, eating patterns, physical activity behaviors, and socioeconomics, are powerful modifiers of the responses to healthcare.

In a narrow sense, transculturalization describes the process of adapting evidence-based clinical recommen-

dations from a source culture to another culture using local thought leaders from both source and target cultures in an interactive setting [10, 11]. From a more pragmatic standpoint, transculturalization is an essential process within precision medicine, which individualizes a care plan to achieve superior clinical outcomes, based on genetic/epigenetic factors, the built (human-made) environment, and culture. The transcultural effect is most pronounced when care is delivered by an HCP of one ethno-cultural background to a patient of another ethno-cultural background. A successful Lifestyle Medicine Center or Clinical Service Line routinely incorporates transcultural medicine approaches. Transcultural recommendations are based on evidence-based white papers (e.g., clinical practice guidelines, algorithms, checklists, and position papers), lifestyle intervention programs, validated anthropometric and biochemical markers cutoffs, and behavioral research. After the transcultural adaptation of evidence-based recommendations, one begins the implementation process [12], represented by the following five steps [13].

1. Clinical practice guidelines production should include cultural adaptations that address physiological and social determinants of health, and not simply language translation [14].
2. Transcultural adaptation is the systematic modification of an evidence-based intervention to incorporate cultural factors and context, and to be compatible with the patient's belief system and way of life [15].
3. Implementation involves the incorporation of transculturalized evidence-based interventions into routine healthcare at clinical, organizational, public health, and/or policy levels.
4. Clinical outcomes following implementation can be analyzed to improve the understanding of what works best

with specific transculturalized interventions, settings, and conditions [16].

5. Clinical effectiveness is achieved when the specific transculturalized intervention realizes the intended patient care objective.

Transcultural Medicine Approach

Diverse ethno-cultural groups are exposed to different SDOH that contribute to their health outcomes [17]. The US Department of Health and Human Services Office of Minority Health describes various epidemiological factors that differ among ethnic populations and chronic disease states (Table 19.1) [18]. Chronic disease categories include (1) cardiometabolic diseases (cardiovascular diseases, obesity/overweight, diabetes, hypertension, and hypercholesterolemia); (2) degenerative/psychiatric diseases (arthritis, osteoporosis, Alzheimer disease, dementia, depression); (3) cancer; (4) kidney and pulmonary diseases (chronic kidney disease, asthma, and chronic obstructive pulmonary disease); and (5) infectious diseases (human immunodeficiency virus/acquired immunodeficiency syndrome and tuberculosis).

Transcultural medicine involves symmetrical relationships between patients who seek therapeutic components that match their beliefs and practices, and HCP who deliver culturally adapted care. For example, the integration of Western and other indigenous medicinal approaches is becoming more accepted in healthcare systems throughout the world. Experiences of this intercultural health initiative have been reported in several Latin American countries (Chile, Ecuador, Suriname, Guatemala, and Colombia) [19] and in Eritrea [20]. Although the Ecuadorian government legalized the State Office of Intercultural Health in 2008, the real-life integration of both health models in Ecuador has been modest [21]. Recorded consultations in rural facilities in Cameroon show that, compared with patients served by Western-medicine Cameroonian HCPs, patients of traditional healers traveled 2.5 times farther, paid 12 times more, and had shorter consultations, with a smaller share of the communication. However, there was a higher percentage of content discussed on lifestyle and psychosocial aspects of care, with information communicated more emotionally. Therefore, contrary to the premise that patients consult traditional healers due to lack of money or geographical inaccessibility to Western style healthcare, a more patient-centered communication style with an emphasis on lifestyle could be the more important driver of popularity of these "alternative" approaches [22].

Different religious beliefs can also influence individual behaviors and the willingness to accept specific lifestyle or behavior changes. People who are more, compared to less, religious/spiritual have better mental health and adapt more quickly to health problems [23]. Monotheistic religions (e.g., Christianity, Judaism, and Islam) incorporate decisions, lifestyle choices, and health behaviors that interact to produce

Table 19.1 Cultural factors by ethnic group and chronic disease[a]

Ethnic group	Cardiometabolic diseases	Degenerative/psychiatric diseases	Cancer	Kidney and pulmonary diseases	Infectious diseases
Native Americans/Alaska Natives	Rates of obesity, diabetes, cardiovascular disease, and metabolic syndrome are higher than other ethnic groups	In 2014, suicide was the second leading cause of death between the ages of 10 and 34	Cancer rates are lower than non-Hispanic white population, with some exceptions in certain types of cancer	Children are 60% more likely to have asthma as non-Hispanic white children	HIV and AIDS rates are twice as compared to the white population
Asian and Pacific Islanders	Lower prevalence of obesity, hypertension, tobacco, and lower rates of heart disease and diabetes than whites	Southeast Asians show high risk for post-traumatic stress disorder after migration to the USA	Lower rate of prostate and breast cancer, but higher of stomach cancer than whites	60% higher risk of end-stage renal disease than non-Hispanic whites	HIV rates are similar than whites
Latino/Hispanic	Latino/Hispanics in the USA have a lower rate of CVD mortality and the longest life expectancy, despite a higher prevalence of CVD risk factors and lower socioeconomic conditions "Hispanic Paradox" [18]	Mental health treatment and suicides are lower in Latino/Hispanics than whites	Latino/Hispanics shows lower incidence of breast and prostate cancer, but higher stomach, liver, and cervical cancer than whites	Latino/Hispanics have higher rates of end-stage renal disease, caused by diabetes	One out of four cases with HIV is Latino/Hispanic
African American	African Americans are 30% more likely to die from heart disease and 60% from stroke than non-Hispanic whites	African Americans are 10% more likely to report having serious psychological distress than Non-Hispanic whites	African Americans have the highest mortality rate of any racial and ethnic group for all cancers combined	African Americans were almost three times more likely to die from asthma-related causes than the white population	Men have 8.6 times and women 18.6 times the AIDS rate than whites

[a]Abbreviations: *AIDS* acquired immunodeficiency syndrome, *CVD* cardiovascular disease, *HIV* human immunodeficiency virus

positive emotions and social connections. The result can be manifested as better mental, immune, endocrine, and cardiovascular function promoting physical health and longevity [23]. The US population has a diverse representation of religions. In a 2016 survey including 173,229 interviews, 48.9% of participants reported being Protestant/Other Christian, 23.0% Catholic, 18.2% None/Atheist/Agnostic, 2.1% Jewish, 1.8% Mormon, 0.8% Muslim, and 2.5% other non-Christian religion [24]. However, despite the contention that different religious beliefs are related with different health behaviors and outcomes, the Nashville REACH 2010 project ($N = 3014$) failed to show any significant relationship, after adjusting for potentially confounding sociodemographic variables [25]. Faith communities should always be taken into account as part of the cultural content to promote healthy behaviors, but socioeconomic status, ethnicity, and cultural backgrounds appear to be stronger predictors of health than religious beliefs per se [25].

A review of meta-analyses on culturally adapted mental health interventions concluded that adapting interventions for a specific culture is better than usual care [26]. However, this analysis was limited by the lack of studies, including active controls or nonculturally adapted treatment arms, as well as methodological heterogeneity with diverse designs, contexts, and criteria used to adapt interventions. This study highlights the importance of developing a common evidence-based framework for cultural adaptations of mental health interventions [26].

Transcultural Adaptation Process

Evidence-based recommendations can be transculturally adapted according to a validated, formal process. The transcultural Diabetes Nutrition Algorithm (tDNA) was developed as a portable tool to facilitate the delivery of evidence-based lifestyle modifications and nutrition therapy in those with prediabetes and T2D for a variety of geographic locations and cultural settings [27]. The tDNA was created and implemented in many countries [28–34], and clinically validated in Malaysia [35].

Continuing with the Arab patient case study, the following formalized transculturalization steps are detailed:

1. *Identify target population.* The Arab population living in a community in Miami is part of a larger Arab community of 15,000 in Miami Dade County and 112,300 in Florida [36], which is the southernmost contiguous state in the USA and the third most populous state with 21 million inhabitants.
2. *Identify the clinical question.* One-third of US adults have prediabetes [37]. The American Diabetes Association rec-

ommends implementing primary prevention (e.g., the Diabetes Prevention Program [DPP]) in those with prediabetes [38]. As an example, the US government created the National DPP, and though available in English and Spanish, this is not a bona fide transculturalization product, and more specifically, is not inclusive of an Arab DPP version.

3. *Create a team of expert HCPs representing the source (National DPP) and target populations (Arab culture).* This team consists of different stakeholders, especially from the target population, conferring leadership in areas of scientific methodology, diabetes and nutrition, primary care, health policy and economics, and governmental and regulatory factors, among others. The mere language translation of the DPP content into Arab is not a cultural adaptation. Cultural, ethnicity, racial, social, and biological health determinants must be included in this formal process. The deliverable of this step is a new, evidence-based, culturally adapted clinical decision-making tool (e.g., guidelines, algorithm, checklist, and brochures) to assist and optimize healthcare for the target population.
4. *Clinical action based on transculturalized decision nodes using a validated framework.* The evidence-based recommendations represented as clinical decision nodes in an algorithm can be interpreted and organized using the Ecological Validity Model (EVM) (Table 19.2) [39]. The EVM taxonomy consists of eight dimensions (language, persons, metaphors, content, concepts, goals, methods, and context) that serve as a guide for developing culturally sensitive interventions [40]. These action steps should be followed by an assessment step on the effectiveness of the intervention [13].

Table 19.2 Dimensions of the ecological validity model

Domain	Definition
Language	Adaptation of materials in a culturally sensitive way, ensuring the message is received as intended
Persons	Patient and provider variables and the relationship between them
Metaphors	Symbols and concepts shared with the target population
Content	Cultural knowledge (i.e., social, economic, historical, and political values, customs, and traditions)
Concepts	Constructs of a theoretical model; how the problem/intervention is conceptualized and communicated to the participant
Goals	Objectives of the intervention, which should be aligned between the healthcare professional and the participant based on the cultural values of the target population
Methods	Procedures for achieving the intervention goals
Context	Consideration of the participant's environment (e.g., economic, political, and developmental) during the intervention

In this example, the lifestyle-related aspects of the Arab culture and relevant Muslim customs must be incorporated for transcultural adaptation. Important differences include diet, ideas of modesty, privacy, touch restriction, and alcohol restriction [41]. The physical exam should be done by a HCP of the same gender. If it is not possible, then a third person should be in the room that is the same gender as the patient [41]. Nutritional recommendations should include culturally specific meal plans. Traditionally, Arabs of the Arabian Peninsula relied heavily on a diet of dates, wheat, barley, rice, meat, and yogurt products, with little variety. A typical dinner can consist of a large platter, shared commonly, with a vast quantity of rice, including lamb or chicken, or both, as separate dishes, with various stewed vegetables, heavily spiced, sometimes with tomato sauce. Tea is a frequent accompaniment of the meal. Islamic (Sharia) law prohibits alcohol consumption, non-Halal animal fats, pork, by-products of pork, and any animals that have not been slaughtered according to Islamic custom [41]. Dietary customs, particularly fasting rules, during Ramadan, and their implications for the management of chronic diseases, such as diabetes, should be considered [42]. In their native countries, the Arab lifestyle involves more physical activity in forms of walking, work activities, and gardening [43]. Traditionally, Arab women will wear a hijab, or covering for modesty and demonstration/expression of their Islamic faith. This should be part of any conversation about physical activity and structured exercise, including team (soccer, softball, and basketball) and individual (boxing, archery, running, swimming, and tennis) sports.

Culture, immigration, and acculturation status can affect health beliefs and lifestyle behaviors, such as physical activity, nutrition, and weight control among Arab Americans [43]. Acculturation describes changes that occur when two or more cultures interact [44]. More acculturated Arab Americans immigrants often adopt the Western lifestyle, which can include less physical activity and the consumption of processed food with high fat and salt content [43]. A similar acculturation pattern associated with greater increases in adiposity over 5 years was described in a Puerto Rican cohort that used more English (than Spanish) for usual daily activities [45]. Acculturation in dietary habits and physical activity has also been found in Arab mothers living in Texas: negative behaviors were associated with children's preferences, less access to traditional foods, low cost of most unhealthy foods, and lack of time to prepare foods; positive behaviors were associated with healthier cooking techniques and food choices, reading nutritional labels, and better availability of healthy choices in the USA [46]. Examples of culturally adapted approaches to improve lifestyle in different cultures are provided in Table 19.3 [47–52].

Table 19.3 International culturally adapted interventions of lifestyle medicine[a]

Adaptation	Population	Design	Components	Results
tDNA: MNT consisting of a structured, low-calorie meal plan, incorporation of one or two diabetes-specific formula servings as meal replacements, and a physical activity prescription [47]	Malaysia $N = 230$ patients with overweight/obesity and T2D	RCT	Usual care vs. tDNA (structured low-calorie meal plan, diabetes specific meal replacements, and increased physical activity) during 6 months	Culturally adapted, structured lifestyle intervention including MNT, motivational interviewing, and physical activity, improved weight loss and metabolic control in patients with overweight/obesity and T2D compared with standard care
Cultural adaptation of a psychoeducational program for cancer survivors was addressed assessing the context and lifestyle preferences of local population to facilitate its adoption [48]	Singaporean Asians $N = 72$ adults	RCT comparing effectiveness of psychoeducation group intervention program with usual care to reduce distress for physical symptom and psychological aspects in breast cancer survivors	Intervention group participated in three educational sessions of the psychoeducation group intervention program; control group booklet on self-management of cancer and treatment-related symptoms	Intervention arm showed reduction in physical symptom distress and fatigue compared with standard care
A culturally adapted DSME intervention [49]	US Marshallese adults $N = 221$ with T2D	RCT comparing standard model DSME with a culturally adapted family model DSME	Adapted DSME included an adapted content, delivered by a Marshallese adult, individually, in patient's home with their family members	Subjects in the adapted DSME group showed lower A1C levels at the end of intervention (0.61%) and 12 months later compared with standard DSME

(continued)

Table 19.3 (continued)

Adaptation	Population	Design	Components	Results
A stepwise approach: (1) identifying cultural needs, (2) evaluating evidence, (3) determining intervention's principles, (4) translating principles into culturally practice, and (5) assessing the content validity [50]	Korean Americans $N = 28$ adults with hypertension	Pre/post intervention	A 10-week of dietary approaches to stop hypertension for Koreans intervention consisted of two structured in-class education sessions with interactive group sessions and individual counseling	After intervention blood pressure and low-density lipoprotein cholesterol decreased significantly. A culturally adapted dietary intervention demonstrated improve dietary pattern and risk factors in Korean Americans
Culturally tailored, community-based CVD prevention using theory of planned behavior and social cognitive theory [51]	US South Asians $N = 23$ participants	Qualitative evaluation	16-week lifestyle intervention including group classes, experiential activities, behavior change counseling, and telephone support	Participants reported that these activities improved their awareness of risk factors and promoted change behaviors
Adaptation of the current children's weight management program delivered in Birmingham, UK, using two theoretical frameworks and evaluation [52]	UK Pakistani and Bangladeshi communities children aged 4–11 years and their families (recruitment goal = 80 children and their families)	Randomized clinical trial allocating culturally adapted program vs existing program	Weight management program includes six sessions delivered to children and parents to improve diet and physical activity, incorporating behavior change techniques; 16 intervention groups were compared with 8 groups of standard care	78.8% of the intervention groups completed the program; the program was highly accepted by children and families

[a]Abbreviations: *A1C* hemoglobin A1c, *DSME* diabetes self-management education, *MNT* medical nutrition therapy, *RCT* randomized controlled trial, *tDNA* transcultural Diabetes Nutrition Algorithm, *T2D* type 2 diabetes, *UK* United Kingdom

Preparing a Lifestyle Medical Center with Transculturalized Care

A Lifestyle Medicine Center must be provided with a set of human (physicians, nurses, nutritionists, exercise physiologists, coaches, psychologists/behavioralists, community healthcare workers, etc.), physical (infrastructure, equipment, and facilities), technological (hardware and software), and specific evidence-based informational resources to optimize the capacity for screening, case finding, prevention, diagnosis, and treatment of chronic diseases for a variety of cultural groups. The scope and breadth of services reflects the cultural diversity of the known catchment area, as well as emergent patient population as the Center operates and evolves over time. For instance, a Lifestyle Medicine Center in a country such as Qatar will, notwithstanding the relatively small geographic size, need more diversified information since 94 different nationalities live there, with only 10.9% of the population are native Qatari [53]. This is in stark contrast with North Korea, which has the lowest immigration rate in the world (0.2% of the total population) [54]. Transcultural elements of the evaluation, diagnosis, and prescription in a Lifestyle Medicine Center are provided in Table 19.4 [6, 55–59].

Staff and Strategies Needed for Cultural Competence

A culturally competent practice recognizes and includes cultural dynamics to improve the interactions between patients and HCPs, and consequently, the effectiveness of healthcare delivery [6]. Personnel should be trained on the three main elements of cultural competency.

1. *Knowledge* about community context, cultural protocols, culturally adapted clinical practice guidelines, and SDOH
2. *Attitudes* toward awareness of cultures and health inequities, education about culture, and respect for cultural differences
3. *Skills* about cross-cultural communication and patient-centered healthcare

These elements can increase patient engagement and acceptance of the service through the perception of respect and cultural safety. Moreover, the elements forge a connection between the patient and HCP, activating the patient for change, and thereby improving chronic care outcomes [6].

Patient-staff interactions depend on language skills. A compassionate and effective staff person must offer the

Table 19.4 Checklist of transcultural resources in the care sequence in a Lifestyle Medicine Center[a]

Transcultural components		Step of the lifestyle medicine evaluation			
		Receiving and attending the patient (A)	Obtaining information (B)	Making the diagnosis (C)	Prescribing lifestyle interventions (D)

Cultural competence (A, B, D)		Staff and HCP training in cultural competence knowledge, attitudes, and skills [6]
		 Cultural competence framework to overcome sociocultural barriers to care at the organizational (leadership/workforce), structural (processes of care), and clinical (HCP/patient encounter) levels [55]
		 Communication strategies according to CLAS standards [56]
		    Staff and HCPs with ethnic-culturally specific communication skills
		    Bilingual staff
		    Language assistant and translation services at no cost and at all points of contact
		    Diversity of HCPs
		 Easily understood patient-related print or multimedia materials and post signage in the languages of the commonly evaluated groups
		 Elaborate in the center's policy handbook
		 Consider ethnic, cultural, and nationality aspects when providing group sessions, education, and prescriptions			

Infrastructure and services (A)		Culturally diverse artwork Distribution of spaces (i.e., separate by gender in Arab cultures) Native music according nationalities of the patients Relaxation spaces Access to regional healthy foods for meals and snacks Restrooms with ethno-cultural considerations Avoid religious symbolism			
Information and software resources	Medical history (B, C)	Health-related social needs and formal SDOH included in the clinical history [57]. Can use the WellRx questionnaire to screen for SDOH (utilities, income, employment, education, food security, housing, transportation, safety, substance abuse, childcare, and abuse) [58]			
	Screening tools and risk scores (B, C)	Culturally customized questionnaires, screening tools, and risk scores for chronic diseases (cardiovascular disease, diabetes, cancer, depression, etc.)			
	Anthropometric and laboratory cutoffs (C)	Software or toolkits containing portable information about anthropometrics, body composition, clinical diagnosis tests, and laboratory/biochemical-specific cutoffs adapted by gender, race, and ethnicity			
	Clinical practice guidelines, algorithms and checklists (C, D)	Clinical practice guidelines and algorithms for screening and decision treatment of chronic diseases with transcultural information Algorithms including physical activity and nutrition Healthy dietary pattern menus classified by caloric content for pertinent ethnic or countries Exercise plans classified by intensity and type considering ethno-cultural particularities and preferences A framework of cultural competence interventions – including minority recruitment into the health professions, development of interpreter services and language-appropriate health educational materials, and HCP education on cross-cultural issues [55]			
	Diagnostic, treatment, and educational tools (D)	Educational programs/curriculum for staff, HCP, patients, and family on cultural aspects of chronic disease and lifestyle medicine Culturally customized and easy to understand educational tools translated to the language needed Real-size food models, including those from specific countries Pedometers and accelerometers to quantify physical activity Informative and educational flyers translated to several languages			
Administrative and organizational (A)		Payment systems (cash payment, direct primary care, fee for service, and concierge) and costs adapted to each country's economy [59] Insurance coverage preferred Strategies to increase accessibility to care and guarantee high quality Culturally adapted clinical protocols. Multidisciplinary approach and efficient use of resources to build and implement outcome-oriented models			

[a]Abbreviations: *CLAS* culturally and linguistically appropriate services, *HCP* healthcare professional, *SDOH* social determinants of health

patient a brief but complete explanation of the evaluation process in a way that is easily understood, and in a manner compatible with health beliefs and practices [56]. The US Department of Health and Human Services Office of Minority Health established National Standards for Culturally and Linguistically Appropriate Services to provide effective, equitable, understandable, and respectful quality care and services that are responsive to diverse cultural health beliefs and practices, preferred languages, literacy, and other communication needs [56].

A multicultural Lifestyle Medicine Center should have at least a few bilingual staff members that speak English and their native language. An inventory for assessing the patient-centered cultural sensitivity of front desk office staff has been proposed [60]. Instruments to enhance communication are discussed in a Brazilian transcultural adaptation developed in Canada (Small Communication Strategies Scale) to improve communicative strategies of caregivers for the elderly with dementia [61].

Infrastructure

The Lifestyle Medicine Center must have basic services that are culturally sensitive and appropriate for a diverse patient population. For example, some non-Arab countries have a significant Muslim population in Europe (e.g., Bosnia-Herzegovina 50.7%), Africa (e.g., Guinea 89.1%), and Southeast Asia (e.g., Indonesia 87.2%) [62]. The restrooms in centers located in these locales should have a bidet to take into account culturally specific toilet rules dictated by Muslim hygiene jurisprudence [63].

Information and Technology

Medical History

A complete medical history should be obtained. Most importantly, this should include SDOH, which can be assessed using standardized screening methods (e.g., the Accountable Health Communities Screening Tool focused on socioeconomics, education, housing instability, food insecurity, transportation, utility needs, and interpersonal safety) [57]. Alternatively, an 11-question instrument (WellRx) can be used [58]. This screening instrument was applied to 3048 patients for SDOH (utilities, income, employment, education, food security, housing, transportation, safety, substance abuse, childcare, and abuse) and piloted in three family medicine clinics over a 90-day period [58]. The WellRx instrument was found to be feasible and capture relevant information. The favorable outcomes with WellRx prompted institutionalization in a university teaching hospital and influenced governmental requirements for

community healthcare workers in health centers to care for Medicaid patients [58].

Screening and Case Finding Tools

In most preventive medicine evaluations, the use of validated screening and aggressive case finding tools are essential. Screening is the process to identify disease risk in subjects at population level (e.g., hypertension, diabetes, and various cancers). Screening tools should be transculturally adapted and validated in different populations to optimize performance. External validations can affirm that various tools can be used in different settings [64]. For example, the Finland Diabetes Risk Score (FINDRISC) is popular worldwide to detect subjects at risk for T2D [65] and has been externally validated in several countries, such as Venezuela [66], Colombia [67, 68], Peru [69], Uruguay [70], Germany [71], New Zealand [72], Belgium [73], Spain [74], Greece [75], and the USA [76–78]. A similar version, only modified by changing waist circumferences to specific cutoffs for the Latino population, has also been validated [68, 79].

On the other hand, aggressive case finding represents a systematic or opportunistic approach to individuals already at risk for a disease to determine the presence of a disease. For example, the FRAX tool (https://www.sheffield.ac.uk/FRAX/; Accessed on March 21, 2020) is implemented in those with risk factors for bone loss and fracture, calibrated to different populations, and based on meta-analyses of large-scale population-based studies, including the descriptors: age, sex, body mass index (BMI), fracture history, parental hip fracture, current smoking, excessive alcohol intake, rheumatoid arthritis, glucocorticoid use, and other forms of secondary osteoporosis [80–83].

Erroneous risk stratifications can be avoided if software with normative data by ethno-cultural groupings is used. This applies to predictors of morbidity and mortality for all relevant chronic disease states encountered by the Lifestyle Medicine Center. Risk classifiers (high, intermediate, low) are based on various anthropometric, biochemical, and clinical descriptors, each of which is defined by ethno-cultural population data. For example, using data from 73 centers worldwide, multi-ethnic reference values for spirometry have been published for those between 3 and 95 years old [84]. Waist circumference has also been customized based on ethno-cultural populations [10, 85]. Region- and ethnic-specific cutoff point values in South Asian, Southeast Asian, and East Asian adults (men ≥85 cm and women ≥74–80 cm), USA and Canada (men ≥102 cm and women ≥88 cm), and Latin America [86] (men >94 cm and women >90 cm) to detect abdominal obesity have been proposed.

Waist circumference and BMI do not accurately capture adiposity risk at all levels of obesity, ethnicity, gender, and age. BMI cutoffs for identifying excess adiposity and the risk of cardiometabolic disease are even lower for some ethnicities. For example, in South Asian, Southeast Asian, and East Asian people, a BMI cutoff between 23.0 and 24.9 kg/m^2 (inclusive) has been proposed for overweight and ≥25 kg/m^2 for obesity. More specifically, the "Asian Indian" phenotype refers to a person with greater insulin resistance, abdominal obesity, and lower ß-cell activity, with increased risk for T2D and cardiovascular disease at lower BMI [87]. In addition, mildly higher BMI (e.g., > 25 kg/m^2) could classify some subjects as lower risk, even though they have abnormal adiposity – particularly adiposity distribution – with body fat localization detected by imaging [88]. Analysis of the Third NHANES [89] and a cohort from Venezuela [90] demonstrate that a BMI 25.0–29.9 kg/m^2 may underestimate the prevalence of obesity by 50% and 21%, respectively, compared with body fat measurements by bioimpedance analysis. Thus, a cutoff >27.5 kg/m^2 to detect obesity can be used in Venezuelans [10, 34, 90]. Body mass index cannot be interpreted in the same way in the Netherlands where the average height in men is the highest in the world (182.5 cm) compared to Guatemalan women born in 1984 with the lowest height globally (140.3 cm) [91]. In this latter population, high BMI values overestimate the real proportion of the obese population. New approaches to conceptualize cardiometabolic-based chronic disease along a continuum, and initialized by primary drivers (genetics, environment, and behavior) and impelled by metabolic drivers (adiposity-based chronic disease and dysglycemia-based chronic disease) have been recently described [92]. These new chronic disease models are part of complications-centric approaches that rely less on numerical definitions that vary among different ethno-cultural populations, and more on pathophysiological correlates and targets for early and sustainable prevention.

Culturally Adapting White Papers

White papers are authoritative documents written by professional organizations on a specific topic, and in medicine, these can take the form of clinical practice guidelines, position papers, conference proceedings, technical reviews, algorithms, and checklists. White papers are portable tools that can be applied from one population to another when evidence-based recommendations are culturally adapted and then readily available for clinical decision-making. Multiple clinical practice guidelines containing lifestyle recommendations have been published for a wide range of chronic diseases including dyslipidemia [93], cardiovascular disease [94, 95], obesity [96], diabetes [97, 98], cancer [99], obstructive sleep apnea [100], menopause [101], osteoporosis [102], arthritis [103], and dementia [104]. Some of these include transcultural adaptations [98], whereas others were developed to present specific transcultural topics. Transcultural aspects of endocrine disorders in Latin America [105] (diabetes, obesity, osteoporosis, and thyroid disease) and recommendations to adapt diabetes management globally have

been developed [13]. Some of these recommendations have been delivered in more portable presentations as algorithms (diabetes [106] and tDNA [27]). More in-depth transcultural information for lifestyle interventions, especially nutrition and physical activity recommendations, has been reviewed elsewhere [10, 11].

Diagnostic and Educational Tools

Real-size food models of typical foods for specific countries, and wearable pedometers or accelerometers to quantify physical activity, are useful tools to have available in a Lifestyle Medicine Center. A software or toolkit containing translations of the food names in different languages and even the name's variations in different countries of the same language is very useful when making nutritional recommendations. Those Lifestyle Medicine Centers with exercise facilities can provide representations of typical exercises using images and videos of humans of different races and ethnicities.

Administrative and Organizational Issues

A Lifestyle Medicine Center must develop an evidence-based structure that provides state-of-the-art care to achieve the highest clinical outcomes, while also optimizing resources in a cost-efficient way to promote sustainability. Clinical protocols and policies need to be developed that consider ethnic, cultural, and other considerations for minority populations to promote universal access to health services, without any of the disparities that currently exist. When considering centers in other countries, costs and administrative issues must be adapted to different economies, currencies, socioeconomics, and political situations. Depending on a variety of operational, economic, and marketing factors, insurance coverage needs to be clarified. Some successful models of reimbursement of lifestyle medicine interventions [107] and recommendations to create Lifestyle Medicine Centers in the USA [59] have been proposed.

Case Studies

Case 1. Japanese Patient in Brazil for Diabetes Risk Screening

Patient Presentation

A 36-year-old Japanese male is evaluated in a healthcare center in São Paulo, Brazil. He wants to know if he has T2D because, ever since arriving in Brazil, his dietary habits have worsened, resulting in weight gain and increased fasting blood sugar.

Cultural Factors

The Japanese population of Brazil is estimated at 1.6 million and is the largest in the world outside of Japan [108]. The attending Brazilian physician interpreted the BMI of 24.3 kg/m² and the waist circumference of 94 cm as normal based on criteria for the Caucasian population. The patient reported a previous fasting blood glucose of 115 mg/dl, but today's blood glucose was 90 mg/dl. As he did not find any other associated risk factor, the doctor recommended a new evaluation in 1 year and gave him a pamphlet with healthy recipes for the Brazilian population. Because the patient's father developed diabetes at age 28, the patient visited another doctor who recommended an oral glucose tolerance test, resulting in a blood glucose level at 2 hours post-challenge to be 234 mg/dl (diagnostic for T2D).

Discussion

What transcultural components were not considered the first encounter? At hemoglobin A1c levels below 7.1%, postprandial hyperglycemia in Asians contributes more to excess hyperglycemia than fasting glycemia [109], contributing to the development of T2D at younger ages and lower degrees of adiposity. Asians are considered to be overweight with BMI ≥23 kg/m² and obesity with BMI ≥25 kg/m² [10]. A specific waist circumference cutoff of 85 cm for men and 90 cm for women was recommended in the Japanese population based on correlation with 100 cm² of visceral fat area obtained by computed tomography scan [110]. According to the adiposity-based chronic disease protocol [96], Asians with a BMI ≥ 23 kg/m² need to be evaluated for weight-related complications, and a checklist consulted for durable care as provided by published clinical practice guidelines [96].

The initial approach should have more diligently pursued management of T2D. A noninvasive diabetes risk score from a Japanese cohort has been developed and its application could have detected a higher risk in this patient [111]. A cross-cultural adaptation of the interventions modeled by the Finnish Diabetes Prevention Study has been developed for South Asians, which could have been used as a framework to implement lifestyle strategies with specific considerations according to the country where he is living [112]. Medical nutritional therapy and the algorithmic steps of screening, case finding, risk stratification, intervention, and follow-up can be applied using the Asian version of the tDNA [28]. In this approach, nutritional recommendations incorporate cultural preferences. Considering the high consumption of dietary rice [28] and prevalence of postprandial hyperglycemia [109] in Asians, a useful recommendation is to reduce consumption of carbohydrates with a high glycemic index, such as "glutinous" short-grain rice and porridge, and replace or mix them with grains and/or pulses with a lower glycemic index [113]. Healthy eating should be coupled with physical activity, and most Asian medical professional organizations recommend 150 min per week of moderate-intensity exercise for patients with diabetes as part of their comprehensive management strategy [28].

Case 2. African American Female in Memphis, Tennessee, for Cardiovascular Risk Reduction

Patient Presentation

A 71-year-old African American woman with multiple chronic conditions and strong family history of heart disease is referred to a Lifestyle Medicine Center to reduce her cardiovascular disease risks. In this center, 27% of the served patients are African American [114]. The patient increased coughing and shortness of breath with a long-standing history of tobacco use (about 1 pack/day for over 50 years), high blood pressure, and weight loss. After her husband passed away 2 years ago, she lives alone, developed major depression, and increased alcohol and tobacco consumption significantly. Her only daughter lives in Chicago.

Cultural Factors

Transcultural factors that are also SDOH were incorporated into the evaluation of this patient. A diligent, compassionate, and culturally competent staff with knowledge, attitudes, and skills received the patient in the center, and the patient perceived respect from all the personnel. The chronic disease model-based protocol included individualized case finding and risk stratification with a detailed history focusing on modifiable cardiovascular risk factors, anthropometric assessment (e.g., weight, height, waist circumference, and % body fat determinations using bioimpedance), physical examination, and biochemical evaluation using validated markers (e.g., hemoglobin A1c, C-reactive protein, and lipids). Noninvasive cardiac testing followed.

A critical part of the transcultural approach for different ethnicities within American society is the formal assessment of SDOH [115]. Questionnaires can be created and presented to patients in the reception area prior to each encounter to capture this information. This patient did not complete high school. Although her house has the benefit of all necessary utilities (water, electricity, gas, etc.), housing instability (e.g., difficulty with rent or mortgage payments, overcrowding, moving frequently, and/or staying with relatives) was detected, and in response to perceptions of isolation and medical risk, her daughter is planning to relocate her to a nursing home facility. Food insecurity, defined both as a limited or uncertain availability of nutritionally adequate and innocuous foods, or the incapacity for acquiring them by socially acceptable means [116], in the last year was also reported. Annual income categorized her in low income/poverty status. She maintains her medical insurance but stopped taking some of her medications because of the lack of transportation to pick up them. Several additional specific questionnaires were applied in this patient: Cognition was intact by Montreal Cognitive Assessment [117], Geriatric Depression Scale (short version 15 items) was consistent with severe depression [118], and a Mini Nutritional Assessment (short version) < 17 categorized her to have protein-calorie malnutrition [119].

The current weight was 48 kg (compared with 66 kg, 2 years earlier); height 1.63 m; BMI 18.1 kg/m² (low); body fat: 13% (low); handgrip strength 14 kg force (low); and blood pressure 125/78 mmHg (normal on lisinopril 40 mg/day). Loss of subcutaneous fat with loss of temporal and supraclavicular muscle was detected. Chest auscultation detected expiratory wheeze and she uses accessory muscles when short of breath. Oral exam reveals tooth loss and periodontal disease. There is no peripheral edema.

Significant laboratory results include Hgb 9.6 g/L (low); total cholesterol 120 mg/dl (low); albumin 3.3 mg/dl (low); creatinine 1.28 mg/dl (high); estimated glomerular filtration rate (eGFR) 52 mL/min/1.73m² (chronic kidney disease 3a for African Americans) [120]; and 25-hydroxyvitamin D 26 ng/ml (low for Caucasian population, but normal for African Americans). Spirometry reported a forced expiratory volume first second (FEV1) of 1.04 L (37% of predictive value for African Americans), forced vital capacity (FVC) of 2.03 L (61% of predictive value for African Americans), and FEV1/FVC of 51% (low; normal >80%) with both obstructive and restrictive findings. Chronic conditions diagnosed during the evaluation included chronic obstructive pulmonary disease, anemia, chronic kidney disease stage 3A due to hypertension, depression, and both tobacco and alcohol use disorder. Based on muscular strength and muscle mass, a sarcopenia diagnosis was also established. Multiple factors for malnutrition were detected: poor dentition, depression, living alone, functional status, multiple chronic diseases, and food insecurity.

The availability of proper information and culturally specific anthropometric and laboratory cutoffs led to higher diagnostic accuracy for risk factors and chronic diseases amenable to lifestyle medicine interventions. Mild cognitive impairment was evaluated with the Montreal Cognitive Assessment, which has demonstrated its cross-cultural applicability [117]. The Geriatric Depression Scale has been widely used in ethno-culturally diverse elderly medical patient populations (i.e., Asians, African Americans, Mexican Americans) and has demonstrated good internal consistency and stability over a 15-month interval in African Americans [118]. The Mini Nutritional Assessment (MNA) has also demonstrated reliability in defining the nutritional state of elderly patients [119] and has been validated in different cultures [121–123]. The predicted percentage body fat measured by dual X-ray absorptiometry for African American women between 60 and 79 years corresponding to a BMI <18.5 is 23% [124]. Therefore, a finding of 13% in this patient corresponds to low energy stores, chronic negative energy balance, and nutritional risk [124]. Vitamin D insufficiency is established from the point at which serum intact parathyroid hormone levels significantly rise [125]. The 25-hydroxyvitamin D thresholds for insufficiency are approximately 20 ng/ml for African Americans versus approximately 30 ng/ml in Caucasians [126]. Thus, in this patient, a level of 25-hydroxyvitamin D of 26 ng/ml is considered normal. If the specific eGFR cut-off point for African Americans had not been considered and a default Caucasian calculation performed, the patient (age 71 years and serum creatinine 1.28 mg/dl) would have been categorized with chronic kidney disease 3b (eGFR 43 mL/min/1.73m²) instigating possible unnecessary therapeutic interventions. Compared with Caucasians, African American females have 13.8% less FEV1 and 14.4% less FVC [84]. In sum, the use of specific ethno-culturally adjusted predictive data is recommended for routine encounters and interpretation of a host of metrics in a Lifestyle Medicine Center.

Discussion

Interventions for all aspects of the lifestyle medicine evaluation must be considered. A physical rehabilitation protocol to stop and overcome sarcopenia and frailty was designed with supervised resistance training, which is demonstrated to improve muscle strength and physical performance [127]. Recommendations for older patients are available [128]. The tDNA [34] includes physical activity recommendations to start at low intensity for this patient: aerobic (slow walking and/or stationary cycling) for a minimum of 10 minutes to increase the pulse rate less than 40% of the maximum heart rate. The progressive resistance training program should initially involve at least three large muscle groups (e.g., quadriceps, biceps, and triceps) with two sets of 10 repetitions per muscle group, performed on three nonconsecutive days per week. Flexibility and balance exercises include stretching to the point of tightness and holding the position for a few seconds on all days that aerobic or muscle-strengthening activity is performed. Balance training exercise should occur two to three times per week. The lack of transportation and living alone (social isolation) are barriers to physical rehabilitation, so the use of an outpatient physiotherapist, wearable technology, and a Center's app are good alternatives while the patient gains autonomy in their daily tasks. Patient's preferences should always be considered. Motivations (e.g., perceived health benefits, social support, and enjoyment) and barriers (e.g., time, physical limitations, peer pressure, family responsibilities, weather, and poor neighborhood conditions) for physical activity have been identified in older African American women [129]. Dancing in groups and other modalities as tai chi or yoga were preferred choices and are easy to customize based on cultural preferences [129].

Medical nutritional therapy is an important component of lifestyle medicine. This patient's preference is African American cuisine, including barbecued meats, sweet cornbread, fried chicken, and desserts. Sides include black-eyed peas, candied yams, macaroni and cheese, and stewed greens. Thus, a nutritional recommendation was made based on detailed conversations between the patient and the nutritionist. An individualized healthy eating plan was fashioned considering physiological changes (poor dentition and less sense of taste), customs, and preferences. Cultural attitudes toward dietary supplements should be explored prior to their prescription. Parenthetically, diabetes-specific formulas should be used in cases of dysglycemia. Sleep hygiene recommendations are routinely providing and should include at least 7 hours of sleep. The management of depression and excessive use of tobacco and alcohol was also addressed.

Conclusion

Globalization creates more racially, ethnically, and culturally diverse societies and medical practices. The USA is projected to become a majority-minority country, and by the year 2044, "minority" populations will become the majority nationwide [130]. This represents a major challenge to HCPs and those interested in building Lifestyle Medicine Centers. The modern healthcare system must provide culturally tailored lifestyle recommendations and avoid health disparities as part of this new Lifestyle Medicine Clinical Service Line. Different cultures, religions, beliefs, and contexts can influence how patients adopt lifestyle recommendations. Lifestyle components need to be adapted to cultures anticipated to be encountered in the Lifestyle Medicine Center. Transculturalization describes the process of how experts can adapt evidence-based information from one culture to another, and frameworks, such as the EVM, provide a checklist to consider all the involved components. The tDNA is a good example of cultural adaptations of lifestyle recommendations for those with dysglycemia and consists mainly of medical nutritional therapy for application to different countries and regions of the world. The relevant recommendation here is that besides considering the scientific evidence concerning management of chronic disease risk factors or complications, the HCP should ask patients about their beliefs and customs, assess cultural factors and SDOH, and together, create strategies and tactics that improve behaviors and realize optimal outcomes.

Glossary

Culture [131]   Belief systems and values that influence customs, standards, practices, and social institutions, including psychological aspects (language, care, practices, media, educational systems) and organizations.

Race [13]   Clustering of only physical or genetic attributes common to a category of people.

Ethnicity [13]   Clustering that incorporates not only culture and race but also emphasizes on genealogy, ancestry, geography (region), linguistics, and political ideology.

Acculturation [13]   Changes in culture that occur when two or more cultures interact.

Deculturation [13]   Process of adapting one culture to another losing the previous culture.

Neoculturation [13]   Process of adapting one culture to another creating a new culture.

Transculturation [13]   Creation of a new culture when two or more cultures merge.

Transculturalization [13] Process of adapting concepts from one culture to another, without changing either culture, through local experts from both source and target cultures in an interactive setting.

Transcultural adaptation [13, 15, 40]   Systematic modification of an evidence-based intervention to consider language, culture, and context to be compatible with the participant's cultural patterns, meanings, and values. Transcultural adaptation offers guidance on how to adapt an intervention to increase its fit for the target population.

Cultural competence [6] A set of consistent behaviors, attitudes, and policies that enable a system, agency, or individual to work within a cross-cultural context or situation effectively.

Implementation research [40, 132] Development and application of scientific methods to promote incorporation of evidence-based interventions into routine healthcare in clinical, organizational, public health, or policy contexts. Answer the question how implementation of an effective program works in specific contexts.

References

1. National Academies of Sciences. The state of health disparities in the United States. In: Baciu A, Negussie Y, Geller A, Weinstein JN, editors. Communities in action: pathways to health equity. Washington, DC: National Academies Press; 2017. https://www.ncbi.nlm.nih.gov/books/NBK425844/. Accessed on 19 Mar 2020.
2. Xierali IM, Nivet MA. The racial and ethnic composition and distribution of primary care physicians. J Health Care Poor Underserved. 2018;29:556–70.
3. Bodai BI, Nakata TE, Wong WT, et al. Lifestyle medicine: a brief review of its dramatic impact on health and survival. Perm J. 2018;22:17–25.

4. Velasquez-Mieyer PA, Cowan PA, Perez-Faustinelli S, et al. Racial disparity in glucagon-like peptide 1 and inflammation markers among severely obese adolescents. Diabetes Care. 2008;31:770–5.

5. Ashton CM, Haidet P, Paterniti DA, et al. Racial and ethnic disparities in the use of health services: bias, preferences, or poor communication? J Gen Intern Med. 2003;18:146–52.

6. Watt K, Abbott P, Reath J. Developing cultural competence in general practitioners: an integrative review of the literature. BMC Fam Pract. 2016;17:158.

7. Checchi F, Warsame A, Treacy-Wong V, et al. Public health information in crisis-affected populations: a review of methods and their use for advocacy and action. Lancet. 2017;390:2297–313.

8. Mitchell T, Weinberg M, Posey DL, et al. Immigrant and refugee health: a Centers for Disease Control and Prevention perspective on protecting the health and health security of individuals and communities during planned migrations. Pediat Clin North Am. 2019;66:549–60.

9. Grabovac I, Smith L, Stefanac S, et al. Health care providers' advice on lifestyle modification in the US population: results from the NHANES 2011-2016. Am J Med. 2019;132:489–97.

10. Hegazi RA, Devitt AA, Mechanick JI. The transcultural Diabetes Nutrition Algorithm: from concept to implementation. In: Watson RR, Dokken BB, editors. Glucose intake and utilization in prediabetes and diabetes implications for cardiovascular disease. Amsterdam: Elsevier Inc.; 2015. p. 269–80.

11. Hamdy O, Mechanick JI. Transcultural applications to lifestyle medicine. In: Mechanick JI, Kushner RF, editors. Lifestyle medicine: a manual for clinical practice. New York: Springer; 2016. p. 183–90.

12. Rabin B, Brownson R. Developing the terminology for dissemination and implementation research. In: Brownson R, Colditz G, Proctor E, editors. Dissemination and implementation research in health: translating science to practice. Oxford University Press: New York, NY; 2012. p. 23–51.

13. Nieto-Martinez R, Gonzalez-Rivas JP, Florez H, et al. Transcultural endocrinology: adapting type-2 diabetes guidelines on a global scale. Endocrinol Metab Clin N Am. 2016;45:967–1009.

14. Mechanick JI, Camacho PM, Garber AJ, et al. American Association of Clinical Endocrinologists and American College of Endocrinology Protocol for Standardized Production of Clinical Practice Guidelines, Algorithms, and Checklists – 2014 Update and the AACE G4G Program. Endocr Pract. 2014;20:692–702.

15. Bernal G, Jiménez-Chafey M, Domenech R. Cultural adaptation of treatments: a resource for considering culture in evidence-based practice. Prof Psychol Res Pract. 2009;40:361–8.

16. Proctor E, Silmere H, Raghavan R, et al. Outcomes for implementation research: conceptual distinctions, measurement challenges, and research agenda. Admin Pol Ment Health. 2011;38:65–76.

17. Center for Disease Control and Prevention (CDC). NCHHSTP Social Determinants of Health. https://www.cdc.gov/nchhstp/socialdeterminants/faq.html. Accessed on 1 Apr 2019.

18. Medina-Inojosa J, Jean N, Cortes-Bergoderi M, et al. The Hispanic paradox in cardiovascular disease and total mortality. Prog Cardiovasc Dis. 2014;57:286–92.

19. Mignone J, Bartlett J, O'Neil J, et al. Best practices in intercultural health: five case studies in Latin America. J Ethnobiol Ethnomed. 2007;3:31.

20. Habtom GK. Integrating traditional medical practice with primary healthcare system in Eritrea. J Complement Integr Med. 2015;12:71–87.

21. Herrera D, Hutchins F, Gaus D, et al. Intercultural health in Ecuador: an asymmetrical and incomplete project. Anthropol Med. 2019;26:328–44.

22. Labhardt ND, Aboa SM, Manga E, et al. Bridging the gap: how traditional healers interact with their patients. A comparative study in Cameroon. Trop Med Int Health. 2010;15:1099–108.

23. Koenig HG. Religion, spirituality, and health: the research and clinical implications. ISRN Psychiatry. 2012;2012:278730. https://doi.org/10.5402/2012/278730.

24. UK Prospective Diabetes Study Group. Effect of intensive blood glucose control with metformin on complications in overweight patients with type 2 diabetes (UKPDS 34). Lancet. 1998;352:854–65.

25. Schlundt DG, Franklin MD, Patel K, et al. Religious affiliation, health behaviors and outcomes: Nashville REACH 2010. Am J Health Behav. 2008;32:714–24.

26. Rathod S, Gega L, Degnan A, et al. The current status of culturally adapted mental health interventions: a practice-focused review of meta-analyses. Neuropsychiatr Dis Treat. 2018;14:165–78.

27. Mechanick JI, Marchetti AE, Apovian C, et al. Diabetes-specific nutrition algorithm: a transcultural program to optimize diabetes and prediabetes care. Curr Diab Rep. 2012;12:180–94.

28. Su HY, Tsang MW, Huang SY, et al. Transculturalization of a diabetes-specific nutrition algorithm: Asian application. Curr Diab Rep. 2012;12:213–9.

29. Joshi SR, Mohan V, Joshi SS, et al. Transcultural diabetes nutrition therapy algorithm: the Asian Indian application. Curr Diab Rep. 2012;12:204–12.

30. Hussein Z, Hamdy O, Chin Chia Y, et al. Transcultural diabetes nutrition algorithm: a Malaysian application. Int J Endocrinol. 2013;2013:679396.

31. Gougeon R, Sievenpiper JL, Jenkins D, et al. The transcultural diabetes nutrition algorithm: a Canadian perspective. Int J Endocrinol. 2014;151068:16.

32. Galvis AB, Hamdy O, Pulido ME, et al. Transcultural diabetes nutrition algorithm: the Mexican application. J Diabetes Metab. 2014;5:1–10.

33. Moura F, Salles J, Hamdy O, et al. Transcultural Diabetes Nutrition Algorithm: Brazilian application. Nutrients. 2015;7:7358–80.

34. Nieto-Martinez R, Hamdy O, Marante D, et al. Transcultural Diabetes Nutrition Algorithm (tDNA): Venezuelan application. Nutrients. 2014;6:1333–63.

35. Winnie S S Chee, Harvinder Kaur Gilcharan Singh, Osama Hamdy, Jeffrey I Mechanick, Verna K M Lee, Ankur Barua, Siti Zubaidah Mohd Ali, Zanariah Hussein, (2017) Structured lifestyle intervention based on a trans-cultural diabetes-specific nutrition algorithm (tDNA) in individuals with type 2 diabetes: a randomized controlled trial. BMJ Open Diabetes Research & Care 5 (1):e000384.

36. Arab American Institute. Accessed on September 15, 2019. Available online: https://www.aaiusa.org/state-profiles.

37. Ali MK, Bullard KM, Saydah S, et al. Cardiovascular and renal burdens of prediabetes in the USA: analysis of data from serial cross-sectional surveys, 1988-2014. Lancet Diabetes Endocrinol. 2018;6:392–403.

38. American Diabetes Association. 3. Prevention or Delay of Type 2 Diabetes: Standards of Medical Care in Diabetes-2020. Diabetes Care. 2020;43(Suppl 1): S32–6.

39. Bernal G, Bonilla J, Bellido C. Ecological validity and cultural sensitivity for outcome research: issues for the cultural adaptation and development of psychosocial treatments with Hispanics. J Abnorm Child Psychol. 1995;23:67–82.

40. Tabak RG, Sinclair KA, Baumann AA, et al. A review of diabetes prevention program translations: use of cultural adaptation and implementation research. Transl Behav Med. 2015;5:401–14.

41. Attum B, Waheed A, Shamoon Z. Cultural competence in the care of muslim patients and their families. Treasure Island, FL: StatPearls Publishing LLC; 2019.

42. Pinelli NR, Jaber LA. Practices of Arab American patients with type 2 diabetes mellitus during Ramadan. J Pharm Pract. 2011;24:211–5.

43. Tailakh AK, Evangelista LS, Morisky DE, et al. Acculturation, medication adherence, lifestyle behaviors, and blood pressure control among Arab Americans. J Transcult Nurs. 2016;27:57–64.
44. Berry J. Acculturation: living successfully in two cultures. Internat J Intercult Relat. 2005;29:697–712.
45. Mattei J, McClain AC, Falcon LM, et al. Dietary acculturation among Puerto Rican adults varies by acculturation construct and dietary measure. J Nutr. 2018;148:1804–13.
46. Tami SH, Reed DB, Boylan M, et al. Assessment of the effect of acculturation on dietary and physical activity behaviors of Arab mothers in Lubbock, Texas. Ethnicity Dis. 2012;22:192–7.
47. Chee WSS, Gilcharan Singh HK, et al. Structured lifestyle intervention based on a transcultural diabetes-specific nutrition algorithm (tDNA) in individuals with type 2 diabetes: a randomized controlled trial. BMJ Open Diabetes Res Care. 2017;5:e000384.
48. Chan A, Gan YX, Oh SK, et al. A culturally adapted survivorship programme for Asian early stage breast cancer patients in Singapore: a randomized, controlled trial. Psycho-Oncology. 2017;26:1654–9.
49. McElfish PA, Long CR, Kohler PO, et al. Comparative effectiveness and maintenance of diabetes self-management education interventions for Marshallese patients with type 2 diabetes: a randomized controlled trial. Diabetes Care. 2019;42:849–58.
50. Kim H, Song H-J, Han H-R, et al. Translation and validation of the dietary approaches to stop hypertension for koreans intervention: culturally tailored dietary guidelines for Korean Americans with high blood pressure. J Cardiovasc Nurs. 2013;28:514–23.
51. Jayaprakash M, Puri-Taneja A, Kandula NR, et al. Qualitative process evaluation of a community-based culturally tailored lifestyle intervention for underserved South Asians. Health Promot Pract. 2016;17:802–13.
52. Pallan M, Griffin T, Hurley KL, et al. Cultural adaptation of an existing children's weight management programme: the CHANGE intervention and feasibility RCT. Health Technol Assess. 2019;23:1–166.
53. Communications PD. Population of Qatar by nationality – 2019 report. http://priyadsouza.com/population-of-qatar-by-nationality-in-2017/. Accessed on 1 Sept 2019.
54. Nations U. Trends in International Migrant Stock: The 2015 Revision. United Nations Department of Economic and Social Affairs, Population Division, 2015. https://www.un.org/en/development/desa/population/migration/data/estimates2/estimates15.asp. Accessed on 1 Sept 2019.
55. Betancourt JR, Green AR, Carrillo JE, et al. Defining cultural competence: a practical framework for addressing racial/ethnic disparities in health and health care. Public Health Rep. 2003;118:293–302.
56. Estrada RD, Messias DK. A scoping review of the literature: content, focus, conceptualization and application of the National Standards for Culturally and Linguistically Appropriate Services in Health Care. J Health Care Poor Underserved. 2015;26:1089–109.
57. Billioux A, Verlander K, Anthony S, et al. Standardized screening for health-related social needs in clinical settings the accountable health communities screening tool. In: Perspectives expert voices in health health care: National Academy of Medicine; 2017. p. 1–9.
58. Page-Reeves J, Kaufman W, Bleecker M, et al. Addressing social determinants of health in a clinic setting: the WellRx pilot in Albuquerque, New Mexico. J Am Board Fam Med. 2016;29:414–8.
59. Braman M, Edison M. How to create a successful lifestyle medicine practice. Am J Lifestyle Med. 2017;11:404–7.
60. Tucker CM, Wall W, Marsiske M, et al. Validation of a patient-centered culturally sensitive health care office staff inventory. Prim Health Care Res Develop. 2015;16:506–12.
61. Delfino LL, Komatsu RS, Komatsu C, et al. Brazilian transcultural adaptation of an instrument on communicative strategies of caregivers of elderly with dementia. Dementia Neuropsychologia. 2017;11:242–8.
62. Islam by country. Accessed on September 15, 2019. Available online: https://en.wikipedia.org/wiki/Islam_by_country#Table.
63. Rizvi SSA. Elements of Islamic Studies. Bilal Muslim Mission of Tanzania 1983, 4th Ed. https://www.al-islam.org/printpdf/book/export/html/30714. Accessed on 19 Mar 2020.
64. Altman DG, Vergouwe Y, Royston P, et al. Prognosis and prognostic research: validating a prognostic model. BMJ. 2009;338:b605.
65. Noble D, Mathur R, Dent T, et al. Risk models and scores for type 2 diabetes: systematic review. BMJ. 2011;343:d7163.
66. Nieto-Martinez R, Gonzalez-Rivas JP, Ugel E, et al. External validation of the Finnish diabetes risk score in Venezuela using a national sample: the EVESCAM. Prim Care Diabetes. 2019;13:574–82.
67. Gomez-Arbelaez D, Alvarado-Jurado L, Ayala-Castillo M, et al. Evaluation of the Finnish Diabetes Risk Score to predict type 2 diabetes mellitus in a Colombian population: a longitudinal observational study. World J Diabetes. 2015;6:1337–44.
68. Nieto-Martinez R, Gonzalez-Rivas JP, Aschner P, et al. Transculturalizing diabetes prevention in Latin America. Ann Glob Health. 2017;83:432–43.
69. Bernabe-Ortiz A, Perel P, Miranda JJ, et al. Diagnostic accuracy of the Finnish Diabetes Risk Score (FINDRISC) for undiagnosed T2DM in Peruvian population. Prim Care Diabetes. 2018;12:517–25.
70. Vignoli DA, Connio E, Aschner P. Evaluation of the Findrisc as a screening tool for people with impaired glucose regulation in Uruguay using a modified score with validated regional cutoff values for abdominal obesity. Poster presented at 8th World Congress on Prevention of Diabetes and its Complications Cartagena, Colombia Poster # 53, 2015.
71. Bergmann A, Li J, Wang L, et al. A simplified Finnish diabetes risk score to predict type 2 diabetes risk and disease evolution in a German population. Horm Metab Res. 2007;39:677–82.
72. Silvestre MP, Jiang Y, Volkova K, et al. Evaluating FINDRISC as a screening tool for type 2 diabetes among overweight adults in the PREVIEW:NZ cohort. Prim Care Diabetes. 2017;11:561–9.
73. Meijnikman AS, De Block CE, Verrijken A, et al. Screening for type 2 diabetes mellitus in overweight and obese subjects made easy by the FINDRISC score. J Diabetes Complicat. 2016;30:1043–9.
74. Soriguer F, Valdes S, Tapia MJ, et al. Validation of the FINDRISC (FINnish Diabetes RIsk SCore) for prediction of the risk of type 2 diabetes in a population of southern Spain. Pizarra Study. Med Clin. 2012;138:371–6.
75. Makrilakis K, Liatis S, Grammatikou S, et al. Validation of the Finnish diabetes risk score (FINDRISC) questionnaire for screening for undiagnosed type 2 diabetes, dysglycaemia and the metabolic syndrome in Greece. Diabetes Metab. 2011;37:144–51.
76. Zhang Y, Hu G, Zhang L, et al. A novel testing model for opportunistic screening of pre-diabetes and diabetes among U.S. adults. PLoS One. 2015;10:e0120382.
77. Zhang L, Zhang Z, Zhang Y, et al. Evaluation of Finnish Diabetes Risk Score in screening undiagnosed diabetes and prediabetes among U.S. adults by gender and race: NHANES 1999–2010. PLoS One. 2014;9:e97865.
78. Kulkarni M, Foraker RE, McNeill AM, et al. Evaluation of the modified FINDRISC to identify individuals at high risk for diabetes among middle-aged white and black ARIC study participants. Diabetes Obes Metab. 2017;19:1260–6.
79. Aschner P, Nieto-Martinez R, Marin A, et al. Evaluation of the FINDRISC score as a screening tool for people with impaired glucose regulation in Latin America using modified score points for waist circumference according to the validated regional cutoff values for abdominal obesity. Minerva Endocrinol. 2012;37:114.

80. Tobias JH. Clinical features of osteoporosis. In: Hochberg MC, Silman AJ, Smolen JS, Weinblatt ME, Weisman MH, editors. Rheumatology. 6th ed. Philadelphia, PA: Elsevier Mosby; 2015. p. 1641–9.

81. Zerbini CA, Szejnfeld VL, Abergaria BH, et al. Incidence of hip fracture in Brazil and the development of a FRAX model. Arch Osteopor. 2015;10:224.

82. Lalmohamed A, Welsing PMJ, Lems WF, et al. Calibration of FRAX 3.1 to the Dutch population with data on the epidemiology of hip fractures. Osteopor Internat. 2012;23:861–9.

83. Grigorie D, Sucaliuc A, Johansson H, et al. Incidence of hip fracture in Romania and the development of a Romanian FRAX model. Calcif Tissue Internat. 2013;92:429–36.

84. Quanjer PH, Stanojevic S, Cole TJ, et al. Multi-ethnic reference values for spirometry for the 3–95-yr age range: the global lung function 2012 equations. Eur Resp J. 2012;40:1324–43.

85. Alberti KG, Zimmet P, Shaw J. The metabolic syndrome--a new worldwide definition. Lancet. 2005;366:1059–62.

86. Aschner P, Buendia R, Brajkovich I, et al. Determination of the cutoff point for waist circumference that establishes the presence of abdominal obesity in Latin American men and women. Diabetes Res Clin Pract. 2011;93:243–7.

87. Bodhini D, Mohan V. Mediators of insulin resistance & cardiometabolic risk: newer insights. Indian J Med Res. 2018;148:127–9.

88. Neeland IJ, Poirier P, Després J-P. Cardiovascular and metabolic heterogeneity of obesity: clinical challenges and implications for management. Circulation. 2018;137:1391–406.

89. Romero-Corral A, Somers VK, Sierra-Johnson J, et al. Accuracy of body mass index in diagnosing obesity in the adult general population. Internat J Obes. 2008;32:959–66.

90. Nieto-Martínez R, Perez Y, Suarez MA, et al. A BMI of 27.5 can improve the detection of obesity in a Venezuelan population. Diabetes. 2013;62:A750.

91. NCD Risk Factor Collaboration. A century of trends in adult human height. elife. 2016;5:e13410. https://doi.org/10.7554/eLife.13410.

92. Mechanick JI, Farkouh ME, Newman JD, Garvey WT. Cardiometabolic-based chronic disease – adiposity and dysglycemia drivers. J Am Coll Cardiol. 2020;75:525–38.

93. Grundy SM, Stone NJ. 2018 Cholesterol Clinical Practice Guidelines: Synopsis of the 2018 American Heart Association/American College of Cardiology/Multisociety Cholesterol Guideline. Ann Intern Med. 2019;170:779–83.

94. Jellinger PS, Handelsman Y, Rosenblit PD, et al. American Association of Clinical Endocrinologists and American College of Endocrinology guidelines for management of dyslipidemia and prevention fo cardiovascular idsease. Endocr Pract. 2017;23:1–87.

95. Rosenzweig JL, Bakris GL, Berglund LF, et al. Primary prevention of ASCVD and T2DM in patients at metabolic risk: an Endocrine Society clinical practice guideline. J Clin Endocrinol Metab. 2019; https://doi.org/10.1210/jc.2019-01338.

96. Garvey WT, Mechanick JI, Brett EM, et al. American Association of Clinical Endocrinologists and American College of Endocrinology comprehensive clinical practice guidelines for medical care of patients with obesity. Endocr Pract. 2016;22 Suppl 3:1–203.

97. Garber AJ, Abrahamson MJ, Barzilay JI, et al. Consensus statement by the American Association of Clinical Endocrinologists and American College of Endocrinology on the comprehensive type 2 diabetes management algorithm – 2019 Executive Summary. Endocr Pract. 2019;25:69–100.

98. Jeffrey I. Mechanick, Stephanie Adams, Jaime A. Davidson, Icilma V. Fergus, Rodolfo J. Galindo, Kevin H. McKinney, Steven M. Petak, Archana R. Sadhu, Susan L. Samson, Rajesh Vedanthan, Guillermo E. Umpierrez, (2019) TRANSCULTURAL DIABETES CARE IN THE UNITED STATES – A POSITION STATEMENT BY THE AMERICAN ASSOCIATION OF CLINICAL ENDOCRINOLOGISTS. Endocrine Practice 25 (7):729-765.

99. Lyman GH, Greenlee H, Bohlke K, et al. Integrative therapies during and after breast cancer treatment: ASCO endorsement of the SIO clinical practice guideline. J Clin Oncol. 2018;36:2647–55.

100. Qaseem A, Holty JE, Owens DK, et al. Management of obstructive sleep apnea in adults: a clinical practice guideline from the American College of Physicians. Ann Intern Med. 2013;159:471–83.

101. Cobin RH, Goodman NF. American Association of Clinical Endocriniologists and American College of Endocrinology position statement on menopause – 2017 update. Endocr Pract. 2017;23:869–80.

102. Camacho PM, Petak SM, Binkley N, et al. American Association of Clinical Endocriniologists and American College of Endocrinology clinical practice guidelines for the diagnosis and treatment of postmenopausal osteoporosis – 2016 Executive Summary. Endocr Pract. 2016;22:1111–8.

103. Singh JA, Saag KG, Bridges SL Jr, et al. 2015 American College of Rheumatology guideline for the treatment of rheumatoid arthritis. Arthritis Rheumatol. 2016;68:1–26.

104. van der Steen JT, Radbruch L, Hertogh CM, et al. White paper defining optimal palliative care in older people with dementia: a Delphi study and recommendations from the European Association for Palliative Care. Pall Med. 2014;28:197–209.

105. Mechanick JI, Harrell RM, Allende-Vigo MZ, et al. Transculturalization recommendations for developing Latin American clinical practice algorithms in endocrinology – proceedings of the 2015 Pan-American workshop by the American Association of Clinical Endocriniologists and American College of Endocrinology. Endocr Pract. 2016;22:476–501.

106. Garber AJ, Abrahamson MJ, Barzilay JI, et al. Consensus statement by the American Association of Clinical Endocrinologists and American College of Endocrinology on the comprehensive type 2 diabetes management algorithm – 2016 Executive Summary. Endocr Pract. 2016;22:84–113.

107. Jensen LL, Drozek DS, Grega ML, et al. Lifestyle medicine: successful reimbursement methods and practice models. Am J Lifestyle Med. 2019;13:246–52.

108. Instituto Brasileiro de Geografia y Estadistica (IBGE). Accessed on September 21, 2019. Available online: https://www.ibge.gov.br.

109. Wang JS, Tu ST, Lee IT, et al. Contribution of postprandial glucose to excess hyperglycaemia in Asian type 2 diabetic patients using continuous glucose monitoring. Diabetes Metab Res Rev. 2011;27:79–84.

110. Oda E. New criteria for 'obesity disease' in Japan. Circ J. 2002;66:987–92.

111. Hu H, Nakagawa T, Yamamoto S, et al. Development and validation of risk models to predict the 7-year risk of type 2 diabetes: the Japan Epidemiology Collaboration on Occupational Health Study. J Diab Invest. 2018;9:1052–9.

112. Wallia S, Bhopal RS, Douglas A, et al. Culturally adapting the prevention of diabetes and obesity in South Asians (PODOSA) trial. Health Promot Int. 2014;29:768–79.

113. Chan EM, Cheng WM, Tiu SC, et al. Postprandial glucose response to Chinese foods in patients with type 2 diabetes. J Am Diet Assoc. 2004;104:1854–8.

114. Velasquez P, Neira C, Velasquez A, et al. Comparison of cardiovascular risk factors in children and adults stratified by age and severity of overweight. Endocr Pract. 2015;21:294–5.

115. Mechanick JI, Adams S, Davidson JA, et al. Transcultural diabetes care in the United States – a position statement by the American Association of Clinical Endocrinologists. Endocr Pract. 2019;25:729–65.

116. FAO 1996. Cumbre Mundial sobre la Alimentación. Declaración de Roma sobre la Seguridad Alimentaria Mundial y Plan de Acción. Roma. http://www.fao.org/3/X2051s/X2051s00.htm. Accessed on 19 Mar 2020.

117. O'Driscoll C, Shaikh M. Cross-cultural applicability of the Montreal Cognitive Assessment (MoCA): a systematic review. J Alzheimers Dis. 2017;58:789–801.

118. Pedraza O, Dotson VM, Willis FB, et al. Internal consistency and test-retest stability of the Geriatric Depression Scale – short form in African American older adults. J Psychopathol Behav Assess. 2009;31:412–6.

119. Vellas B, Guigoz Y, Garry PJ, et al. The Mini Nutritional Assessment (MNA) and its use in grading the nutritional state of elderly patients. Nutrition. 1999;15:116–22.

120. Levey AS, Bosch JP, Lewis JB, et al. A more accurate method to estimate glomerular filtration rate from serum creatinine: a new prediction equation. Modification of Diet in Renal Disease Study Group. Ann Intern Med. 1999;130:461–70.

121. Hailemariam H, Singh P, Fekadu T. Evaluation of mini nutrition assessment (MNA) tool among community dwelling elderly in urban community of Hawassa city, Southern Ethiopia. BMC Nutr. 2016;2:11.

122. Ghimire S, Baral BK, Callahan K. Nutritional assessment of community-dwelling older adults in rural Nepal. PLoS One. 2017;12:e0172052-e.

123. Kabir ZN, Ferdous T, Cederholm T, et al. Mini Nutritional Assessment of rural elderly people in Bangladesh: the impact of demographic, socio-economic and health factors. Public Health Nutr. 2006;9:968–74.

124. Gallagher D, Heymsfield SB, Heo M, et al. Healthy percentage body fat ranges: an approach for developing guidelines based on body mass index. Am J Clin Nutr. 2000;72:694–701.

125. Mosekilde L. Vitamin D and the elderly. Clin Endocrinol. 2005;62:265–81.

126. Wright NC, Chen L, Niu J, et al. Defining physiologically "normal" vitamin D in African Americans. Osteopor Int. 2012;23: 2283–91.

127. Cruz-Jentoft AJ, Landi F, Schneider SM, et al. Prevalence of and interventions for sarcopenia in ageing adults: a systematic review. Report of the International Sarcopenia Initiative (EWGSOP and IWGS). Age Ageing. 2014;43:748–59.

128. Mora JC, Valencia WM. Exercise and older adults. Clin Geriat Med. 2018;34:145–62.

129. Gothe NP, Kendall BJ. Barriers, motivations, and preferences for physical activity among female African American older adults. Gerontol Geriat Med. 2016;2:2333721416677399.

130. United States Census Bureau. US Department of Commerce. Economics and Statistics Administration. Accessed on May 29, 2020. Available online: https://www.census.gov/content/dam/Census/newsroom/releases/2015/cb15-tps16_graphic.pdf.

131. American Psychological Association. Guidelines on multicultural education, training, research, practice, and organizational change for psychologists. Am Psychol. 2003;58:377–402.

132. Eccles MP, Foy R, Sales A, et al. Implementation science six years on – our evolving scope and common reasons for rejection without review. Implement Sci. 2012;7:71. https://doi.org/10.1186/1748-5908-7-71.

Spirituality

Zorina Costello, Brittney Henry, and Vanshdeep Sharma

Abbreviations

CHA	Community Health Advisors
FBO	Faith-based organization
FICA	Faith, Importance/Influence, Community, Action/Address
HCP	Healthcare professional
HEAL	Health Through Early Awareness and Learning
MICAH	Multi-faith Initiative on Community and Health
R/S	Religious/spiritual
SDOH	Social determinants of health

Introduction

In the last three decades, there has been an increased focus on understanding the associations among religion, spirituality, and physical and mental health. Despite a voluminous literature, the terms "religion" and "spirituality" are still used inconsistently. In general, spirituality is considered to be a multi-dimensional construct, whereas religion is seen as a subset of spirituality. A 2009 US conference reached consensus on a definition of spirituality as, "the aspect of humanity that refers to the way individuals seek and express meaning and purpose and the way they experience their connectedness to the moment, to self, to others, to nature, and to the significant or sacred" [1]. A similar consensus process at a European conference in 2010 defined spirituality as " the dynamic dimension of human life that relates to the way persons (individual and community) experience, express, and/or seek meaning, purpose, and transcendence, and the way they connect to the moment, to self, to others, to nature, to the significant, and/or the sacred" [2]. In secular societies, a related construct is an existential orientation, which consists of concepts that do not require a belief in a transcendent reality. These include personal values, moral beliefs, responsibility to others, and freedom [3].

Religion is seen as a set of beliefs and rituals shared within a community in the search for God [4]. Religion has been described as "a subset of spirituality, encompassing a system of beliefs and practices observed by a community, supported by rituals that acknowledge, worship, communicate with, or approach the Sacred, the Divine, or God (in Western cultures), or Ultimate Truth, Reality or Nirvana (in Eastern cultures)" [5]. A common thread within all of these constructs is the attempt by human beings to make meaning of their lives. A "meaning systems" or "meaning-making" framework has been proposed and includes cognitive and affective components geared toward global beliefs and goals [6, 7]. Due to a lack of clear distinction between these constructs, and the continuing debate as to which construct is most relevant [8–10], the term "religious/spiritual" (R/S) beliefs is used to represent these constructs.

Religion as a Social Determinant of Health

In the United States, 74–77% of Americans believe in God and slightly more than 70% identify religion as one of the most important influences in their lives (Table 20.1) [11–13]. In recent years, the association between R/S beliefs and physical and mental health has been firmly established, although a preponderance of research on R/S beliefs and health is related to mental health. This is not surprising since

Z. Costello (✉)
Center for Spirituality and Health, Mount Sinai Health System, Icahn School of Medicine, New York, NY, USA
e-mail: zorina.costello@mountsinai.org

B. Henry
Mount Sinai Hospital, Population Health Science & Policy, New York, NY, USA

V. Sharma
Center for Spirituality and Health, Mount Sinai Hospital, Department of Psychiatry, New York, NY, USA

© Springer Nature Switzerland AG 2020
J. I. Mechanick, R. F. Kushner (eds.), *Creating a Lifestyle Medicine Center*, https://doi.org/10.1007/978-3-030-48088-2_20

Table 20.1 Religious groups in the United States by tradition, family, and denomination[a]

Christian 65%	
Evangelical Protestant 25%	
Mainline Protestant 12%	
Historically Black Protestant 6%	
Catholic 20%	
Mormon 2%	
Orthodox Christian 0.5%	
Jehovah's Witness 1%	
Other Christian 0.5%	
Unaffiliated (religious "nones") 26%	
Atheist 4%	
Agnostic 5%	
Nothing in particular 16%	
Non-Christian Faiths 8%	
Jewish 2%	
Muslim 1%	
Buddhist 1%	
Hindu 1%	
Other faiths 3%	
Don't know 1%	

[a]See Ref. [11]

mental health and R/S beliefs share social, behavioral, and psychological aspects more so than physical health. Moreover, the impact on physical health is most likely through these psychosocial and behavioral factors [14, 15]. It has been shown that R/S beliefs can be impacted by illness such that individuals may have positive or negative coping styles of their R/S beliefs, particularly in the context of spiritual struggles of an individual. Positive styles encompass a sense of being closer to God who provides comfort and support, whereas negative styles manifest in being angry with God, doubting that God loves them or God does not want to help them [16].

There are many studies that show an inverse relationship between R/S beliefs and the presence of depression, anxiety, substance abuse, and suicidality [17–19]. More recently, a meta-analysis found an inverse relationship between R/S beliefs and positive physical markers of health, such as lower body mass index, inflammatory markers, kidney disease markers, hypertension, and diabetes risk markers, among others [20]. Conversely, a growing number of studies have shown a direct correlation between R/S beliefs and coping with adversity, meaning and purpose, and optimism [21–23]. R/S beliefs have also been conceptualized as a social determinant of health (SDOH). A faith-based organization (FBO) affects health status by providing social support to their congregants and others, by establishing norms and the social control of behavior, especially health-related behaviors. While it is known that many effects of R/S coping styles tend to improve health, it has also been shown that some negative R/S coping styles have a deleterious effect, such as depres-

sion, anxiety, and feelings of hopelessness [24, 25]. Faith-based organizations and positive R/S practices may also indirectly mitigate or enhance the effects of some of the other SDOH, such as poverty, economic inequality, social deprivation, and lack of access to health care [26].

Chaplains in the Community

Racial and ethnic health inequalities in minority groups across America are well documented, along with mistrust of the health organizations by the disenfranchised communities [27, 28]. Enhancing community and individual health resources, implementing evidence-based practices, and providing racially and ethnically relevant health information are critical elements in reducing these inequalities and engendering trust [29]. Community engagement to increase access to care by providing outreach between communities and healthcare systems is essential. FBOs can play an important role in disseminating health information, providing health-related social support, and effectively reducing racial/ethnic inequality [30–33]. At present, church settings are popular venues for community health education and promotion, as well as access to care [34–36].

Prior work has demonstrated that a hospital's community outreach program utilizing a healthcare chaplain can improve certain indices, such as healthcare costs and readmission rates, that are related to public health [37]. While there are many programs that work with FBOs to promote health, there is a paucity of literature that incorporates a medical center's healthcare chaplain in a key role for community outreach. The use of FBOs in the Harlem community in New York City is an example [38]. Briefly, the Center for Spirituality and Health in the Icahn School of Medicine at Mount Sinai created this program, named the Multi-faith Initiative on Community and Health (MICAH) Project, which was initiated in 2015 and is presently under the direction of a healthcare chaplain (Z.C.), who is very familiar with the Harlem areas served by the Mount Sinai Health System. This project was then expanded by including training of Community Health Advisors (CHAs) based on the Health through Early Awareness and Learning (HEAL) program. The CHAs were identified and selected by church leaders. The chaplain who oversaw the MICAH Project was again chosen to be the liaison for the training of the CHAs in the MICAH HEAL project, since she had been responsible for developing such strong partnerships. As liaison, she worked directly with the FBOs regarding what health topics were their priorities and managed the scheduling of the training program.

The choice of a chaplain to oversee community outreach was made because chaplains are trained to be sensitive to the role of faith in medical decision-making, the importance that congregations place on promoting health, and the use of scripture that may be relevant to health education. As an example, a scriptural reference in the Bible that is used to encourage people to become more proactive about their health states that "I can do all this through him who gives me strength, Philippians 4:13" [39]. The scripture is discussed in reference to a health concern where early screening can be used as a preventive measure, such as in encouraging a patient to get a colonoscopy. Introducing sacred text can also empower patients to use health information to reflect cognitively between taking the next steps to improve lifestyle management. Another example of appealing to the human faith experience used in the Project HEAL Lifestyle Medicine Module was developed by Dr. Jeffrey Mechanick, where the chaplain integrated a scriptural reference from the Bible with a health imperative. For example, introducing the idea of eating more vegetables was integrated with "Please test your servants for ten days: Give us nothing but vegetables to eat and water to drink. Then compare our appearance with that of the young men who eat the royal food, and treat your servants in accordance with what you see, Daniel 1:12–15" [39]. Similarly, other holy texts, such as the Quran, make references to the importance of health promoting behaviors, including diet and nutrition: "We have brought it (the Earth) to life and brought forth from it grain, and from it they eat, Surat Ya-Sin 36: 33" and "Let man reflect upon the food he eats, Surat Abasa 80:24" [40, 41]. Among Jewish texts, the Torah points out the importance of exercise and physical activity, "As long as a person exercises and exerts himself … sickness does not befall him and his strength increases … But one who is idle and does not exercise … even if he eats healthy foods and maintains healthy habits, all his days will be of ailment and his strength will diminish, Mishneh Torah, 'De'ot' 4:14–15" [42].

This MICAH HEAL project was able to establish the ability to translate, adapt, and implement an evidence-based CHA training program with FBOs. This was accomplished by demonstrating how healthcare systems can use existing partnerships, or develop new partnerships, with FBOs as a platform for health education, and moreover, how healthcare chaplains can play important roles for such programs [38].

Chaplains in Healthcare Settings

Chaplains who work in major medical hospital/academic medical settings must have a seminary degree from an accredited institution, such as a Master of Divinity (M.Div.). Many chaplains also have varying doctoral degrees, such as a Doctor of Ministry (D.Min.), Doctor of Education, (E.D.) Doctor of Theology (Th.D.), or a Ph.D. in a related disci-

pline. Some of the areas of concentrated focus of study are Pastoral Care, Pastoral Theology, Pastoral Counseling, and others. The studies are inclusive of psychology, sociology, religious anthropology, and human development, as well as world religions. The Chaplains' ability to meet the spiritual and emotional needs of patients and community members is informed by their training, which emphasizes attentiveness to active listening, empathy, non-judgmental stance, and appreciation for existential themes such as human connectedness, transcendence, isolation, despair, and hope. In major medical centers, chaplain training programs consist of helping to address patients' spiritual and emotional needs using interfaith methods.

While respecting individual faith/belief systems, chaplains can spend time at both the bedside and in outpatient facilities offering spiritual counseling, which helps patients to feel understood and respected. Prayer and other ceremonial interactions are offered upon request. There is a certain pace to the listening, a cadence of presence, and the ability to be drawn into the patient's narrative without being overwhelmed by it in order to maintain objectivity. In this way, the chaplain can also offer vital insight as part of the interdisciplinary team in order to address best practices in communicating with patients about care plans. In cases where patients have particular religious needs, chaplains are trained to seek consultation with a cleric from that particular faith. This is similar to a medical doctor asking for a consultation from a specialist in another service. For example, if the patient is Catholic, and the chaplain is not authorized to give a requested sacrament, such as "holy communion," the chaplain would call upon the services of a Eucharistic Minister or a Catholic Priest. If the patient is of the Hindu faith, the interfaith chaplain would call a Hindu Priest for specific prayers and ceremonies when needed. Jewish patients may request the services of a Rabbi and that request would be honored. Muslim patients who feel more comfortable with an Imam or Muslim liaison are offered these services as well. In a case where a cleric from a particular faith is not an employee of the hospital, it is recommended to establish relationships with local religious communities, as with a Buddhist Monk who can be vetted as a volunteer for the healthcare system to offer services from the faith tradition.

The chaplain must remain alert and sensitive to the needs of patients of all faiths or emotional needs of those who do not express a faith. Finally, as HCPs and chaplains attune with patient's S/R expressions by being able to articulate their own spiritual beliefs around love, meaning, connectedness, and compassion, they learn to integrate spiritual care in the overall care plan. However, the awareness of a clinician knowing when to refer a patient to a chaplain for spiritual care is also excellent clinical practice.

Chaplains as Members of the Interdisciplinary Team

The chaplain is an important member of the interdisciplinary team in meeting the R/S needs of patients. Chaplains are also involved in providing staff support to members of the interdisciplinary teams in the form of debriefing and defusing sessions. Chaplains are seen as spiritual care specialists whereas the other members of the team are spiritual care generalists. Although other members of the interdisciplinary team are capable of meeting some of patients' R/S needs, there are several barriers to this. A recent study describes a national survey of physicians in which 65% of physicians believe that it is good clinical practice for physicians to address patients' R/S needs, especially as part of end of life care. Additionally, physicians who were more religious were more likely to believe that spiritual care is essential to good medical practice and believed that was appropriate to encourage patients to talk to a chaplain. A majority of the physicians (55%) stated that, if asked, they would join the family and patient in prayer. Physicians' willingness to join ranged from 67% (when there was concordance between the physician's and the patient's religious affiliation) to 51% (when there was discordance) [43]. The findings of this study are consistent with those of several others [44, 45]. However, despite this willingness, very few physicians or nurses actually engage in providing R/S care. Patient reports frequently describe that they desire their physicians to inquire about their spiritual beliefs and practices, and yet most physicians do not ask those questions. The authors also found that 41% of inpatients wished to have a conversation with their doctor about spiritual concerns, but only half of the patients actually had such a conversation [44].

Various reasons have been given for this disconnect. Balboni et al. [46] found that the most frequently stated reason for not being able to provide R/S care was a "lack of time," followed by other barriers, such as "lack of adequate training," physicians felt that it was "not my professional role," and that there was a "power inequity with patients." Interestingly, those physicians who had lower R/S beliefs were less willing to engage in R/S training or engage with patients around these concerns [46]. It is also the case that physicians, in general, do not have any formal training in R/S care while in medical school or during residency training [47]. Most training is informal in nature and is informed by the physician's own R/S beliefs. Inadequate training is one of the main reasons why physicians do not refer patients to chaplains for spiritual care [48]. Studies have shown that medical students who have had an opportunity to shadow a chaplain in the hospital had a better understanding of the role of spirituality in health care, the role of the chaplain in a hospital setting, a better idea about how to utilize the expertise of the chaplain, and experiencing an enhanced doctor-patient relationship [49, 50]. It has been suggested that familiarity with the spirituality literature as part of a residency educational curriculum may help break down barriers to addressing R/S needs with patients [51, 52].

Spiritual Assessment

In 1999, the Association of American Medical Colleges published outcome goals and learning objectives for medical schools on spirituality and health [53]. Since then, many efforts have been made to introduce R/S training in medical schools and residency educational curricula. Some of these efforts have involved interprofessional teams (e.g., physicians, social workers, and chaplains) co-leading spirituality groups, with opportunities for medical students to shadow chaplains. There are several screening tools that have been developed to provide a clear understanding of a patient's spiritual history, and baseline assessments can, and should, be, conducted by physicians and/or other HCPs. Among these screening tools, the *F*aith, *I*mportance/Influence, *C*ommunity, *A*ction/Address in Care (FICA) Spiritual History Tool© was one of the first scales developed to help HCPs address spiritual needs and concerns of patients, as well as identify their spiritual resources of strengths (Table 20.2) [54, 55]. Furthermore, the FICA tool probes how a person is coping, how they connect to their spirituality, and how their spirituality shapes their purpose.

The FICA tool serves as a guide for conversation in both the in- and outpatient clinical settings, and feedback from the physicians has shown that there is a deeper doctor-patient connection when the FICA tool was incorporated [56]. While

Table 20.2 FICA tool[a]

F – Faith, Belief, Meaning	Do you consider yourself spiritual or religious? Do you have spiritual beliefs that help you cope with stress? What gives your life meaning?
I – Importance and Influence	What importance does your faith or belief have in your life? On a scale of 0 (not important) to 5 (very important), how would you rate the importance of faith/belief in your life? Have your beliefs influenced you in how you handle stress? What role do your beliefs play in your health care decision-making?
C – Community	Are you a part of a spiritual or religious community? Is this of support to you and how? Is there a group of people you really love or who are important to you?
A – Address in Care	How would you like your healthcare professional to use this information about your spirituality as they care for you?

[a]See Refs. [54, 55]

the FICA tool has become quintessential to HCPs who focus on palliative care, the tool itself can be used with all patients. Obtaining a clearer understanding of the role of spirituality in a patient's way of life can create a level of intimacy, while also maintaining the necessary formality [57].

Conclusion

Chaplains have come a long way from when they were lay members of clergy who simply visited their parishioners to being employed by hospitals and becoming an integral part of the healthcare team, working full time providing R/S care for patients (Table 20.3) [58–69]. More recently, an internal study conducted at the Mount Sinai Hospital examined the role of chaplains as providers of R/S care for hospital staff and faculty, helping them to cope with increasing levels of burnout and compassion fatigue in the staff. A newer development in the field has been the emerging role of chaplains in the community and interacting with clergy leaders, while improving access to care for members of the community. As community members proactively request more healthcare information to prevent, delay, or cure disease, the healthcare chaplain can become an anchor of trust to respective faith communities. Consequently, the healthcare chaplain becomes a vital resource to HCPs who sometimes struggle with ways in which to communicate more effectively with patients and families to achieve improved healthcare outcomes. Sustainable patient-HCP relationships come about when the patient feels understood and is trusting. The impor-

Table 20.3 Broad guidelines for clinicians in outpatient settings attending to religious/spiritual needs[a]

Religion/ spiritual context	Health and wellness	Illness	Death/dying
Judaism	Belief in one omnipotent God Degrees of adherence to religion and tradition vary Cultural aspects include traditions that provide connections and acceptance Identity is personal	Provide active listening Provide compassionate care Provide access to opportunity for prayer and meditation Honor religious rituals as needed Facilitate referral to community/faith-leader as needed Example of a prayer to offer: "El Na Refah Nah La." "Oh Lord Heal her" (Numbers 12:13)	Body seen as a holy vessel carrying a soul Practices honor the dead and help ease the transition for survivors Family/community gather for Shemirah and Tahara Prayers and Psalms recited
Christianity	Belief in one omnipotent God Followers of the Bible's New Testament teachings of Christ who is understood to be the Messiah. Degrees of belief in a triune God as Father, Son, and Holy Spirit following the Ascension of Christ after death Possibilities for forgiveness, mercy, and redemption offer hope	Provide active listening Provide compassionate care Attention to cultural aspects of patient and family life Access to prayer support, sacred text, and religious rites, such as "Holy Communion" and "Sacrament of the Sick," brings comfort There are many denominations with variance in religious practices Example of a prayer to offer: "Heal me, Lord and I shall be healed, save me and I shall be saved, for you *art* my praise" (Jeremiah 17:14)	Faith is a source of strength with a belief that everlasting life of the person's soul can be obtained through following the teachings and practices of Jesus Funeral services arranged by family or friends Burial or cremation is acceptable There is a need for a religious leader such as a priest, reverend, or church elder
Islam	Culture and values and religion closely tied Belief in Allah the only deity Collectivists with family and community supports Ritual prayers 5 times a day Women may wear traditional clothing Family roles are complimentary Keeping the Fast of the Holy Month of Ramadan	Provide active listening Provide compassionate care During an illness, cross-gender care concerns may be expressed Attention to and concern for traditional modesty Be open to discussing spiritual beliefs Facilitate referral to a community/faith leader. Provide privacy for prayers and reading of the Qu'ran Example of a prayer to offer: "Truly distress has seized me, but You are Most Merciful of those that are merciful" (Qu'ran 21:83–84)	Patient prefers to die at home Muslims pray toward Mecca and bed is positioned for this purpose preferably in the home Help patient with prayers in combination with visitors and relatives Religious requirement to bury the dead as soon as possible Family distress is minimized if community gathers in a timely fashion for the funeral

(continued)

Table 20.3 (continued)

Religion/ spiritual context	Health and wellness	Illness	Death/dying
Buddhist	Foundational teachings explore life of Buddha, life problems, and solutions The Four Noble Truths provide a philosophy to live by: 1. There is Dukkha or suffering which is a part of life experiences of discomfort 2. There is a cause to stress and a craving for more pleasant experiences. With this truth underlying causes can be explored 3. The cessation of Dukkha is possible 4. The Path to Cessation of Dukkha The practice of mindfulness and meditation are prominent	Provide active listening and compassionate care, and peaceful health care environment Patients may seek the paths of Metta (gentleness) for self and others: loving kindness in response to suffering, compassion, appreciative joy, equanimity, which is a mind and heart seeking balance Variety in practice across cultures which may include use of art, meditation, sounds, symbolism, tea, and mantra recitation Patients may study and identify aspects of Buddha for purposes of seeking body equilibrium to alleviate illness Example of a Prayer to offer: "At the foot of the Bodhi tree, beautifully seated, peaceful and smiling, the living source of understanding and compassion, to the Buddha I go for refuge" (The Refuge Chant, Excerpt)	Family and community gather to support patient Customs vary between traditions and geographic locations Clinical staff can benefit from consulting with Spiritual leaders from sect of patient An altar may be displayed along with a portrait of the deceased with offerings of candles, incense, flowers, incense, and fruit Funeral service with rites performed often by monks Family/community wears white, chants or sings sutras (prayer) Cremation preferred Meaning-making results from reflecting on the virtues of the deceased and other life affirming teachings
Hindu	Practice and belief of hymns, meditations and prayers, noise, and music Moral Law and Karma tied together through knowledge or insight Moksha attained by being detached from all feeling tying one to the world God, religious leaders, and philosophies help to guide worship and festivals The practice of Ayurveda medicine promotes good health and longevity via a healthy lifestyle, including nutrition A shrine in the home to make offerings and prayer at the altar is meaningful for seeking well-being for the family	Provide active listening and compassionate care During illness, patients may seek cultural/ spiritual opportunities for healthy balance, as in Yoga Desire a minimal level of invasive medical interventions Spiritual goals encompass being free from equating ill health with spiritual beliefs of consequences from acts committed in a previous life Plant-based remedies may be considered a healing option alone or in concert with valued medical practice Example of a prayer to offer: "Where faith prevails, there can be no failure. Even a brief glimpse of the truth protects the seeker from the greatest fear of all – the fear of death" (Bhagavad Gita 2:40)	Prayers, rituals, mantras, and sacred chants are entered into at home, in the temple, and at the bedside of the patient Patients prefer to die at home when possible Family may seek the guidance of Temple Priest or leader at the time of eminent death Typically it is important to the family to have a funeral within 24 hours The body is then cremated. The belief in reincarnation provides solace to surviving family members

[a]See Refs. [58–69]

tance of clear communication, coupled with easily accessible literature (print or web-based), demonstrates that HCPs are invested in the relationship. Inquiring about the faith or belief system of the patient can furnish insight as to how to approach health topics and sustainable treatment plans for the patient. HCPs who are willing to go out into the community to give health talks and do basic screenings in faith-based or other community settings can also derive a better sense of the milieu and coping techniques of the patient. In addition, as healthcare systems adjust to new methods of value-based purchasing, healthcare chaplains can add value in communicating with the community and teaching HCPs how to build innovative methodologies that improve clinical outcomes.

References

1. Puchalski C, Ferrell B, Virani R, et al. Improving the quality of spiritual care as a dimension of palliative care: the report of the consensus conference. J Palliat Med. 2009;12:885–904.
2. Nolan S, Saltmarsh P, Leget CJW. Spiritual care in palliative care: working towards an EAPC task force. Eur J Palliat Care. 2011;18:86–9.
3. la Cour P, Hvidt NC. Research on meaning-making and health in secular society: secular, spiritual and religious existential orientations. Soc Sci Med. 2010;71:1292–9.
4. Zinnbauer BJ, Pargament KI, Cole B, et al. Religion and spirituality: unfuzzying the fuzzy. J Sci Study Relig. 1997;36:549–64.
5. Koenig HG. Medicine, religion, and health: where science & spirituality meet. West Conshohocken: Templeton Foundation Press; 2008.

6. Park CL. Religiousness/spirituality and health: a meaning systems perspective. J Behav Med. 2007;30:319–28.

7. Park CL. Religion as a meaning-making framework in coping with life stress. J Soc Issues. 2005;61:707–29.

8. Hall DE, Koenig HG, Meador KG. Conceptualizing "religion": how language shapes and constrains knowledge in the study of religion and health. Perspect Biol Med. 2004;47:386–401.

9. Breitbart W. Who needs the concept of spirituality? Human beings seem to! Palliat Support Care. 2007;5:105–6.

10. Salander P. Who needs the concept of 'spirituality'? Psychooncology. 2006;15:647–9.

11. In U.S., Decline of Christianity continues at rapid pace: an update on America's changing religious landscape. Pew Research Center, Washington D.C. 2019. https://www.pewforum.org/2019/10/17/in-u-s-decline-of-christianity-continues-at-rapid-pace/. Accessed on 21 Mar 2020.

12. The Harris Poll®. Americans' belief in god, miracles and heaven, 2013. https://theharrispoll.com/new-york-n-y-december-16-2013-a-new-harris-poll-finds-that-while-a-strong-majority-74-of-u-s-adults-do-believe-in-god-this-belief-is-in-decline-when-compared-to-previous-years-as-just-over. Accessed on 21 Mar 2020.

13. Pew Research Center. Religious landscape study. Pew Research Center, Washington, DC. 2015. https://www.pewforum.org/religious-landscape-study/. Accessed on 21 Mar 2020.

14. Koenig HG. Religion, spirituality, and health: the research and clinical implications. ISRN Psychiatry. 2012;278730. https://doi.org/10.5402/2012/278730.

15. Bonelli RM, Koenig HG. Mental disorders, religion and spirituality 1990 to 2010: a systematic evidence-based review. J Relig Health. 2013;52:657–73.

16. Pargament KI, Koenig HG, Perez LM. The many methods of religious coping: development and initial validation of the RCOPE. J Clin Psychol. 2000;56:519–43.

17. Bonelli R, Dew RE, Koenig HG, et al. Religious and spiritual factors in depression: review and integration of the research. Depress Res Treat. 2012;2012:962860.

18. Rasic DT, Belik SL, Elias B, et al. Spirituality, religion and suicidal behavior in a nationally representative sample. J Affect Disord. 2009;114:32–40.

19. Rasic D, Robinson JA, Bolton J, et al. Longitudinal relationships of religious worship attendance and spirituality with major depression, anxiety disorders, and suicidal ideation and attempts: findings from the Baltimore epidemiologic catchment area study. J Psychiatr Res. 2011;45:848–54.

20. Shattuck EC, Muehlenbein MP. Religiosity/spirituality and physiological markers of health. J Relig Health. 2018;59:1035. https://doi.org/10.1007/s10943-018-0663-6.

21. Schuster MA, Stein BD, Jaycox L, et al. A national survey of stress reactions after the September 11, 2001, terrorist attacks. N Engl J Med. 2001;345:1507–12.

22. Park CL. Meaning making in the context of disasters. J Clin Psychol. 2016;72:1234–46.

23. Koenig HG, Berk LS, Daher NS, et al. Religious involvement is associated with greater purpose, optimism, generosity and gratitude in persons with major depression and chronic medical illness. J Psychosom Res. 2014;77:135–43.

24. Park CL, Smith PH, Lee SY, et al. Positive and negative religious/spiritual coping and combat exposure as predictors of posttraumatic stress and perceived growth in Iraq and Afghanistan veterans. Psychol Relig Spiritual. 2017;9:13–20.

25. Bowland S, Edmond T, Fallot RD. Negative religious coping as a mediator of trauma symptoms in older survivors. J Relig Spiritual Aging. 2013;25:326–43.

26. Idler E, editor. Religion as a social determinant of public health. New York: Oxford University Press; 2014.

27. Wheeler SM, Bryant AS. Racial and ethnic disparities in health and health care. Obstet Gynecol Clinics. 2017;44:1–11.

28. Story L, Hinton A, Wyatt SB. The role of community health advisors in community-based participatory research. Nurs Ethics. 2010;17:117–26.

29. Williams DR, Purdie-Vaughns V. Needed interventions to reduce racial/ethnic disparities in health. J Health Polit Policy Law. 2016;41:627–51.

30. Van Olphen J, Schulz A, Israel B, et al. Religious involvement, social support, and health among African-American women on the east side of Detroit. J Gen Intern Med. 2003;18:549–57.

31. Tucker CM, Wippold GM, Williams JL, et al. A CBPR study to test the impact of a church-based health empowerment program on health behaviors and health outcomes of black adult churchgoers. J Racial Ethn Health Disparities. 2017;4:70–8.

32. Matthews AK, Sellergren SA, Manfredi C, et al. Factors influencing medical information seeking among African American cancer patients. J Health Commun. 2002;7:205–19.

33. Holt CL, Lewellyn LA, Rathweg MJ. Exploring religion-health mediators among African American parishioners. J Health Psychol. 2005;10:511–27.

34. Fallon EA, Bopp M, Webb B. Factors associated with faith-based health counselling in the United States: implications for dissemination of evidence-based behavioural medicine. Health Soc Care Community. 2013;21:129–39.

35. Baig AA, Mangione CM, Sorrell-Thompson AL, et al. A randomized community-based intervention trial comparing faith community nurse referrals to telephone-assisted physician appointments for health fair participants with elevated blood pressure. J Gen Intern Med. 2010;25:701–9.

36. Baruth M, Wilcox S, Laken M, et al. Implementation of a faith-based physical activity intervention: insights from church health directors. J Community Health. 2008;33:304–12.

37. Cutts T, Baker B, Gunderson G. Church-health system partnership facilitates transitions from hospital to home for urban, low-income African Americans, reducing mortality, utilization, and costs. Agency for Healthcare Research and Quality. 2012. https://innovations.ahrq.gov/profiles/church-health-system-partnership-facilitates-transitions-hospital-home-urban-low-income. Accessed on 21 Mar 2020.

38. Marin DB, Costello Z, Sharma V, et al. Adapting health through early awareness and learning program into a new faith-based organization context. Prog Community Health Partnersh. 2019;13:321–9.

39. Zondervan J. Life application Bible: new international version. Wheaton: Tyndale House Publishers, Inc.; 1997.

40. King Saud University. The Holy Quran. King Saud University Electronic Moshaf Project. 2013. http://quran.ksu.edu.sa/index.php?l=en. Accessed on 21 Mar 2020.

41. Aboul-Enein BH. Health-promoting verses as mentioned in the Holy Quran. J Relig Health. 2016;55:821–9.

42. Chabad.org. Mishneh Torah, De-ot - chapter four. https://www.chabad.org/library/article_cdo/aid/910344/jewish/Deot-Chapter-Four.htm. Accessed on 21 Mar 2020.

43. Smyre CL, Tak HJ, Dang AP, et al. Physicians' opinions on engaging patients' religious and spiritual concerns: a national survey. J Pain Symptom Manage. 2018;55:897–905.

44. Williams JA, Meltzer D, Arora V, et al. Attention to inpatients' religious and spiritual concerns: predictors and association with patient satisfaction. J Gen Intern Med. 2011;26:1265–71.

45. Berg GM, Crowe RE, Budke G, et al. Kansas physician assistants' attitudes and beliefs regarding spirituality and religiosity in patient care. J Relig Health. 2013;52:864–76.

46. Balboni MJ, Sullivan A, Enzinger AC, et al. Nurse and physician barriers to spiritual care provision at the end of life. J Pain Symptom Manage. 2014;48:400–10.

47. Rasinski KA, Kalad YG, Yoon JD, et al. An assessment of US physicians' training in religion, spirituality, and medicine. Med Teach. 2011;33:944–5.

48. Balboni MJ, Sullivan A, Amobi A, et al. Why is spiritual care infrequent at the end of life? Spiritual care perceptions among patients, nurses, and physicians and the role of training. J Clin Oncol. 2013;31:461–7.

49. Graves DL, Shue CK, Arnold L. The role of spirituality in patient care: incorporating spirituality training into medical school curriculum. Acad Med. 2002;77:1167.

50. Puchalski CM. Spirituality and medicine: curricula in medical education. J Cancer Educ. 2006;21:14–8.

51. Saguil A, Fitzpatrick AL, Clark G. Is evidence able to persuade physicians to discuss spirituality with patients? J Relig Health. 2011;50:289–99.

52. Saguil A, Fitzpatrick AL, Clark G. Are residents willing to discuss spirituality with patients? J Relig Health. 2011;50:279–88.

53. Association of American Medical Colleges. Contemporary issues in medicine: communications in medicine: report III. Washington, DC: Medical School Objectives Project; 1999.

54. Borneman T, Ferrell B, Puchalski CM. Evaluation of the FICA tool for spiritual assessment. J Pain Symptom Manage. 2010;40:163–73.

55. Puchalski CM. The FICA spiritual history tool #274. J Palliat Med. 2014;17:105–6.

56. Puchalski C, Romer AL. Taking a spiritual history allows clinicians to understand patients more fully. J Palliat Med. 2000;3:129–37.

57. Vermandere M, De Lepeleire J, Smeets L, et al. Spirituality in general practice: a qualitative evidence synthesis. Br J Gen Pract. 2011;61:e749–60.

58. Version KJ. Holy Bible. p. Jeremiah 17:4.

59. Torah p. Numbers 12:3.

60. Ali AY. The Holy Qu'ran. Saeed International (Pvt) Ltd.; 2015. p. 21:83–84.

61. Krishna BS. Bhagavad Gita. New York: Chintamani Books; 2015. p. 40.

62. Brownstein T. The interfaith prayer book. Lake Worth: Lake Worth Interfaith Network; 2001.

63. Berkeley Center for Religion Peace & World Affairs. Hinduism on health and illness. 2020. https://berkleycenter.georgetown.edu/essays/hinduism-on-health-and-illness. Accessed on 21 Mar 2020.

64. Bowker J. World religions: the great faiths explored & explained. London: DK Publishing; 2003.

65. Sheikh A. Death and dying--a Muslim perspective. J R Soc Med. 1998;91:138–40.

66. Sue DW, Sue D. Counseling the culturally diverse: theory and practice. Hoboken: John Wiley & Sons, Inc; 2013. p. 451–2.

67. Hatim IM. Caregiving to Muslim: A guide for Chaplains, Counselors, Healthcare and Social Workers. Jerusalem: Muhammad Hatim; 2017. p. 35–40.

68. Goldstein HR. Being a blessing: 54 ways you can help people living with illness. H Rafael Goldstein; 2009. p. 187–9.

69. Sockolov M. Basic Buddhist teachings and practices; March 21, 2019. https://oneminddharma.com/buddhist-teachings/. Accessed on 21 Mar 2020.

Community Engagement to Improve Health

21

John B. Wetmore and Deborah B. Marin

Abbreviations

BMI	Body mass index
CARES	Community Awareness, Reach, & Empowerment for Screening
CDC	Centers for Disease Control and Prevention
CHA	Community health advisor
CTQ	Courage to quit
EPIC	Encourage, Practice, and Inspire Change
HCP	Healthcare professional
HEAL	Project Health Through Early Awareness and Learning
HIV	Human immunodeficiency virus
MSM	Men who have sex with men
SHAPP	Stroke and Heart Attack Prevention Program
WISEWOMAN	Well-Integrated Screening and Evaluation in Women Across the Nation

Introduction

The primary and secondary objectives of prevention in public health include implementing interventions to prevent the onset of disease and conducting screening to identify disease in its earliest stages, respectively [1]. According to the Centers for Disease Control and Prevention (CDC), commu-

J. B. Wetmore
Icahn School of Medicine at Mount Sinai, Population Health and Health Policy, New York, NY, USA
e-mail: john.wetmore@mountsinai.org

D. B. Marin (✉)
Center for Spirituality and Health, Icahn School of Medicine at Mount Sinai, New York, NY, USA
e-mail: deborah.marin@mssm.edu

nity engagement encourages healthier behaviors, educates community members, and promotes screening programs, and is therefore a fundamental component of these prevention strategies [1]. Specifically, community engagement is defined as actions "involving communities in decision-making and in the planning, design, governance, and delivery of services" [2]. Community engagement is necessary for the success of healthcare professionals' (HCPs) outreach to their respective catchment areas.

There are a wide variety of approaches that exist in the planning and deployment of community engagement programs that focus on lifestyle and medicine, such as smoking cessation, diet, and exercise programs [2]. Through the direct involvement of community members in the delivery of interventions, some programs seek to enhance their efficacy [2]. On the other hand, some programs are directly planned and deployed by community members themselves in order to target identified health needs [2]. Both of these models of community engagement work together to enable people who are socioeconomically disadvantaged to gain control over their lives, thereby improving their own health. Underserved populations are often the audience for community engagement programs because they experience more barriers to healthcare [3].

Barriers and Facilitators to Community Engagement Programs

In order to overcome these barriers, partnerships between community engagement programs and local organizations are essential. Yancey et al. [4] implemented a physical activity intervention in a multi-ethnic urban population and evaluated the ability of multiple types of local organizations to host the community engagement intervention program. They laid out seven important organizational characteristics for effective program promotion and determined that organizations with less than four of these seven characteristics did not have

© Springer Nature Switzerland AG 2020
J. I. Mechanick, R. F. Kushner (eds.), *Creating a Lifestyle Medicine Center*, https://doi.org/10.1007/978-3-030-48088-2_21

the organizational capacity to host the intervention program [4]. These characteristics are site leadership commitment, an "in-group" site contact, a captive audience, communication mechanisms, pre-existing group cohesiveness, a shared mission, and a preexisting and trusting relationship between the organization and the program [4]. However, recent research further refines these findings. Sly et al. [5] conducted interviews of leadership personnel from 32 program sites of a colorectal cancer education program in a greater metropolitan area. Using thematic content analysis, it was determined that organizational capacity, an "in-group" site contact, a captive audience, communication mechanisms, and shared mission are the most relevant characteristics of partnerships between community engagement programs and local organizations [5].

Firstly, having the support of site leadership can help the program succeed through space allocation, a desire to cooperate, and flexibility [4, 6]. Therefore, organizations that have defined hierarchical structures have a greater capacity to host and maintain community engagement programs because of their ability to provide ample space, coordinate events, and promote events within the organization and in the general public [5]. Limited services, difficulty in sustaining change, and the substantial time required are all barriers to maintaining a community engagement program [7, 8]. Ongoing follow-up, focusing on the positive effects of change, utilizing electronic media, and the incorporation of community services have all been identified as facilitators of program sustainability [8].

Secondly, the recruitment and retention of community members in a program may be facilitated by [1] a site contact who actively promotes the program and recruits participants and [2] effective communication mechanisms within the organization to advertise events [4, 5]. According to a study that conducted focus groups and interviews with adolescents, parents, and community stakeholders, barriers to recruitment also involve stigma, difficulty in defining unhealthy lifestyles, and broader social factors. However, strategic marketing, a positive approach, and subsidizing program costs can enhance recruitment [8]. Ensuring that a program's events are well publicized is an important step to securing and increasing attendance at events. Using local avenues of communication, such as radio talk shows, social media, and hard-copy advertisements, can contribute to a more comprehensive and inclusive engagement program [9]. Similarly, partnering with other organizations and taking part in larger events, such as health fairs, can drastically increase the visibility of a community engagement program [9].

Barriers to retention include location, timing, commitment, and social factors [8]. In order to combat these barriers, guides for effective community engagement recommend the provision of support for attendance and avoiding exclusion-

ary practices [9]. Hosting events at a convenient time and place within a partner organization is essential to creating a captive audience [4, 5]. One successful strategy might be to host events before, during, or after other events at the organization [4], while another may be to hold events at a time when there is not a naturally-occurring group [5]. Moreover, each community will require its own unique type of support. For example, elderly populations may need meetings to be held in handicap-accessible locations, while programs targeted at young couples may need to supply day care for their children. It is important to consider these unique needs in order to be as inclusive as possible. Also, during the process of conducting a program, the feedback supplied by participants and coordinators allows for both the development of more appropriate educational materials and the garnering of greater community support [7].

Beyond organizational capacity and participant recruitment and retention, trust is key to any program's success [4]. Underserved communities may be wary of outside organizations that do not understand their cultural values [10]. The history of mistrust memorialized by the Tuskegee experiments, implicit and explicit racial biases by HCPs, and language and culture barriers between patients and HCPs can discourage minority populations from seeking out healthcare [10]. Therefore, it is essential for community engagement programs to have a shared mission with an organization and to incorporate local racial/ethnic minority heritages (cultural adaptation) in their content and delivery in order to create a mutually beneficial and fruitful partnership [4, 5, 10, 11].

Examples of Successful Community Engagement Programs

Various successful community engagement programs, as part of a larger lifestyle medicine approach, have focused on cancer prevention; nutrition, obesity, and diabetes; hypertension and cardiovascular disease; smoking cessation; and human immunodeficiency virus (HIV) prevention. Successful examples of these types of programs are described in detail below.

Project HEAL

Project Health through Early Awareness and Learning (HEAL) successfully employed a community-based participatory research model in order to train community health advisors (CHAs) to implement a series of breast, prostate, and colorectal cancer screening educational workshops in African American churches [12]. With the help of an advisory panel composed of community stakeholders, the project team branded and tailored these evidence-based interventions to the community [12]. This faith-based and faith-placed intervention program included a Health Ministry Guide to introduce organizational leadership to the program and its mission, CHA training either in-person or online, CHA certification exams, workshop materials and PowerPoint slides that incorporate excerpts of religious scripture, and a community resource guide that lists local HCPs [12]. The program had an adoption rate of 42% at the organizational level (15 out of 36 churches) [13]. Most churches completed the three-workshop series in a timely manner, and on average, participants reported attending most workshops and reading more than half of the distributed educational reading materials [13]. Community health advisors also reported a positive rating of the intervention itself, high levels of participant engagement, and a strong sense of familiarity with the workshop material [13].

Project HEAL's program showed acceptable sustainability, as almost 40% of the initial sample attended follow-up workshops 12 and 24 months later, and around 90% said they shared information from Project HEAL with family and friends [14]. The program also reported partnership-level sustainability with the churches, church-level sustainability with the development of health ministries within the churches, sustained attention to health issues among the churches and CHAs, and community-level sustainability as other churches requested Project HEAL training materials after hearing about the program by word of mouth [14]. Two years after the program's pilot run was complete, organizational capacity assessments were completed by church leadership, and tailored reports were given to each of the participating churches in order to provide recommendations to partners for sustainability in health-related events or programs [15].

The Witness Project

The CHA model, which has been acknowledged as a promising mitigator of health disparities, is also a large part of The Witness Project, a national evidence-based community intervention program that focuses on increasing breast and cervical cancer screening rates in African American women [16–19]. Through this faith-based program, CHAs discuss breast and cervical cancer screening in addition to teaching how to perform a breast self-examination [17]. Cancer survivors are also part of this intervention program; they bear witness to their experiences with cancer, address the fears and mistrust surrounding cancer and medical care, and empower other African American women to seek out screening and/or treatment [17, 19]. It has been shown that women who participate in The Witness Project programs had significant increases in seeking out mammograms and performing breast

self-examinations [17, 19]. It was also shown that the program was both culturally appropriate and effective in reaching low-income minority women [17]. The Witness Project has been effectively replicated in over 40 sites throughout the United States and continues to improve screening rates among African American women [6, 17].

Based on The Witness Project, the Witness Community Awareness, Reach, & Empowerment for Screening (CARES) program was developed to address high incidence and mortality rates of colorectal cancer among African Americans [20]. In a randomized control trial, two types of videos were tested: [1] a didactic video in which information regarding colorectal cancer screening was delivered to the participants and [2] a narrative video in which two African Americans discussed colorectal cancer, their fears and feelings regarding colonoscopies, and their experiences [20].

Esperanza y Vida (Hope and Life)

Esperanza y Vida is another peer-led program that presents educational materials regarding breast and cervical cancer to participants and that provides navigation for screening [21]. After cultural adaptation of The Witness Project model and materials, Esperanza y Vida addressed Latino perspectives on gender roles and healthcare as well as culture-specific barriers and facilitators to cancer screening [21, 22]. Similar to The Witness Project, CHAs provide information regarding breast and cervical cancer, while the cancer survivors share their own stories about their diagnosis, treatment, and recovery [21]. CHAs and survivors were recruited from the community; these volunteers were required to be fluent in Spanish and to attend a 2-day training session [23]. The training session included discussions about volunteers' roles and responsibilities, breast and cervical cancer, female anatomy, the art of teaching and storytelling, local screening and cancer resources, and how to teach breast self-examination [23]. Pre-and post-testing revealed that volunteer knowledge of breast and cervical cancer was significantly higher after the training session, except for the survivors who displayed greater knowledge about breast cancer during the pre-test [23].

A randomized control trial was used to determine the efficacy of this community engagement program; participants were allocated either to the intervention or to a control group that discussed diabetes [21, 24]. After 2 months, follow-up revealed that rates of clinical breast exams, breast self-examination, and pap testing were significantly higher among the intervention group [24]. Demonstrating its replicability, Esperanza y Vida was conducted in three unique locations with different Latino populations [21].

The Stroke and Heart Attack Prevention Program

The Stroke and Heart Attack Prevention Program (SHAPP) employs nursing staff at clinics throughout Georgia to educate and offer direct services in low-income communities [25, 26]. This program provides screening, referrals, diagnosis, and treatment for hypertension, as well as lifestyle counseling, medication, and education [25, 26]. Given the high mortality rate of cardiovascular disease in Georgia, this program has also been instrumental in improving health outcomes for Georgians and has served over 15,000 patients thus far, most of whom are middle-aged and African American [25]. Based on the Chronic Care Model, SHAPP individually pairs patients with nurse case managers who coordinate each patient's care and are responsible for monitoring the patients' progress and adherence [26]. When interviewed, administrators and clinic staff who participated in the SHAPP program reported that participants displayed greater knowledge of high blood pressure and its causes and effects, better adherence to medication, and an increased likelihood of keeping their appointments [25]. As a result, SHAPP has not only been shown to reduce the burden associated with the costs of adverse events when compared to no treatment and typical treatment scenarios, but also to increase blood pressure control rates and improve health outcomes when compared to no treatment or treatment offered at the average level expected nationally [26]. According to the CDC, SHAPP was successful in improving blood pressure control rates through easy enrollment into the program, nonjudgmental and supportive care, continuous patient monitoring by HCPs, and low-to-no cost medications [25].

The WISEWOMAN Project

Similarly, the Well-Integrated Screening and Evaluation in Women Across the Nation (WISEWOMAN) project provides risk factor screenings and promotes healthy behaviors to reduce the risk of heart disease and stroke among low-income middle-aged women with limited or no healthcare coverage [27–31]. This program combines lifestyle education programs, individual health counseling, and other community resources to promote heart health [31]. Examples of these resources include educational training sessions, supporting community-based farmers' markets and other sources of healthy food options, encouraging smoking cessation and physical activity, and engaging participants' HCPs in the monitoring and remediation of high blood pressure and other risk factors for heart disease and stroke [31]. Over the course of several studies, the WISEWOMAN project has been shown to improve dietary outcomes, rates of physical activity, and body mass index (BMI), in addition to helping women take control of their blood pressure, total cholesterol, and blood glucose levels [27–30].

The Mpowerment Project

Through the development of a safe community in which gay and bisexual men can share their experiences, the Mpowerment Project is an intervention program that seeks to promote HIV prevention at the community-level in addition to decreasing risky sexual behaviors among men who have sex with men (MSM) [32, 33]. After conducting focus groups with young gay/bisexual men, the program developers realized that promoting social interactions among these men would incentivize them more, rather than relying on a fear of HIV to increase participant attendance [32]. As such, this socially-focused intervention program aimed to create social networks among their participants, in addition to providing a safe space for these men to build a community [32]. Moreover, the peer-based, sex-positive Mpowerment Project was designed to empower young gay/bisexual men [32]. The organizational structure of this community engagement program is 2–4 program coordinators, 15–20 diverse community members who serve as the "Core Group" and design the project's activities, volunteers who are matched with committees and tasks, and an advisory board composed of community members and outside professionals who offer ideas and advice [32, 33]. Program members engage participants through formal peer outreach in the form of team performances and hosted events, small "M-group" sessions that provide information about safe sex and social issues, informal outreach through casual conversations and safer-sex information/incentive packages, and publicity through newspaper articles and flyers [32, 33]. After hiring project coordinators, the Mpowerment Project focused on gaining an understanding the community by conducting a community assessment, organizing the program through the Core Group, cultivating supportive relationships with other HIV prevention-related organizations in the area, and tailoring their intervention program to the unique social and cultural environment of the community they are serving [32]. Declared by the CDC as one of the country's model HIV prevention programs, the Mpowerment Project has been shown to significantly reduce rates of unprotected anal intercourse among young gay/bisexual MSM communities [32, 33].

d-up: Defend Yourself

Another community-level intervention designed to reduce HIV incidence in black MSM communities is d-up: Defend Yourself, a program that recruits and trains local opinion leaders to have risk reduction conversations with their friends and acquaintances in order to change the social norms surrounding condom use [34]. Opinion leaders are identified using ethnographic techniques at well-defined community venues frequented by Black MSM, such as local nightclubs, and trained in HIV risk reduction by prevention specialists over a period of four 2-hour sessions [34]. These sessions cover a wide range of topics, including the local HIV/AIDS epidemiology, the facts and myths surrounding HIV/AIDS, and the keys to an effective risk reduction conversation [34]. By the end of the four sessions, the local opinion leaders have been shown to increase awareness of the negative social and cultural factors that impact Black MSM risky sexual behaviors and to promote a more positive self-worth among their friend groups through risk reduction conversations [34]. After the initial trainings, opinion leaders held small group weekly sessions to further improve their own skills, gain confidence in their techniques, and share/receive feedback regarding their experiences [34].

Courage to Quit

Evidence-based programs are also employed to promote smoking cessation. One such program, Courage to Quit (CTQ), conducted smoking cessation intervention sessions at community sites, including health centers and faith-based organizations, that serve a racially diverse and low income population [35]. This program is comprised of an orientation and psychoeducation session, two weekly sessions prior to the participants' assigned quit date, and four weekly sessions after the quit date [35]. In these sessions, program facilitators incorporate cognitive, behavioral, and motivational smoking intervention strategies [35]. Some examples of modules that are employed are identifying triggers, coping with craving, and managing stress [35]. Program facilitators were recruited from a variety of backgrounds, had to attend a 1-day onsite training and certification course, and had to be current non-smokers for at least the past 6 months [35]. In order to accommodate their host sites' needs, the CTQ program also offered a shorter three-session format and was translated into several different languages [35]. Overall, the full-length program was shown to be more efficacious in achieving cessation among completers than the shortened program, and those using smoking cessation medication were shown to be more likely to quit smoking than those who did not use any medication [35].

Project Joy

Project Joy was a trial of three different interventions focused on improving nutrition and physical activity among African American women in order to promote cardiovascular health [36]. These three lifestyle interventions were: [1] weekly educational sessions on nutrition and physical activity that followed a "standard" group behavioral model, [2] the "standard" model with an added spiritual and church cultural component, and [3] a non-spiritual self-help group that served as the control group [36]. The church-culture intervention also included group prayers, health messages enriched with scripture, and physical activities including gospel music and praise and worship dance [36]. Based on focus group and additional in-depth interviews, the intervention was designed and implemented in one church over 20 weeks as a pilot program; a community expert panel was also assembled to further refine the intervention [36]. The final product was an educational intervention program that discussed nutrition topics, such as portion size and sodium intake, and exercise topics, such as heart rate and long-term exercise maintenance [36]. Each "standard" intervention session, which was led by formally trained lay leaders, consisted of weigh-ins, group discussions, the nutrition education modules, and 30 minutes of moderate intensity aerobic activity [36]. While there were no statistically significant differences between the "standard" and church-culture interventions, intervention participants overall had lower body weight, waist circumference, systolic blood pressure, dietary energy, dietary total fat, and sodium intake; the self-help control group showed no changes [36].

The LIFE Project

The LIFE Project, a 10-week weight loss intervention program, offered both spiritually-based and non-spiritually-based interventions centered on promoting nutrition and physical activity among women at rural African American churches to prevent chronic conditions related to obesity and diabetes [37]. This program was created in direct response to concerns expressed by African American women during local community forums [37]. Diabetes, hypertension, and obesity were identified as major health issues among the community, and there was interest in an education program regarding nutrition and physical activity [37]. The LIFE Project's curriculum was based on Project Joy and focused on the "3Ds": Dietary practices, Daily physical activities, and Discussions with HCPs [36, 37]. Ensuring a consistent experience for those in the spiritual and non-spiritual groups, the county extension educator was trained in both curricula and led all sessions [37]. Analysis of pre- and post-physiological measures demonstrated a statistically significant reduction in weight and systolic blood pressure in both the spiritual and non-spiritual intervention groups [37]. Moreover, statistically significant decreases in BMI and increases in both physical activity and communication with HCPs were found among the spiritual group [37]. Given the success of the LIFE Project, the authors concluded that community member involvement prior to the development of a community engagement program can facilitate health interventions and improve the capacity of host organizations [37].

The EPIC Kids Study

Children have also been the focus of community engagement programs, as seen in the Encourage, Practice, and Inspire Change (EPIC) Kids study conducted by Hingle et al. [38]. These researchers tested a family-focused, YMCA-based type 2 diabetes prevention program for children aged 9–12 and their families to promote nutrition, exercise, and supportive home environments [38]. This feasibility study examined two different interventions: [1] a face-to-face lifestyle intervention led by a coach and [2] an alternative face-to-face and digitally delivered intervention [38]. Both interventions, which included structured physical activity and hands-on practice with food preparation, were designed and refined by YMCA administrators, YMCA youth members, and an expert advisory board [38]. This 12-week intervention program included topics such as promoting time outside rather than inside with computers and televisions, purchasing healthier options from the grocery store, and practicing healthy exercise and sleep routines [38]. While there were no significant differences between either intervention group, there were statistically significant decreases in children's BMI scores and positive changes in healthy home environments with respect to home nutrition and physical activity [38].

Conclusion

Opportunities for community engagement allow HCPs and health educators the ability to reach out to and improve the health and knowledge among disadvantaged populations. Community engagement programs train volunteers from the community to provide peer-based health education, offering direct services to participants, fostering community building, and/or responding to the direct needs of a community (Table 21.1) [12–15, 17–38]. These programs can be leveraged through the implementation process when planning, building, and operating a Lifestyle Medicine Center (Table 21.2). Through the use of community engagement programs, barriers like medical mistrust may be overcome in order to improve health outcomes for many topics related to lifestyle and medicine in a wide variety of community settings.

Table 21.1 Key points from successful community engagement programs

Author and reference	Name	Program content	Methodology	Outcomes
Holt et al. [12–15]	Project HEAL	Breast, prostate, and colorectal cancer screening	Community health advisors hold faith-based educational workshops	Adoption rate of 41% at the organizational level 90% of participants said they shared information from Project HEAL with family and friends
Erwin et al. [17–20]	The Witness Project	Breast and cervical cancer screening in African American women	Faith-based educational workshops led by peer health educators	Significant increases in seeking out mammograms and performing breast self-examinations
Erwin et al. [21–24]	Esperanza y Vida	Breast and cervical cancer screening in Latina women	Culturally-competent educational workshops led by peer health educators	Rates of clinical breast exams, breast self-examination, and pap testing were significantly higher among the intervention group
SHAPP [25, 26]	The Stroke and Heart Attack Prevention Program	Cardiovascular disease in low-income communities	Screening, referrals, diagnosis, and treatment for hypertension as well as lifestyle counseling, medication, and education	Participants displayed greater knowledge of high blood pressure and its causes and effects, better adherence to medication, and an increased likelihood of keeping their appointments Reduced the burden associated with the costs of adverse events when compared to no treatment and typical treatment scenarios Increased blood pressure control rates and improved health outcomes when compared to no treatment or treatment offered at the average level expected nationally
The WISEWOMAN Project [27–31]	The WISEWOMAN Project	Heart disease and stroke among low-income middle-aged women with limited or no healthcare coverage	Lifestyle education programs, individual health counseling, and other community resources	Improved dietary outcomes, rates of physical activity, and body mass index Helped women take control of their blood pressure, total cholesterol, and blood glucose levels

Table 21.1 (continued)

Author and reference	Name	Program content	Methodology	Outcomes
Kegeles et al. [32, 33]	The Mpowerment Project	HIV prevention among young gay/bisexual men	Formal and informal peer outreach, educational group sessions, and flyers	Reduced rates of unprotected anal intercourse
Jones et al. [34]	d-up: Defend Yourself	HIV prevention among black MSM communities	Risk reduction conversations	35.2% reduction in unprotected insertive anal sex 44.1% reduction in unprotected receptive anal sex 23.0% increase in condom usage for insertive anal sex 30.3% increase in condom usage for receptive anal sex 40.5% reduction in number of active partners for unprotected receptive anal sex
Asvat et al. [35]	Courage to Quit	Smoking cessation	Educational workshops and weekly group meetings	Those using smoking cessation medication were shown to be more likely to quit smoking than those who did not use any medication
Yanek et al. [36]	Project Joy	Nutrition and physical activity among African American women to promote cardiovascular health	Weekly education sessions, group behavioral modeling, group exercise, spiritual and church cultural components	Intervention group participants had lower body weight, waist circumference, systolic blood pressure, dietary energy, dietary total fat, and sodium intake
Parker et al. [37]	The LIFE Project	Nutrition and physical activity among women at rural African American churches	Educational sessions focusing on dietary practices, daily physical activities, and discussions with healthcare professionals	Reduction in weight and systolic blood pressure Decreases in body mass index Increases in both physical activity and communication with healthcare professionals
Hingle et al. [38]	The EPIC Kids Study	Family-focused, YMCA-based type 2 diabetes prevention program for children ages 9–12 years	Educational intervention sessions that included structured physical activity and hands-on practice with food preparation	Decreases in children's body mass index scores Positive changes in healthy home environments with respect to home nutrition and physical activity

Table 21.2 Implementing community engagement as part of a Lifestyle Medicine Center

Steps	Examples
1. Establish relationships in the community and/or partner with community-based organizations	Identify and meet with community leaders to introduce your organization and develop a trusting relationship Create a community advisory board to get feedback from the leaders and to show what you have to offer as a healthcare professional
2. Determine a community need	Obtain feedback from community leaders to identify the issues they face and their needs
3. Propose program models that fit with these needs	Health education workshops Smoking cessation programs Exercise and diet programs
4. Design the intervention program	Peer education Direct services
5. Obtain feedback to optimize the program	Review the proposed program with community leaders and focus groups to determine feasibility and acceptability
6. Take into account community feedback	Change content, length, date, or time of a program to facilitate success
7. Devise ways to monitor program progress and success	Sign-in sheets to monitor the frequency of events and the reach of the program Be available at the start of the program implementation Attend programs to ensure consistency across sites and educators Conduct participant surveys
8. Have ongoing relationships with the community	Meet with stakeholders on a regular basis to discuss progress

References

1. Health NCfE. Preveention. In: Prevention CfDCa, editor. Picture of America. Centers for Disease Control and Prevention; 2017. p. 1–9.
2. Brunton G, Thomas J, O'Mara-Eves A, Jamal F, Oliver S, Kavanagh J. Narratives of community engagement: a systematic review-derived conceptual framework for public health interventions. BMC Public Health. 2017;17(1):944.
3. O'Mara-Eves A, Brunton G, McDaid D, Oliver S, Kavanagh J, Jamal F, et al. Community engagement to reduce inequalities in health: a systematic review, meta-analysis and economic analysis. Southampton: Public Health Research; 2013.
4. Yancey AK, Miles O, Jordn AD. Organizational characteristics facilitating initiation and institutionalization of physical activity programs in a multiethnic urban community. J Health Educ. 1999;30:9.
5. Sly JR, Henry B, Morgan G, Erwin D, Kiviniemi M, Jandorf L, et al. Promoting colorectal cancer education in the African American community: a qualitative evaluation of academic-community partnerships 2019.
6. Shelton RC, Charles TA, Dunston SK, Jandorf L, Erwin DO. Advancing understanding of the sustainability of lay health advisor (LHA) programs for African-American women in community settings. Transl Behav Med. 2017;7(3):415–26.
7. Carter MW, Tregear ML, Lachance CR. Community engagement in family planning in the U.S.: a systematic review. Am J Prev Med. 2015;49(2 Suppl 1):S116–23.
8. Smith KL, Straker LM, McManus A, Fenner AA. Barriers and enablers for participation in healthy lifestyle programs by adolescents who are overweight: a qualitative study of the opinions of adolescents, their parents and community stakeholders. BMC Pediatr. 2014;14:53.
9. Crew. A guide to effective community engagement 2015.
10. Muncan B. Cardiovascular disease in racial/ethnic minority populations: illness burden and overview of community-based interventions. Public Health Rev. 2018;39:32.
11. Mechanick JI, Adams S, Davidson JA, Fergus IV, Galindo RJ, McKinney KH, et al. Transcultural diabetes care in the United States – a position statement by the American Association of Clinical Endocrinologists. Endocr Pract. 2019;25(7):729–65.
12. Holt CL, Tagai EK, Scheirer MA, Santos SL, Bowie J, Haider M, et al. Translating evidence-based interventions for implementation: experiences from Project HEAL in African American churches. Implement Sci. 2014;9:66.
13. Santos SL, Tagai EK, Scheirer MA, Bowie J, Haider M, Slade J, et al. Adoption, reach, and implementation of a cancer education intervention in African American churches. Implement Sci. 2017;12(1):36.
14. Scheirer MA, Santos SL, Tagai EK, Bowie J, Slade J, Carter R, et al. Dimensions of sustainability for a health communication intervention in African American churches: a multi-methods study. Implement Sci. 2017;12(1):43.
15. Holt CL, Shelton RC, Allen JD, Bowie J, Jandorf L, Zara Santos SL, et al. Development of tailored feedback reports on organizational capacity for health promotion in African American churches. Eval Program Plann. 2018;70:99–106.
16. Shelton RC, Dunston SK, Leoce N, Jandorf L, Thompson HS, Crookes DM, et al. Predictors of activity level and retention among African American lay health advisors (LHAs) from The National Witness Project: implications for the implementation and sustainability of community-based LHA programs from a longitudinal study. Implement Sci. 2016;11:41.
17. Erwin DO, Ivory J, Stayton C, Willis M, Jandorf L, Thompson H, et al. Replication and dissemination of a cancer education model for African American women. Cancer Control. 2003;10(5 Suppl):13–21.
18. Shelton RC, Dunston SK, Leoce N, Jandorf L, Thompson HS, Erwin DO. Advancing understanding of the characteristics and capacity of African American women who serve as lay health advisors in community-based settings. Health Educ Behav. 2017;44(1):153–64.
19. Erwin DO, Spatz TS, Stotts RC, Hollenberg JA. Increasing mammography practice by African American women. Cancer Pract. 1999;7(2):78–85.
20. Ellis EM, Erwin DO, Jandorf L, Saad-Harfouche F, Sriphanlop P, Clark N, et al. Designing a randomized controlled trial to evaluate a community-based narrative intervention for improving colorectal cancer screening for African Americans. Contemp Clin Trials. 2018;65:8–18.
21. Sudarsan NR, Jandorf L, Erwin DO. Multi-site implementation of health education programs for Latinas. J Community Health. 2011;36(2):193–203.
22. Erwin DO, Johnson VA, Feliciano-Libid L, Zamora D, Jandorf L. Incorporating cultural constructs and demographic diversity in the research and development of a Latina breast and cervical cancer education program. J Cancer Educ. 2005;20(1):39–44.
23. Saad-Harfouche FG, Jandorf L, Gage E, Thelemaque LD, Colon J, Castillo AG, et al. Esperanza y Vida: training lay health advisors and cancer survivors to promote breast and cervical cancer screening in Latinas. J Community Health. 2011;36(2):219–27.
24. Jandorf L, Bursac Z, Pulley L, Trevino M, Castillo A, Erwin DO. Breast and cervical cancer screening among Latinas attending culturally specific educational programs. Prog Community Health Partnersh. 2008;2(3):195–204.
25. Promotion NCfCDPaH. The Stroke and Heart Attack Prevention Program (SHAPP) fact sheet 2014.
26. Rein DB, Constantine RT, Orenstein D, Chen H, Jones P, Brownstein JN, et al. A cost evaluation of the Georgia Stroke and Heart Attack Prevention Program. Prev Chronic Dis. 2006;3(1):A12.
27. Hayashi T, Farrell MA, Chaput LA, Rocha DA, Hernandez M. Lifestyle intervention, behavioral changes, and improvement in cardiovascular risk profiles in the California WISEWOMAN project. J Womens Health (Larchmt). 2010;19(6):1129–38.
28. Homan SG, McBride DG, Yun S. The effect of the Missouri WISEWOMAN program on control of hypertension, hypercholesterolemia, and elevated blood glucose among low-income women. Prev Chronic Dis. 2014;11:E74.
29. Keyserling TC, Samuel Hodge CD, Jilcott SB, Johnston LF, Garcia BA, Gizlice Z, et al. Randomized trial of a clinic-based, community-supported, lifestyle intervention to improve physical activity and diet: the North Carolina enhanced WISEWOMAN project. Prev Med. 2008;46(6):499–510.
30. Khare MM, Cursio JF, Locklin CA, Bates NJ, Loo RK. Lifestyle intervention and cardiovascular disease risk reduction in low-income Hispanic immigrant women participating in the Illinois WISEWOMAN program. J Community Health. 2014;39(4):737–46.
31. Promotion NCfCDPaH. WISEWOMAN overview 2018.
32. Hays RB, Rebchook GM, Kegeles SM. The Mpowerment Project: community-building with young gay and bisexual men to prevent HIV1. Am J Community Psychol. 2003;31(3–4):301–12.
33. Kegeles SM, Hays RB, Coates TJ. The Mpowerment Project: a community-level HIV prevention intervention for young gay men. Am J Public Health. 1996;86(8):1129–36.

34. Jones KT, Gray P, Whiteside YO, Wang T, Bost D, Dunbar E, et al. Evaluation of an HIV prevention intervention adapted for Black men who have sex with men. Am J Public Health. 2008;98(6):1043–50.

35. Asvat Y, Cao D, Africk JJ, Matthews A, King A. Feasibility and effectiveness of a community-based smoking cessation intervention in a racially diverse, urban smoker cohort. Am J Public Health. 2014;104(Suppl 4):S620–7.

36. Yanek LR, Becker DM, Moy TF, Gittelsohn J, Koffman DM. Project Joy: faith based cardiovascular health promotion for African American women. Public Health Rep. 2001;116(Suppl 1):68–81.

37. Parker VG, Coles C, Logan BN, Davis L. The LIFE project: a community-based weight loss intervention program for rural African American women. Fam Community Health. 2010;33(2):133–43.

38. Hingle MD, Turner T, Going S, Ussery C, Roe DJ, Saboda K, et al. Feasibility of a family-focused YMCA-based diabetes prevention program in youth: The E.P.I.C. Kids (Encourage, Practice, and Inspire Change) Study. Prev Med Rep. 2019;14:100840.

Simin Liu and Kenneth Lo

Value of Epidemiological Scientific Evidence for Optimizing Lifestyle Medicine

> Epidemics appear, and often disappear without traces, when a new culture period has started; thus with leprosy, and the English sweat. The history of epidemics is therefore the history of disturbances of human culture. – Rudolph LK Virchow [1]

Not long after the above statement made by the German pathologist and founding father of the modern science of pathology did cardiovascular diseases emerge as mankind's No. 1 killer epidemic of the twentieth century. Now with the second decade of a new millennium, 382 million people had diabetes mellitus (DM), and the number will probably rise to 592 million by the next two decades and fast becoming yet another No. 1 epidemic of our time [2]. This pandemic is especially severe in fast developing countries such as China and India. Type 2 diabetes is the leading cause of end-stage renal disease [3], preventable amputations [4], and blindness [5]. The incidence of major cardiovascular events is increased two- to fourfold by diabetes, with women and minorities disproportionately bearing the largest burden [6].

Set against this backdrop in descriptive epidemiology are the many breathtaking discoveries and technological advances that also are unprecedented in the history of biomedical sciences. Genomes and proteomes of human beings can be assayed *en masse* yielding experimental insights at the nanoscale [7]. Yet, cardiovascular disease is arguably 100% lifestyle or environmental (note that because of gene-environment interaction, there is no upper limit in determining attributable risk). How can the major advances in biomedical sciences be harnessed to conquer what appears to be the public health nemesis of the present time? Prevention strategies need to be developed that are precise, personal-

ized, and with outcomes that are predictable when they are implemented to the general population with good public policies. However, many important questions in the molecular pathogenesis, related metabolic consequences, and respective diagnostic/therapeutic/preventative strategies in many facets of obesity and diabetes remain poorly understood.

The main justification and rationale for the development of integrative research and training in major academic health science centers is to apply specialized expertise and resources to not just one scientific study but a program of scientific studies. In the past two decades, a systematic approach using the "6 P.I.G. strategy" has been developed in a lifestyle medicine program so that evidence from observational epidemiology and clinical interventions can be evaluated in the context of their totality, consistency, and quality. To improve both individual and population health outcomes globally, the 6 PIG strategy clearly spells out the "What?" (6Ps), "How?" (6Is), and "Why?" (6Gs) in scientific inquiry for chronic disease:

- *P* – Prediction, Precision, Prevention, Personalized, Population, and Policy
- *I* – International, Interdisciplinary, Interpretation, Integration, Innovation, and Implementation
- *G* – Good will, good food, good environment, good choice, good deed, and common goods

In brief, a systems approach to prevention across the lifespan and generations is needed. This would use effective prevention efforts at each phase of time-dependent processes in the development of cardiometabolic disorders. The approach would also implement them in all appropriate populations, described by diverse racial and ethnic backgrounds. Approximately 40 years ago, the noted English epidemiologist Geoffrey Rose articulated the principles and ramifications of the population strategy (in contrast to the traditional intervention strategy for high-risk individuals) for cardiovascular disease prevention. Rose argues that preven-

S. Liu (✉) · K. Lo
Center for Global Cardiometabolic Health, Brown University, Epidemiology, Medicine and Surgery, Providence, RI, USA
e-mail: simin_liu@brown.edu; kenneth_lo@brown.edu

© Springer Nature Switzerland AG 2020
J. I. Mechanick, R. F. Kushner (eds.), *Creating a Lifestyle Medicine Center*, https://doi.org/10.1007/978-3-030-48088-2_22

tive and lifestyle medicine must embrace both strategies to improve public health and calls for control strategies that carefully distill epidemiological observation into meaningful changes in health care delivery. To be sure, the significant impact of diabetes, obesity, and related cardiometabolic disorders on human societies everywhere now demands that biomedical scientists and policy makers alike be well versed in issues ranging from molecular genetics to public health sciences concerning these devastating phenotypes. Nevertheless, improving the health of the population goes beyond simply translating basic science discoveries into clinical practice. Both directions – from the laboratory to the individual patients and population at risk to the individual patient require well-funded resources and well-trained investigators capable of conducting sound research that integrate the entire continuum from "sick" molecules to "sick" populations. However, talented young people well trained in the concepts, strategies, and advanced tools of both population and lab-based research remain a rarity. This is true in the field of cardiometabolic disease, and particularly true in establishing and sustaining the necessary academic infrastructure and human resources in epidemiology, quantitative sciences, information technology, pathology, and the other medical specialties.

How to Assemble the Necessary Infrastructure

Due to its multidisciplinary nature, epidemiology is the discipline inherently capable of integrating concepts and strategies from multiple population- and laboratory-based sciences. At UCLA, for example, the range of resources and faculty expertise in both laboratory and population sciences (including physiological sciences, pathology, biostatistics, genetics, and epidemiology) provide a fertile ground for nurturing and developing talented young investigators. Basic, clinical, and population studies addressing biomedical problems provide excellent opportunities for training, since a productive collaboration has already been established. During the formation of the Program on Genomics and Nutrition at the School of Public Health (http://www.ph.ucla.edu/epi/faculty/liu/index.htm, accessed 08 Dec 2019), abilities to bring collective experiences and expertise were demonstrated in integrative training and research. This greatly expanded peer and faculty interactions with trainees interested in the disciplines of molecular epidemiology and the programmatic field of metabolic diseases. There was a continual flow of excellent trainees, eager to work in population sciences and molecular epidemiology. The dedicated group of faculty mentors and trainees must be active in their respective area of research. The most important aspect in securing the success of this type of program is the intellectual resource.

There were many questions in diabetes research that needed to be addressed through epidemiology. Examples include appropriate criteria for defining dysglycemia; effective strategies for screening, aggressive case finding, diagnosing, and predicting complications in diverse populations; and how to integrate genomic, proteomic, and environmental variables to better understand multi-dimensional interactive forces as potential causes for metabolic diseases in human populations. Whereas effective treatments exist, these treatments often require prolonged clinical trials to determine relative benefit and cost effectiveness. Tools of population-based and laboratory-based can address these high-impact questions. In this regard, faculty members from diverse departments and disciplines at UCLA were already quite prominent in studying the use of nutritional and dietary approaches in cardiometabolic outcomes of interest. What is necessary is some dedicated effort to bring the commitments of these existing faculty members together to form a critical mass with incentives to attract the best possible trainees to their work while maintaining high visibility and institutional support at the highest level. Moreover, a focus was created on extensive cross-departmental and cross-school collaborations, integrated via the 6 PIG platform, and using epidemiologic methodology. The proposed training program based on this focus fits squarely into the educational mission at UCLA.

Program Mission, Specific Features, and Administration

Program directors diligently craft a program mission statement with short, intermediate, and long-term goals. The Program on Genomics and Nutrition program is tasked to develop high quality science (both population- and laboratory-based) to [1] assess the impact of genes and their interactions with behavior, nutrition, and the environment on health and diseases, and [2] critically and systematically evaluate the significance of genetic and dietary variations within populations and applying that knowledge to improve public's health. This cohesive set of goals is set forth to bring together trainees of diverse academic background ranging from biology to social and quantitative sciences. The skill sets of these groups differ: lab-based scientists cannot simply "pick up" expertise in the design and analysis of large epidemiologic cohorts, and epidemiologists benefit from more direct contact with the clinical and laboratory aspects of their chosen diseases.

There is a unique culture of the UCLA consisting of in-depth expertise in a specific area of research, while also being exposed to broad areas of cardiometabolic health outcomes based on the 6 PIG strategy. This is conducted in an interactive environment with a set of regular conferences and lectures spaced quarterly over a year that nurture lifelong "self-directed" learning habits. The culture encourages a continued self-identification of deficiencies in knowledge.

From an administrative standpoint, this research program in areas of lifestyle medicine took advantage of existing structures of Ph.D. programs in the participating degree-granting departments. The recruitment of trainees and research mentors on faculty were the responsibility of the program directors. The research mentors involved each trainee in lab- and population-based sciences, theoretical concepts, and the practical designs of their research projects. In so doing, a new office was created, jointly administered by the Department of Pathology and Laboratory Medicine at the UCLA School of Medicine and the Department of Epidemiology at the UCLA School of Public Health, where the co-directors were responsible for the dayto-day operation of the Training Program, with guidance from Steering Committee and Advisory Committee. All participating faculty can nominate suitable candidates to the program for consideration by the Steering Committee.

Institutional Commitments and Necessary Infrastructure

It is important to obtain the highest institutional leadership commitment as early as possible for research initiatives and execution in lifestyle medicine. This can be accomplished by demonstrating data-driven, evidence-based deliverables for proposed programmatic work and that fits squarely in the core University mission. When successful, this process safeguards a program's long-term success in the academic University setting. In this section, another exemplar is explored. Brown University subsequently provides the infrastructure for population studies on cardiometabolic outcomes. This component is housed within the School of Public Health at Brown University: The Center for Population Health and Clinical Epidemiology, the Center for Statistical Sciences, Survey Center, and Molecular Epidemiology and Nutrition Laboratory. Members of this Center are epidemiologists, physicians, and social scientists who combined state-of-the-art research methods with expertise in specific diseases. The Center provides support to its faculty for pilot studies, professional development, and administrative support for research-related activities. The financial support structure allows for protected time for research with salary support. Physical resources, such as office space, conference rooms, teleconference equipment, computer resources, and support staff, have been allocated to the investigator's research efforts. Close physical proximity and shuttle service to the Women & Infants Hospital provides easy access to the participants, clinicians, and researchers collaborating on this project.

Network and Computing Infrastructure

All offices are connected into a single virtual local area network by the central Brown Computing and Information Services group. Servers are in a physically secured, temperature-controlled environment. The operations staff work in proximity to the server core allowing for easy support of the hardware. All external network access is limited to a single gateway. Network traffic is filtered by type, and if deemed a major security risk, disallowed. The servers themselves are likewise defended by protocol filters, which limit the nature and type of network traffic. These machines host a complete suite of Internet-working facilities as well as data storage and backup. The Center uses a variety of security techniques including firewalls and antivirus software to maintain a secure and reliable computer environment. Additionally, the Center for Computation and Visualization maintains a powerful supercomputing environment that is extended to faculty for high-performance, large platform computational and statistical processing. The Center maintains a robust and highly flexible computing environment, drawing on both local and remote resources. An aggregate of approximately 7TB of online storage supports all of the Center's centralized operations and is backed up on a regular basis.

Data Confidentiality

Data containing person-identifiers is considered highly sensitive. By policy, such data is only stored within the virtual memory system (VMS) cluster. Access is controlled by the VMS access control lists mechanism, allowing read-only access to a small group of specific users and read-write access to an even smaller group. Internet access (e.g., via Web server) is disallowed for such storage areas. Network access is tightly controlled to allow anonymous access only to a small amount of read-only data; all "risky protocols" are disallowed from Internet access. For any given study with person-identifying information, such data is stripped before the data is made accessible to staff not authorized to access such identifiers. In those cases where the data is longitudinal, a non-reversible encryption of the person's identity is performed. This provides a unique person identity that is not traceable to the underlying person.

The specific algorithm used for any given set of data is stored in the same fashion and given the same security as the data itself. To make data use simpler, hierarchical "trees" of directories are given consistent access controls tied to a unique identifier, which is then granted to staff authorized to use such data. Programming staff authorized to make individual-level data available to staff not authorized to access the person-identifying components routinely copy the "encrypted" versions from the more-secured tree to a less-secured tree. Security controls are thus relatively automatic, based on the propagation of rights based on the location of a file within the file system and the identity of the user attempting to access it. All data is, by policy, controlled by Windows Management Instrumentation tools, allowing read-only access to a small group of specific users and read-write access to an even smaller group, and disallowed internet access to prevent data leakage. Windows security controls determine permissions for users, since some data is acquired on Windows-specific media. The necessity to grant/revoke access to any data, user groups, or any other security-relevant event data is continuously logged and analyzed in the Windows Domain. Network access is tightly controlled to allow anonymous access only to a small amount of read-only data.

Computational Resources

The current UNIX computational systems consist of the following Sun Microsystems servers: an x4600 with 8 Dual Core Advanced Micro Devices 64-bit Central Processing Unit (CPU) with 32GB Random Access Memory (RAM), and a x4275 with 2 quad core Intel Xeon processors and 48GB RAM. These systems are configured with SAS, R, SPlus, MatLab, and other research software, some of which are provided by University-wide site license. Automatic systems are used to alert updates and security patches, in order to make sure that these servers are actively maintained and promptly updated.

Data Storage

Network storage consists of two fiber-channel disk arrays, which are configured with 1.8 Terabytes and 7.4 Terabytes of usable disk space. This appliance is designed to be easily upgraded to provide all needed storage requirements for both the Windows desktops and the UNIX systems, and is maintained by redundant Sun Microsystems T2000 SPARC 8 core 64bit CPU servers. Database storage consists of three Sun Microsystems x2200 servers configured as a high availability failover cluster. This cluster is connected to a Dell MiniDisc 1000 SAS disk array through a perc5 Redundant Array of Independent Disks controller.

Network and Data Security

The Center implements a Netscreen SSG 550M firewall providing network security for the entire domain. This configuration gives us full control over who has access to the network and systems, creates full logs of all access to the

network, and provides the security needed for acquiring confidential data and keeping it secure. In addition, all servers, backup devices, disk storage devices, and other related hardware are kept in a private operating area within a locked steel cage inside a secured room employing a separate backup air conditioning unit and power generator, as well as extremely restricted key card access through two steel doors. All devices are connected to uninterruptible power supplies.

It is helpful to have the expertise of the Director of Computing at the highest levels of the University who has experience or completed specialized training in network security. A state-of-the-art telephone call center is also necessary to conduct quantitative and qualitative computer-assisted telephone interviews in multiple languages, with Enterprise Call Recorder software that records all telephone interviews and allows for question-by-question monitoring and quality control. The call center should operate 7 days a week to maximize survey completions. E-mail integration is provided, so survey participants can be automatically contacted as appropriate, with the system optionally tracking failed e-mail contact attempts. Web data entry can also be used for local transcription or in telephone interviewing settings, depending upon the needs of the project, and a remote data entry module has been licensed so field staff can collect data using a local copy of a survey on a laptop disconnected from the Internet. Technical support, as well as feature upgrades, is provided by contract with Datstat, Inc.

Sample Storage and Handling

Some capacity should be built in to accommodate the handling, preparation, and storage of research specimens. This space can be used to house −84 °C freezers or nitrogen tanks equipped with advanced temperature monitoring alarms where biospecimens are stored; two refrigerators; and lab benches with equipment to process biological samples. The research group's Molecular Epidemiology and Nutrition Laboratory is equipped with appropriate analytical and molecular biological instrumentation, as well as appropriate bio-containment hoods for extraction of human biologic materials. These labs have the capacity for three main functions: [1] to serve as a flexible repository for sample storage, [2] to conduct small-scale molecular work, and [3] to evaluate new technologies and bioinformation, and then generate pilot-study data in a timely fashion.

A Research Study Example: Nutritional Intervention During Pregnancy

Available epidemiologic and experimental evidence indicates that magnesium (Mg)-rich diets may improve glucose tolerance and lower the risk for type 2 diabetes and metabolic syndrome.

Magnesium is a biologically active constituent found abundantly in green leafy vegetables, beans, and nuts and involved in hundreds of enzymatic reactions in the body. A large body of literature has reported that dietary patterns high in Mg were favorably associated with lower plasma fasting concentrations of insulin and glucose [8, 9], markers of systemic inflammation [10–12], and reduced risk of metabolic syndrome and type 2 diabetes [13, 14]. Several mechanistic pathways may be affected by Mg, including glucose and insulin homeostasis, lipid metabolism, vascular contractility, and endothelial, immune, and other hemodynamic functions (Fig. 22.1).

One research question is whether increased Mg intake in pregnant women who are overweight can improve maternal metabolic profiles and birth outcomes. This topic has not been studied comprehensively and no clinical trials to date have directly compared the efficacy of Mg from diet and supplements for short- and long-term effects on maternal and fetal outcomes in both mothers and their offspring. However, a recent meta-analysis of seven studies concluded that Mg treatment prior to the 25th week of gestation was associated with lower frequencies of preterm birth [relative risk (RR) = 0.73 (0.57–0.94)], low birth weight [RR = 0.67 (0.46–0.96)], and small for gestational age infants [RR = 0.70 (0.53–0.93)] [15]. If effective, dietary and/or supplementary Mg could be easily implemented in any clinical setting and could be added safely to prenatal vitamins (the majority of prenatal vitamins contain no Mg) and/or emphasized in nutritional guidelines for pregnant women, especially for low socioeconomic status minority populations.

Recruitment and Enrollment

A provider-based recruitment strategy has been developed at Women & Infants Hospital of Rhode Island (WIH), the major provider of obstetric and gynecologic services in the State of Rhode Island and southeastern Massachusetts. Women were given information about this study by research staff members who work closely with healthcare professionals (obstetricians, residents, and midwives) at the Women's Primary Care Center.

Expertise and Experience of Multidisciplinary Team of Investigators

In order to maximize the potential scientific output and to achieve all specific aims in the proposed work, a team of investigators was organized with exceptional expertise and resources in study design methodology, nutrition, molecular genetics, reproductive and women's health, perinatal physiology, pediatrics, and biostatistics. The skills and experiences brought together in this dynamic, interactive team of investigators, all at the forefront of their respective substantive areas, achieve the ambitious goal of this randomized controlled trial.

Demonstrating Feasibility

It is important to conduct preliminary/pilot studies to demonstrate the feasibility of larger clinical trials and efforts within a research program. In several large prospective studies conducted in this research project of middle-aged women and men, the direct relationships between Mg intake and risks of type 2 diabetes, hypertension, and CVD have been demonstrated. Among initially healthy women followed for 6 years in the Women's Health Study, Mg intake was inversely associated with type 2 diabetes risk [8]. This inverse association was stronger among overweight women

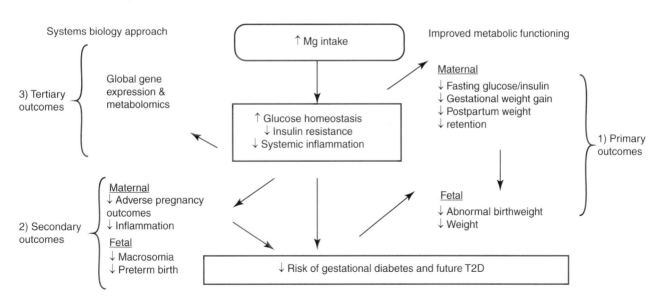

Fig. 22.1 Magnesium and hypothesized influence on primary, secondary, and tertiary outcomes in the proposed randomized trial

(BMI ≥ 25 kg/m^2) where an analysis of 349 women without type 2 diabetes also showed an inverse relation between Mg intake and levels of fasting insulin [8]. The multivariable-adjusted geometric mean insulin levels in the lowest quartile of Mg intake was 53.5 pmol/L as compared with 41.5 in the highest quartile ($p = 0.03$ for trend) [8]. In 10 years of follow-up, higher intake of dietary Mg also appeared to lower risks of hypertension and stroke [16], as well as the risk of the metabolic syndrome [17]. These findings indicate that Mg intake may exert early beneficial effects on metabolic defects common to the initiation of atherosclerosis and type 2 diabetes pathogenesis.

Magnesium homeostasis in the human body is tightly regulated [18]. To further understand the role of genetic mechanisms underlying cellular magnesium homeostasis, genes encoding the two highly selective Mg ion channel proteins, as well as the transient receptor potential membrane melastatin 6 and 7 (TRPM6 and TRPM7) responsible for intestinal and renal Mg absorption in type 2 diabetes development, were investigated. In a comprehensive analysis of common single-nucleotide polymorphisms across TRPM6 and TRPM7, carriers of the two rare alleles leading to two amino acid substitutions in the TRPM6 gene (Val1393Ile in exon 29 [rs3750425] and Lys1584Glu in exon 30 [rs2274924]) were found to have a significantly increased risk of type 2 diabetes when their Mg intakes were inadequate (<250 mg/day) [19]. In a 4-week randomized controlled crossover trial of Mg citrate supplementation (providing 500 mg elemental Mg daily) among overweight, but otherwise healthy young adults [20], Mg treatment was found to significantly decrease fasting C-peptide levels and fasting insulin (data from the trial was used to generate Fig. 22.2). Down-regulation of several genes related to metabolic and inflammatory pathways was also observed. Results from urine proteomic profiling

showed several proteins with significantly altered expression in response to Mg treatment.

Another feasibility study was completed where the aim was to determine metabolic and clinical effects of Mg in pregnant women with overweight/obesity. A total of 28 pregnant women with overweight/obesity were enrolled in a double-blinded, placebo-controlled pilot study where they were randomized to one of the three treatment arms: magnesium supplementation (300 mg elemental Mg), placebo, or nutritionist counseling about magnesium rich foods. Results show significant differences in vascular endothelial growth factor receptor 2 and TRPM6 placental mRNA expression (varied by several orders of magnitudes) across treatment groups of patients (Fig. 22.3). Hemoglobin A1c (A1C) levels and Interleukin-6 levels at 24–28 weeks displayed a statistically significant difference between groups. This pilot study provided valuable information on logistical aspects for this study, suggesting that a larger scale study with intervention endpoint beyond the second trimester with a larger set of biomarkers is necessary.

Study Design of the Mg Supplementation Trial

This study was a randomized, controlled, three-arm parallel trial comparing: [A] 300 mg/day of elemental Mg in the form of Mg citrate plus typical diet (A arm), [B] placebo plus Mg-enriched diet with 300 mg/day of produce package for 1 week once per month (B arm), versus [C] a control group consisting of placebo plus a typical diet. Women in all study arms were additionally counseled to follow the USDA dietary guidelines for pregnant women. Pregnant women with BMI ≥ 25 kg/m^2 between the ages of 18 and 40 years in their first trimester of pregnancy were eligible for the study

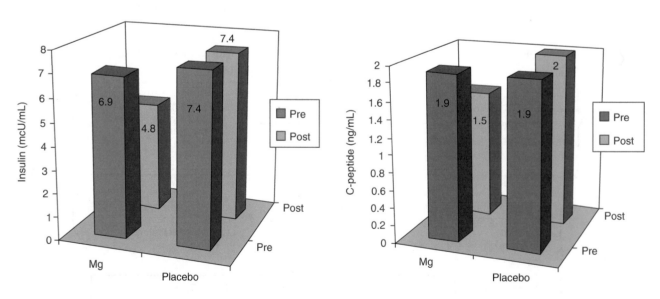

Fig. 22.2 Randomized controlled trial of magnesium supplementation among overweight individuals

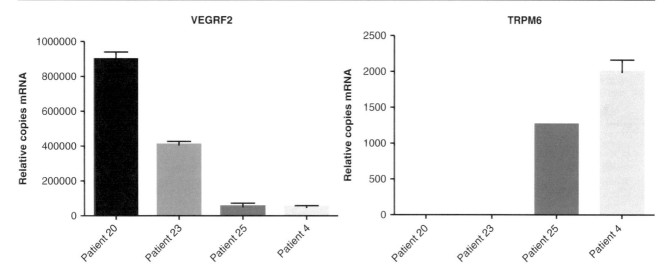

Fig. 22.3 *TRPM6* and *VEGFR2* mRNA expression in placental samples from our pilot study

and were in generally good health, mobile, and able to give complete informed consent.

Outcome Ascertainment

Multiple maternal and neonatal outcomes were targeted for ascertainment (Table 22.1).

Timeline of the Mg Supplementation Trial

The first quarter of Year 1 was dedicated to develop and standardize the study protocol, train the research staff, and obtain IRB approval (Fig. 22.4). This time was also used to prepare for the recruitment process.

Statistical Management of Experimental and Epidemiological Data

Standardized procedures in handling research data will provide high quality findings with reproducibility. This will also enhance synergy with upcoming research projects when encountering similar analytic plans. Components for appropriate data management are outlined in Table 22.2.

Mining the Existing Medicine Literature

Apart from analyzing experimental and epidemiological data, appropriate methods in mining literature will be necessary to conduct comprehensive systematic reviews and meta-analyses. Research team will get the most updated research evidence, which will provide inspiration for upcoming projects and publications. Essential steps and tools for conducting literature review are provided in Table 22.3

Table 22.1 Timing of baseline/outcome assessment

	Week's gestation			Postpartum		
	<13	24–28	36–40	6 weeks	6 months	12 months
Primary maternal outcome						
Metabolic biomarkers	X	X	X	X	X	X
Gestational weight gain	X	X	X			
Postpartum weight retention				X	X	X
Primary neonatal outcome						
Birthweight/ weight			X	X	X	X
Secondary/tertiary maternal outcome						
Pregnancy complications	X	X	X			
Inflammatory/ hormonal markers	X	X	X	X	X	X
Genomic/ metabolomics analysis	X		X		X	
Secondary/tertiary neonatal outcome						
Macrosomia/ preterm birth			X	X	X	X
Head circumference			X			
Apgar score			X			
Cord blood			X			

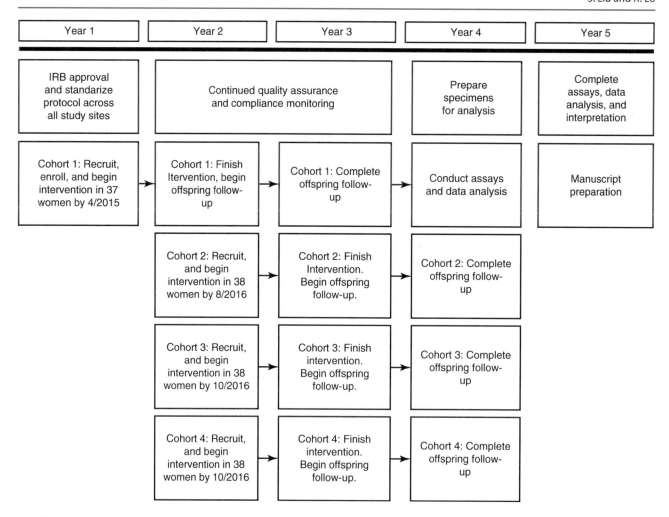

Fig. 22.4 Study timeline among 150 pregnant women with low socioeconomic status and overweight plus their offspring

Table 22.2 Procedures in managing experimental and epidemiological data

Procedures	Remarks
Data collection	Prior to data collection, protocols for the study should be registered in recognized registries (e.g., clinicaltrials.gov) and/or published in peer-reviewed journals that accept study protocols (e.g., Trials, BMJ Open, BMC Public Health). Study procedures should be performed strictly according to protocols. Amendments of procedures during the study should be documented, with changes being submitted to the registries
Data management	All data should be stored at safe space that only the research team and principal investigator have access. Data files should be locked with passwords, with data managers in the research team responsible for data cleaning. Data managers have to convert raw data into standardized forms for analysis
Data analysis	Analysis for clinical trials is preferably performed by biostatisticians being blinded to the randomization status. For all study designs, codes and strategies for data analysis should be documented and being cross-checked by independent researchers in the team to ensure high data quality. Common statistical softwares for data analysis include R, SAS, STATA, SPSS, etc.
Data reporting	The results of statistical analyses, as well as the whole report should be reported according to corresponding guidelines, e.g., CONSORT (Consolidated Standards of Reporting Trials) for clinical trials and STROBE (STrengthening the Reporting of OBservational studies in Epidemiology) for observational studies

Table 22.3 Procedures in mining the existing medicine literature

Procedures	Remarks
General	Researchers are suggested to adhere to guidelines of Cochrane Handbook, PRISMA (Preferred Reporting Items for Systematic Reviews and Meta-Analyses), and AMSTAR (A Measurement Tool to Assess Systematic Reviews) to ensure their work is conducted in high quality. Protocols for systematic reviews and meta-analyses should also be registered in recognized registries (e.g., PROSPERO and clinicaltrials.gov) before starting
Data Sources	Describe all information sources (e.g., databases with dates of coverage, contact with study authors to identify additional studies) in the search and date last searched. Literature search should be conducted in at least two data sources (e.g., PubMed, Medline)
Study Selection	Abstracts for potentially eligible studies should be selected with predefined criteria, then undergo full-text evaluation. Study selection has to be performed by two independent reviewers, and resolve the discrepancy of selection by the third reviewer
Data Extraction	Two independent researchers reviewed and extracted relevant data from each included studies in standardized formats. Whenever relevant data is missing from the included studies, researchers should contact the authors to retrieve the data
Data Analysis	State the principle summary measures (e.g., risk ratio, difference in means) and describe the methods of handling data and combining results of studies (with the use of fixed or random effects model), with measures of consistency (e.g., Cochran's Q-statistics) for each meta-analysis. Common statistical softwares for meta-analyses include Review Manager, R, STATA, SAS, etc. Assessment for publication bias (e.g., funnel plot and Egger's test) is also essential
Grading of the evidence	The overall certainty of the evidence should be evaluated using the GRADE approach (https://gradepro.org/), AACE methodology (https://web.aacei.org/), and/or assessment tools for risk of bias (e.g. Cochrane risk-of-bias tool for randomized trials). That will help readers to understand how the quality of studies may affect the cumulative evidence

Glossary

1. Virtual memory system: a multi-user, multiprocessing virtual memory-based operating system (OS) designed for use in time-sharing, batch processing, and transaction processing.
2. Windows Management Instrumentation: a set of extensions that provides an operating system interface through which instrumented components provide information and notification.
3. UNIX computational system: a family of multitasking, multiuser computer operating systems.
4. High availability failover cluster: groups of computers that support server applications that can be reliably utilized with a minimum amount of time that computers are out of action or unavailable for use.

References

1. Colditz GA. Cancer culture: epidemics, human behavior, and the dubious search for new risk factors. Am J Public Health. 2001;91:357–9.
2. Guariguata L, Whiting DR, Hambleton I, Beagley J, Linnenkamp U, Shaw JE. Global estimates of diabetes prevalence for 2013 and projections for 2035. Diabetes Res Clin Pract. 2014;103:137–49.
3. Narres M, Claessen H, Droste S, et al. The incidence of end-stage renal disease in the diabetic (compared to the non-diabetic) population: a systematic review. PLoS One. 2016;11:e0147329.
4. Humphries MD, Brunson A, Hedayati N, Romano P, Melnkow J. Amputation risk in patients with diabetes mellitus and peripheral artery disease using statewide data. Ann Vasc Surg. 2016;30:123–31.
5. Hippisley-Cox J, Coupland C. Diabetes treatments and risk of amputation, blindness, severe kidney failure, hyperglycaemia, and hypoglycaemia: open cohort study in primary care. BMJ. 2016;352:i1450.
6. Emerging Risk Factors Collaboration, Sarwar N, Gao P, et al. Diabetes mellitus, fasting blood glucose concentration, and risk of vascular disease: a collaborative meta-analysis of 102 prospective studies. Lancet. 2010;375:2215–22.
7. Pang L, Li Q, Li Y, Liu Y, Duan N, Li H. Urine proteomics of primary membranous nephropathy using nanoscale liquid chromatography tandem mass spectrometry analysis. Clin Proteomics. 2018;15:5.
8. Song Y, Manson JE, Buring JE, Liu S. Dietary magnesium intake in relation to plasma insulin levels and risk of type 2 diabetes in women. Diabetes Care. 2004;27:59–65.
9. Fung TT, Manson JE, Solomon CG, Liu S, Willett WC, Hu FB. The association between magnesium intake and fasting insulin concentration in healthy middle-aged women. J Am Coll Nutr. 2003;22:533–8.
10. Liu S, Manson JE, Stampfer MJ, et al. Dietary glycemic load assessed by food-frequency questionnaire in relation to plasma high-density-lipoprotein cholesterol and fasting plasma triacylglycerols in postmenopausal women. Am J Clin Nutr. 2001;73:560–6.
11. Song Y, Li TY, van Dam RM, Manson JE, Hu FB. Magnesium intake and plasma concentrations of markers of systemic inflammation and endothelial dysfunction in women. Am J Clin Nutr. 2007;85:1068–74.
12. Chacko SA, Song Y, Nathan L, et al. Relations of dietary magnesium intake to biomarkers of inflammation and endothelial dysfunction in an ethnically diverse cohort of postmenopausal women. Diabetes Care. 2010;33:304–10.
13. Liu S. Intake of refined carbohydrates and whole grain foods in relation to risk of type 2 diabetes mellitus and coronary heart disease. J Am Coll Nutr. 2002;21:298–306.
14. Liu S, Manson JE, Stampfer MJ, et al. A prospective study of whole-grain intake and risk of type 2 diabetes mellitus in US women. Am J Public Health. 2000;90:1409–15.
15. Makrides M, Crosby DD, Bain E, Crowther CA. Magnesium supplementation in pregnancy. Cochrane Database Syst Rev. 2014;(4):CD000937.
16. Song Y, Sesso HD, Manson JE, Cook NR, Buring JE, Liu S. Dietary magnesium intake and risk of incident hypertension among middle-aged and older US women in a 10-year follow-up study. Am J Cardiol. 2006;98:1616–21.

17. Song Y, Ridker PM, Manson JE, Cook NR, Buring JE, Liu S. Magnesium intake, C-reactive protein, and the prevalence of metabolic syndrome in middle-aged and older U.S. women. Diabetes Care. 2005;28:1438–44.

18. Schlingmann KP, Weber S, Peters M, et al. Hypomagnesemia with secondary hypocalcemia is caused by mutations in TRPM6, a new member of the TRPM gene family. Nat Genet. 2002;31:166–70.

19. Song Y, Hsu YH, Niu T, Manson JE, Buring JE, Liu S. Common genetic variants of the ion channel transient receptor potential membrane melastatin 6 and 7 (TRPM6 and TRPM7), magnesium intake, and risk of type 2 diabetes in women. BMC Med Genet. 2009;10:4.

20. Chacko SA, Sul J, Song Y, et al. Magnesium supplementation, metabolic and inflammatory markers, and global genomic and proteomic profiling: a randomized, double-blind, controlled, crossover trial in overweight individuals. Am J Clin Nutr. 2011;93:463–73.

Lifestyle Medicine Centers: Introduction to Case Studies

Jeffrey I. Mechanick and Robert F. Kushner

Introduction

Many times in healthcare, an idea is presented based on theory, perceived needs, and anticipated successes. However, in practice, realizing these ideas in a way that can be implemented to achieve initial and emergent goals is generally very difficult. This difficulty in translating theory to practice primarily results from economic obstacles, political pressures, subjective fears, decreased confidence, or unforeseen events. Building a Lifestyle Medicine Center, or Lifestyle Medicine Clinical Service Line, within a sponsoring healthcare system is a great example of how these difficulties arise and can be overcome. Unfortunately, the nascent field of lifestyle medicine is riddled not only with research and knowledge gaps, but also practice gaps — disappointingly minimal instances of successful buildouts, operations, and financially sustainable enterprises. In other words, the concept of a Lifestyle Medicine Center can be substantiated based on epidemiological and clinical data, but it is the instantiation of a working and successful physical entity along with the reification of the idea over the long haul with organic growth and adaptation, that lends relevance and promise to a struggling healthcare system. The purpose of this brief chapter is to set the stage for the individual case studies that follow so the reader can discern features and actions along a broad range of concepts and aspirations that resonate with different lifestyle medicine trajectories and targets. A series of existing Lifestyle Medicine Centers are selected to showcase diversity in terms of scope, design, infrastructure, and maturity.

J. I. Mechanick (✉)
The Marie-Josée and Henry R. Kravis Center for Cardiovascular Health at Mount Sinai Heart, and the Division of Endocrinology, Diabetes and Bone Disease, Icahn School of Medicine at Mount Sinai, New York, NY, USA
e-mail: jeffrey.mechanick@mountsinai.org

R. F. Kushner
Departments of Medicine and Medical Education, Northwestern University, Chicago, IL, USA

Rationale for Building a Lifestyle Medicine Center

Providing a rationale for the investment in a Lifestyle Medicine Center is critical to the formulation of the strategic plan (including Mission and Vision statements), which serves as the backbone for the business plan (to demonstrate profit/loss expectations toward profitability, revenue neutrality, fiscal soundness, or other endpoints that can support the strategic plan and ongoing operations). Subsequent infrastructure (physical and human resources), logistics and operations, adaptations for future growth and scalability, and long-term sustainability features are then configured (Fig. 23.1). Justifications to build a Lifestyle Medicine Center can be prompted by newly recognized problems or shortcomings, regulatory mandates, financial opportunities or need to compete better, changes in leadership or strategies, or simply available funds.

Each case study is tasked with identifying an interpretation of the lifestyle medicine problem, or set of problems, to be addressed with the construction and operation of a Lifestyle Medicine Center. The scope of the problem will be expressed in terms of prevalence, demographics, morbidity, and mortality on scales relevant to the catchment area of the Center: local, state, national, or global. In addition, the case study authors are asked to provide a general practice paradigm for the particular focus of the Center, in terms of disease or condition. In particular, the impact of lifestyle medicine on these particular diseases or conditions will be outlined.

Logistics

Once the development and physical building processes have been approved and funded, there is a sequence of steps that must occur. For each of the case studies, the authors will provide context as to whether the Centers are part of an academic

Fig. 23.1 Framework to
develop a Lifestyle Medicine
Center*. *Funding is in most
cases an initial and necessary
criterion for the development
process

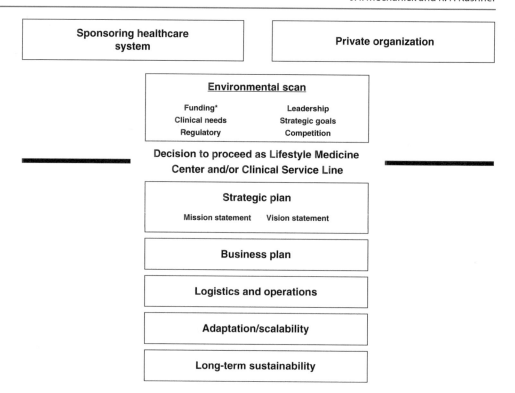

or private setting, and whether they are freestanding or function as clinical service lines that are part of a sponsoring
healthcare organization/corporation. The market will be
described, particularly if it is highly competitive or saturated,
or whether the Center will be a first of its kind in the region,
and how this would influence operations.

Other unique aspects of infrastructure and environment
may be included. For instance, will the Center be comprised
of different programs, such as primary care or clinical specialty care, nutritional counseling with a Registered Dietitian
or Registered Dietitian Nutritionist, medical fitness and/or
cardiac/pulmonary rehabilitation with exercise physiologists
and/or physical therapists, education and community engagement, and/or utilization of wearable technologies?

Moreover, for a Center with different programs, how will
administrative support and staffing be allocated and managed? Will there be vertical management, horizontal management, or a combination of both? Vertical management
structures are more typical, described as a formal "top-down"
multilevel structure, where each employee (healthcare professional or staff person) is accountable to their superior, but
not always responsible for making organizational decisions.
In this structure, decision-making and execution may be
slower. In contrast, horizontal management structures are
"flat," where employees are empowered to make decisions
more autonomously and according to organizational goals,
and communication flows more freely and faster due to networking effects and collaboration. In general, routine operations in a Lifestyle Medicine Center are managed vertically
for greater accountability, but there may be times when criti-

cal problem solving is needed, or are preferred, such as during transitions or major infrastructural change. Case studies
will describe how team members interact with one another in
the models presented.

Human resources depend on the mission, programs, and
management structure of the Center. The case studies will
provide information about staffing, positions and titles, team
members, number and allocation of full-time employees, and
roles and responsibilities. Programs should have policies and
protocols (or clinical care pathways), and in many of the case
studies, these details are provided.

The physical space is another variable that will be apparent when each of the different case studies is reviewed. Floor
plans are provided in some of the case studies and space
design and utilization (square footage, rooms and décor,
equipment and furnishings, and location in a healthcare system), in relation to Center operations and programs, can be
reviewed. Readers may wish to consider whether the space is
sufficiently "immersive" to motivate engagement, and conducive to promote a "high-touch" patient experience.

Operations are described in the case studies and include
patient flow (number of patients seen as new consults or
follow-ups; how they are navigated in the Center) and bill-
ing/payment structures. The economics are particularly
important, since in many cases, these are the major determinants of sustainability (as opposed to success, which should
be based on clinical outcomes). Other aspects worthy of
mention are the expanded roles and responsibilities of
employees, specific role of the Center in the healthcare system, available community resources, educational programs

within and outside of the Center, research capabilities, and staff development. Lastly, are there opportunities for patients to provide feedback to leadership to improve the facility and even guide decision-making for scaling-up (adding more services and programs) and/or scaling-out (across a geographic area with multiple Centers)?

Discussion

The purpose of providing case studies is to assist with the formulation, design, and operation of a Center in such a way that it can be uniquely fashioned to the needs of leadership and produce desirable clinical outcomes with financial viability and sustainability. Case studies allow thought experiments by the reader to consider whether a certain plan would work according to the goals and constraints at play. More specifically, each case scenario can be reverse-engineered by the reader to see how it works, in order to inform and engineer new strategic and business plans. Case studies can reveal which components are responsible for successes, or even failures or difficulties. In short, the reader should review each of the case studies, which complements clinical evidence and technical advice already presented, to create a roadmap for a new tailored Lifestyle Medicine Center.

James M. Rippe

The Rationale for Rippe Lifestyle Institute Approach to Lifestyle Medicine

Addressing the Issue

When Rippe Lifestyle Institute (RLI) was established in 1993, the RLI team was already deeply involved in many aspects of physical activity, nutrition, and weight management, and their impact on both short- and long-term health and quality of life. While the evidence base, even back in 1993, was very robust showing that these modalities had profound benefits, having a firm evidence base was deemed necessary for the field of lifestyle medicine to grow, prosper, and assume a rightful place in mainstream medicine.

The scientific evidence for physical activity, nutrition, and weight management, and other aspects of positive lifestyle in the management of chronic disease can be identified in multiple disciplines, but detailed information was generally difficult to access for most healthcare professionals (HCPs). Notwithstanding this challenge, HCPs still believed that proper nutrition, regular physical activity, and maintaining a healthy body weight were very important to preserving or enhancing health. Unfortunately, most HCPs had only a passing familiarity of the robust literature connecting behavior and health. Therefore, considerable knowledge and practice gaps existed in healthcare, setting the stage for the emergence of an evidence-based Lifestyle Medicine Center, not to mention the champions motivated and formally trained by such a Center.

General Approach

In order to establish the strongest level of evidence for the positive impact of lifestyle medicine modalities, a general approach was adopted involving 4 separate and intertwined strands of work.

- A vigorous, academic research program was established to explore each of the major areas of lifestyle medicine. This has resulted in the publication of over 500 academic abstracts and research papers, as well as 53 books: 35 for physicians and other HCPs, and 18 for the general public [1]. Specifically, the RLI publishing program includes editing a major lifestyle medicine textbook (*Lifestyle Medicine*, now in its third edition, CRC Press, Boca Raton, FL, 2019) and launching and editing the first and only peer-reviewed journal in the area of lifestyle medicine (*The American Journal of Lifestyle Medicine*, SAGE Publications).
- A clinical program was developed, involving executive health services and clinical research trials.
- A counseling program for patients in the cardiovascular clinic was created to focus on the importance of lifestyle as part of an overall approach to health.
- A high level of credibility was maintained through continued immersion in traditional medical services (e.g., participation with the cardiac catheterization laboratory and coronary care unit).

The Impact of Lifestyle Medicine Components

There is no longer any serious doubt that regular physical activity, proper nutrition, and weight management exert profound effects on chronic disease risk factor mitigation, as well as short- and long-term health and quality of life. While there are many studies that support these concepts, two that drive the point home derive from the large databases maintained at

J. M. Rippe (✉)
Rippe Lifestyle Institute, Shrewsbury, MA, USA
e-mail: jrippe@rippelifestyle.com; bgrady@rippelifestyle.com

© Springer Nature Switzerland AG 2020
J. I. Mechanick, R. F. Kushner (eds.), *Creating a Lifestyle Medicine Center*, https://doi.org/10.1007/978-3-030-48088-2_24

Harvard Medical School. In the Nurses' Health Trial, females who adopted 5 measures related to positive lifestyle, including regular physical activity (30 minutes of moderate intensity physical activity on most, if not all days), proper nutrition (more fruits and vegetables, two fish meals/week, and more whole grains), healthy weight management (body mass index between 19 and 25 kg/m^2), not smoking cigarettes, and consuming one alcoholic beverage/day reduced the risk of cardiovascular disease by 84% and diabetes by 91% [2]. Similar findings were also true in the male population, as published in the Health Professionals' Follow-up Study [3]. Many other studies have corroborated and expanded these findings; the impact of these lifestyle measures is profound and consistent. These data are further underscored by their inclusion in virtually every evidence-based, national and international guideline for the reduction of risk factors or treatment of metabolically related diseases (Table 24.1) [4].

Table 24.1 Sampling of guidelines that incorporate lifestyle recommendations for the prevention of chronic disease[a]

Guidelines	Website
ACC/AHA guidelines for the prevention, detection, evaluation and management of high blood pressure in adults	https://www.acc.org/latest-in-cardiology/ten-points-to-remember/2017/11/09/11/41/2017-guideline-for-high-blood-pressure-in-adults
National academies workshops on obesity and nutrition	https://sparck.nationalacademies.org/vivisimo/cgi-bin/query-meta?query=obesity&v%3Aproject=uweb_proj_ext
Dietary guidelines for Americans 2015–2020	https://health.gov/dietaryguidelines/2015/guidelines/
Guidelines from the American Academy of Pediatrics for heart disease risk factor reduction in children	https://pediatrics.aappublications.org/content/128/Supplement_5/S213
American Heart Association strategic plan for 2020	https://www.aha.org/strategy
Preventing cancer, cardiovascular disease and diabetes: A common agenda for the American Cancer Society, the American Diabetes Association and the American Heart Association	https://www.ncbi.nlm.nih.gov/pubmed/15220271
Defining optimal brain health in adults: A presidential advisory from the AHA/ASH	https://www.ahajournals.org/doi/full/10.1161/STR.0000000000000148
2013 AHA/ACC/TOS guideline for the management of overweight and obesity in adults	https://ahajournals.org/doi/full/10.1161/01.cir.0000437739.71477.ee
2018 physical activity advisory committee scientific report	https://health.gov/paguidelines/second-edition/report/

[a]All websites accessed on 24 Mar 2020

Rippe Lifestyle Institute Research, Clinical Activities, and Publishing

Rippe Lifestyle Institute researchers have conducted and published numerous studies in the area of physical activity and health. The RLI laboratory developed the first field test of walking to estimate aerobic capacity [5], and published 5 books [6–10] and numerous academic papers and abstracts [1, 11–13] related to walking and health. While other forms of physical activity have been investigated by RLI, walking remains the core research effort in the area of physical activity. In fact, findings from RLI research was foundational to the earliest guidelines from the American College of Cardiology and the American College of Sports Medicine with their published *Guidelines for Physical Activity and Health* [14], and served as the driving force behind the initial American Heart Association "Walk with your Doc" program, which ultimately grew into the current "Walk with a Doc" program [15].

In the area of nutrition, RLI has explored a wide variety of approaches to good health. These have included specific research projects in the areas of increased fiber, fruit, and vegetable consumption, as well as low fat dietary strategies [16–20]. RLI research protocols are consistent with American Heart Association [21] and Dietary Guidelines for Americans [22], and incorporate principles from both the Mediterranean [23] and the Dietary Approaches to Stop Hypertension (DASH) Diets [24].

Clinicians at RLI have also conducted research and published widely in the area of healthy approaches to weight management [25–27]. Examples include how weight loss and weight management impact on a variety of risk factors for cardiovascular disease, diabetes, and the metabolic syndrome, as well as high blood pressure, dyslipidemia, distribution of body fat, and inflammatory responses. Three books specifically related to weight management [28–30] were published by RLI authors and incorporated advice about weight management and/or weight loss.

Vision

While considerable progress has been made in lifestyle medicine, there are still knowledge and practice gaps to close. For example, numerous studies including the American Heart Association Strategic Guidelines for 2020 [31] and the Behavioral Risk Surveillance System [32] have shown that only 5% or less of American adults adopt all of these positive lifestyle measures. Furthermore, within the medical community, less than 40% of physicians routinely counsel their patients in these areas [33]. The vision at RLI is to target these metrics through evidence-based decision-making, conveyed not only to the medical community, but also to the public at large.

Development and Organization of Rippe Lifestyle Institute

Infrastructure and Environment

Since inception, RLI has had relationships with various academic medical centers and teaching hospitals. The relationship with academic medical centers was important since it provided access to additional expertise in a variety of disciplines. The relationship with teaching hospitals was also important since it afforded access to multiple, high level, expensive technologies which would be very difficult to establish within the Center. Many of these technologies are important for increasingly sophisticated metabolic measurements that are needed in lifestyle medicine assessments. These are outlined in Table 24.2.

Private Research Laboratory

As the RLI staff grew, it became apparent that physical space needs could not be accommodated within a traditional academic medical center. Thus, a private research laboratory was established and was moved offsite, though proximate to affiliated academic medical centers and teaching hospitals including the University of Massachusetts Medical School, Florida Hospital, and the University of Central Florida Medical School. The initial RLI facility was 9000 square feet of administrative, publishing, and research space, which was housed approximately one-half mile from the affiliated academic medical center.

Publishing Infrastructure

RLI has been the source of multiple publications, so in order to facilitate a large number of contacts, a publishing infrastructure was fashioned to involve a fulltime Publishing Director, Office Assistant, and other administrative staff.

Executive Health Program

The Executive Health Program was established in coordination with a teaching hospital. Several hundred executives were seen each year for their annual health and fitness evaluations. The teaching hospital supplied some of the resources to support this, while the vast majority of clinicians working in the Executive Health Program were employed by RLI.

Amenities for the Executive Health Program include access to an indoor swimming pool, as well as a comprehensive fitness center, both of which were owned by the teaching hospital affiliated with RLI (Florida Hospital). Services within the Executive Health Program included a comprehensive physical examination, exercise tolerance test with direct measurement of VO2 max, 3-day food records and nutritional consultation, and dual X-ray absorptiometry scanning to determine lean muscle mass and body fat. Selected patients were also offered a coronary computerized tomography, as well as computerized tomography of the head, abdomen, and lungs on an as-needed basis for individuals who were at high risk for various malignancies or coronary heart disease. Follow-up with our nutrition team and exercise physiologists was provided for individuals who needed and requested these services.

Table 24.2 Various technologies employed by the Rippe Lifestyle Institute[a]

Technology	Clinical applications/ rationale	Population
Serum measurements	Baseline measurements on all patients	All patients Selected research subjects
Metabolic panel	Baseline values	
Complete blood count	36-hour measurements to determine metabolic response to various nutritional interventions	
Insulin		
Leptin		
Ghrelin		
Exercise tolerance test with VO2 max measurement	Precise measurement of aerobic fitness	All patients
DXA scanning	Body composition including lean muscle mass and adiposity	All patients and selected research subjects in weight loss studies
Coronary artery imaging	Determination of level of plaque and atherosclerosis	Selected patients at high risk for CHD
CT scans of abdomen, chest, and head	Screening for malignancies	Selected patients
Functional MRI Brain Liver	Cerebral response to various nutritional interventions Liver fat in response to various nutritional interventions	Selected research subjects Selected research subjects

[a]Abbreviations: *CHD* coronary heart disease, *CT* computerized tomography, *DXA* dual X-ray absorptiometry, *MRI* magnetic resonance imaging, *VO2* = maximal oxygen consumption

Process and Approach

Research

Rippe Lifestyle Institute collaborates with many research sponsors in the fitness arena, the packaged goods space, and the pharmaceutical industry, as well as trade associations. For each research contract, a specific business plan is constructed, which outlines the tasks that RLI researchers will accomplish, including traditional research approaches, outline of hypotheses, power calculations and other statistical issues, timetable, and budget. In each of these settings, a budget is established and agreed upon with the research sponsor. This enables annual financial projections for the entire RLI organization based on various revenue streams.

Partnerships

For each project, research sponsors are aware that while RLI has ultimate control of what is published, relationships are viewed as ongoing collaborative partnerships. This has been very important to all of our research sponsors. The RLI team has had the pleasure of working with multiple research sponsors in the packaged goods and nutrition arena, as well as multiple fitness equipment companies and pharmaceutical companies.

Publishing

A larger pool of individuals is available to help with publishing, since there are personnel in RLI for clinical and research activities. Rippe Lifestyle Institute publications are supported by a Director who deals with hundreds of academic researchers each year, as well as interfacing with textbook and journal publishers. The infrastructure for receiving and accepting papers is handled by commercial publishing partners, while generation and review of manuscripts, both for book chapters and journal articles, is handled internally by an RLI Director, Office Assistant, and Institute Director. Budgets that guide the publication of internally generated scientific data, as well as fund presentations and derivative activities, are incorporated into institutional research business plans. Books are also written for the general public and coordinated by the Publishing Director [1]. These publishing efforts generate their own independent revenue streams.

Executive Health Program

The RLI Executive Health Program was designed to run in conjunction with a teaching hospital. A business plan was therefore devised with this institution, which included projected revenues and expenses. The teaching hospital provided the infrastructure for billing and accounting. The RLI Executive Health Program did not accept insurance, so revenue was generated from either the individuals who came through the program themselves or the companies that they worked for. RLI established contracts to supply annual executive health evaluations for Fortune 500 companies in the Central Florida area. RLI also established contracts with other local businesses, as well as serving as a site for multinational companies who had offices in the Central Florida area. Individual Executive Health Programs were also developed for individuals whose companies had this as a "key individual" benefit or for individuals who sought this service on their own.

Physical Space

Space needs for the RLI have been consistent over time. When started, RLI was located in an academic medical center at the University of Massachusetts Medical School and had approximately 1000 square feet of space. However, the Institute quickly outgrew this space as staff expanded and relocation offsite became necessary. A 9000 square foot research space – a publishing and administrative space near an academic medical center in Massachusetts – was subsequently procured and occupied. Subsequently, RLI moved the research and clinical facilities to a teaching hospital in Florida, and as staff increased further in that setting, another two offsite facilities were established. These moves established additional clinic and research space. Within these two facilities were two metabolic wards, where overnight studies could be conducted for up to six individuals at a time, as well as laboratory and office space, six private counseling rooms, a small clinic, and storage and freezer rooms for various blood samples and other products for various protocols. Administration and finance functions remained at the RLI facility in Massachusetts, which was decreased in size to 4000 square feet to accommodate administrative and publishing staff. The move of our major clinical and research facility to Florida occurred in conjunction with the building of a new, state-of-the-art hospital and clinical compound by Florida Hospital on Disney property in the town of Celebration Health, outside of Orlando.

Human Resources

Staffing

Many of the RLI staff members are active in both research and clinical work. In the research area, Master- and Doctorate-level exercise physiologists, research nurses, Master-level research nutritionists (e.g., Master of Science [M.Sc.,M.S.], Registered Dietitian Nutritionist [R.D.N.]), one or two full-time recruiters (depending on the number of studies that we have had in progress at any given time) , and a full-time Marketing and Client Services Director to interface with public and research sponsors have been employed. Within the publishing area, there is a full-time Publishing Director and full-time Administrative Assistant interfacing with multiple authors/contributors/editors, as well as publishers. Both research and publishing teams are actively involved in the generation of academic papers and abstracts, as have been the two full-time Executive Assistants (one in Massachusetts and one in Florida). There is also a full-time Chief Financial Officer for the entire organization.

In the Executive Health Program, there is a Clinic Director and several other clinical specialists, in the areas of exercise physiology and nutrition. A part-time psychologist is also employed to supervise issues, such as stress reduction and anxiety counseling. Physicians in RLI handle issues related to tobacco cessation and sleep hygiene, among others. There is also a full-time receptionist to handle logistical issues related to Executive Health Program patients, and also a Marketing and Client Services Director to coordinate issues among individuals, their companies, and RLI. Billing and finance have been handled through the teaching hospital.

Patient and Research Subject Flow

The RLI research laboratories typically handle 200–500 research subjects at a given time, depending on the particular research trials and their duration. These subjects typically reside in free living environments (typically their homes) or occasionally a nearby hotel, and come to our facilities for counseling and testing, although there is the capability of studying 3–6 individuals at a time for 1–2 overnight stays in two metabolic wards. The Executive Health Program patients range from 2 to 6 per day and typically are seen by 1–2 physicians. The treatment care facilities vary according to the needs of research trials, specific procedures being undertaken, and clinical offerings at the Executive Health Program. Executive health patients can be seen in the research facility, although it is preferred that they are seen in the clinic in collaboration with the teaching hospital.

Billing and Payment Structure

Research billing is based on the number of procedures performed and the amount of staff time required for counseling and other procedures. Blood samples for research subjects are sent to an outside certified laboratory. For the Executive Health Program, blood samples are sent either to an outside certified laboratory, or when these patients are seen in conjunction with the teaching hospital, the blood work is sent to that facility's in-house laboratory. Billing is based on the agreed upon research contract with outside research sponsors. Executive Health Program billing occurs according to contracts with companies who have sent their executives through the RLI research program, or is directly billed to the executive who was seen. The RLI does not participate with any insurance plans. Billing for publishing work is based on contracts with various publishers and is based on a pre-specified fee structure for work by HCPs or RLI staff. A rough depiction of sources of revenue for RLI is found in Fig. 24.1.

Expanded Roles and Responsibilities

In the area of publishing, great pride is taken in the ability to not only publish academic books and research papers, but also to present research and educational content at scientific and medical meetings. Abstracts are typically presented by various RLI staff members or the Research Director [1].

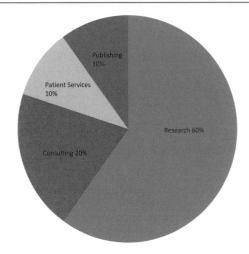

Fig. 24.1 Average percentage of revenue coming from various sources for the Rippe Lifestyle Institute (varies from year to year)

Due to the RLI infrastructure, symposia can be organized in a variety of settings in the United States, Europe, South America, and Asia [1]. A unique aspect of RLI is the long-standing track record of communicating through various channels to HCPs, media, and the general public. Budgets for these activities are typically included in research proposals, although in some instances there have been separate budgets for communications.

Discussion

The RLI employs an academic medical model of lifestyle medicine that combines research, education, and clinical services. This vision has spawned a relatively large and multicenter resource for lifestyle medicine. As a result of this core philosophy, various drivers for success can be identified. First, personnel are attracted to RLI because of the ability to perform both research and clinical practice in an emerging field – lifestyle medicine. Second, other organizations that actively seek out intellectually stimulating collaborations gravitate toward RLI and facilitate the broad range of research projects that directly and indirectly support the other facets of enterprise: education, publication, and clinical practice. Third, RLI can be interpreted as an incubator for the training and maturation of champions in lifestyle medicine; this is a critical implementation science factor for the expansion of interest in this field. And fourth, by having each of these components in play, a culture of learning, caring, and promulgation of knowledge arises, which can ultimately guide the development of other Lifestyle Medicine Centers and close the gaps that have challenged population-based adoption of lifestyle medicine. The future is bright for RLI as current efforts with the largest, self-insured healthcare organization in the State of Massachusetts are underway to develop programs that incorporate lifestyle medicine. The goal of this partnership is to improve patient outcomes and satisfaction, control expenses, and perhaps even reduce physician burnout.

References

1. Rippe Health. https://www.rippehealth.com/index.htm. Accessed on 29 May 2019.
2. Carey V, Walters E, Colditz G, et al. Body fat distribution and risk of non-insulin dependent diabetes mellitus in women: the nurses' health study. Am J Epidemiol. 1997;145:614–9.
3. Chiuve S, McCullough M, Sacks F, et al. Healthy lifestyle factors in the primary prevention of coronary heart disease among men: benefits among users and nonusers of lipid-lowering and antihypertensive medications. Circulation. 2006;114:160–7.
4. Rippe JM. Lifestyle medicine: the health promoting power of daily habits and practices. Amer J Lifestyle Med. 2018;12:499–512.
5. Kline G, Porcari J, Hintermeister R, et al. Estimation of VO2 max from a one mile track walk, gender, age and body weight. Med Sci Sports Exerc. 1987;19:253–9.
6. Sweetgall R, Rippe J, Katch F. Fitness walking. New York: Putnam; 1985.
7. Kashiwa A, Rippe J. Fitness walking for women. New York: Putnam; 1987.
8. Ulene A, Rippe J. Art Ulene's fitness walking book. New York: Random House; 1988.
9. Rippe J, Ward A. The Rockport walking program. New York: Prentice Hall Press; 1989.
10. Rippe J, Ward A. The complete book of fitness walking. New York: Prentice Hall Press; 1990.
11. Rippe J, Ward A, Porcari J, et al. Walking for health and fitness. JAMA. 1988;13:259–72.
12. Ward A, Malloy P, Rippe J. Exercise prescription guidelines. Cardiol Clin. 1987;5:197–210.
13. Rippe JM, Ward A, Freedson P. Walking for health and fitness: Encyclopedia Britannica Health Annual; 1988.
14. Pate R, Pratt M, Blair S, et al. Physical activity and public health: a recommendation from the Centers for Disease Control and Prevention and the American College of Sports Medicine. JAMA. 1995;273:402–7.
15. Walk with a Doc. https://walkwithadoc.org. Accessed on 31 May 2019.
16. Lichtenstein A, Ornish D, Rippe J, et al. The best diet for healthy adults? Patient Care, November 15, 1999.
17. Rippe JM. Challenges and opportunities of communicating nutrition in the information age. Nutr Today. 2000;35:1–3.
18. Dwyer J, Rippe J. Lifestyle nutrition. London: Blackwell Science; 2000.
19. Rippe J. Nutrition in lifestyle medicine. New York: Humana Press; 2016.
20. Rippe JM. Lifestyle strategies for risk reduction, prevention and treatment of cardiovascular disease. Am J Lifestyle Med. 2018;13:204–12.
21. Lichtenstein A, Appel L, Brands M, et al. Diet and lifestyle recommendations revision 2006 a scientific statement from the American Heart Association Nutrition Committee. Circulation. 2006;114:82–96.
22. U.S. Department of Health and Human Services and U.S. Department of AGRICULTURE. 2015–2020 dietary guidelines for Americans. 8th Edition. 2015. http://health.Gov/dietaryguidelines/2015/guidelines/. Accessed on 30 Dec 2019.
23. Estruch R, Ros E, Salas-Salvadó J, et al. Primary prevention of cardiovascular disease with a Mediterranean diet. N Engl J Med. 2013;368:1279–90.
24. Obarzanek E, Sacks F, Vollmer W, et al. Effects on blood lipids of a blood pressure-lowering diet: the Dietary Approaches to Stop Hypertension (DASH) trial. Am J Clin Nutr. 2001;74:80–9.
25. Melanson K, McInnis K, Rippe J, et al. Obesity and cardiovascular disease risk: a research update. Cardiol Rev. 2001;9:202–7.
26. Rippe J, McInnis K, Melanson K. Physician involvement in the management of obesity as a primary medical condition. Obes Res. 2001;9:302S–11S.
27. Melanson K, Summers A, Nguyen V, et al. Body composition, dietary composition, and components of metabolic syndrome in overweight and obese adults after a 12 week trial on dietary treatments focused on portion control, energy density, or glycemic index. Nutrition J. 2012;11:57.
28. Foreyt J, Poston W, McInnis K, et al. Lifestyle obesity management. London: Blackwell Science; 2003.
29. Rippe J. Weight loss that lasts: break through the 10 big diet myths. Hoboken: John Wiley & Sons; 2004.
30. Rippe J, Angelopoulos T. Obesity: prevention and treatment. Boca Raton: CRC Press; 2012.
31. Lloyd-Jones D, Hong Y, Labarthe D, et al. Defining and setting national goals for cardiovascular health promotion and disease reduction: the American Heart Association's strategic impact goal through 2020 and beyond. Circulation. 2010;121:586–613.
32. Behavioral risk factor surveillance system. https://www.cdc.gov/brfss/index.html. Accessed on 3 June 2019.
33. Kelly J. High intensity therapeutic lifestyle change. In: Rippe J, editor. Lifestyle medicine. 3rd ed. Boca Raton: CRC Press; 2019.

Robert F. Kushner and Holly R. Herrington

Abbreviations

ABOM	American Board of Obesity Medicine
AVS	After visit summary
BMI	Body mass index
CLM	Center for Lifestyle Medicine
DHC	Digestive Health Center
EHR	Electronic health record
FSM	Feinberg School of Medicine
HCP	Healthcare professional
MNT	Medical nutrition therapy
NCD	Non-communicable disease
NM	Northwestern Medicine
NMG	Northwestern Medical Group
RDN	Registered dietitian nutritionist

Introduction

The Northwestern Medicine Center for Lifestyle Medicine (CLM) is a specialty referral center for the treatment of obesity. The rationale for creation of the Center was based on four principles: [1] the population prevalence and burden of obesity has reached epidemic levels [2]; there is an insufficient response to management of obesity by healthcare professionals (HCPs) [3]; the foundational treatment of obesity is focused on lifestyle modification; and [4] a new field of obesity medicine has emerged.

R. F. Kushner (✉)
Departments of Medicine and Medical Education,
Northwestern University, Chicago, IL, USA
e-mail: rkushner@northwestern.edu

H. R. Herrington
Northwestern Memorial Hospital, Center for Lifestyle Medicine,
Chicago, IL, USA

The Population Prevalence and Burden of Obesity

In 2016, approximately 40% of adults and 18% of children had excess body weight worldwide, equating to almost 2 billion adults and 340 million children [1]. Currently, most of the world's population live in countries where overweight and obesity kills more people than underweight [2]. The US prevalence rates for obesity are roughly similar [3] and are particularly alarming among certain subpopulations, including those with severe (class III, body mass index [BMI] ≥ 40 kg/m^2) obesity where overall age-adjusted prevalence rates are 5.5% and 9.9% for men and women, respectively, and 16.8% for non-Hispanic women. Based on scientific advancements over the past several decades, obesity is now recognized as a disease by multiple national organizations [4–6] and is included among the global non-communicable disease (NCD) targets identified by the World Health Organization [7]. Obesity is a risk factor for an expanding set of chronic diseases, including cardiovascular disease, type 2 diabetes, chronic kidney disease, nonalcoholic fatty liver disease, gastroesophageal reflux disease, metabolic syndrome, and many cancers, among other comorbid conditions. Obesity is considered to result from the complex interplay of environmental, social, behavioral, genetic, and biological determinants that result in a dysregulation of calorie balance.

Insufficient Response to Manage Obesity by the Medical Community

Despite the medical, social, and economic impact of obesity, the disease is insufficiently addressed in the primary care setting. For example, among 9827 patients in a Mayo Clinic primary care database, just 5% of all patients received a diagnosis of obesity, despite 26% having recorded BMIs greater than 30 kg/m^2 [8]. A 2013 analysis of electronic health record (EHR) data from 25 primary care practices found that

J. I. Mechanick, R. F. Kushner (eds.), *Creating a Lifestyle Medicine Center*, https://doi.org/10.1007/978-3-030-48088-2_25

one-third of patients did not have BMI information recorded [9]. Among those whose BMI were recorded, only 17% of patients with a BMI > 25 kg/m² received a formal diagnosis of overweight and just 30% of patients with BMI > 30 kg/m² had a formal obesity diagnosis documented in the EHR. A 2013 systematic review found that most physicians only prescribe 1–2 interventions to their patients, rather than offering counseling on the range of treatment options, and rarely refer to dietitians or obesity specialists [10]. The review found that current weight counseling fixates on general education, such as informing of the risks of obesity or the benefits of weight loss, rather than specific behavioral guidance. Finally, data from the National Ambulatory Medical Care Survey from 2008 to 2013 showed that, despite emerging national recommendations and policies over the intervening years, obesity counseling significantly declined from 33% to 21%, a suboptimal response to the obesity epidemic [11]. For these reasons, there is a role for a more systematic approach to obesity that includes referral to a specialty program, such as a Lifestyle Medicine Center.

The Foundational Treatment of Obesity Focuses on Lifestyle Modification

The primary foundational concept in obesity care is to guide and assist patients in making healthier dietary, physical activity, and behavioral choices that will lead to net negative energy balance, and then support life-long changes to maintain a healthy body weight. Multiple studies have demonstrated the impact of lifestyle management in reducing body weight, enhancing quality of life, and improving the disease burden associated with obesity such as diabetes, hypertension, and dyslipidemia [12–14]. In patients who are overweight or have obesity, there is a dose-response relationship between the amount of weight loss and metabolic benefits achieved [15]. Weight loss has also been demonstrated to improve other obesity-related comorbid complications, such gastroesophageal reflux disease, urinary incontinence, and obstructive sleep apnea. More recently, data have emerged that other lifestyle factors, such as sleep hygiene and stress, are also important in the development and treatment of obesity [16, 17]. Thus, a comprehensive approach to obesity that targets lifestyle medicine factors is essential in the treatment paradigm.

The New Field of Obesity Medicine

Obesity medicine is a nascent discipline that was born out of the need to develop an expanded workforce to combat the rising epidemic of obesity and its associated disease burden. It contains a unique body of knowledge that is not typically included in other disciplines of medicine. The American Board of Obesity Medicine (ABOM) was created in 2011 to provide certification to physicians who want to achieve a higher level of recognized competency in the care of patients with obesity [18]. According to the ABOM, a diplomat is described as:

- A physician with expertise in the field of obesity medicine; this field requires competency in and a thorough understanding of the treatment of obesity and the genetic, biologic, environmental, social, and behavioral factors that contribute to obesity.
- A physician who employs certain therapeutic interventions to manage obesity, including diet, physical activity, behavioral change, and pharmacotherapy.
- A physician who utilizes a comprehensive approach to obesity, which may include additional resources such as nutritionists, exercise physiologists, psychologists, and bariatric surgeons as indicated to achieve optimal results.
- A physician who maintains competency in providing pre-, peri-, and postoperative care of patients undergoing a bariatric procedure; promotes the prevention of obesity; and advocates for those who suffer from obesity.

As of 2020, 4152 physicians have been certified as diplomats of the ABOM with the majority stemming from Internal Medicine and Family Medicine specialties (www. abom.org [Accessed on May 23, 2020]). Physicians wishing to lead a Lifestyle Medicine Center focusing on obesity care should consider the education and rigor required to become a Diplomat of the ABOM.

General Practice Treatment Paradigm for Obesity

Several obesity treatment guidelines have been published as a resource for clinicians (Table 25.1). These guidelines should be considered when establishing the lifestyle medicine treatment paradigm for the Center. Despite the diversity of published guidelines, there is a near uniformity in their recommendations. Several general concepts are consistent among the guidelines:

- Obesity is a chronic disease requiring long-term management.
- Patients should be appropriately screened for obesity.
- Healthcare professionals should understand and be prepared to address obesity using a collaborative, shared decision-making approach.
- Use of appropriate treatment modalities should be considered, as indicated.
- Multicomponent interventions are preferred over individual treatments.

Table 25.1 Obesity treatment guidelines[a]

Guideline	URL
American Gastroenterological Association Practice guide on obesity and weight management, education and resources (POWER) (2017)	https://www.gastro.org/practice-guidance/practice-updates/obesity-practice-guide
American Heart Association (AHA)/American College of Cardiology (ACC)/The Obesity Society (TOS) Guideline for the Management of Overweight and Obesity in Adults (2013)	https://www.ahajournals.org/doi/10.1161/01.cir.0000437739.71477.ee
American Obesity Association (OMA) Obesity Management Algorithm (Updated 2019)	https://obesitymedicine.org/obesity-algorithm/
The American Society of Clinical Endocrinologists (AACE) and the American College of Endocrinology (ACE) Clinical Practice Guidelines for Comprehensive Care of Patients with Obesity (2016)	https://journals.aace.com/doi/full/10.4158/EP161356.ESGL
AACE/ACE/TOS/American Society for Metabolic and Bariatric Surgery (ASMBS)/American Society of Anesthesiologists (ASA) Clinical Practice Guidelines for the Perioperative Nutrition, Metabolic, and Nonsurgical Support of Patients Undergoing Bariatric Procedures – 2019 Update	https://www.aace.com/disease-state-resources/nutrition-and-obesity/clinical-practice-guidelines/clinical-practice-1
European Practical and Patient-Centered Guidelines for Adult Obesity Management in Primary Care (2019)	https://www.karger.com/Article/FullText/496183
Pharmacological Management of Obesity guidelines from the Endocrine Society (2015)	https://academic.oup.com/jcem/article/100/2/342/2813109
U.S. Preventive Services Task Force (USPSTF): Weight Loss to Prevent Obesity-Related Morbidity and Mortality in Adults: Behavioral Interventions	https://www.uspreventiveservicestaskforce.org/Announcements/News/Item/us-preventive-services-task-force-issues-final-recommendation-statements-for-screening-for-obesity-and-counseling-to-promote-a-healthful-diet-and-physical-activity-in-adults

[a]All websites access on December 8, 2019

Table 25.2 Proposed standards of care for obesity for healthcare professionals[a]

1. Should be competent to address the role of social determinants of obesity and its outcomes
2. Should consider an individual's genetic background and ethnicity when considering the risk associated with body mass index and/or waist circumference
3. Should assess patients for obesity-associated comorbidities
4. Should educate patients about the relationship between excess body fat and health risks
5. Should employ evidence-based counseling techniques to facilitate behavioral change
6. Should jointly decide with patients on obesity care options that include behavior modification, pharmacotherapy, and/or bariatric procedures
7. Should refer patients to an evidence-based program or recommend an evidence-based dietary strategy, considering individual preference and the potential health benefit of diet composition
8. Should recommend appropriate levels of physical activity and/or refer patients to programs that include physical activity counseling
9. Should minimize the use of medications that may cause weight gain and preferentially consider those that are weight neutral or associated with weight loss
10. When appropriate, should discuss and/or prescribe obesity medications
11. When appropriate, should discuss and/or refer patients for bariatric procedures
12. Should be knowledgeable about long-term nutritional and medical needs of patients who have had a bariatric procedure

[a]Adapted from Ref. [19]

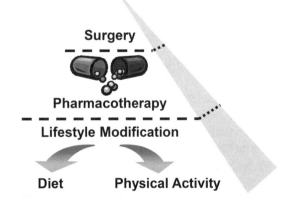

Fig. 25.1 Obesity treatment paradigm. Treatment rests on a foundation of lifestyle management consisting dietary and physical activity counseling. If indicated, treatment is intensified to include pharmacotherapy and bariatric procedures

Additional considerations for Lifestyle Medicine Centers are to establish a standard of obesity care for all Center HCPs [19] and utilize published obesity competencies to ensure that staff is competent in the assessment, prevention, and treatment of obesity [20]. Although published only as a pro-

posal, the standards for clinical HCPs set a benchmark for professionalism and minimal competence (Table 25.2).

Furthermore, considering obesity as a chronic medical disease state helps to frame the concept of using a stepped intensification of care approach to weight management (Fig. 25.1). In this progression of care, all patients are provided a foundation of lifestyle therapy. If the patient is not able to achieve the desired weight and health goal by lifestyle alone and meets the indications for medication management, then addition of adjunctive pharmacotherapy should be considered. As a third step, bariatric procedures can be considered for patients with more severe disease and who meet its indications. Using this medical-surgical paradigm, clinicians and patients can advance through increasing intensities of treatment using shared decision-making to discuss the benefits and risks of each option.

Development and Organization of the Northwestern Medicine Center for Lifestyle Medicine

Infrastructure and Environment of Northwestern Healthcare System

Northwestern Medicine (NM) links Northwestern Memorial Health (NMH) system and Northwestern University's Feinberg School of Medicine (FSM). The total NM enterprise consists of 30,000 staff members, 5783 aligned physicians, 2390 students and trainees, and an additional 5000 nonclinical researchers and staff at FSM. Nearly 2 million patients were served in calendar year 2018. Northwestern Medical Group (NMG) comprises the fully salaried physicians at NM that work in more than 25 outpatient care locations spread across Chicago and the northern suburbs, offering primary, specialty, and immediate care within and surrounding the communities where people live and work. All NM physicians hold an academic position at FSM.

Center for Lifestyle Medicine

The Center for Lifestyle Medicine (CLM) was created in 2008 after a reorganization of the Wellness Institute (1998–2007) into the Center for Integrative Medicine. A shift in direction from an obesity-focused lifestyle risk reduction and prevention program to integrative medicine was due, in large part, to a funding opportunity and desire by administrative officials to establish a presence in integrative medicine in the Chicago market. Thus, a new Center was established and renamed the CLM in accordance to this newly emerging field in medicine. Administrative support for the CLM is shared between FSM (University) and NM (Medical Group). Only the physicians and health psychologists who hold advanced degrees have faculty positions at the University. Their salaries and productivity benchmarks are determined by their respective departments or divisions. On the other hand, employment contracts, salaries and compensation structures, and productivity benchmarks of other ancillary staff members, along

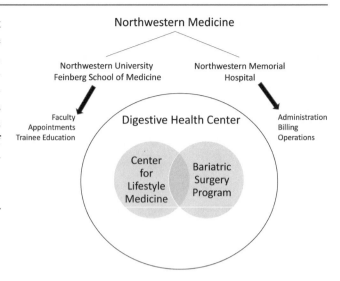

Fig. 25.2 Organizational structure of the Center for Lifestyle Medicine within the Northwestern Medicine Healthcare System

with daily operations of the Center, are the responsibility of NM administrators. Despite these administrative differences, the staff works seamlessly together to provide patient care.

Since the CLM is a consultative practice, all patients are referred or self-referred. The majority of patients are referred by HCPs within the Northwestern healthcare system. This is typical of the majority of medical and surgical subspecialty clinical service lines within NM. Additional referrals stem from specialty programs, most notably orthopedics, obstetrics/gynecology, oncology, and cardiology. Referrals to the center and CLM staff are facilitated by placing an order in the electronic health record (EHR).

Physical Setting

The CLM is co-located with the Bariatric Surgery program within the Digestive Health Center (DHC) of NM. This was deliberately chosen to facilitate a more streamlined patient care experience for patients who are electing to pursue bariatric surgery and would provide foundational pre-and post-bariatric surgery support. The organization structure of the CLM within the NM healthcare system is depicted in Fig. 25.2.

All CLM HCPs are located in one hallway within the DHC. Although there is no distinct designation of the Center, rooms that are allocated for the CLM are specially equipped with large examination tables, benches for patient seating, large gowns, and large adult blood pressure cuffs (Fig. 25.3). A privately located broad-based foot scale that weights up to 800 lbs. and a wall-mounted stadiometer (height scale) is used by all staff. The scale is calibrated by the NM Maintenance Engineering Department using free weights for accuracy every 3 months. Discipline-specific HCPs share rooms to maximize room efficiency, e.g., medical HCPs share examination rooms whereas registered dietitian nutritionists

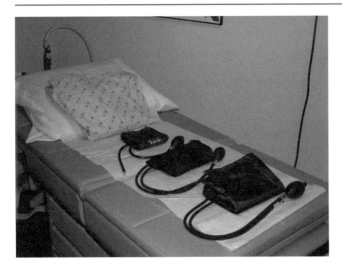

Fig. 25.3 The exam room should include a wide based, bariatric exam table, appropriately sized blood pressure cuffs (including normal, large, and thigh cuffs), and extra-large gowns

(RDN) share consultation rooms. Overall, on a typical day, the CLM has access to 3 examination rooms, 3 RDN consultation rooms, and 3 health psychologist consultation rooms. There is also shared staff workspace for computer charting. Recommendations and considerations for appropriately furnishing a Center that primarily cares for patients with obesity are displayed in Table 25.3 [21]. Although these unique features present an additional startup cost, they are important for patient comfort, respect, and dignity. All of these program elements are essential features of a prepared obesity practice.

Human Resources

A comprehensive obesity care team usually consists of medical HCPs, RDNs, and mental HCPs. Other disciplines may include health coaches, exercise specialists, and social workers. The CLM employs 4 medical HCPs (2 physicians, a nurse practitioner, and physician assistant), 4 RDNs (2.25 FTE), and 3 health psychologists (2.0 FTE). The DHC also provides registration staff for patient check in/check out, and a medical assistant to facilitate administrative support for drug prior approval calls, patient reminder calls, and monitoring of patient schedules. Billing, coding, and payment services are provided by NM.

Pathway

The CLM uses an individualized, fee-for-service model of care. New patient appointments to the program begin with a 60-minute visit scheduled with one of the medical HCPs. Patients are directed to complete an 8-page new visit patient questionnaire that is available to complete and download from the dedicated website (https://www.nm.org/conditions-and-care-areas/center-for-lifestyle-medicine [Accessed on November 28, 2019]) prior to their initial visit. This pre-visit questionnaire is consistent with the chronic care model,

Table 25.3 Equipping an appropriate clinic environment for obesity care

	Recommendations	Considerations
Furniture	Wide-base, higher-weight-capacity chairs (preferably armless) in waiting area, patient areas, and clinic rooms; provide seating that can support and fit larger individuals. Provide floor-mounted toilets with weight capacity of at least 1000-lbs; toilet seat height should be 17″ to 19″; wheelchair-accessible bathrooms. Door width. Wide based, bariatric examination tables	Prevent stigmatization by integrating bariatric furniture with regular seating; select a variety of seating alternatives. Pedestal toilets, rather than wall-mounted; consider having clinic rooms and waiting areas close to the bathroom, avoid making patients walk long distances; consider placing sinks away from toilets so that patients do not use sink for support when standing or sitting; equip bathrooms with handrails near toilet. Allow 4–6 feet door width for wheelchairs and turning room. Provide comfort for patients with severe obesity
Clinic room equipment	Large-sized or thigh-sized blood pressure cuffs. High-capacity weighing scales (ideally >500 lbs). Step stool for the exam table. Extra-large gowns	Avoid "miscuffing" and obtaining a spurious blood pressure. Consider placing scales in a private are to avoid patient discomfort
RDN equipment	Food models. Fat/muscle models	Layout of the RDN office or clinic room should be open, no barriers between patient and HCP
Staff	Educated about obesity and weight bias	Certification and board certification in weight management and obesity

Adapted from Ref. [21]
Abbreviations: *RDN* registered dietitian nutritionist, *HCP* healthcare professional

which posits that optimal care is delivered when the patient is informed and activated, and the practice team is prepared and proactive [22]. In addition to obtaining traditional medical information, the questionnaire specifically asks patients about their diet, physical activity, lifestyle habits, and weight history. The questionnaire is used to guide the encounter and provides a more in-depth and comprehensive overview of the patient's history. In addition to obtaining an obesity-focused history, the initial encounter also entails performing a complete physical examination and obtaining laboratory tests and diagnostic procedures as indicated. For example, patients with symptoms of obstructive sleep apnea may be referred for a polysomnogram, or those with an elevated liver ALT/AST ratio may have a liver imaging study obtained. Management of obesity-related complications is often co-managed in concert with the patients' primary care HCP.

Based on information obtained from the medical visit, patients are provided a personalized treatment plan that includes lifestyle recommendations and when indicated, discussion of pharmacotherapy or a bariatric procedure. Multiple patient care handouts to facilitate counseling are available on the CLM homepage for printing in the after-visit summary (AVS). Although the frequency of the 20- to 30-minute follow-up visits with the medical HCP varies based on patient need and program capacity, they usually occur every 6–12 weeks. A decision to refer the patient to one of the RDNs for medical nutrition therapy (MNT) and/or one of the health psychologists for psychological and behavioral counseling is determined by shared decision-making between the patient and the medical HCP. Common indications for referral to the RDN include diet and nutrition education, meal planning and preparation, and behavioral counseling. Common indications for referral to the clinical psychologist include mood or eating disorders, body image disturbance, or behavioral inertia (the tendency to do nothing or to remain unchanged). The roles and responsibilities of lifestyle medicine team members have been described [23]. During the initial 60-minute dietary visit, the RDN reviews the medical visit in the EHR for background information and continuity of care. Thirty-minute follow-up visits are scheduled on an individual basis and typically occur every 8–12 weeks. Health psychology visits are 45 minutes in length with a variable follow-up schedule depending on need and program capacity. All three HCPs use a templated note that is specific for their discipline (Tables 25.4, 25.5, and 25.6). This uniformity among HCPs is important for efficiency, continuity, and completeness.

Although treatment pathways are individually determined, they all are based on a foundation of healthy living that emphasizes diet, physical activity, and behavioral change. Examples of patient care handouts that are accessible on the CLM homepage and printed in the AVS are displayed in Table 25.7. Patients that are seeing more than one HCP, e.g., medical HCP, RDN, and health psychologist, typically alternate appointments among the HCPs. Review of patient notes along with informal conversations in the hall are all used to ensure a continuity of care.

For patients that need or desire intensification of treatment beyond lifestyle treatment alone, a decision to use adjunctive pharmacotherapy is based on shared decision-making, US Food and Drug Administration indications, and treatment guidelines. Selection of which agent to prescribe is based on the patient's comorbidities, contra-indications, drug-drug interactions, cost and insurance coverage, and patient preference. Patients are continuously monitored for drug safety and effectiveness at each visit.

Patients that elect to pursue a bariatric procedure enter a separate pathway within the CLM. As a first step, they are all asked to attend a free orientation session that is led by one

Table 25.4 New patient electronic health record template for medical healthcare professional

Chief complaint	Obesity, associated medical problems
Weight history	Onset, precipitating events, quality of life, remedial interventions setting, temporal pattern
Patient expectations	Weight goals, improvement in physical and mental health
Past medical history	Review of obesity-related comorbid conditions
Past surgical history	Impact on nutritional health and functionality
Current medications	Special attention to weight-gaining medications
Supplements	Vitamins, minerals, and herbs taken for weight management
Allergies	Particular attention to drug allergies that may be considered for treatment
Social history	Living environment, employment, community
Habits	Tobacco, alcohol, recreational drug use, sleep hygiene
Family history	Obesity and obesity-related comorbid conditions
Nutritional history	Meals, snacks, beverages, dietary pattern, food composition, nutritional literacy
Physical activity	Current exercise pattern, barriers to exercise
Review of systems	Attention to obesity-related conditions, signs and symptoms
Physical exam	Including height, weight, waist circumference
Labs	Complete blood count, chemistry panel, lipid panel, hemoglobin A1c
Assessment and plan	Summary of causation and contributing factors of obesity, evaluation of obesity status and associated burden, discussion of treatment plan through shared decision-making
Follow-up	Scheduled return visit with multidisciplinary staff

Table 25.5 New patient electronic health record template for registered dietitian nutritionist

Initial dietitian visit reason	Wellness, overweight/obesity, underweight, food allergy/intolerance, other
Past medical history	Overweight/obesity, diabetes, cardiovascular disease, cancer, other
Weight history	Current weight, weight class, highest weight, lowest weight, goal weight
Diet recall	Meals, snacks, beverages, frequency of restaurant meals, food allergies/intolerances
Supplements	Prescribed/not prescribed by healthcare professional, indication, dosing, duration, effects
Sleep	Hours/night, quality
Physical activity	Activities of daily living, types of exercise/activity, barriers to exercise
Diet recall/food log	Inadequate, excessive, patient goals for visit, weight and diet history, prior RDN visits, most weight lost from any prior diet attempt, current eating pattern, grocery shopping, meal, preparation habits, food safety, biggest challenges with eating, emotional eating, timing of eating
Assessment and plan	Diet (nutrition needs and goals), physical activity, behavior

Table 25.6 New patient electronic health record template for health psychologist

Behavioral observation	Orientation, rapport, appearance, speech, judgment
Presenting problem	Weight management, mood disturbance, behavioral change, eating disorder
Contributing factors	Emotional eating (e.g., assess binge purge symptoms), greatest success with weight loss (e.g., when and how much), how long sustained, what got you off track?
Marital status, significant others, living arrangements	Household members, relationship history, supports for change, status of relationships, social support
Employment status	How do they like the work, what is the work environment, boundaries around work time, financial stability
Substance abuse history	Alcohol, nicotine, addictive substances, past treatments
Medical issues	Presence of diseases and conditions that may impact treatment
Stress	Impact on behavior change, associations with past relationships, current life stressors, what is weighing the most? coping strategies
Psychiatric history and treatment	Family history, treatment history, current treatment
Motivation/confidence for change on 0–10 scale	Anticipated obstacles for change
Sleep	Hours/night, quality, pattern
Physical Activity	Activities of daily living, types of exercise/activity, barriers to exercise
Impression	Knowledge, motivation, psychosocial health, diagnosed mental health disorders
Recommendations	Cognitive behavioral therapy, multidisciplinary team involvement, stress reduction training

Table 25.7 Selected patient care handouts available on the Center for Lifestyle Medicine homepage[a]

Building Your Own Calorie-Controlled Meals 1200–1500 Calories
Building Your Own Calorie-Controlled Meals 1200–1500 Calories
Building Your Own Calorie-Controlled Meals 1500–1800 Calories
Chair Exercises
Ethnic Eating
Exercise Prescription
Fast Food Facts
Health Eating On-the-Go
Healthy Snack Guide: 100–200 Calories Each
Meal Delivery Programs
Meal Replacement for Weight Loss
Menu Replacement for Weight Loss
Menu and Ordering Tips
Physical Activity Basics
Starting Physical Activity
Weight Management Tracking Tools

[a]See https://www.nm.org/conditions-and-care-areas/center-for-life-style-medicine (Accessed on March 26, 2020)

of the bariatric surgeons. During this session, two surgical procedures – Roux-en-Y gastric bypass and vertical sleeve gastrectomy – are reviewed, along with the benefits and risks of each procedure. This bariatric surgery pathway is also reviewed in detail, which includes 4 preparation group classes led by an RDN, and an individual consultation visit with the bariatric surgeon. Pre- and postoperative medical and nutritional care are provided by the CLM staff.

Billing and Coding

Since the CLM functions within an academic Medical Center, billing and coding is consistent with other consultative services. Medical HCPs use ICD-10 codes for obesity and other presenting obesity-related comorbid conditions as indicated (Table 25.8). If the patient is referred

Table 25.8 ICD-10 diagnostic and billing codes for obesity

International Classification of Diseases (ICD) – 10 diagnostic codes	
E66.9	Obesity not otherwise specified
E66.01	Obesity, extreme or morbid
E66.0	Obesity due to excess calories
E66.01	Morbid (severe) obesity due to excess calories
E66.09	Other obesity due to excess calories
E66.1	Drug-induced
E66.2	Morbid (severe) obesity with alveolar hypoventilation
E66.3	Overweight
E66.8	Other obesity
E66.9	Obesity, unspecified
Z68.41	Morbid obesity with BMI 40.0–44.9 adult
Z68.42	Morbid obesity with BMI 45.0–49.9 adult
Z68.43	Morbid obesity with BMI 50.0–59.9 adult
Z68.44	Morbid obesity with BMI 60.0–69.9 adult
Z68.45	Morbid obesity with BMI 70.0 and greater
Z71.3	Dietary counseling and surveillance
Z71.82	Exercise counseling
Z72.9	Problem related to lifestyle, unspecified

Current Procedural Terminology (CPT) billing codes for medical nutrition therapy (MNT)[a]			
97802	Initial	Individual	15-minute increments
97803	Reassessment	Individual	15-minute increments
97804	-----	Group	30-minute increments

[a]Coverage is allowed for up to 4 visits per calendar year and must be provided by a Licensed Registered Dietitian or nutrition professional meeting certain requirements

by another HCP, a time-based consultation code is used for the initial visit. Health psychologists use health and behavior assessment and intervention codes for services that treat behavioral, social conditions, and psychophysiological conditions for the treatment or management of physical health problems. The RDNs use MNT coding in 15-minute increments. In contrast to medical HCPs and health psychologists, insurance coverage varies widely for RDN visits and is usually a hybrid between self-pay and a covered benefit.

Expanded Role and Responsibilities

Northwestern Medicine is an academic Medical Center affiliated with the Northwestern University FSM that provides undergraduate and graduate medical education. As such, the CLM is actively involved in medical education, clinical research, and wellness programs within the Medical Center. Every member of the CLM is expected to participate in the educational programs. Having trainees is important for several reasons: teaching allows staff to reflect on the uniqueness of their own profession; teaching provides an opportunity to develop educational skills; and teaching builds team unity.

Undergraduate education A lifestyle medicine curricular thread was introduced into the medical school in 2014. Over the first 2 years of medical school, students are introduced to the components of lifestyle medicine that include diet, physical activity, behavioral change, sleep health, substance misuse, tobacco, stress reduction, and weight management. A description of the nutrition component has been published [24]. Beginning in 2019, all third-year medical students rotate through the CLM for a half-day shadowing experience where students have an opportunity to observe patient-HCP interactions with a medical HCP and an RDN. The learning objectives for the rotation are to:

1. Describe the obesity-focused history, physical examination, and care plan.
2. Observe patient-centered counseling that incorporates multiple elements of the lifestyle medicine thread, including diet, physical activity, and behavioral change.
3. Recognize the inter-professional working relationship among team members.

The CLM is also an elective training site for the Northwestern Physician Assistant program, where students will spend a half-day shadowing the on-site Physician Assistant.

Graduate education Since 2015, the CLM has been a training site for both Family Medicine and Internal Medicine residents. Second-year Family Medicine residents spend 4 half-day sessions per week for an entire month working with all members of the CLM team. The goal is to achieve minimal competency in the provision of comprehensive obesity care that they can implement in their primary care clinics. In contrast, the Internal Medicine residents spend a 2-week block in the center, allowing time off for their own clinic and night float responsibilities.

Clinical research The CLM actively participates in clinical research for obesity studies. It has served as a clinical site for several multicenter pharmacological and device trials along with principle investigator-initiated studies. Participating in clinical research is important for staying abreast of cutting-edge therapies, contributing to the science and practice of obesity, providing the opportunity for Center staff to gain experience in clinical research, and varying the monotony of daily patient care.

Staff education Continuing medical education for staff is essential for a state-of-the-art Center. In addition to weekly team meetings for administrative and patient care issues, as well as discussion of relevant published articles, team members attend regional and national meetings for continuing education. Each discipline has its own requirements for CME. Additionally, staff are encouraged to seek additional certifications, such as the ABOM (for physicians), and the Academy of Nutrition and Dietetics (AND) Interdisciplinary Obesity and Weight Management Certification or the Certified Diabetes Educator (CDE) for RDNs. Staff members are also encouraged to co-author articles and book chapters to further their writing skills and professional development.

How Does the Center for Lifestyle Medicine Succeed?

There are several aspects of the program that are important for success. These include hiring highly qualified staff, practicing up-to-date evidence-based care, and providing individualized and patient-centered encounters.

Highly Qualified Staff

When hiring new staff members for an obesity program, key criteria to assess include "people skills" (compassion, empathy, approachability, and humility), professionalism, education, and experience. Whereas the first 3 listed qualifications are a necessity, experience can be acquired through on-the-job training, as long as the staff member is inquisitive and interested in learning. Other qualities include teamwork and ambition.

Practice Up-To-Date and Evidence-Based Care

As a consultative Center, it is essential to keep abreast of and deliver up-to-date and evidence-based care. Obesity is a multifactorial chronic disease that includes multiple treatment approaches. Treatment continues to evolve and incorporate new approaches to lifestyle therapies along with emerging pharmacological and procedural interventions. New information is acquired through reading the literature and attending conferences.

Individualized and Patient-Centered Encounters

Similar to other consultative programs that provide specialty care, patients expect that their treatment will be customized to their individual needs. The philosophy of the CLM is that each patient presents with his or her own unique weight history, with psychosocial and behavioral issues that require an individualized approach to treatment. This individualized care incorporates shared decision-making in all aspects of care.

Other Attributes

In addition to the factors noted above, the key attributes of the Center that support success are embracing a shared philosophy, teamwork and mutual respect, and professionalism. All CLM members view obesity as a chronic relapsing disease that is best managed by employing an interdisciplinary, medically based approach that incorporates lifestyle management, pharmacotherapy, and bariatric procedures when indicated. The teamwork entails coordination and delegation of tasks among HCPs and staff. Starfield [25] defines a patient care team as "a group of diverse clinicians who communicate with each other regularly about the care of a defined group of patients and participate in that care." A sense of "groupness," defined as the degree to which the group practice identifies itself and functions as a team [26], is also fundamental to daily operations and enhances the quality and efficiency of patient care

Take-Home Points

The following take-home points are important for establishing and maintaining a successful Lifestyle Medicine Center for obesity care.

1. Due to the high prevalence of obesity, associated disease burden, and insufficient attention at the primary care

level, all Medical Centers should consider establishing a specialized obesity management program.
2. Financial viability, patient referral pathways, and treatment paradigms need to be determined early in the process.
3. The program and delivered clinical service line must be embedded within the sponsoring Medical Center to strengthen its importance and viability.
4. It is essential to support staff members regarding their continued education and career growth to maintain excellence in patient care and avoid burnout.
5. The Center should actively participate in the educational mission of the Medical Center and University in order to advocate for and promote the importance of lifestyle medicine and obesity care.

What Are the Challenges for the Center for Lifestyle Medicine?

The unique challenges of the CLM ironically relates to success. Since the CLM is the only program that provides comprehensive obesity care within the NM system, timely patient access and availability for new and return appointments is difficult. Furthermore, as more HCPs identify patients with obesity that would benefit from weight loss services, there is an increased volume of uncomplicated obesity referrals that should be managed in the primary care setting prior to being seen in a specialty program, e.g., provision of diet and physical activity counseling and recommendations for self-monitoring. This increased volume of patients with uncomplicated obesity displaces other patients that require a more intensive, team-based approach. Finally, despite the increased demand for services, there is a lack of physical space for growth within the Medical Center. These challenges are not unique to a Lifestyle Medicine Center. Solutions will require administrative leadership and a population-based healthcare system approach to this unmet need. When building an obesity-focused Lifestyle Medicine Center, these scalable factors should be considered *a priori* and continually revisited as the program grows.

References

1. NCD Risk Factor Collaboration. Worldwide trends in body-mass index, underweight, overweight, and obesity from 1975 to 2016: a pooled analysis of 2416 population-based measurement studies in 128·9 million children, adolescents, and adults. Lancet. 2017;390:2627–42.
2. World Health Organization. https://www.who.int/news-room/fact-sheets/detail/obesity-and-overweight. Accessed on 6 Oct 2019.

3. Hales CM, Carroll MD, Fryar CD, et al. Prevalence of obesity among adults and youth: United States, 2015–2016. NCHS Data Brief. 2017;2017(288):1–8.

4. AMA Report of the Council on Science and Public health. http:// www.ama-assn.org/assets/meeting/2013a/a13-addendum-ref-comm-d.pdf#page=19. Accessed 6 Oct 2019.

5. Jastreboff AM, Kotz CM, Kahan S, et al. Obesity as a disease: the obesity society 2018 position statement. Obesity. 2019;27:7–9.

6. Bray GA, Kim KK, Wilding JPH, World Obesity Federation. Obesity: a chronic relapsing progressive disease process. A position statement of the World Obesity Federation. Obes Rev. 2017;18:715–23.

7. Kontis V, Mathers CD, Rehm J, Stevens GA, et al. Contribution of six risk factors to achieving the 25×25 non-communicable disease mortality reduction target: a modelling study. Lancet. 2014;384:427–37.

8. Bardia A, Holtan SG, Slezak JM, Thompson WG. Diagnosis of obesity by primary care physicians and impact on obesity management. Mayo Clin Proc. 2007;82:927–32.

9. Baer HJ, Karson AS, Soukup JR, et al. Documentation and diagnosis of overweight and obesity in electronic health records of adult primary care patients. JAMA Intern Med. 2013;173:1648–52.

10. van Dillen SME, van Binsbergen JJ, Koelenc MA, et al. Nutrition and physical activity guidance practices in general practice: a critical review. Patient Educ Couns. 2013;90:155–69.

11. Fitzpatrick SL, Stevens VJ. Adult obesity management in primary care, 2008–2013. Prev Med. 2017;99:128–33.

12. Franz MJ, Boucher JL, Rutten-Ramos S, et al. Lifestyle weight-loss intervention outcomes in overweight and obese adults with type 2 diabetes: a systematic review and meta-analysis of randomized trials. J Acad Nutr Diet. 2015;115:1447–63.

13. Whelton PK, Carey RM, Aronow WS, et al. 2017 ACC/AHA/ AAPA/ABC/ACPM/AGS/APhA/ASH/ASPC/NMA/PCNA guideline for the prevention, detection, evaluation, and management of high blood pressure in adults: executive summary: a report of the American College of Cardiology/American Heart Association task force on clinical practice guidelines. Circulation. 2018;138:e426–83.

14. Van Horn L, Carson JA, Appel LJ, et al. Recommended dietary pattern to achieve adherence to the American Heart Association/ American College of Cardiology (AHA/ACC) guidelines: a scientific statement from the American Heart Association. Circulation. 2016;134:e505–29.

15. Jensen MD, Ryan DH, Apovian CM, et al. 2013 AHA/ACC/ TOS guideline for the management of overweight and obesity in adults: a report of the American College of Cardiology/ American Heart Association task force on practice guidelines and the obesity society. Circulation. 2013;129(25 Suppl 2):S102–38.

16. Reutrakul S, Van Cauter E. Sleep influences on obesity, insulin resistance, and risk of type 2 diabetes. Metabolism. 2018;84:56–66.

17. Proper KI, Picavet HS, Bogers RP, et al. The association between adverse life events and body weight change: results of a prospective cohort study. BMC Public Health. 2013;13:957.

18. Kushner RF, Brittan D, Cleek J, ABOM Board of Directors, et al. The American Board of Obesity Medicine: five-year report. Obesity. 2017;25:982–4.

19. Dietz WH, Gallagher C. A proposed standard of care for all providers and payers. Obesity. 2019;27:1059–62.

20. Kushner RF, Horn DH, Butsch WS, et al. Development of obesity competencies for medical education: a report of the Obesity Medicine Education Collaborative. Obesity. 2019;27:1063–7.

21. Kahan S. Practical strategies for engaging individuals with obesity in primary care. Mayo Clin Proc. 2018;93:351–9.

22. Bodenheimer T, Wagner EH, Grumbach K. Improving primary care for patients with chronic illness. JAMA. 2002;288:1775–9.

23. Arena R, Lavie CJ. The healthy lifestyle team is central to the success of accountable care organizations. Mayo Clin Proc. 2015;90:572–6.

24. Kushner RF, Van Horn L. Teaching nutrition in the context of lifestyle medicine. Med Sci Educ. 2018;28:9–12.

25. Starfield B. Primary care concepts, evaluation, and policy. New York: Oxford University Press; 1992.

26. Crabtree BF, Miller WL, Aita VA, et al. Primary care practice organization and preventive services delivery: a qualitative analysis. J Fam Pract. 1998;46:404–9.

Lifestyle Medicine Center for Brain Aging and Neurodegenerative Diseases

Mark P. Mattson

Abbreviations

AD	Alzheimer's disease
BDNF	Brain-derived neurotrophic factor
GABA	Gamma aminobutyric acid
IF	Intermittent fasting
LMC-BAND	Lifestyle Medicine Center for Brain Aging and Neurodegenerative Diseases
MRI	Magnetic resonance imaging
PD	Parkinson's disease
PET	Positron emission tomography

Rationale for Lifestyle Medicine Centers for Brain Aging and Neurodegenerative Disorders

Because of advances in the early diagnosis and treatment of diabetes, cardiovascular disease, and cancers, an increasing number of people are living well into their 70s, 80s, and 90s, which are the decades where they become very likely to suffer from Alzheimer's disease (AD), Parkinson's disease (PD), or stroke. Unfortunately, there are currently no effective treatments for any of these brain disorders of aging. However, emerging evidence suggests that lifestyle modifications can prevent or reduce the risk of developing AD, PD, or a stroke and may improve brain function in those already affected by a brain disorder of aging. The three lifestyle interventions for which sufficient data exist to justify broad incorporation into risk reduction and treatment plans are exercise programs, eating behavior modification (diet composition and intermittent fasting [IF]), and intellectual challenges.

M. P. Mattson (✉)
Department of Neuroscience, Johns Hopkins University School of Medicine, Baltimore, MD, USA
e-mail: mmattso2@jhmi.edu

Scope of the Problem: Alzheimer's and Parkinson's Diseases and Stroke

Aging is the major risk factor for AD, PD, and stroke, and the numbers of elderly people are rapidly increasing in countries throughout the world. The Global Burden of Disease Study group found that in 2016 there were approximately 44 million people worldwide living with AD/dementia which is twice as many as there were in 1990. In the United States, there are currently approximately 6 million people with AD, and by 2030 this number will double [1]. From 2010 to 2030, there will be approximately an 80% increase in the number of people with PD in the United States [2]. Worldwide, in 2010, approximately 16 million people suffered a stroke, and there were 6 million stroke-related deaths [3, 4]. The dramatic increases in brain disorders of aging are the result of increased life expectancy and the fact that advances in the early diagnosis and treatment of cardiovascular disease and cancers have enabled people who would have died from these diseases to live into the "danger zone" age range for AD, PD, and stroke (65–90 years old). The sustained intensive care that patients suffering from AD, PD, or stroke require places major psychological and financial burdens on their families and contributes substantially to the increasing cost of healthcare.

Current Clinical Diagnosis and Patient Care

A diagnosis of probable AD is based on a standardized battery of cognitive tests that provide quantitative measures of short-term memory. Borderline performance on cognitive tests is consistent with a diagnosis of mild cognitive impairment, which is often a prodrome of AD [5]. Evidence of atrophy of the hippocampus, and frontal, parietal, and temporal lobes, and ventricular enlargement support a diagnosis of AD. As the disease progresses, AD patients exhibit impaired language, reasoning, judgment, and insight, with

J. I. Mechanick, R. F. Kushner (eds.), *Creating a Lifestyle Medicine Center*, https://doi.org/10.1007/978-3-030-48088-2_26

irritability, agitation, and aggression also occurring in many patients. However, a final diagnosis of AD requires postmortem analysis of brain tissue sections which must exhibit agreed upon threshold amounts of beta-amyloid plaques and neurofibrillary tangle-bearing neurons. Approximately 20% of patients diagnosed with AD do not reach threshold levels of plaques and tangles but nevertheless have extensive loss of neurons in the hippocampus and functionally connected brain regions [6].

A diagnosis of PD is ascribed to patients that exhibit a resting tremor of the hands that disappears with movement, muscle rigidity, and slowed body movements [7]. The diagnosis can be further validated by positron emission tomography (PET) brain imaging using a radiolabeled tracer for the neurotransmitter dopamine. Dopamine-producing neurons in the substantia nigra degenerate in PD, which is reflected by a large reduction in the PET signal in this brain region. In addition to progressively worsening motor symptoms, patients with PD often develop cognitive impairment in the latter stages of the disease. Moreover, emerging findings suggest that gastrointestinal dysfunction (chronic constipation) attributable to degeneration of neurons in the brainstem that innervate the gut via axons in the vagus nerve often occurs prior to the diagnostic motor symptoms [8].

AD and PD are progressive neurodegenerative disorders that culminate in death. Typically, a patient with AD will first experience short-term memory impairment, which worsens over a period of several years during which time somewhat normal activities of daily living can still be performed. As the neurodegenerative process spreads, the patient's learning and memory will become completely disabled, and they will be unable to care for themselves and so will require the constant care of a relative or professional caregiver. The usual time period from diagnosis to death is from 6 to 12 years. In 2016, the estimated cost of caring for patients with AD was $220 billion [9]. The annual cost of care for patients with PD was nearly $15 billion in 2013 [10] and for patients with stroke, over $70 billion [11].

A stroke is caused either by a clot blocking blood flow in an artery in the brain (ischemic stroke) or by rupture of a cerebral blood vessel (hemorrhagic stroke). People who suffer a stroke typically have a sudden partial paralysis on one side of their body (the side opposite the side of the brain where the stroke occurred) and often exhibit slurred speech [12]. Depending upon which cerebral artery is affected, and how severely blood flow is disrupted, a stroke can result in immediate or delayed (hours to weeks) death. Stroke survivors often have permanent disabilities ranging from mild to severe.

Lifestyle Risk Factors for Neurodegenerative Disorders and Stroke

Aging is the major risk factor for AD, PD, and stroke. The molecular and cellular changes that occur in neurons, glial cells, and blood vessel cells in the brain during aging have been reviewed recently [13]. These adversities of aging include an impaired ability of neurons to acquire and utilize glucose; dysfunction of mitochondria; accumulation of proteins, DNA, and membranes damaged by free radicals; impaired ability to repair or remove the damaged molecules (impaired lysosome function and autophagy); a compromised ability of neurons to respond adaptively to stress; aberrant neuronal network activity resulting, in part, from damaged gamma aminobutyric acid (GABA)-ergic inhibitory neurons; inflammation; and senescence of stem cells [14]. As is true for blood vessels in the heart and other organ systems, cerebral vessels exhibit arteriosclerosis (stiffening) and atherosclerosis (local inflammation and accumulation of lipid-laden plaques) during aging, which predispose to reduced blood flow and stroke [15]. Lifestyle factors that accelerate these aging-related processes have a detrimental impact on brain function and predispose to AD, PD, and stroke [13, 16].

Major modifiable lifestyle risk factors for stroke are well-established and include excessive calorie intake, diets high in saturated fat and cholesterol, diets devoid of vegetables and fruits, and being sedentary. Being overweight or obese, smoking, or having hyperlipidemia (low-density lipoprotein cholesterol and triglycerides), hypertension, insulin resistance, or diabetes increases one's stroke risk [17]. Lifestyle risk factors for AD and PD are emerging from recent studies and include a sedentary lifestyle, excessive calorie intake, and diets rich in processed foods, simple sugars, and saturated fats [18, 19]. Compared to normal-weight people, those who are obese perform more poorly on various cognitive tests, including those that evaluate visuospatial memory and executive function [16]. Remarkably, people who are obese have (on average) reduced volumes of several brain regions that play key roles in learning and memory, including the hippocampus and prefrontal cortex. Of particular concern are recent studies showing that even children and adolescents that are obese have relatively poorer cognition and reduced brain sizes compared to their normal-weight classmates [16]. Reversal of the metabolic morbidity (overweight, obesity, and insulin resistance) that results from such lifestyles should be a major focus of any brain health center.

Additional lifestyle risk factors for poor brain outcomes during aging have emerged from studies of human populations and animal models. People with a low level of education, and with occupations and lifestyles that lack intellectual challenges, are at increased risk for AD [20]. Laboratory animals that live in "impoverished" environments and/or are subjected to chronic psychological stress are unable to maintain their cognitive abilities as they age and exhibit accelerated cognitive impairment in models of AD [21, 22]. Another risk factor for AD and PD is traumatic brain injury, particularly with a history of multiple concussions [23]. There is also evidence that exposure to environmental toxins, especially pesticides that impair the function of mitochondria, may increase the risk of PD [24].

Diet, Exercise, and Intellectual Challenges for Prevention and Treatment

How often, how much (in terms of calories), and what kinds of food and drinks one consumes throughout life are increasingly recognized as having a major impact on the structure and function of the brain during aging. These lifestyle factors also affect one's risk of being afflicted with AD, PD, or stroke later in life. Moderation in calorie intake helps to maintain body weight within a low normal level and can also improve cognition [25, 26]. Recent findings suggest that IF eating patterns may be particularly beneficial for brain health [27, 28]. Intermittent fasting involves frequent periods of fasting sufficient to deplete liver glucose stores and mobilize fatty acids and ketone production (typically 16–24 hours of fasting). Similar to exercise, IF eating patterns reduce levels of anxiety and improve cognition by mechanisms involving increased production of the brain-derived neurotrophic factor (BDNF) and enhancement of GABAergic inhibitory neurotransmission [26, 27, 29–32].

In general, diets that include a variety of vegetables, fruits, nuts, whole grains, yogurt, olive oil, and fish are beneficial for brain health during aging. Simple sugars and diets high in saturated animal fats should be consumed only in small amounts or avoided entirely. The data supporting these dietary recommendations are based on epidemiological findings and on evidence from studies of animal models of aging, AD, PD, and stroke [33–35]. Consumption of fruits and vegetables that contain chemicals that elicit adaptive cellular stress responses in neurons may be particularly beneficial for brain health [36, 37].

Exercise improves cognition, reduces levels of anxiety, and protects against depression in humans and other animals [38]. Regular aerobic exercise during adult and later life reduces stroke risk [39] and may also reduce the risks of AD [40] and PD [41]. Exercise has also been shown to improve quality of life in AD, PD, and stroke patients [42, 43]. The underlying mechanisms include stimulation of the production of neurotrophic factors such as BDNF, formation of new synapses and strengthening of existing synapses, increased production of new neurons from stem cells (neurogenesis), stimulation of mitochondrial biogenesis (increased numbers of mitochondria) in neurons, and bolstering of resistance of brain cells to stress [13, 44].

Finally, considerable evidence suggests that people who regularly engage in intellectually challenging and social endeavors throughout their life are more resistant to AD, compared to those who live more mundane lifestyles [45]. The mechanisms by which cognitive challenges protect against neuronal degeneration during aging appear similar to the mechanisms by which exercise enables maintenance of muscle mass during aging. Thus, animals maintained in enriched physical and social environments exhibit greater numbers of synapses in their hippocampus [46]. Evidence is also emerging from animal and human studies that suggest that environmental enrichment in early life improves brain health outcomes later in life and, conversely, that early life deprivation or stressful conditions predispose to poor brain health outcomes [47].

The take-home message is that brain health is improved, and the risks of AD, PD, and stroke reduced, by lifestyles that include moderation in energy intake, IF, heart-healthy diets (rich in vegetables, fruits, nuts, fish, and healthy oils), regular aerobic exercise, and daily cognitive challenges. Based on these evidence-based strategies, a needs analysis is fashioned and tactical challenges of building a successful Lifestyle Medicine Center for Brain Aging and Neurodegenerative Diseases (LMC-BAND) identified.

Organization of the Lifestyle Medicine Center for Brain Aging and Neurodegenerative Diseases

The primary purposes of an LMC-BAND are education, counseling, and facilitation of lifestyle changes. A full-service LMC-BAND would include both outpatient and live-in (haven) components (Fig. 26.1). The LMC-BAND would serve patients with AD, PD, and stroke, as well as patients with lifestyles that increase their risk for these age-related neurological disorders. An LMC-BAND could be viewed as a dedicated Clinical Service Line within a sponsoring University School of Medicine, private hospital, independent dedicated Center, or larger healthcare system.

Physical Setting and Environment

The setting for the outpatient LMC-BAND would be in a location accessible by public transportation (if possible) and

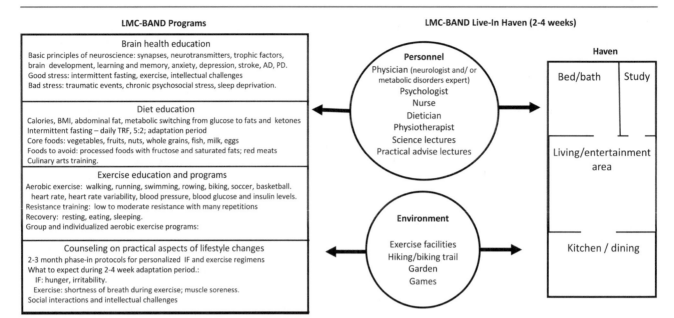

LMC-BAND Programs

Brain health education
Basic principles of neuroscience: synapses, neurotransmitters, trophic factors, brain development, learning and memory, anxiety, depression, stroke, AD, PD.
Good stress: intermittent fasting, exercise, intellectual challenges
Bad stress: traumatic events, chronic psychosocial stress, sleep deprivation.

Diet education
Calories, BMI, abdominal fat, metabolic switching from glucose to fats and ketones
Intermittent fasting – daily TRF, 5:2; adaptation period
Core foods: vegetables, fruits, nuts, whole grains, fish, milk, eggs
Foods to avoid: processed foods with fructose and saturated fats; red meats
Culinary arts training.

Exercise education and programs
Aerobic exercise: walking, running, swimming, rowing, biking, soccer, basketball.
   heart rate, heart rate variability, blood pressure, blood glucose and insulin levels.
Resistance training: low to moderate resistance with many repetitions
Recovery: resting, eating, sleeping.
Group and individualized aerobic exercise programs:

Counseling on practical aspects of lifestyle changes
2-3 month phase-in protocols for personalized IF and exercise regimens
What to expect during 2-4 week adaptation period.:
   IF: hunger, irritability.
   Exercise: shortness of breath during exercise; muscle soreness.
Social interactions and intellectual challenges

LMC-BAND Live-In Haven (2-4 weeks)

Personnel
Physician (neurologist and/ or metabolic disorders expert)
Psychologist
Nurse
Dietician
Physiotherapist
Science lectures
Practical advise lectures

Environment
Exercise facilities
Hiking/biking trail
Garden
Games

Haven
Bed/bath | Study
Living/entertainment area
Kitchen / dining

Fig. 26.1 Organization of a Lifestyle Medicine Center for Brain Aging and Neurodegenerative Diseases. The major purposes of the LMC-BAND are education, facilitation, and counseling in a pleasant environment where participants work together to achieve lifestyle changes that will result in enduring improvements in their brain health. The LMC-BAND would include both outpatient and live-in components with both groups of participants being offered the same educational opportunities. The facilities would be staffed with one or more physicians, psychologists, nurses, dieticians, and physiotherapists. A regular series of lec-

tures by experts on specific aspects of brain health, diet, and exercise would be offered. Ideally, the LMC-BAND would be located in a natural setting with opportunities for activities outdoors. Live-in quarters would be located and constructed so that each room receives natural light with minimal noise pollution. Abbreviations: *AD* Alzheimer's disease, *LMC-BAND* Lifestyle Medicine Center for Brain Aging and Neurodegenerative Diseases, *PD* Parkinson's disease, *TRF* time-restricted feeding

would provide sufficient parking space for patients that drive to the facility. The physical dimensions of the facility would be appropriate for the expected numbers of patients and would consist mainly of staff offices, larger meeting rooms for small groups, and a larger conference room equipped with furniture and audiovisual equipment to accommodate lectures and videos. The facility would also include a space, equipment, and resources for exercise and medical fitness training, including apparatus for both aerobic and strength/resistance training activities.

The setting for the LMC-BAND havens would be urban or rural with proximity to a city. It may or may not be in the same location as the outpatient Center. Ideally, the havens would be located adjacent to a park with trails for hiking and biking. The living quarters for each patient would be approximately 600 square feet with a living room, bedroom, study, and kitchen and dining area.

Equipment for Participant Evaluation

Onsite medical equipment would include scales, sphygmomanometers, thermometers, equipment for drawing blood, and computers outfitted with software for testing cogni-

tive function. Advanced Centers would include a magnetic resonance imaging (MRI) instrument, which would be used for MRI analysis of brain regional volumes and analysis of neuronal network activity. Blood work would typically be outsourced.

Human Resources: Staffing, Positions and Titles, Team Members, and Responsibilities

A Director with experience in managing healthcare facilities would oversee all aspects of the LCM-BAND. Each facility would employ at least two full-time physicians. Ideally, one would be a neurologist, and another would have expertise in metabolic disorders and preventative medicine. The physicians would perform patient evaluations and prescribe lifestyle interventions in consultation with other healthcare professionals, such as psychologists, dietitians, and physiotherapists. Patients and their caregivers would attend a core set of live and/or videotaped lectures aimed at educating the patient on the basics of how the brain works and what goes awry in stroke, AD, and PD. The psychologist, dietitian, and physiotherapist would focus on informing the patient as to what they can expect during the time period when they are changing their eating pattern and diet composition and during the period when they are incorporating exercise into their daily and weekly routines. Depending upon the size of the outpatient and haven facilities, one or more administrators handle financial and insurance transactions and personnel salaries. Additional staff might include a full- or part-time human resources person. If the outpatient facility and havens are located at the same site or close to each other, then some personnel can serve both facilities.

Patient Care and Flow: Outpatients and Inpatients

The LCM-BAND outpatient facility treats patients that have recently been diagnosed with mild cognitive impairment, early AD or PD, and stroke with mild to moderate levels of disability. The outpatient Center also treats patients at risk for an age-related brain disorder as a consequence of their family history and/or metabolic state (e.g., obesity, insulin resistance, and diabetes). In addition, the outpatient Center provides educational materials to anyone interested in brain health and aging. Patients are initially seen by a physician who will perform a clinical evaluation and become familiar with the patient's medical history. Baseline measurements are recorded including body weight, height, waist circumference, body mass index, blood pressure, heart rate, blood glucose, insulin, triglycerides, and ketone concentrations. Tests of cognition, strength, balance, and coordination are also performed. The dietitian gathers information on the patient's usual eating pattern and types of food they consume. The physiotherapist gauges the patient's fitness. Alternatively, the LCM-BAND haven facility houses patients for extended time periods of 2–4 weeks depending upon the patient and their ability to adapt to IF and exercise regimens.

Expanded Roles and Responsibilities

Ideally, LMC-BANDs are incorporated into national and regional organizational structures, with regional Directors and committees comprised of a broad spectrum of expertise within the realms of medical education, neurology, preventative medicine, and healthcare provision. There would be annual national and regional meetings aimed at exchanging information and developing novel approaches to proliferate brain healthy lifestyles in communities throughout the region and country. Working groups would be tasked with developing uniformity in educational materials, protocols, and prescriptions among LMC-BANDs.

The Centers would contribute to the training of medical students and physicians on the science and application of nutrition, IF, and exercise in clinical practice. In the case of IF, trainees would learn how to prescribe specific IF eating patterns, such as daily time-restricted eating and twice weekly modified fasts [28]. The importance of the 2- to 4-week adaptation period should be emphasized so that patients understand that improvements in general health, mood, and cognition will not be immediate. As with an exercise program, students and physicians will learn how to monitor the effects of IF on health indicators (e.g., glucose regulation, blood pressure, and abdominal fat). National or private healthcare insurance systems would cover outpatient and inpatient programs in which patients can be "coached" on how to change their eating pattern to IF.

The LMC-BANDs would provide public outreach, as well as outreach to major employers in the region. Through advertisements and outreach, the centers would encourage healthy lifestyles in their employees and accommodate IF eating patterns by allowing employees to, for example, arrive and begin work 1 hour earlier than usual and then allow the employees a 90-minute period midday when they can exercise and then eat.

Local, state, and national governments would be expected to discourage big agriculture and encourage production of a wide range of vegetables, fruits, whole grains, and nuts to be sold to the consumer without further processing. The propaganda of the processed food (including the breakfast food) industries and the pharmaceutical industries that encourage unhealthy food consumption and lifestyles should be reigned-in by government-enforced limitations on advertisements (Fig. 26.2). Lifestyle Medicine Centers, including those for BANDs, could help disseminate accurate information concerning lifestyles and health. This includes messages that emphasize the suffering and expense resulting from lifestyles dominated by overconsumption of highly processed foods and little or no exercise.

Specific prescriptions for lifestyle changes that improve brain health can be effectively applied to patients at risk for a neurodegenerative disorder and/or stroke based upon their family history/genetics, metabolic profile, and/or cognitive status. Novel approaches for implementing such prescriptions are being developed as first-line interventions for the prevention and treatment of neurodegenerative disorders and stroke. The four pillars of such prescriptions for brain health are (1) patient education, (2) graded transition with flexible stepwise goals, (3) frequent evaluation of progress, and (4) coaching with positive reinforcement. In the examples presented below, it is expected that the patients that will benefit most are those with current lifestyles characterized by three meals plus snacks every day with a predominance of highly processed foods, a low level of physical activity, and an occupation and home environment that are intellectually unchallenging.

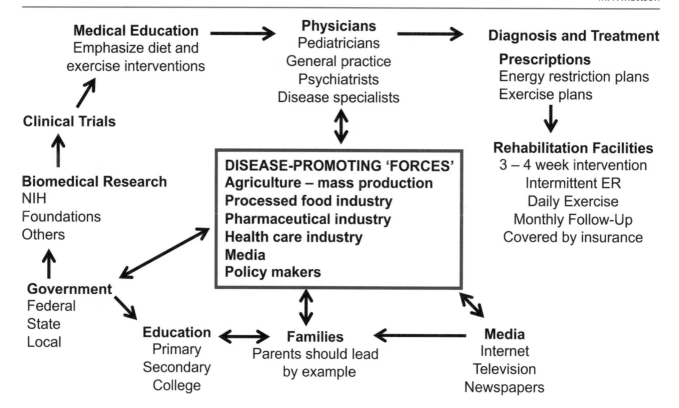

Fig. 26.2 Overview of American institutions that contribute to poor brain health and the institutions that could work to improve brain health. Agriculture is dominated by production of corn, soybeans, and wheat. Those grains are processed into highly palatable – even addictive – products that are extensively marketed. The pharmaceutical industry and much of the healthcare industry have no interest in facilitating lifestyle interventions because fewer sick people translates into less income for these industries. Media companies profit from advertisements from the processed food, pharmaceutical, and healthcare industries. Policymakers are influenced by lobbyists for these "disease-promoting forces" and so can be considered as contributing to the proliferation of unhealthy lifestyles. Education of parents and their children, government officials, medical school students, and practicing physicians must occur to achieve a reversal of the current situation in which healthy lifestyles are de-emphasized. Abbreviation: ER energy restriction, NIH National Institutes of Health

Eating and Exercise Patterns

The general goal is to facilitate the patient's transition to an eating pattern that includes frequent periods of ketosis. In a sedentary person, this requires fasting for at least 14–16 hours. Examples of two prescriptions for IF eating patterns are shown in Fig. 26.3. In the first example, the goals are to compress the patient's daily total eating time period to 8 hours every day (fasting for 16 hours every day) and to walk for at least 1 hour 4 days/week and engage in high-intensity exercise for 30 minutes, 2 days/week. In the second example, the goals are to eat no more than 700 calories on 2 days every week and to walk for at least 1 hour 4 days/week and engage in high-intensity exercise for 30 minutes, 2 days/week. For both prescriptions, the goals would be accomplished in a gradual manner during a 3-month time period. The patient can choose which prescription best fits their daily and weekly schedules. At the first office visit, the patient is presented with an over-view of how a sedentary lifestyle food intake throughout the day adversely affects body and brain health and how IF and exercise enhance mood, cognition, and physical health and protect against diabetes, cardiovascular disease, stroke, and neurodegenerative disorders. The patient will then be shown a few examples of how they can change their lifestyle over a period of several months. It is expected that this initial patient education session would require a minimum of 1 hour. Upon choosing specific eating pattern and exercise goals, the patient is provided with one or more means of communicating with the physician. This might entail a dedicated website or cell phone application or text messaging. The patient would be expected to visit the physician's office biweekly during the first 2 months of the intervention and bimonthly during the remainder of the first year of the lifestyle intervention. Evaluations at these visits would include measurements of body weight, blood pressure, blood ketones (i.e., beta-hydroxybutyrate), glucose, and hemoglobin A1c concentrations.

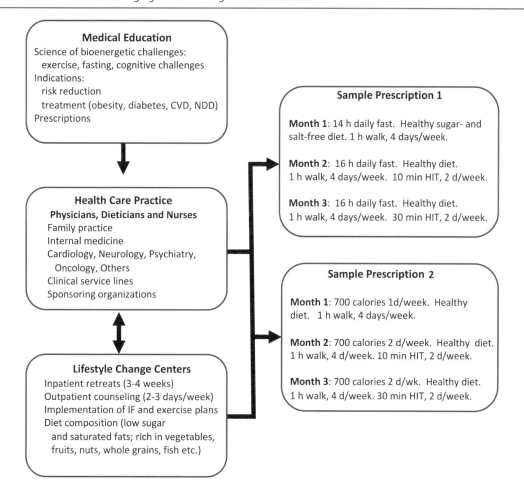

Fig. 26.3 Example of how lifestyle modification prescriptions might be incorporated into the healthcare system. Medical students should be taught about how diet and exercise impact health and disease processes and that prescriptions for lifestyle modifications should be the first-line interventions for people with or at risk for metabolic morbidity (e.g., insulin resistance and abdominal obesity) and associated diseases including stroke and neurodegenerative disorders. All physicians that treat patients with disorders that can benefit from lifestyle modification should be required to document their efforts to prescribe and implement specific lifestyle modifications. Lifestyle Medicine Centers could provide the expertise and resources for patients who are unable to comply with the doctor's lifestyle change prescription in the first instance. Two sample prescriptions that establish specific goals for eating patterns and exercise routines are shown at the right of the illustration. Abbreviations: CVD cardiovascular disease, HIT high-intensity (Interval) training, IF intermittent fasting, NDD neurodegenerative diseases

Intellectual Challenges

Cognitive function and the prevention of chronic disease of the brain are emerging areas of lifestyle medicine. Evidence from longitudinal studies has consistently shown that people who regularly engage in intellectually engaging activities are better able to maintain their cognitive functioning as they age [48]. Many occupations require daily intellectual challenges – learning and remembering new information, integrating and analyzing data/information, and decision-making. Examples include scientists, engineers, doctors, teachers, lawyers, and musicians. People in such occupations have a reduced risk for AD, and for them, it is important to keep intellectually engaged even after they retire. Other occupations may be less intellectually challenging including

retail sales, housekeeping, factory work, and truck driving. People in such occupations have a higher risk for AD and could be offered suggestions and opportunities for intellectually engaging hobbies outside of their work environment. There is evidence that continuing education can reduce one's risk for AD [49]. One can readily find books, magazines, websites, and smart phone apps with "brain training games." However, people who play such games only improve their performance on those games and not in other cognitive tasks. On the other hand, there is emerging evidence that structured tasks can be developed that improve overall cognitive functioning; such tasks require executive coordination of skills and task switching [48]. Using emerging evidence-based findings, the LMC-BAND can provide patients with numerous examples of options for intellectually demanding endeavors that include continuing education and tasks that "exercise" broad networks of cerebral cortical neuronal circuits.

Use of Electronic Communication

Mobile or electronic health (m-health/e-health) is the use of smart phones and other personal devices in medical care. There are two general applications of electronic technologies to the goals of a LMC-BAND: communication of Center staff with outpatients and patient's self-monitoring of their progress [50, 51]. Because the first few months are critical for a patient's success in achieving a major modification such as IF and exercise regimens, frequent communication of the LMC-BAND staff and patient is critical during this time period. Continuing communication over periods of years is also likely to prove valuable for the patient. Smart phones and social media are increasingly used to communicate with patients who are participating in clinical trials, and those same approaches can be used for LMC-BAND staff to communicate with patients who have questions about or help with their brain health-related lifestyle issues.

Self-monitoring devices, the Internet, and smart phones are providing new opportunities for facilitating lifestyle changes that improve lifelong brain health. Many health-conscious people use wearable technologies that measure their activity levels (steps and distance traveled), heart rate, and sleep. Smart phone apps that help organize eating patterns and diet composition are increasingly available. In addition to providing their patients with specific prescriptions for diet, exercise, and intellectual challenges, the LMC-BAND can provide information on these wearable technologies that can help them achieve their lifestyle change goals.

Education and Outreach: From K–12 to MD

A major function of an LMC-HAND is education, not only of patients referred to the Center but also of children and adults in the community and of practicing physicians at large. This outreach requires making contacts at area public and private schools, senior centers and retirement communities, and clinics. The nature and extent of such outreach efforts will depend upon the size of the LMC-BAND and how long it has been in existence.

Summary

As the number of people who reach their 7th, 8th, and 9th decades of life increases, so too does the number of elderly people with AD, PD, or stroke. There are currently no treatments that are effective in stopping or even slowing the progression of AD and PD and no treatments that reverse the brain damage in stroke patients. Because of the complexity of the mechanisms involved in neuronal dysfunction and degeneration in these brain disorders, it is unlikely that there will be any drugs in the near future that stop or reverse the disease processes. However, because there is considerable evidence that diet, exercise, and intellectual challenges can reduce the risk of AD, PD, and stroke, the potential of LMC-BANDs to help people modify their lifestyles in a brain-healthy manner is considerable.

The goals of an LMC-BAND are patient education, graded transition with flexible stepwise goals, frequent evaluation of progress, and coaching with positive reinforcement. To accomplish these goals, the Center staffing should include a Director with expertise in healthcare provision, a neurologist and a physician with expertise in the areas of metabolism and preventative medicine, one or more psychologists, a physiotherapist and/or personal trainer, a dietitian, and a financial manager. After evaluations by a physician, dietitian, and psychologist, a specific plan for intervention will be developed. Depending upon the patient's metabolic state and other risk factors, the plan may include only outpatient prescriptions or a 2-week to 1-month live-in treatment plan. Such prescriptions would include those for eating pattern modification (e.g., IF), diet composition modification, exercise, and/or intellectual challenges. The progress of outpatients can be evaluated by staff that communicates with the patient via electronic devices and by self-monitoring by the patient.

Challenges

The first challenge in the establishment of a LMC-BAND is to acquire data to determine the feasibility of the Center with regard to financial considerations, location and construction plans, and projected patient numbers and flow. These fundamental issues can be readily addressed at a medical school or large hospital that already has experience in establishing new Centers and by LMCs that are expanding. They will likely be able to draw upon existing personnel to begin to staff the center. A LMC-BAND created de novo would require raising sufficient capital to justify moving forward. The next challenges are designing, constructing, and staffing the Center. Other challenges include the implementation of educational protocols and intervention plans tailored for specific categories of patients, as well as outreach to the community.

Fortunately, lifestyle medicine is a rapidly expanding Clinical Service Line within healthcare systems, and a newly developed LMC-BAND can draw upon the tools and resources of local and regional organizations and clinics that serve patients with AD, PD, or stroke and their families. Such organizations include:

- National Institute on Aging Alzheimer's Disease Research Centers (https://www.nia.nih.gov/health/alzheimers-disease-research-centers)
- Alzheimer's Association (https://www.alz.org)
- Parkinson's Foundation (https://www.parkinson.org)
- American Stroke Association (https://www.strokeassociation.org)
- American College of Lifestyle Medicine (https://www.lifestylemedicine.org)
- Rhode Island Lifestyle Medicine Group (https://www.lifespan.org) (all websites accessed on March 27, 2020)

Take-Home Messages

The exponential increase in the numbers of elderly people with AD, PD, and stroke warrants a rapid instillation of society-wide interventions aimed at reducing everyone's risk of these devastating disorders. The scientific evidence that lifestyle factors are the major risk factors for these brain disorders of aging is cogent. Risk is increased in people of all ages who are sedentary, over-consume energy-dense processed foods, and lead intellectually unchallenging lives. Accordingly, risk is reduced by regular exercise, restriction of unhealthy foods, IF, and intellectual challenges. The purpose of an LMC-BAND is to facilitate enduring lifestyle modifications through education and implementation of specific prescriptions. Increasing evidence suggests that with appropriate education, and vigorous counseling and encouragement, LMC-BANDs can be effective in enabling patients to achieve their lifestyle change goals.

References

1. GBD 2016 Dementia Collaborators. Global, regional, and national burden of Alzheimer's disease and other dementias, 1990–2016: a systematic analysis for the Global Burden of Disease Study 2016. Lancet Neurol. 2019;18:88–106.
2. Dorsey ER, George BP, Leff B, et al. The coming crisis: obtaining care for the growing burden of neurodegenerative conditions. Neurology. 2013;80:1989–96.
3. Bennett DA, Krishnamurthi RV, Barker-Collo S, Global Burden of Diseases, Injuries, and Risk Factors 2010 Study Stroke Expert Group, et al. The global burden of ischemic stroke: findings of the GBD 2010 study. Glob Heart. 2014;9:107–12.
4. Krishnamurthi RV, Moran AE, Forouzanfar MH, Global Burden of Diseases, Injuries, and Risk Factors 2010 Study Stroke Expert Group, et al. The global burden of hemorrhagic stroke: a summary of findings from the GBD 2010 study. Glob Heart. 2014;9:101–6.
5. Petersen RC. Clinical practice. Mild cognitive impairment. N Engl J Med. 2011;364:2227–34.
6. Mattson MP. Late-onset dementia: a mosaic of prototypical pathologies modifiable by diet and lifestyle. NPJ Aging Mech Dis. 2015;1. pii: 15003. https://doi.org/10.1038/npjamd.2015.3. Epub 2015 Sep 28.
7. Nutt JG, Wooten GF. Clinical practice. Diagnosis and initial management of Parkinson's disease. N Engl J Med. 2005;353:1021–7.
8. Breen DP, Halliday GM, Lang AE. Gut-brain axis and the spread of α-synuclein pathology: vagal highway or dead end? Mov Disord. 2019;34:307–16.
9. Alzheimer's Association. 2016 Alzheimer's disease facts and figures. Alzheimers Dement. 2016;12:459–509.
10. Kowal SL, Dall TM, Chakrabarti R, et al. The current and projected economic burden of Parkinson's disease in the United States. Mov Disord. 2013;28:311–8.
11. Ovbiagele B, Goldstein LB, Higashida RT, American Heart Association Advocacy Coordinating Committee and Stroke Council, et al. Forecasting the future of stroke in the United States: a policy statement from the American Heart Association and American Stroke Association. Stroke. 2013;44:2361–75.
12. van der Worp HB, van Gijn J. Clinical practice. Acute ischemic stroke. N Engl J Med. 2007;357:572–9.
13. Mattson MP, Arumugam TV. Hallmarks of brain aging: adaptive and pathological modification by metabolic states. Cell Metab. 2018;27:1176–99.
14. Zhang P, Kishimoto Y, Grammatikakis I, et al. Senolytic therapy alleviates Aβ-associated oligodendrocyte progenitor cell senescence and cognitive deficits in an Alzheimer's disease model. Nat Neurosci. 2019;22:719–28.
15. Grinberg LT, Thal DR. Vascular pathology in the aged human brain. Acta Neuropathol. 2010;119:277–90.
16. Mattson MP. An evolutionary perspective on why food overconsumption impairs cognition. Trends Cogn Sci. 2019;23:200–12.
17. Bronner LL, Kanter DS, Manson JE. Primary prevention of stroke. N Engl J Med. 1995;333:1392–400.
18. Luchsinger JA. Adiposity, hyperinsulinemia, diabetes and Alzheimer's disease: an epidemiological perspective. Eur J Pharmacol. 2008;585:119–29.
19. Serrano-Pozo A, Growdon JH. Is Alzheimer's disease risk modifiable? J Alzheimers Dis. 2019;67:795–819.
20. Barnes DE, Yaffe K. The projected effect of risk factor reduction on Alzheimer's disease prevalence. Lancet Neurol. 2011;10:819–28.
21. Carroll JC, Iba M, Bangasser DA, et al. Chronic stress exacerbates tau pathology, neurodegeneration, and cognitive performance through a corticotropin-releasing factor receptor-dependent mechanism in a transgenic mouse model of tauopathy. J Neurosci. 2011;31:14436–49.
22. McEwen BS, Getz L. Lifetime experiences, the brain and personalized medicine: an integrative perspective. Metabolism. 2013;62(Suppl 1):S20–6.
23. Perry DC, Sturm VE, Peterson MJ, et al. Association of traumatic brain injury with subsequent neurological and psychiatric disease: a meta-analysis. J Neurosurg. 2016;124:511–26.
24. Ascherio A, Schwarzschild MA. The epidemiology of Parkinson's disease: risk factors and prevention. Lancet Neurol. 2016;15:1257–72.
25. Singh R, Lakhanpal D, Kumar S, et al. Late-onset intermittent fasting dietary restriction as a potential intervention to retard age-associated brain function impairments in male rats. Age (Dordr). 2012;34(4):917–33.
26. Liu Y, Cheng A, Li YJ, et al. SIRT3 mediates hippocampal synaptic adaptations to intermittent fasting and ameliorates deficits in APP mutant mice. Nat Commun. 2019;10:1886.

27. Mattson MP, Moehl K, Ghena N, et al. Intermittent metabolic switching, neuroplasticity and brain health. Nat Rev Neurosci. 2018;19:63–80.

28. De Cabo R, Mattson MP. Impact of intermittent fasting on health, aging and disease. New Engl J Med. 2019;381:2541–51.

29. Yu ZF, Mattson MP. Dietary restriction and 2-deoxyglucose administration reduce focal ischemic brain damage and improve behavioral outcome: evidence for a preconditioning mechanism. J Neurosci Res. 1999;57:830–9.

30. Duan W, Mattson MP. Dietary restriction and 2-deoxyglucose administration improve behavioral outcome and reduce degeneration of dopaminergic neurons in models of Parkinson's disease. J Neurosci Res. 1999;57:195–206.

31. Halagappa VK, Guo Z, Pearson M, et al. Intermittent fasting and caloric restriction ameliorate age-related behavioral deficits in the triple-transgenic mouse model of Alzheimer's disease. Neurobiol Dis. 2007;26:212–20.

32. Arumugam TV, Phillips TM, Cheng A, et al. Age and energy intake interact to modify cell stress pathways and stroke outcome. Ann Neurol. 2010;67:41–52.

33. Larsson SC, Wallin A, Wolk A. Dietary approaches to stop hypertension diet and incidence of stroke: results from 2 prospective cohorts. Stroke. 2016;47:986–90.

34. Chen X, Maguire B, Brodaty H, et al. Dietary patterns and cognitive health in older adults: a systematic review. J Alzheimers Dis. 2019;67:583–619.

35. Maraki MI, Yannakoulia M, Stamelou M, et al. Mediterranean diet adherence is related to reduced probability of prodromal Parkinson's disease. Mov Disord. 2019;34:48–57.

36. Mattson MP. What doesn't kill you…. Sci Am. 2015;313:40–5.

37. Lee J, Jo DG, Park D, et al. Adaptive cellular stress pathways as therapeutic targets of dietary phytochemicals: focus on the nervous system. Pharmacol Rev. 2014;66:815–68.

38. Hearing CM, Chang WC, Szuhany KL, et al. Physical exercise for treatment of mood disorders: a critical review. Curr Behav Neurosci Rep. 2016;3:350–9.

39. Kramer SF, Hung SH, Brodtmann A. The impact of physical activity before and after stroke on stroke risk and recovery: a narrative review. Curr Neurol Neurosci Rep. 2019;19:28.

40. McGurran H, Glenn JM, Madero EN, et al. Prevention and treatment of Alzheimer's disease: biological mechanisms of exercise. J Alzheimers Dis. 2019;69:311–38.

41. Fang X, Han D, Cheng Q, et al. Association of levels of physical activity with risk of parkinson disease: a systematic review and meta-analysis. JAMA Netw Open. 2018;1:e182421.

42. Archer T, Fredriksson A, Johansson B. Exercise alleviates Parkinsonism: clinical and laboratory evidence. Acta Neurol Scand. 2011;123:73–84.

43. Groot C, Hooghiemstra AM, Raijmakers PG, et al. The effect of physical activity on cognitive function in patients with dementia: a meta-analysis of randomized control trials. Ageing Res Rev. 2016;25:13–23.

44. Mattson MP. Energy intake and exercise as determinants of brain health and vulnerability to injury and disease. Cell Metab. 2012;16:706–22.

45. Kivipelto M, Mangialasche F, Ngandu T. Lifestyle interventions to prevent cognitive impairment, dementia and Alzheimer disease. Nat Rev Neurol. 2018;14:653–66.

46. Stuart KE, King AE, Fernandez-Martos CM, et al. Mid-life environmental enrichment increases synaptic density in CA1 in a mouse model of Aβ-associated pathology and positively influences synaptic and cognitive health in healthy ageing. J Comp Neurol. 2017;525:1797–810.

47. Sale A, Berardi N, Maffei L. Environment and brain plasticity: towards an endogenous pharmacotherapy. Physiol Rev. 2014;94:189–234.

48. Hertzog C, Kramer AF, Wilson RS, et al. Enrichment effects on adult cognitive development: can the functional capacity of older adults be preserved and enhanced? Psychol Sci Public Interest. 2008;9:1–65.

49. Matyas N, Keser Aschenberger F, Wagner G, et al. Continuing education for the prevention of mild cognitive impairment and Alzheimer's-type dementia: a systematic review and overview of systematic reviews. BMJ Open. 2019;9:e027719.

50. Faiola A, Papautsky EL, Isola M. Empowering the aging with mobile health: a mhealth framework for supporting sustainable healthy lifestyle behavior. Curr Probl Cardiol. 2019;44:232–66.

51. Kampmeijer R, Pavlova M, Tambor M, et al. The use of e-health and m-health tools in health promotion and primary prevention among older adults: a systematic literature review. BMC Health Serv Res. 2016;16(Suppl 5):290.

The Marie-Josée and Henry R. Kravis Center for Clinical Cardiovascular Health at Mount Sinai Heart

Janet H. Johnson, Mohamed Al-Kazaz, and Jeffrey I. Mechanick

Abbreviations

A1C	Hemoglobin A1c
ABCD	Adiposity-based chronic disease
AHA	American Heart Association
BMI	Body mass index
CHD	Coronary heart disease
CVD	Cardiovascular disease
DBCD	Dysglycemia-based chronic disease
EHR	Electronic health record
HCP	Healthcare professional
MetS	Metabolic syndrome
T2D	Type 2 diabetes

Rationale for a Cardiometabolic Risk Mitigation Lifestyle Medicine Center

Scope of the Problem

Cardiovascular disease (CVD) produces tremendous burden on the health of individuals and on the economy in the USA and globally. Cardiovascular disease is the leading cause of death globally. It causes significant morbidity and mortality [1]. It has been considered as the primary cause of death for almost a third of the deaths in the USA in 2016. That means it is responsible for the demise of more lives than all forms of cancer combined. Globally, CVD accounts for the death of >17 million individuals in 2016 with expected increased >23 million by 2030.

The prevalence rate of CVD (comprising coronary heart disease [CHD], heart failure, stroke, and hypertension) in adults ≥20 years of age is approximately 50% (or 120 million people), based on 2013–2016 National Health and Nutrition Examination Survey data. In 2016, CHD was the leading cause of deaths in the US related to CVD (over 40%), followed by stroke (~17%), hypertension (~10%), heart failure (~9%), and diseases of the arteries (3.0%) [1]. These figures are concerning and deserving of action: someone in the USA will have a heart attack in every 40 seconds. Each heart attack confers many health and economic consequences for the patient and healthcare system. In addition to heart failure and CHD, many patients suffer from rhythm problems. For example, atrial fibrillation impacts 2.7–6.1 million people in the USA, and this is expected to increase with the aging population. Moreover, atrial fibrillation is a major risk factor for thromboembolic disease [2]. According to 2014–2015 statistics, CVD incurred an estimated cost of $351.2 billion. In 2016, the American Heart Association (AHA) estimated that the total costs of CVD care would reach $1.1 trillion in 2035 [1]. CVD and stroke accounted for 14% of total health expenditures in 2014–2015. This is more than any other group of diseases and therefore requires scrutiny.

CVD is driven by cardiometabolic risk factors such as hypercholesteremia, diabetes, obesity, smoking, unhealthy dietary patterns, and physical inactivity. Using data from 2013 to 2016, diabetes and hypercholesteremia impacted 26 million (9.8%) and 92.8 million (38.2%) adults in the USA, respectively. Obesity is an epidemic impacting 93 million adults based on a national survey in 2015–2016. From 1999–2000 through 2015–2016, there was an increasing trend in obesity that was observed among different age

J. H. Johnson
The Mount Sinai Hospital, Marie-Josée and Henry R. Kravis Center for Cardiovascular Health at Mount Sinai, New York, NY, USA
e-mail: Janet.johnson@mountsinai.org

M. Al-Kazaz (✉)
Icahn School of Medicine at Mount Sinai, Department of Cardiology, New York, NY, USA
e-mail: Mohamed.al-kazaz@mountsinai.org

J. I. Mechanick
The Marie-Josée and Henry R. Kravis Center for Cardiovascular Health at Mount Sinai Heart, and the Division of Endocrinology, Diabetes and Bone Disease, Icahn School of Medicine at Mount Sinai, New York, NY, USA
e-mail: jeffrey.mechanick@mountsinai.org

© Springer Nature Switzerland AG 2020
J. I. Mechanick, R. F. Kushner (eds.), *Creating a Lifestyle Medicine Center*, https://doi.org/10.1007/978-3-030-48088-2_27

groups involving adults and youth [3]. This could reflect the impact of socioeconomic status and healthcare disparities. The estimated annual cost of obesity in 2008 was ~$150 billion with an individual with obesity costing the system at least $1400 per year more than an individual without obesity [4].

Genetic, environmental, and behavioral factors are primary drivers of abnormal adiposity and dysglycemia, which in turn are metabolic drivers of CVD. New multi-morbidity chronic care models, such as adiposity-based chronic disease (ABCD) and dysglycemia-based chronic disease (DBCD), can identify patients at early stages of the disease spectrum and allow for early and sustainable intervention, prevention, and benefit [5, 6]. Within these models, lifestyle medicine offers the advantage of exerting a broad set of network-based interventions. Lifestyle medicine plays a central role in combating CVD and cardiometabolic risk factors.

There is an urgent need to rally efforts and resources in preventive measures to reduce the burden of CVDs [7]. Early and sustainable durable preventative strategies are better and more cost-effective than relying on eventual tertiary prevention once advanced disease manifests. Lifestyle medicine can marshal different types of evidence-based prevention (primordial, primary, secondary, and tertiary), alone or in combination, with every patient encounter. However, the physical and human resources need to be readily available, organized, and primed for engagement.

The Standard of Care Is to Address Component Cardiovascular Risks with Medicines and Procedures

Metabolic syndrome (MetS) is a pathophysiological state defined by a cluster of certain component risk factors for CVD, which are also associated with dysfunction in many other organs. The diagnostic criteria for MetS encompass traditional risk factors, such as abnormal adiposity (waist circumference >102 cm in men and 80 cm in women), dyslipidemia (triglycerides ≥150 mg/dL and/or high-density lipoprotein cholesterol <40 mg/dL in men and <50 mg/dL in women), blood pressure (≥130/80), and fasting glucose ≥100 mg/dL. Unfortunately, MetS remains underdiagnosed [8]. Besides MetS traits, tobacco use is another component risk factor for CVD.

In the USA, most patients who suffered from a myocardial infarction had at least one cardiovascular risk factor. The standard of care for these traditional risk factors revolves around observation, pharmacological interventions, and procedures. Various American and European professional medical societies have issued guidelines for nutritional and physical activity, but the main focus remains on medications or procedural interventions. For instance, the standard of

care for type 2 diabetes (T2D) is still primarily targeting blood glucose and hemoglobin A1C levels with pharmacotherapy [9]. Even though there is a newfound recognition of the critical importance of early prevention of cardiovascular complications in patients with T2D, the emphasis is squarely on new pharmaceuticals and innovative noninvasive and invasive procedures.

Hypercholesterolemia management is driven by risk prediction models (e.g., atherosclerotic cardiovascular disease risk estimator), imaging (e.g., coronary artery calcium score), and various biomarkers (e.g., lipid profiles and high-sensitivity C-reactive protein) that stratify patients to guide decision-making about lifelong cholesterol-lowering medications (e.g., statins). Hypertension, which is a leading cause of CVD morbidity and mortality, is typically managed by setting thresholds for treatment and goals of therapy that guide the initiation and escalation of blood pressure-lowering drugs. Even obesity management, which fortunately enjoys recognition as a disease that requires durable lifestyle change, also requires pharmacological and bariatric procedural interventions in many patients not responding to lifestyle medicine interventions alone. So, the question arises: Do failures to respond to lifestyle medicine result from biological reasons or merely from an inability to provide lifestyle medicine in an effective way?

Impact of Lifestyle Medicine on Residual Cardiovascular Risks

When component risk factors are absent or effectively treated and patients remain at risk for a chronic disease, such as CVD, the remaining risk is termed residual risk. There are many residual risk factors that are believed to interact with each other, and with component risk factors, in a complex way. These residual risk factors include insulin resistance, elevated apolipoprotein B, various adipokines, the prothrombotic state, endothelial dysfunction, and other aspects of low-grade inflammation [10, 11]. Residual risk is also driven by genetic, environmental, and behavioral factors and varies among individuals and populations. Some are modifiable and others are not. However, long-term exposure to residual risk increases the likelihood and burden of CVD [12].

Lifestyle medicine is first-line therapy for all component risk factors for CVD [8], though pharmacotherapy and procedures are commonly employed at late and even early states. More importantly, lifestyle medicine, particularly healthy dietary patterns, physical activity, and stress reduction, is highly suited for the management of residual risk. The scientific substantiation of beneficial effects of lifestyle medicine on CVD risk (component and residual) mitigation serves to anchor the rationale for building a Lifestyle Medicine Center.

Development of the Lifestyle Medicine Center at Mount Sinai Heart

Infrastructure and Environment

The Marie-Josée and Henry R. Kravis Center for Clinical Cardiovascular Health at Mount Sinai Heart ("the Center") opened in March 2017 as a clinical service line that offers a range of integrated and comprehensive programs promoting cardiovascular health and aiming to prevent CVD. The Center is part of Mount Sinai Heart, which also houses the Cardiovascular Institute in the Mount Sinai Health System. The Center is currently located at a "Mount Sinai Doctors" site in the Upper East Side of New York City. The Center has several programs, of which the two largest are the Cardiology/Endocrinology Clinical Practice and Cardiac Rehabilitation/Medical Fitness. The patients are either self-referred or referred by their primary care providers, primary cardiologist, inpatient services, and the community. These programs are staffed by faculty from the sponsoring health system – Mount Sinai – and share administrative leadership with The Mount Sinai Hospital. The Center's programs are depicted in Table 27.1 and management structure in Fig. 27.1.

There were two key drivers for the creation of the Center: first and most significant, the impetus originating from Dr. Valentin Fuster, Director of Mount Sinai Heart and Physician-in-Chief of The Mount Sinai Hospital, who championed the prime importance of early and sustainable prevention at all levels and aspects of CVD [13], and, second, the incorporation of strategies from *Lifestyle Medicine: A Manual for Clinical Practice* [14] co-edited by Drs. Mechanick and Kushner.

The Center is regarded as a Lifestyle Medicine Clinical Service Line within the Mount Sinai Health System with specific mission and vision statements (Table 27.2). Since there are many other entities in the region that have similar missions and visions, it is important that the Center can distinguish itself. Briefly speaking, the Center integrates clinical cardiology, endocrinology, and nutrition, with exercise physiology and dietetics, in a dedicated and durable high-touch/high-tech immersive environment, to optimize cardiovascular health. This is different from a primary care, preventive medicine, diagnostic, or wellness center. Since the Center focuses on cardiovascular health, it is also differentiated from the typical, more generalized Lifestyle Medicine Center.

Business Model

The Center is a clinical service line developed within a sponsoring academic health system. The business model focuses on value, with the goal to optimize a patient's cardiovascular

Table 27.1 Programs at the Center*

Name	Description
Cardiology Clinical Practice	Evidenced-based, state-of-the-art cardiovascular and lifestyle medical care
	Clinical cardiology
Endocrinology, Metabolism, and Nutrition Support Clinical Practice	Evidenced-based, state-of-the-art metabolic lifestyle medical care
	Diabetes care (type 1, type 2, gestational, and atypical)
	Obesity care
	General endocrinology
	Neck ultrasound and fine-needle aspiration biopsy of the thyroid/parathyroid
	Home parenteral and enteral nutrition
Internal Medicine Clinical Practice	Evidenced-based, state-of-the-art lifestyle medical care
	General internal medicine
	Infectious diseases
	HIV medicine
	Travel medicine
Clinical Nutrition and Dietetics	Individual consults and group sessions provided by registered dietician
Cardiac Rehabilitation Phase II	Medically supervised exercise and education program for patients with certain cardiovascular diagnoses for secondary prevention
Cardiac Rehabilitation Phase III	Supervised exercise sessions for patients with cardiovascular disease for secondary prevention
Medical Fitness	Personalized exercise program designed on patient's individual needs and medical condition for primary and secondary prevention
Wearable Technologies	Continuous glucose monitoring, insulin pumps, pedometers/accelerometers, patient education and dedicated lifestyle medicine App

*Programs are components of the Lifestyle Medicine Center and Clinical Service Line

health within budgetary constraints and an objective to develop an economic self-sustained program. The economic strategy is still evolving, but during the early stages of development, revenue streams are considered for each program and then financial success and viability considered for the aggregated clinical service line. Therefore, each program is analyzed using unit economics and reviewed with Mount Sinai Heart finance personnel on a monthly basis.

Revenue streams result from services billing Medicare, Medicaid, and other commercial insurance plans and self-pay. Uniform policies are in place to guide exceptions and adjustments to out-of-pocket requirements; these are on a case-by-case basis and in accordance with existing regulatory guidelines in order to assure care can be delivered to all patients in the Center, despite socioeconomic constraints. No doubt, these and other economic factors pose the greatest challenge to achieving the Center's mission and vision.

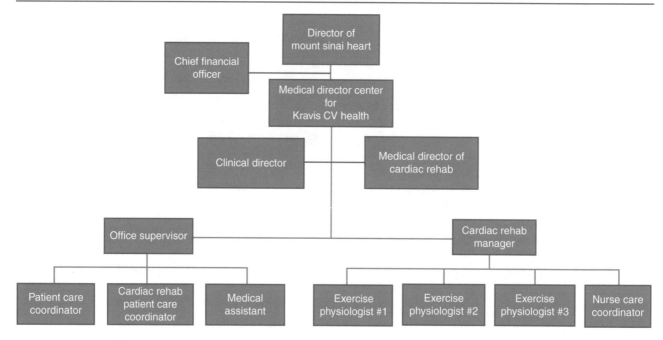

Fig. 27.1 Organizational chart of Center. Center management is primarily vertically organized with small horizontal features (red lines). This provides a more agile, hybrid management system that prioritizes accountability and deliberation in routine circumstances but is able to rapidly adapt and exert control in more fluid or urgent circumstances. *Abbreviation*: CV cardiovascular

Table 27.2 Mission statement and vision

Mission	To prevent and treat chronic cardiovascular disease in individual patients, creating a new culture of cardiovascular health across populations and generations. The Center focuses on lifestyle medicine, including programs in healthy eating, physical activity, stress reduction, sleep hygiene, behavioral science, tobacco cessation, alcohol moderation, and community engagement
Vision	To demonstrate clear success after 2 years at a single site, using validated measures of health and disease prevention, and then scale up and out across the Mount Sinai Health System; after 5 years, to demonstrate clear success on a large population with a working registry containing molecular, biochemical, clinical, and demographic data to drive research and discovery and optimize further lifestyle medicine and preventive cardiology care

Clinical and Economic Targets

Clinical targets are for 80% of patients to meet pre-established cardiometabolic targets within the first 90 days after initial consultation. These include achieving a hemoglobin A1c (A1C) of $\leq 7.0\%$ or a decrease of 0.5%; body mass index of <25 kg/m^2 or decrease by 5%; and low-density lipoprotein cholesterol ≤ 100 mg/dl or decrease by 10%. Achieving these targets is also a performance metric used in physician contracts. Subsequent, durable, and realistic clinical targets are currently being developed and will apply to all Center patients, requiring a comprehensive, integrative, multimodality care plan.

Economic targets are also necessary, and not just sufficient, for the success of the Center. Philanthropy is a continuing effort on the part of leadership to enhance programmatic resources, but organic growth, marketability, and sustainability are the goals. The economic targets are considered as aggregated figures comprising all the programs (clinical practice, registered dietitian (RD), Cardiac Rehabilitation, Medical Fitness, diabetes technology, education, research, etc.) and to be sustainable for current and hopefully future enhanced operations. These targets are feasible when certain patient encounter and utilization benchmarks are reached, after analysis by Mount Sinai Heart financial teams. These metrics are analyzed on a regular basis, and adjustments are subsequently introduced and implemented.

Physical Setting

The Center occupies the lower level of a building owned by the Mount Sinai Health System approximately 20 city blocks from the main campus where The Mount Sinai Hospital is located. A preliminary tour of the empty space was initially conducted with Drs. Fuster and Mechanick, along with the architect and representatives from building services, and after several organizational meetings with other stakeholders, a final floor plan (Fig. 27.2) and architectural renderings were developed and approved. The new facility housed clinical practice suites, a gym for Cardiac Rehabilitation and

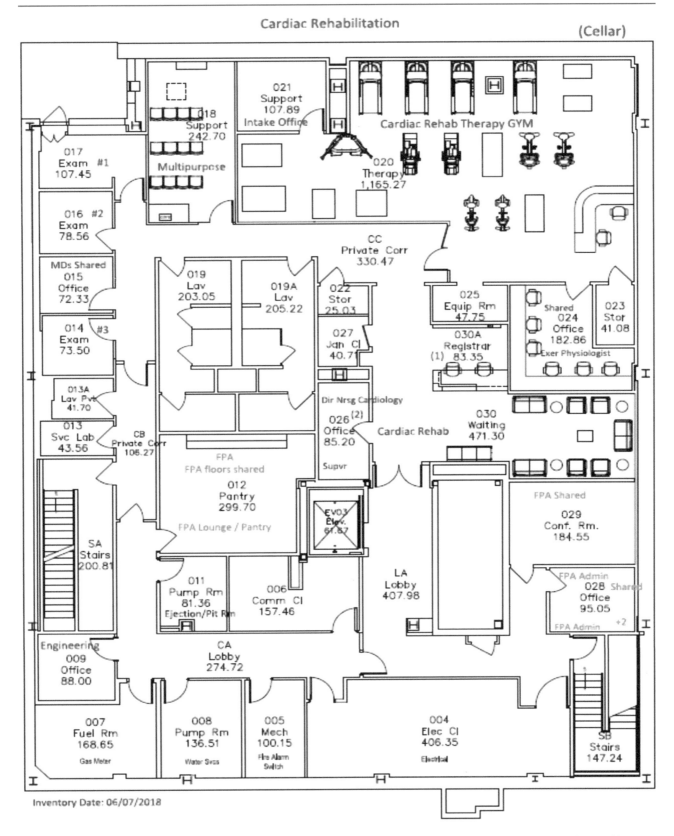

Fig. 27.2 Kravis Center floor plan. Patients enter the lower level of the Center by stairs or elevator and step in the waiting area. Walking past the register, to the right is the gym, exercise physiologist team room, and intake room. To the left of the register is the hallway leading to the multipurpose room, exam rooms, and physician work area. Square footage of work and patient flow areas (not including lavatories, storage, equipment rooms, and other common areas for building): waiting room 471.3; registrar 83.35; front office 85.20; gym 1165.27; intake room 107.89; team room 182.86; multipurpose room 242.7; 3 exam rooms 258.34 (72.33 + 78.56 + 107.45); physician charting room 72.33; total 2669.24

Medical Fitness, a multipurpose room, and usual reception, work, and storage spaces for a total of 2390-square footage. Important considerations at this stage of planning were budget, spatial dimensions, scale of service, need for integrative programs, efficiency, patient flow, and an immersive patient experience.

Patients enter by the staircase from the main lobby or elevator. The staircase is explicitly encouraged and promoted using robust signage (Fig. 27.3a). As the elevator opens, directly in front of the patients are the Center name and an electronic monitor, which presents the photographs and credentials of Center leadership and healthcare professionals (HCPs). A donor plaque is mounted next to the monitor.

After a short left, the foyer opens up to a waiting area that has warm surroundings with cool color tones and artwork depicting a serene landscape (Fig. 27.3b, c). The supervisor and patient coordinators staff the front desk, greet each patient, and assist with registration, which can be via a kiosk computer system for those with frequent appointments (e.g., cardiac rehabilitation) (Fig. 27.3d).

A multipurpose room was imagined and developed to provide bandwidth for all the different programs considering space constraints, unforeseen scheduling logistics, and other special needs. Current activities conducted in this room include educational lectures for HCPs, patients, and community members; staff meetings and team huddles; patient encounters with the RD, certified diabetic educator, exercise physiologist, clinical director, or other HCPs; movement and culinary classes; group and individual clinical sessions; and miscellaneous activities. The multipurpose room accommodates up to 15 attendees and was situated in the center of the facility but also strategically in the main hallway so visitors and patients can witness some of the educational activities conducted with an open door, contributing further to the immersive experience (Fig. 27.4a). The multipurpose room has a cork floor to accommodate dance, yoga, exercise, and other movement classes. The front monitor is wired for health system-wide broadcast and live visual and auditory interaction, as well as storing content for enduring educational use for patients and HCPs, through the web or a dedicated

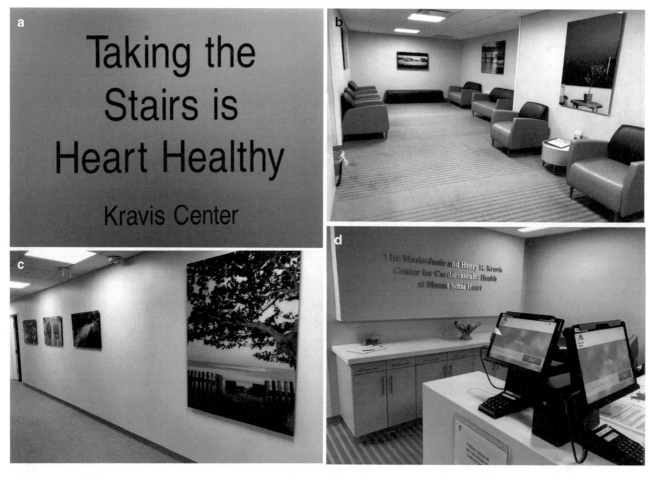

Fig. 27.3 Kravis Center immersive design and culture. Panel (**a**) Signage by stairs; Panel (**b**) waiting room; Panel (**c**) main hallway between gym and exam rooms; Panel (**d**) reception area

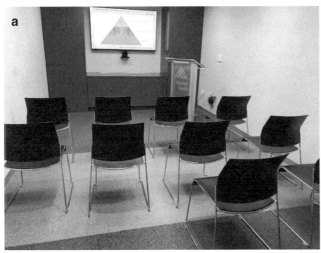
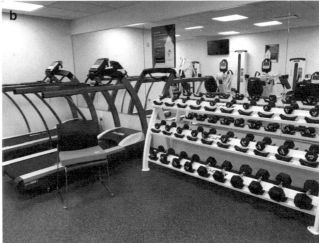
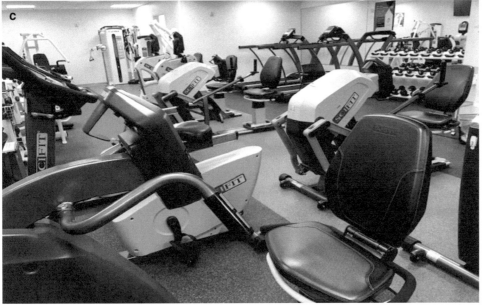

Fig. 27.4 Multipurpose room and gym. Panel (**a**) multipurpose room for conferences, educational and physical activities, and group sessions. Panel (**b**, **c**) Gym room for cardiac rehabilitation, exercise physiolo- gists, medical fitness, strength and aerobic training. Not shown are a body composition device (Health O Meter®) and exam room for intake history and physical

app. Participants who cannot attend lectures in-person can have access to the lecture via the Mount Sinai broadcast system.

Three physician exam rooms, one physician charting room, and a laboratory for specimen handling are clustered at one end of the Center. The multipurpose room and a wom- en's and men's bathroom are located off the main hallway. The men and women's restroom also serves as the locker room for the gym with a shower, changing area, and 15 lock- ers. The gym with telemetry monitoring station and dedi- cated charting room are at the opposite end of the Center. The 1100-square foot gym has the capacity for 16 partici- pants exercising at one session during a Cardiac Rehabilitation or Medical Fitness class (Table 27.3; Fig. 27.4b, c). Other

areas within the gym include an interview room for admis- sion intakes, which doubles as a close observation room for any Cardiac Rehabilitation patient that becomes unstable during exercise, or a consult room used by the RD. There is a balance training space for patients who are at risk for falls. There are also free weights and cardio equipment, positioned so some are facing mirrors, while others face two mounted large screen monitors. Educational videos on cardiovascular risk reduction are played at the start of each class on these monitors. Classes are scheduled either 2 or 3 days a week in morning and afternoons (Fig. 27.5).

Emergency equipment, oxygen, and a glucose meter are readily available. The crash/code cart, Zoll pads for defibril- lation if needed, emergency medications (e.g., nitroglycerin

Table 27.3 Exercise and medical fitness programs in the Center*

Name	Description	Resources Needed
Cardiac Rehab Phase II	A 6–18 week medically supervised program that provides an individualized exercise plan to increase work capacity. Education for heart-healthy living and counseling to reduce stress also provided. Covered by Medicare and most insurance with appropriate diagnosis. Capacity is 16 patients/session	Full gym with telemetry monitoring capacity. Staff: cardiac rehab manager, four certified exercise physiologists, one registered nurse, and a dedicated Cardiac Rehabilitation patient coordinator. ACLS-certified physician readily available for emergencies
Cardiac Rehab Phase III	Maintenance program for Phase II graduates and Medical Fitness patients. Supervised exercise session with exercise physiologist 3 times/week. Blood pressure, weight, blood sugar, perceived rate of exertion followed. Monthly fee self-pay program	One certified exercise physiologist with class enrollment limited to 16 per scheduled timeslot
Cardiac Rehab Phase IV	Ongoing maintenance program of independent exercise and conditioning. Exercise physiologist available on request. Monthly fee self-pay program	One certified exercise physiologist
Medical Fitness	One-on-one tailored exercise plan based on individualized goals and medical diagnosis. Referrals for primary prevention of CVD include overweight/obesity, prediabetes/T2D, prehypertension/HTN, and family history of T2D, among others. Secondary prevention diagnoses include early/asymptomatic CVD, peripheral vascular complications, obesity, T2D, HTN, dysautonomia, osteoporosis and frailty, and cognitive dysfunction. Additional referrals are for primary prevention in specific scenarios and wellness and secondary prevention for other specific debilitations	One certified exercise physiologist

*Abbreviations: ACLS advanced cardiac life support, CVD cardiovascular disease, T2D type 2 diabetes, HTN hypertension

SL), oxygen tank, and glucose meter are checked every morning per hospital quality control standards. If a patient's capillary blood glucose is <100 mg/dl, then the patient is given 15–30 g of carbohydrate. Glucose level is re-measured in 10–15 minutes. If glucose rises to 100 mg/dl or more, exercise can start. If capillary glucose levels are >300 mg/dl, patient will not be permitted to exercise. Discussion is held with the patient to determine why glucose level is elevated, and the referring physician is notified [15]. A folding stretcher is mounted on the wall for transporting patients. A body composition scale using bioelectrical impedance analysis (Health O Meter Scientific, Valhalla Scientific) is located in a private space within the gym. A health risk assessment and body composition profile is generated for every patient seen in the Center at no extra charge. This procedure not only provides valuable body weight, body mass index, % body fat, and calculated estimates of resting energy expenditure but also serves as a motivator that initiates patient interest in health promotion. This scale is calibrated every month per Center protocol.

Start and ending times of exercise sessions are determined by availability of coverage by a cardiologist (faculty or clinical fellow), who has to be readily available for emergencies, which is required by Center for Medicare and Medicaid. Three afternoons a week, the Cardiac Rehabilitation Phase 3 is held. This program is a maintenance program for Phase 2 graduates and Medical Fitness patients. The Medical Fitness program is funded by a self-pay monthly subscription by the patient that provides continued use of the gym for non-telemetry-monitored exercise but with the supervision of an exercise physiologist, with blood pressure and weight checks. Initial Medical Fitness consults are at a price point approximately ½ the average of cost of a private personal trainer in the region. Individuals are evaluated on a case-by-case basis if there are financial challenges.

Human Resources

There is a wide range of personnel involved with the daily operations of the Center (Table 27.4). As the Center was being developed, the selection of leadership, staff, and HCPs was critical to success. It was important that each member of the team, regardless of specific role and responsibility, was completely dedicated to the mission and vision of the Center, namely, to optimize the health of all patients regardless of their state of wellness or illness and to do this with a focus on lifestyle medicine. The goal was to fill the clinical director position with a highly experienced advanced practice provider (nurse practitioner) with additional qualifications as a certified diabetes educator, researcher with preferably a doctorate degree, and administrator. Since the intent by the medical director was to establish a primarily vertical management structure, the new clinical director was then tasked to identify other personnel for vetting, including ongoing searches as needed due to attrition. As a result of this deliberate strategy, a culture of collaboration and consistency in messaging was created. This has proved to be a great asset for Center scalability.

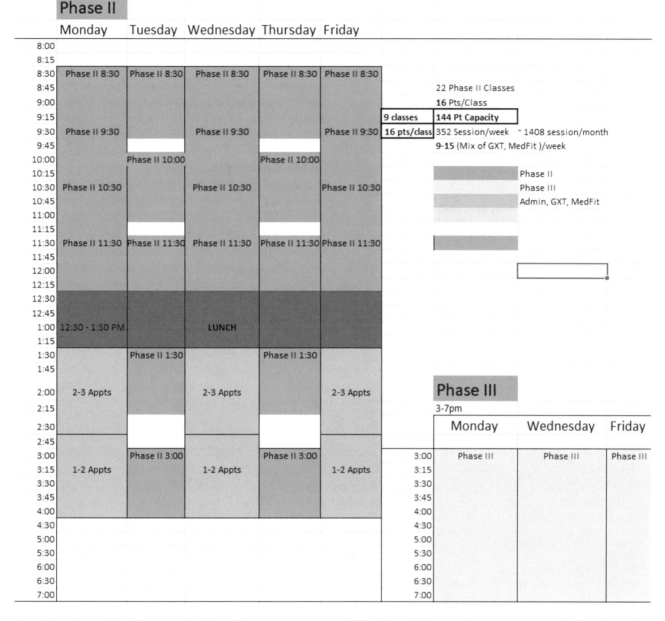

Fig. 27.5 Cardiac Rehabilitation schedule. *Abbreviations*: Appts appointments; Pts/Class patients per class; *GXT* graded exercise testing; Medfit medical fitness consult; Blue Phase II cardiac rehab classes; Red staff lunch break; Green new intake appointments for Phase II, medical fitness consult, or graded exercise testing; Yellow Phase III cardiac rehab

Patient Care and Flow Integration

The Center incorporates a high-touch implementation tactic with expanded roles and responsibilities of human resources. This creates a "safe" place by design (physical and nonphysical) for patients to receive their medical care. This also means that there is no judgment made on whether or not the patient achieves their numerical goals. Rather, the philosophical imperative is attainment, improvement, and optimization of health. In the Center, "health" is defined consistently among all HCP and staff to all patients as a triumvirate of achieving evidence-based clinical and biochemical metrics, low symptom burden, and happiness (Table 27.5). In addition, health messaging is delivered in a positive context ("do this," "you did well," "I will help you," etc.) instead of a negative context ("don't do this," "you didn't do well," "I can't help you," etc.). Regular meetings among HCPs and staff ensure this consistent positive attitude and behavior toward patients, family members, and visitors.

Table 27.4 Human Resources

Description	Personnel
Administrative	1 Medical director 1 Clinical director 1 Office supervisor
Clinical Practice	1 Endocrinologist 3 Preventive cardiologists 1 Internist 1 Advanced practice provider 1 Medical assistant
Cardiac Rehabilitation	1 Medical director 1 Clinical manager 4 Exercise physiologists 1 Registered nurse 1 Cardiac Rehabilitation patient coordinator
Medical Fitness	Shared resources with cardiac rehab Avatar program for exercise instructions
Nutrition	1 Registered dietician
Diabetes Education and Technology	1 Certified diabetes educator
Staff	1 Supervisor 2 Patient care coordinators 1 Medical assistant

Practically, dedicated discussions are held to determine what motivates the patient, specifically using motivational interviewing techniques [16]. Besides expressions of positivity, success is celebrated even in small increments, with accompanying dialogues and discussions. Every patient encounter with a team member provides an opportunity, or human touch, to further patient engagement. A series of human touches defines the patient flow and creates a therapeutic culture in the Center, as elaborated below.

Touch 1. Reception

Patients arrive at the front desk and are greeted by the patient coordinator. Necessary paperwork is completed by the patient with the assistance of the coordinator, with or without use of the kiosk. A brief survey is also completed. The waiting room experience provides an opportunity for patients to relax after the commute to the facility within a large busy metropolitan area. Since the waiting area is separated from the other facility practices in the building, the atmosphere is calm. The color palate of the furnishings, walls, and artwork was specifically created to reflect tranquility. Oversized seating is utilized to accommodate those with an increased body

Table 27.5 What is cardiometabolic health?*

	Guidelines and definitions	Examples

Metrics	ACC/AHA ASCVD 10-year risk calculator
	AHA physical activity guidelines of adults
	AACE type 2 diabetes glucose management goals
	2019 ACC/AHA Guidelines on the Primary Prevention of Cardiovascular Disease
	Healthy eating patterns
		Estimation the 10-year primary risk of atherosclerotic cardiovascular disease among patients without pre-existing CV disease
		150 minutes of moderate-intensity aerobic activity and 2 or more days of muscular-strengthening activity
		Optimal blood pressure 120/80
		LDL < 100
		A1C $\leq 6.5\%$ for most
		BMI 18.5–24.9 kg/m^2 (or ethnicity-adjusted cutoffs)
		Waist circumference:
		  Men ≤ 40 inches
		  Women ≤ 35 inches (or ethnicity-adjusted cutoffs)
		minimum # servings of fresh fruits and vegetables daily = 5–7

Symptoms	DALY – measure of overall disease burden QALY – generic measure of disease burden, including both the quality and the quantity of life lived	DALY – sum of the YLL due to premature mortality in the population and the years lost due to disability (YLD) for people living with the health condition or its consequences: DALY = YLL + YLD QALY – multiply the utility value associated with a given state of health by the years lived in that state. A year of life lived in perfect health is worth 1 QALY (1 year of life ×1 utility value). A year of life lived in a state of less than perfect health is worth less than 1 QALY
Happiness	Definition – state of well-being characterized by emotions ranging from contentment to intense joy. Related to life satisfaction, appreciation of life, and moments of pleasure, but overall it has to do with the positive experience of emotions. Each person has their own way of defining their individual happiness. Optimism – the tendency to think that good things will happen in the future	*Case example:* 60-year-old female seen for management of obesity. Understand the impact of the disease on her well-being and emotional response, and study her psychosocial factors impacting obesity including depression and anxiety Plan intensify lifestyle interventions with focus as well on emotions and addressing depression/anxiety with help of specialists if needed BMI 35–26.4 WC 42 inches to 36 inches Physical activity none to 150 minutes/week Assess the impact of lifestyle intervention on her well-being before and after the interventions. There is usually a positive improvement with weight loss and healthy lifestyle

*Abbreviations: *AHA* American Heart Association, *AACE* American Association of Clinical Endocrinologists, *ACC* American College of Cardiology, *CV* cardiovascular, *LDL* low-density lipoproteins, *A1C* glycated hemoglobin, *BMI* body mass index, *DALY* disability-adjusted life year, *QALY* quality-adjusted life year, *YLL* years of life lost, *YLD* years lost due to disability, *WC* waist circumference

mass index (BMI). Educational content is displayed on the waiting room TV and available with magazines on the side tables. Copies of the monthly educational class schedule are at the front desk along with other Center brochures and announcements.

Touch 2: The Medical Assistant

Patients are greeted again by the medical assistant at the front desk and navigated into the gym to use the body composition scale. This scale is in a private space strategically placed within the gym so that all patients can directly observe exercise sessions in progress as they move to and from this area. This is a critical part of the deliberate immersive experience design of the Center. Patient navigation continues with the medical assistant, who can answer questions about the gym and Center activities, past the multipurpose room where an educational class could be in session, to the examination room. Additional measurements, interviewing, and health risk assessments occur at this point (waist circumference, blood pressure, heart rate, pulse oximeter, and capillary blood glucose).

Touch 3: The Physician

The physician provides a high-impact touch using culturally sensitive and humanistic approaches, focusing on behavior. A "Seven-Plus" lifestyle screening tool is routinely applied at the beginning of the encounter and includes embedded rooming information (e.g., vitals and anthropometrics) and specific questions about modifiable cardiovascular risk factors (adiposity, dysglycemia, dyslipidemia, hypertension, healthy eating [number of servings/day fresh fruits/vegetable, beans/lentils, whole grains, and other healthy foods; consumption of fast- or unhealthy foods], physical activity [aerobic and strength training], and tobacco/alcohol/substance use/abuse) (Table 27.6). This structured tool identifies areas of interest to focus on for improvement and praise during the current encounter. As a result of this conversation, further discussions may involve explanations of mechanisms and even storytelling. This leads to greater patient activation for change, which is a critical cognitive-behavioral step to decrease risks in the chronic care model. The physician then

performs a physical examination and necessary procedures. After completion of the history, physical examination, procedures, and discussion of assessment, the plan is formulated, which may consist of further tests, optimization of the lifestyle medicine approach, and/or judicious pharmacotherapy and procedures. These processes are discussed in plain language with the patient further encouraging engagement and empowerment in the durable care plan.

Touch 4. Medical Assistant

After the physician has left the room, the medical assistant returns to perform any in-office procedures ordered by the physician (e.g., phlebotomy) or necessary coordination of care. Additional questions that may arise are transmitted from the medical assistant to the physician or the nurse practitioner.

Touch 5. Warm Handoff

The physician navigates the patient directly to the nurse practitioner, registered dietitian, or exercise physiologist with verbal introductions and discussion of important points delivered in a private manner. This provides the opportunity for same-day appointments for physician appointments (consult or follow-up), nutrition counseling with the RD, medical fitness consult with the exercise physiologist, and care coordination with the nurse practitioner. The final touch with the nurse practitioner consists of a review of the encounter and care plan. Most importantly, there is a process of repeating the physician recommendations and plan and providing ample time for the patient to ask more questions to maximize understanding. This touch also provides opportunity to verify electronic health record (EHR [Epic]) accuracy and coordinate consults inside and outside the Center, labs, procedures, and other processes (e.g., pre-authorizations, communications with other HCPs, and payment issues). Wearable technologies, such as glucose sensors, insulin pumps, pedometers, and other apps are set up with the patient as needed.

Other Resources

The Mount Sinai Health System has an electronic patient portal that can empower patients and heighten engagement through ease of HCP contact and accessibility to lab results and other clinical information. Many patients are computer illiterate, naïve, or simply averse and are unfamiliar with the portal technology. Extra coaching for the use of the portal is sometimes required and then provided by personnel in the Center. Medical Fitness participants are prescribed a comprehensive exercise program through a Fitness app where they have access to written instruction and a high-quality, high-definition rendered exercise animation to optimize the

Table 27.6 Seven-plus modifiable cardiometabolic risk factors

Standard seven*	Plus**
Adiposity-based chronic disease	Alcohol/substance abuse
Dysglycemia-based chronic disease	Unhealthy behavior
Hypertension	Sleep hygiene problems
Dyslipidemia	Stress level/mood
Tobacco smoking	Poor community engagement
Unhealthy eating pattern	Naïve to wearable technologies
Physical inactivity	Activation for change

*See Refs. [6, 11, 15]
**See Ref. [16]

experience. In fact, leveraging a broad range of technology through education and practical experience is a lifestyle skill that can contribute to better health [17].

Medical nutrition therapy is a dietary intervention that is used to prevent or treat chronic health conditions, particularly diabetes and obesity that are caused or made worse by unhealthy eating habits. The RD provides individual consults and group session and also participates in Cardiac Rehabilitation education classes. Specific medical scenarios amenable to consultation with the RD include diabetes (type 1, type 2, gestational, and atypical), overweight/obesity, food sensitivities (including gluten), malabsorption, malnutrition (especially transitioning off home parenteral nutrition and the use of supplements and/ or meal replacements), wellness to optimize health, and others. Medicare will cover 3 hours of nutrition education for patients with a diagnosis of diabetes, chronic kidney disease, or a kidney transplant (in the last 36 months); otherwise, the service is self-pay. The self-pay price point was set at approximately ½ the average cost of a private along a broad range of socioeconomic factors. 30-minute follow-up, phone, group, and Skype sessions are also available at reduced rates.

The Center has also cultivated a network of off-site referrals to various HCPs. These include a dedicated behaviorist, medical consultants (gastrointestinal, vascular, pulmonary, renal, ophthalmology, etc. throughout the Mount Sinai Health System), diabetes technology resources (e.g., additional certified diabetes educators, insulin pump and glucose sensor vendors), and infusion suites (e.g., for intravenous bisphosphonates).

Medical Education

Academy of Learning

As part of ongoing medical education for HCP and staff members, weekly lectures on lifestyle medicine topics were established. One of the main reasons for this program was to bring everyone's knowledge base to the same minimally required level, especially since this is a relatively new branch of clinical medicine. One of the physicians has the responsibility of creating the curriculum for the upcoming year and then scheduling each weekly lecture topic with expert presenters. Past topics included smoking cessation, cognitive-behavioral therapy for eating and weight disorders, transculturalization of care, lifestyle medicine, lipids, CVD (e.g., coronary heart disease, atrial fibrillation, and heart failure), and digital health strategy.

Daily Lectures for the Cardiac Rehabilitation Program

Multiple educational lectures and small group discussions are offered each noon during the work week for Cardiac Rehabilitation participants and any other patients and their families in the Center. Support is offered on making and sustaining healthy lifestyle changes and coping with anxiety related to illness. Education is done before or after the daytime classes for convenience of the participants. In addition, a monthly Q&A session with a cardiologist and a session with a social worker are available.

Extramural Lectures

Team members provide expert lectures and content on lifestyle intervention in response to requests by local, national, and international organizations. Dissemination of information, experience, and original data not only contribute to advancing the field of lifestyle medicine but also brand recognition for the Center.

Patient Newsletter

A monthly newsletter, the *Healthy Gazette*, is published online, which reaches over 500 past and present Cardiac Rehabilitation participants. A paper version is also available in the waiting room. This newsletter provides evidence-based information on lifestyle interventions, nutrition, and exercise written by Kravis Center staff. Also included are healthy recipes and a monthly calendar of events and classes held at the Kravis Center.

Community Engagement

Lifestyle medicine lectures for the community are provided each Thursday evening free of charge (Table 27.7). These are primarily attended by the Center patients, their families, members of the hospital community, and local community in the Upper East Side of New York. Advertisement for lectures is done through the monthly calendar emailed to all past and present Cardiac Rehabilitation participants, flyers at the front desk in the Center, and other physical materials distributed through the medical building. The classes are also listed in "Broadcast News" which is a weekly online employee update of happenings in hospital and on the "Community Board 8" website calendar. Examples of lectures include nutrition for diabetes, weight loss, yoga, mindfulness, Tai Chi, and even belly dancing. Instructors for these classes are hospital employees that work in different departments with acquired expertise or certification in these areas.

Team members participate in hospital activities held for the community such as "Go Red for Women" and "Stroke Awareness day" by providing an informational table that promotes and provides education on the importance of physical activity and increased awareness of services at the Center.

The Center has also collaborated with local gyms to promote activities and provide information, such as high sodium awareness or healthy eating patterns. An informational table on services provided at the Center has been provided for a "Harlem Hearts" symposium. The Center has also partnered

Table 27.7 Community engagement examples*

New Horizons for Cardiovascular Health at the Mission conference in Harlem. Provided information on services offered at the Center
GO RED AHA at hospital main campus – exhibit table emphasizing importance of exercise and education with the American Heart Association recommendations for weekly exercise
Diabetes Awareness Day at hospital main campus. Exhibit table displaying services at the Center including diabetes and prediabetes classes
Stroke Awareness Day at hospital main campus. Exhibit table displaying services at the Center including cardiovascular risk reduction
Harlem Community Center lecture in Harlem on diabetes
Equinox Gym for blood pressure screening table at health fair
Healthy Lifestyle Screening at Center included stations monitoring of blood pressure and BMI, exercise consult, ASCVD risk and nutrition/diabetes assessment, smoking cessation and second-hand smoking hazards, and final consult with healthcare professional
The M.I.C.A.H. Project HEAL (*Health through Early Awareness and Learning*). Exercise physiologist provided attendees warm-up or stretching exercises at the start of and mid points during the meeting. Lecture on lifestyle intervention
AHA Wall Street Heart Walk and Run. Team "Rhythm Runner"
Lectures open to the community on Thursday evening. Topics on diabetes, prediabetes, nutrition, importance of exercise, mindfulness, and healthy eating pattern
Manhattan Community Board 8 meeting to provide information on services at the Center

Abbreviations: *AHA* American Heart Association, *BMI* body mass index, *ASCVD* atherosclerotic cardiovascular disease, *MICAH* multifaith initiative community and health

with the hospital Ministry which is a faith-based organization active in training programs for leaders and dissemination of health-related information in the local Harlem churches and Community Health Advisors (CHAs). The CHAs use scripture and religious spiritual themes to teach the health message about lifestyle intervention and risk reduction.

Dedicated Apps and Wearable Technologies

The Center has a dedicated App, which was developed with the Sinai AppLab, a collaborative hub within the Icahn School of Medicine at Mount Sinai. The Sinai AppLab builds and evaluates digital health solutions to improve patient outcomes and aid research initiatives. The guiding principles of this App development are improvement in health, reduction of pharmacological use, and contribution to a financially sustainable model through patient engagement and data acquisition. The App is cloud-based and accessible with a smartphone. Other wearables managed in the Center include pedometers/accelerometers, glucose sensors, and insulin pumps.

Successes and Challenges

The success of the Center depends on mission, vision, design, implementation, and adaptation. The Center is focused on lifestyle medicine and cardiometabolic risk mitigation but also incorporates pharmacological interventions adherent with published clinical practice guidelines. Metrics of success for the Center's clinical service line are clinical, economic, and existential in the sense that the sponsoring health system must value the contributions as part of the overall health care mission. Key features that contribute to favorable metrics are having core resources on-site and at the ready; passionate leadership; a multidisciplinary team with shared philosophy, mutual respect, and high level of professionalism; technology and technology education; and mechanisms to audit performance and implement corrections and optimizations.

Successes and challenges are inexorably connected, since it is by addressing and overcoming challenges, which are part of ambitious endeavors, that successes emerge. For the most part, the challenges encountered during the development and operation of the Center were anticipated.

Human Resources

Creating a culture among HCPs and staff was challenging in the early stages of developing the Center as new concepts needed to be introduced and adopted. However, over time, with vigorous education and training, attrition, and introduction of new personnel, the desired culture was realized. A close relationship was developed between Center personnel and upper management (e.g., Human Resources, Labor Relations, and Recruitment) to foster a proactive stance for managing routine and exceptional circumstances. Filling new positions required interaction with the sponsoring health system and provision of a clear demonstration of need, description of services, and economic feasibility regarding a potential employee. The need to maintain adequate coverage of services, especially the Cardiac Rehabilitation program, was also a particular challenge. Shared responsibilities among staff alleviated many of these issues as they arose. For instance, two of the front desk personnel were also medical assistants and could therefore enable a workable rotation for lunches and other breaks, as well as sick- or personal-day absences.

Inefficient Work Processes

Early in the development process, a priority was to increase the patient census for some of the programs based on financial targets. One example was that referrals and utilization of the Cardiac Rehabilitation program was initially low. Fixes were re-allocating human resources to patient callbacks, appointments, and other follow-ups, as well as expediting new referrals in order to shorten the wait list. Mechanisms to accomplish this included integration of an automatic referral system in the EHR; engaging referring programs (e.g., the cardiac catheterization lab, cardiac surgery, and cardiology units), with face-to-face meetings and conferences in specific areas of The Mount Sinai Hospital; and distribution of printed materials (e.g., posters and brochures). Physician and RD encounters were also increased by debugging protocols that resulted in

no-shows (e.g., optimizing directions to the Center, clearer parking instructions, and restructured call center messaging).

Growth

Over the past 2.5 years since inception, the monthly number of patients referred to Cardiac Rehabilitation increased 70%, admissions increased by 18%, exercise sessions increased 47%, and medical fitness consults increased by 60%. This occurred with an overall cardiac rehabilitation attendance rate of 85% (Figs. 27.6a, b and 27.7). The relatively low

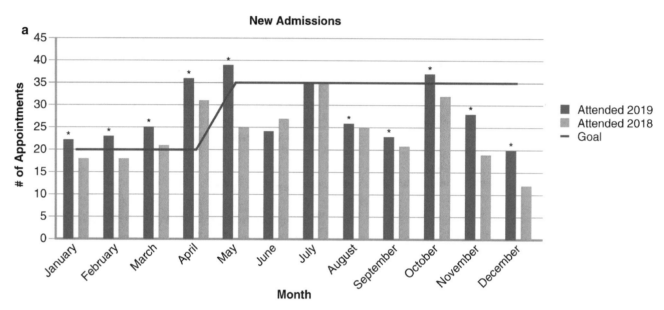

*These months indicate growth from previous year, Increased staffing allowed for increase number of appointments that could be scheduled per month

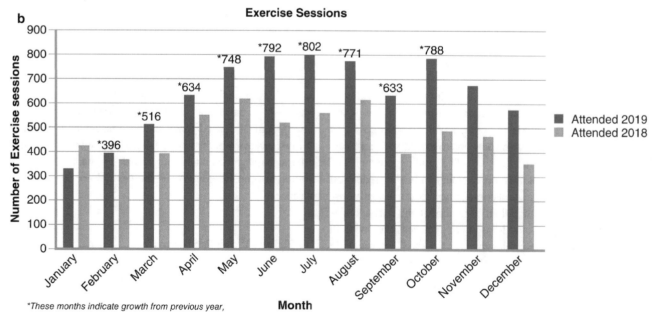

*These months indicate growth from previous year,

Fig. 27.6 Cardiac Rehabilitation Phase II volume. Panel (**a**) admissions to program; Panel (**b**) actual exercise sessions. ∗Indicates growth from 2018 to 2019

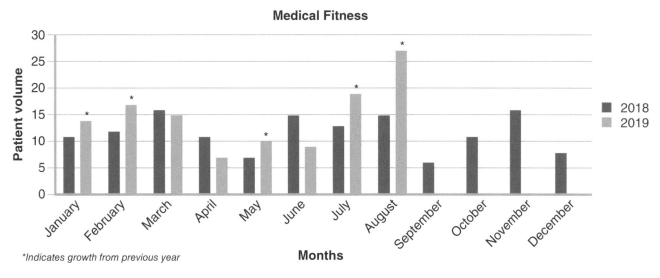

Fig. 27.7 Medical Fitness consults 2018–2019

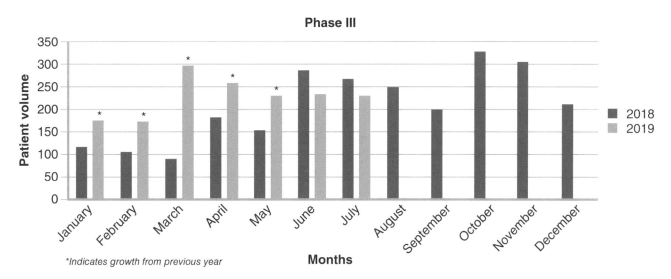

Fig. 27.8 Cardiac Rehabilitation Phase III attendance 2018–2019

growth for Medical Fitness was another distinct challenge but not unexpected since this represented a novel concept with an exclusively private pay model (there is currently no third-party reimbursement for medical fitness as part of health promotion). Alternative economic solutions are currently being explored, such as subscription or bundled fee structures, along with promotion of the Phase III cardiac rehab which is a self-pay program (Fig. 27.8).

With the increase in demand of both Cardiac Rehabilitation and Medical Fitness, there is currently a waiting list of 3+ weeks for an admission appointment. This has sparked interest in scaling up and out these programs within the clinical service line, namely, building out a new larger physical space in another geographic location within the Mount Sinai Health System, increasing staff, and adding additional services (e.g., physical therapy). In addition, one of the requirements for medical coverage for cardiac rehabilitation limits hours

of operation. To address the need for more hours to accommodate the increased number of interested patients, extended hours in the evenings and on weekends are being developed with appropriate staffing. This is yet another challenge but can be solved by hiring a physician off-hours, including moonlighting house staff that are accredited for this work.

Total patient volume for services of endocrinology, cardiology, and internal medicine/infectious disease in the center has grown as a result of improved patient scheduling process, increase in number of faculty, and use of individualized templates for providers appointment (Fig. 27.9).

Reimbursement

At present, the Cardiac Rehabilitation program as outpatient has a relatively low level of reimbursement. Economic sus-

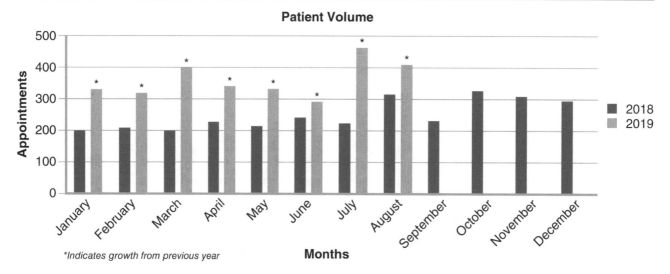

Fig. 27.9 Total patient volume in the Center: Growth includes all services – endocrinology, cardiology, internal medicine/infectious disease, and nutrition (2018–2019)

tainability using this structure has not been possible due to the high fixed overhead costs and mandated compliance with rules and regulations. Even when considered as part of an aggregated figure that includes all Center programs, the adverse economics of cardiac rehabilitation were insurmountable. However, a possible solution is to change to a different location in or near one of the hospitals in the Mount Sinai Health System, which will enable higher reimbursements (i.e., as a designated Article 28 public healthcare facility).

Referral Volume for Nutrition

Referrals for nutrition counseling by the RD have also been targeted for improvement. The goal is 27 sessions/week for economic sustainability for this program. Efforts to increase this have focused on networking with the other faculty practices at the same location, meetings with medical directors of specialty practices, partnering with a local gym to provide services to their customers, advertising and community board flyers, and inclusion in the hospital newsletter. For patients that have expressed their inability to fully pay out-of-pocket for services, discounted rates, shorter sessions, and group sessions are offered.

Community Programs Attendance

Attendance at the evening community programs held in the multipurpose room in the Center has been variable, from 2 to 15 participants per class. Analysis of the issue revealed that there is competition within the local area with multiple community programs offered through churches associations,

community centers, and gyms. The time of evening programs was also a deterrent to our elderly population. Some initiatives that were successful were advertising within the hospital system, using an online link, placing flyers at the front reception desk, and announcing weekly classes at the start of each Cardiac Rehabilitation session. Some classes were changed to during the day and others moved up 30 minutes to 1 hour for the evening classes. A loyal following is developing for each class with return participants; this has resulted in a slow increase in attendance numbers.

Vertical Versus Horizontal Management

The Center requires use of both vertical and horizontal management strategies.

With vertical management, there are clearly defined roles and responsibilities. The medical director and clinical director receive directives from Mount Sinai Heart leadership and transmit decisions and ideas down the chain of command. They rely on managers (in Cardiac Rehabilitation and the office supervisor) to communicate and implement their directives. Managers use organizational rules to understand how much authority they have. To some degree, managers are responsible for all staff below them in the vertical structure. At the bottom levels, managers directly supervise the work of their workers. This is seen in assigning patient care duties and administrative tasks and follow-up on these tasks. Challenges are if middle-level managers do not accurately assign the workload or do not follow-up on tasks and then work is not performed efficiently or at all. For example, when it was discovered that certain metrics (e.g., body composition, waist circumference, and capillary blood glucose) were not in the HER, the medical assistant was interviewed, and root causes for these omissions at the time of rooming were elucidated (e.g., crowding in the private area of the gym, missing tape measures, and shared use of the glucose meter). As a result, corrective actions were instituted. Furthermore, proactive chart reviews were done, and the office supervisor was asked to set up a tracking system where potential shortcomings could be monitored on a periodic basis. The Center's culture is one of continuous improvement and monitoring that leads to shared transparency, initiative, and pride.

In contrast, in horizontal management strategies, a culture of trust needs to occur, in which staff feels respected and where the structural boundaries do not deter the flow of ideas and communication. Staff needs to be accountable to each other, guided to continue to learn, and take action toward a shared performance goal. New ideas need to be encouraged and innovative thoughts rewarded. Small-scale examples of horizontal management have been embedded in a primarily vertically managed Center operation. At the leadership level, the Mount Sinai Heart chief financial officer works with the Mount Sinai Heart director but also provides guidance to the Center's medical and clinical directors. Also, the medical director of the Cardiac Rehabilitation program works closely with the Center's medical and clinical directors. At lower management levels, this type of embedded horizontal management is seen in the weekly Cardiac Rehabilitation strategy meeting for the Center. The Center's clinical director, cardiac rehabilitation manager, and patient coordinator meet to discuss the weekly statistics, the exercise session schedule, patient discharge dates from the program, admission appointments, medical hold patients, and any other problems concerning referrals or admissions into the program. Another example of this type of horizontal management is the team meetings to develop the Center's dedicated App. All team members have input on what information should go into the app and then assist in developing the content and evaluating the final product. In short, the hybrid model of vertical > horizontal management provides necessary accountability, agility, and individuality for optimal performance.

References

1. Benjamin EJ, Muntner P, Alonso A, et al. Heart disease and stroke statistics – 2019 update: a report from the American Heart Association. Circulation. 2019;139:e56–e528.

2. January CT, Wann LS, Alpert JS, et al. 2014 AHA/ACC/HRS guideline for the management of patients with atrial fibrillation: executive summary: a report of the American College of Cardiology/American Heart Association Task Force on practice guidelines and the Heart Rhythm Society. Circulation. 2014;130:2071–104.

3. Hales CM, Fryar CD, Ogden CL. Prevalence of obesity among adults and youth: United States, 2015–2016. NCHS data brief, no 288. Hyattsville: National Center for Health Statistics; 2017.

4. Finkelstein EA, Trogdon JG, Cohen JW, et al. Annual medical spending attributable to obesity: payer-and service-specific estimates. Health Aff (Millwood). 2009;28:w822–31.

5. Mechanick JI, Hurley DL, Garvey WT. Adiposity-based chronic disease as a new diagnostic term: the American Association of Clinical Endocrinologists and American College of Endocrinology position statement. Endocr Pract. 2017;23:372–8.

6. Mechanick JI, Garber AJ, Grunberger G, et al. Dysglycemia-based chronic disease: an American Association of Clinical Endocrinologists position statement. Endocr Pract. 2018;24:995–1011.

7. Arnett DK, Khera A, Blumenthal RS. ACC/AHA guideline on the primary prevention of cardiovascular disease: part 1, lifestyle and behavioral Factors. JAMA Cardiol. 2019;4(10):1043–4. https://doi.org/10.1001/jamacardio.2019.2604.

8. Sperling LS, Mechanick JI, Neeland IJ, et al. The CardioMetabolic Health Alliance: working toward a new care model for the metabolic syndrome. J Am Coll Cardiol. 2015;66:1050–67.

9. Arnett DK, Blumenthal RS, Albert MA, et al. 2019 ACC/AHA guideline on the primary prevention of cardiovascular disease: executive summary: a report of the American College of Cardiology/American Heart Association Task Force on Clinical Practice Guidelines. Circulation. 2019;140:e563–95.

10. Yudkin JS, Juhan-Vague I, Hawe E, et al. Low-grade inflammation may play a role in the etiology of the metabolic syndrome in patients with coronary heart disease: the HIFMECH study. Metabolism. 2004;53:852–7.

11. Mechanick JI, Zhao S, Garvey WT. The adipokine-cardiovascular-lifestyle network: translation to clinical practice. J Am Coll Cardiol. 2016;68:1785–803.

12. Efstathiou SP, Skeva II, Zorbala E, et al. Metabolic syndrome in adolescence: can it be predicted from natal and parental profile? The prediction of metabolic syndrome in adolescence (PREMA) study. Circulation. 2012;125:902–10.

13. Turco JV, Inal-Veith A, Fuster V. Cardiovascular health promotion: an issue that can no longer wait. J Am Coll Cardiol. 2018;72:908–13.

14. Mechanick J, Kushner R, editors. eLifestyle medicine: a manual for clinical practice. New York: Springer; 2016.

15. Williams MA, Roitman JL. American Association of Cardiovascular and Pulmonary Rehabilitation. Guidelines for cardiac rehabilitation and secondary prevention programs. 5th ed. Champaign: Human Kinetics; 2013. p. 227–8.

16. Elwyn G, Dehlendorf C, Epstein RM, et al. Shared decision making and motivational interviewing: achieving patient-centered care across the spectrum of health care problems. Ann Fam Med. 2014;12:270–5.

17. Sorondo B, Allen A, Fathima S, et al. Patient portal as a tool for enhancing patient experience and improving quality of care in primary care practices. EGEMS (Wash DC). 2016;4:1262.

Building a Prostate Cancer Lifestyle Medicine Program

28

Zach Seth Dovey and Ash K. Tewari

Abbreviations

BF	Body fat
BMI	Body mass index
HCP	Healthcare professional
HRQOL	Health-related quality of life
IIEF	International Index of Erectile Function
IPSS	International Prostate Symptom Score
LOS	Length of stay
MBSR	Mindfulness-based stress reduction
MRI	Magnetic resonance imaging
PCa	Prostate cancer
PCP	Primary care physician
PSA	Prostate-specific antigen
RARP	Robotic-assisted radical prostatectomy
TRUS	Targeted and systematic transrectal ultrasound

Rationale for a Lifestyle Medicine Center for Prostate Cancer

Scope of the Problem

The National Cancer Institute figures show there are approximately 1.7 million men with a diagnosis of prostate cancer (PCa) in the United States. Globally, 1.1 million new cases were diagnosed in 2012, with incidence highest in Australasia, North America, and Western and Northern Europe (age standardized rates per 100,000 of 111.6, 97.2, 94.9, and 85, respectively) [1, 2]. In the United States, nearly 30,000 men die each year of the disease, and 230,000 men are newly diagnosed with PCa. Mortality rates do not vary in the same way as incidence and are similar across different continents, although there is ethnic variation. Men of African American descent have a lifetime risk of PCa of 1 in 6, and specific mortality of 1 in 23 [3], whereas by comparison, Caucasians have a lifestyle risk of PCa of 1 in 8, and specific mortality of 1 in 42 [3].

General Principles for Investigation and Treatment

Positive family history and racial background play a role, although in reality only about 9% of patients have hereditary PCa [4], defined as two or more relatives with early-onset disease (under 55 years) or three or more affected relatives of any age [4]. Genome-wide association studies have found 100 PCa susceptibility genes, accounting for nearly 40% familial risk [5, 6], with almost 12% of these genes involved in DNA repair processes [7]. Identification of BRCA1/2 and HOXB13 genes as risk carriers offers the potential for familial screening [8, 9]. Other risk factors are age, with biopsy incidence being less than 5% for men in their 30s, rising to nearly 60% for men in their late 70s [10], as well as environmental factors. Metabolic syndrome [11, 12], diabetes [13], obesity [14], high alcohol intake [15], smoking [16], dairy proteins [17], fried food [18], cadmium [19], high and low vitamin D [20], and vitamin E and selenium [21] have all been studied with reference to possible associations with increased PCa risk. In contrast, both lycopenes [22] and phytoestrogens [23] have been found to be associated with a reduced risk.

As PCa awareness rises in the general male population and the etiology is understood in more detail, lifestyle changes are becoming an increasingly important part of the preventive and management process. Population-based screening for PCa as a means of early diagnosis with reduc-

Z. S. Dovey (✉) · A. K. Tewari
Department of Urology, Icahn School of Medicine at Mount Sinai, New York, NY, USA
e-mail: Zachary.dovey@mountsinai.org

© Springer Nature Switzerland AG 2020
J. I. Mechanick, R. F. Kushner (eds.), *Creating a Lifestyle Medicine Center*, https://doi.org/10.1007/978-3-030-48088-2_28

tion in mortality has been thoroughly investigated but remains one of the most controversial topics in Urology. A recent statement from the US Preventive Services Task Force in 2017 recommended that healthcare professionals (HCPs) explain the pros and cons of prostate specific antigen (PSA) screening to men between the ages of 55 and 69 years, based on evidence of survival benefit [24]. The largest European trial on the use of PSA screening for PCa (European Randomized Study of Screening for Prostate Cancer [ERSPC]) screened over 162,000 patients with mortality reduction at 9 years' follow-up of 21% (29% after adjustment for noncompliance [25]. The number needed to screen and the number needed to treat were 1410 and 48, respectively [25, 26]. Interestingly at 13 years' follow-up, the ERSPC showed the mortality reduction remained the same, but the number needed to screen and treat was falling, now below the number needed to screen for breast cancer trials [25, 26], suggesting a formal public PSA screening program, analogous to breast cancer screening, may be beneficial longer term. Currently, patient referrals involve men over age 40 years with elevated PSAs, who have already undergone opportunistic screening by their primary care physician (PCP) or local urologists. Sometimes, patients will have had abnormal digital rectal exams and occasionally abnormal magnetic resonance imaging (MRI) of the prostate or, alternatively, been investigated and diagnosed with PCa by their local urologists and referred for treatment. The Mount Sinai Program diagnostic process after presenting with an elevated PSA includes a full history, examination, and 4 K test, a multi-parametric MRI of the prostate leading to a targeted and systematic transrectal ultrasound (TRUS) guided prostate biopsy. The 4 K test incorporates not only a PSA but four kallikrein proteins in a blood assay, in combination with the digital rectal exam and biopsy history to produce a percentage score that indicates a more accurate risk of clinically significant PCa [27]. Once the diagnosis has been made, patients are seen in the clinic to discuss treatment options. The mainstay of treatment for early disease (localized cancer) is surgical excision of the prostate gland (radical prostatectomy, either open, laparoscopic, or robotic [RARP]). Other treatment options for localized PCa with curative intent include external beam radiation therapy and interstitial brachytherapy.

Preoperative counseling is an important part of patient management and, by nature, a multidisciplinary process. Patients are strongly encouraged to engage in lifestyle changes that maximize treatment recovery in what has become known as "prehabilitation" [28–30]. This begins as soon as patients make a decision to proceed with surgery and incorporate healthy dietary changes, increased physical activity, specific pelvic floor muscle therapy, and education so they are better prepared when the recovery process begins. Prehabilitation may include consultations with multiple spe-

cialties, including urologists with specific expertise in recovery from RARP, endocrinologists for nutritional support and advice about weight loss, and radiation and medical oncologists for advice about what potential additional treatments may be necessary. Consultations from cardiologists, neurologists, and pulmonologists and other subspecialties are also sought for significant medical problems not directly managed by the PCP. Education is important so that patients are aware of the potential adverse effects of treatment. Whichever treatment is chosen will inevitably impact patients' health-related quality of life (HRQOL), and as a result, patients may select less invasive treatments depending on comparable efficacy. Individual treatments differ in side effect profiles (e.g., sexual dysfunction and urinary symptoms such as urinary incontinence) and their impact on HRQOL. For more advanced disease, management may be multimodal, incorporating many of the above treatments. Medical oncologists will play a crucial role advising about additional hormonal therapy, chemotherapy, and the rapidly emerging field of immunotherapy.

Impact of Lifestyle Medicine Components on Prevention and Treatment

The Mount Sinai Urology Prostate Cancer Lifestyle Program offers integrative and complementary medicine to PCa patients, helping them find holistic treatments across different specialties aimed at maintaining health and wellness. Offering this program under the umbrella of a Urology Department with more traditional subspecialty services (e.g., Uro-Oncology, Endo-Urology, Female and Reconstructive Urology) has occurred in parallel with the emergence of a new subspecialist interest termed "Integrative Urology." This new discipline of Urology incorporates complementary therapies into urological practice and emphasizes the importance of nutrition, acupuncture, herbal and supplementary medicines, and mind-body treatments to maximize the benefits of mainstream urological treatments [31]. The mission of the Program is to care for the person as a whole, using proven and individualized treatment approaches, including holistic therapies focused on the entire person – mind, body, and spirit; educating men about lifestyle changes to prevent disease progression; as well as helping them cope with treatments they are undergoing. The goal of the program is to offer the most efficacious treatments available, build strong patient-HCP relationships, and assist patients in staying healthy and active throughout their treatment journey.

Prostate cancer lends itself to Integrative Urology. With the widespread use of PSA, the majority of patients are diagnosed with localized disease, many of which will be low risk and enter into active surveillance programs. Accordingly, patients establish a long-term relationship with the HCP

[21]. Moreover, active surveillance programs, with regular ongoing visits to the clinic, can create anxieties that an effective Integrative Urology program can address using mind/body-based activities to improve patients' state of mind. Patients with metastatic disease are also living much longer lives, and because of the adverse effects of hormone therapy, as well as the goal of limiting disease progression, they benefit significantly from the advice and support offered by an Integrative Urology program. Taking a broader view, the Program with its long-term relationship provides an opportunity to improve patients' overall health and reduce the risk of other comorbidities. Cardiovascular mortality still remains the leading cause of death for both sexes in this age group, and it is increasingly recognized that "heart healthy" is "prostate healthy" [32]. Avoiding obesity; staying physically fit; paying attention to a healthy diet to reduce the risk of diabetes, hypertension, and lipid abnormalities; and stopping smoking and limiting alcohol intake all maximize heart health [32]. It is now clear that this approach also may reduce PCa risk and potentially aggressive forms of the disease [32].

Establishing a Prostate Cancer Lifestyle Medicine Program

Lifestyle

The Program's lifestyle, consisting of healthy eating and plenty of physical activity, focuses on helping patients with increased adiposity lose weight and better prepare themselves for treatment (a body mass index [BMI] ≥ 40 kg/m^2 is an absolute contraindication to surgery), not only to maximize recovery but also to improve their overall health by decreasing risks for other chronic diseases. Those patients with overweight/obesity are encouraged to achieve weight loss that reduces the BMI to <35 kg/m^2 and are referred to an endocrinologist to help them achieve this goal. The Program also provides stress reduction and relaxation techniques, such as massage, acupressure, acupuncture, and reflexology. Physical activity regimens are guided by current fitness levels and comorbidity status. Pending PCP or, for example, Cardiology clearance, a recommendation is made for moderate-intensity exercise, 3–4 times a week, dividing their exercise time between aerobic and resistance exercise. Patients are encouraged to take advice from a personal trainer and also participate in home-based exercise sessions [28–30].

There is a similar approach for patients in the active surveillance program, optimizing health outcomes with changes in diet, improved physical activity regimes, and mind-body techniques to reduce stress. For patients with advanced disease, there is an emphasis on helping other symptoms that may arise, including fatigue, pain, hot flashes, neuropathy, and digestive symptoms. Overall, it is important not to underestimate the benefits of improved general health for patients after treatment, whether it be surgery or radiotherapy, in order to create long-term wellness aims and provide supportive care for any patient needs that may arise.

Nutrition

Epidemiological research has shown that obesity is linked to poorer outcomes in men with PCa, especially more advanced disease [21]. Systemic inflammation may underlie this process [21, 33], and men with obesity have higher levels of inflammatory cells and cytokines derived from adipose tissue, believed to facilitate disease progression [33]. Moreover, high-fat diets and obesity change the immune landscape of the tumor microenvironment, altering levels of myeloid-derived suppressor macrophages, myeloid-derived suppressor cells, neutrophils, B cells, and complement which may further contribute to disease progression [33]. On the basis of these findings, interventions aimed at reducing obesity to prevent systemic and/or local inflammation have been suggested as viable therapies for PCa [33].

There is a myriad of conflicting and ambiguous advice on eating patterns for patients with PCa. A plant-based diet has traditionally been recommended because of the association of PCa with milk and dairy products, red meat and animal fats, and alcohols and sugar [34, 35]. However, the World Cancer Research Fund and American Institute for Cancer Research suggest the dairy and meat evidence is weak [21, 34, 35]. The addition of fish is also recommended based on the ability of omega-3 fatty acids to reduce inflammation [25]. Specific dietary recommendations include increased consumption of lycopenes (e.g., in tomatoes) [34], cruciferous vegetables [36, 37], soy (for isoflavones that are phytoestrogens), green tea (for polyphenols), and pomegranate (for polyphenols) [21]. Specifically, both lycopenes and green tea polyphenols have activity against PCa lines, both in vitro and in animal models [21]. The role of the integrative urologist is to keep abreast of the evidence for and against these recommendations and provide informed guidance to the patient. From a practical standpoint, this requires regular surveillance of the molecular nutrition literature as it applies to PCa.

Supplements

The current evidence base for dietary supplements for PCa is inconsistent. In the Program, Zyflamend™ (www.newchapter.com/products/zyflamend-whole-body/ [accessed on February 9, 2020]) and Pomi-T™ (www.pomi-t.com [accessed on February 9, 2020]) are used routinely.

Zyflamend™ contains green tea, turmeric, ginger, basil, rosemary, barberry, oregano, Hu zhang, Chinese goldthread, and Baikal skullcap and is routinely used based on demonstrable anti-inflammatory activity [21]. Zyflamend™ has been shown to have activity against human PCa cell lines in culture as well as potentially delaying progression to PCa in patients diagnosed with high-grade prostatic intraepithelial neoplasia with the only significant adverse effect being dyspepsia [21, 38]. Pomi-T™ contains extracts of pomegranate, green tea, turmeric, and broccoli and has been shown to produce a significant PSA response compared to placebo in men on active surveillance and post-local treatment [39]. Sulforaphane from cruciferous vegetables and citrus pectin from citrus fruit peels have shown promising results in the context of biochemical recurrence after local treatment, either delaying the rise or reducing PSA values [40, 41], and so may also have a place in supplemental treatments. The SELECT study showed no benefit from vitamin E or selenium supplementation [22]. The association of vitamin D levels with PCa is complex [21]. High levels of vitamin D may carry an increased risk of developing PCa, but low levels are associated with increased risk of metastasis in those with established disease [42, 43]. On the basis of these data, patients should avoid low levels or over-supplementation with vitamin D_3, aiming to achieve blood levels of 25-hydroxyvitamin D of 40–50 ng/ml [21].

Complementary Therapies

The Mount Sinai Hospital Integrative Urology Program has developed a variety of Western and Eastern complementary therapies that are used in different management approaches. This includes acupuncture and other traditional eastern practices, PCa directed dietary supplement advice, mind-body techniques (e.g., Qigong, meditation, yoga, and Tai chi), physical activity education, and techniques for home-based massage therapy, all of which can be incorporated into an overall lifestyle change.

Mind-Body

Mindfulness-based stress reduction (MBSR) includes a program of yoga, meditation, and relaxation designed to be done at home on a daily basis. Carlson et al. [44] studied the use of MBSR in breast and PCa patients over a year of follow-up. Both groups of patients demonstrated reduced stress and improved quality of life, lowered blood pressure, and decreased cortisol and pro-inflammatory cytokines [44]. Another randomized, controlled, feasibility pilot study used MBSR in PCa patients during active surveillance. With nearly half of patients agreeing to participate, they showed reduced anxiety as well as improved global mental health and anxiety tolerance [45].

Development and Organization of the Center

The Mount Sinai Urology Prostate Cancer Lifestyle Program is based at 625 Madison Avenue, New York, and is a clinical service line that is part of the Mount Sinai Health System. As an academic institution, the clinical service line is competing with other PCa services across New York City. Mount Sinai Urology, led by Dr. Ash Tewari, also has national and international reach, with referrals out of state and across the globe.

The revenue generated by the program is directly based on patient care, including consultations and procedures. Targeted patient cohorts include those at risk, diagnosed preoperative and high-risk patients, patients on hormones, survivorship cohorts, and those on active surveillance. In 2018, Dr. Tewari saw over 1000 new patients, 398 of which underwent prostate biopsy, and 379 were offered robotic prostatectomy, with a parallel active surveillance program of 318 patients. There is information on the Mount Sinai Department of Urology website, but patient referrals mainly come from a network of trusted PCPs and urologists, locally, out of state, and internationally. These patient cohorts are offered diagnostic assessments including BMI; exercise tolerance; inflammatory, metabolic, and endocrinology assessment; and % body fat (BF) assessments, calculated as total mass of fat divided by total body mass, multiplied by 100 [29]. Following their assessment, patients are provided with recommendations for specific interventions highlighted above, including dietary advice, physical activity regimes, anti-inflammatory management, and mind and body management, such as meditation.

The physical setting for the Program is based at the Midtown Offices, with six clinic rooms, four procedure rooms, and various administrative offices. The earliest stage of development requires recruitment of personnel specifically trained in the field of urology and associated services. Key staff in the Lifestyle Medicine Program include a nutritionist, an integrative urology physician, reconstructive urologists for sexual and pelvic floor rehabilitation, cardiologists for cardiovascular health, a mind and body wellness expert, anesthesiologists, endocrinologists for metabolic health, geneticists, uro-oncological surgeons, and radiation and medical oncologists. Supporting staff include medical assistants and physician assistants.

Care pathways are determined based on the patient's health status and clinical stage of the disease. The diagnostic pathway includes laboratory testing for PSA, 4 K test, and MRI of the prostate, leading to a shared decision-making process between clinician and patient, about whether to perform a TRUS prostate biopsy. If a prostate biopsy is performed and demonstrates PCa, treatment pathways are determined by disease stage. Low-risk disease may be managed by active surveillance, the details of follow-up varying from Center to Center, but generally requiring up to four clinic visits per year for examination and PSA testing, one MRI prostate per year, and TRUS prostate biopsy every 2–3 years [46]. Intermediate- and high-risk diseases are managed by either surgery or radiotherapy, with or without hormonal therapy, and advanced disease with hormonal therapy, with or without chemotherapy and immunotherapy. The program is supported by additional diagnostics, such as genomics, and front office administrative services for scheduling and appointments. This includes a multidisciplinary clinic that occurs once a month and takes place in a seminar room at the 625 Madison Avenue facility, where patients have the opportunity for an extended interaction with a panel of experts in the specialties listed above. This affords patients and their families the opportunity to discuss their management options face-to-face with different clinicians in a less formal setting and has contributed significantly to helping patients make the difficult decisions about their treatment.

Public Outreach and Community Services

Public education is an important part of the Mount Sinai Urology Prostate Cancer Lifestyle Program. There are planned public engagement exercises through various channels, such as a recent PSA screening event in Harlem (where public members were offered a PSA test), online education campaigns via the Mount Sinai Urology website, as well as on social media. These activities serve to disseminate information about the program and the importance of a healthy lifestyle and diet for the prevention and management of PCa. Moreover, Dr. Tewari invites all his patients to the annual Prostate Cancer and Uro-Oncology International Symposium that takes place every autumn at The Mount Sinai Hospital. Although this is primarily aimed at clinicians, patients also attend and benefit from many of the speakers' talks and information.

Discussion

Specific Attributes of the Program

The Lifestyle Program has clearly defined goals and targets. These include the reduction of PCa incidence through public education and engagement, efficient diagnosis partnered with early dietary assessment and nutritional advice, reducing inflammation and slowing disease progression, reducing

perioperative and long-term surgical morbidity, and effective radiation and adjuvant treatments. The ultimate aim of these efforts is to minimize morbidity and support the patients' overall health and mental well-being throughout their clinical journey. These outcomes are assessed by a number of ongoing research projects that patients are invited to participate in, as well as by an ongoing patient database.

Lifestyle programs of this type are gaining increasing support with a growing level of scientific substantiation, with research conclusively demonstrating benefit. In fact, one group created a clearly defined protocol incorporating all the aspects of a modern prostate cancer lifestyle program [47]. In this study, 93 men with low- or intermediate-risk PCa were randomly assigned to an experimental or control group. The experimental group followed the "Ornish Protocol," which required a vegan diet (with 10% of calories from fat) supplemented by vitamin C (2 g daily), soy, vitamin E (400 I.U. daily), fish oil (3 g daily), and selenium (200 mcg daily) [47]. Other lifestyle changes included yoga, progressive relaxation, breathing and meditation, walking as exercise 30 minutes × 6 days a week, and a weekly support group to provide advice and support on how to adhere to the protocol [21, 47]. The experimental group showed benefits not seen in the control group, including an average 4% drop in PSA, significantly reduced requirement for treatment intervention, and improved weight status, blood pressure, and cholesterol profile [47]. Interestingly, they also showed reduced expression of genes involved in PCa oncogenesis [48] and, after 5 years' follow-up, showed increased telomerase activity, with a relative increase in telomere length from baseline in the experimental group, compared to a decrease in the control group [49].

Overall, these findings suggest a comprehensive broad-based lifestyle program can produce significant long-term benefits to patients. Moving forward, a process of continual assessment is important to ensure goals are being met, and this benefit to patients is being realized. Fundamental to this is the development of a database, with a database manager, for the purposes of audit and research, and at Mount Sinai Urology, there are currently two Department of Defense-funded trials in active surveillance patients, who have much to gain from comprehensive lifestyle programs. One of these trials is exploring the interplay between the family and patient and the other the role of ethnicity in the decision-making process for treatment, compliance, and other HRQOL factors for patients with low-risk PCa.

Building upon the work of the Ornish programs [47–49], further developing and validating an evidence-based universal lifestyle program incorporating all aspects that have been described above will benefit HCPs and patients alike. Importantly, this will require further research and support from the oncological community [21].

Conclusion

There is still much to learn in the field of men's health and lifestyle in relation to PCa incidence and disease progression, with newly discovered genomic links to obesity, hypertension, and metabolic syndrome. Ethnic disparities in PCa incidence and prognosis are an emerging challenge, and new immunotherapies are coming to the forefront of treatment planning in neoadjuvant, adjuvant, and advanced disease settings. As discussed, underpinning this is the knowledge that a more holistic approach to treatment has genuine benefits in terms of clinical outcomes and avoidance of treatment-related complications. With that in mind, the Mount Sinai Urology Prostate Cancer Lifestyle Program is supported enthusiastically by all the staff involved and will continue to engage in relevant clinical trials, incorporate emerging technologies and diagnostic techniques, and promote effective health interventions.

References

1. Ferlay J, et al. Cancer incidence and mortality worldwide: sources, methods and major patterns in GLOBOCAN 2012. Int J Cancer. 2015;136:E359. https://www.ncbi.nlm.nih.gov/pubmed/25220842.
2. Haas GP, Delongchamps N, Brawley OW, et al. The worldwide epidemiology of prostate cancer: perspectives from autopsy studies. Can J Urol. 2008;15:3866–71.
3. Mottet N, Bellmunt J, Briers E, et al. Members of the EAU – ESTRO – ESUR –SIOG Prostate Cancer Guidelines Panel. EAU – ESTRO – ESUR – SIOG Guidelines on Prostate Cancer. Edn. presented at the EAU Annual Congress Copenhagen. EAU Guidelines Office: Arnhem, The Netherlands. 2018. 978-94-92671-02-8.
4. DeSantis CE, Siegel RL, Sauer AG, et al. Cancer statistics for African Americans, 2016: progress and opportunities in reducing racial disparities. CA Cancer J Clin. 2016;66:290–308.
5. Hemminki K. Familial risk and familial survival in prostate cancer. World J Urol. 2012;30:143–8.
6. Eeles RA, Olama AA, Benlloch S, et al. Identification of 23 new prostate cancer susceptibility loci using the iCOGS custom genotyping array. Nat Genet. 2013;45:385–91.
7. Amin Al Olama A, et al. Multiple novel prostate cancer susceptibility signals identified by fine mapping of known risk loci among Europeans. Hum Mol Genet. 2015;24:5589–602.
8. Pritchard CC, et al. Inherited DNA-repair gene mutations in men with metastatic prostate cancer. N Engl J Med. 2016;375:443–53.
9. Ewing CM, et al. Germline mutations in HOXB13 and prostate-cancer risk. N Engl J Med. 2012;366:141–9.
10. Lynch HT, et al. Screening for familial and hereditary prostate cancer. Int J Cancer. 2016;138:2579–91.
11. Bell KJ, et al. Prevalence of incidental prostate cancer: a systematic review of autopsy studies. Int J Cancer. 2015;137:1749–57.
12. Blanc-Lapierre A, et al. Metabolic syndrome and prostate cancer risk in a population-based case control study in Montreal. Canada BMC Public Health. 2015;15:913.
13. Esposito K, et al. Effect of metabolic syndrome and its components on prostate cancer risk: meta analysis. J Endocrinol Invest. 2013;36:132–9.
14. Preston MA, et al. Metformin use and prostate cancer risk. Eur Urol. 2014;66:1012–20.
15. Vidal AC, et al. Obesity increases the risk for high-grade prostate cancer: results from the REDUCE study. Cancer Epidemiol Biomarkers Prev. 2014;23:2936–42.
16. Zhao J, et al. Is alcohol consumption a risk factor for prostate cancer? A systematic review and meta-analysis. BMC Cancer. 2016;16:845.
17. Islami F, et al. A systematic review and meta-analysis of tobacco use and prostate cancer mortality and incidence in prospective cohort studies. Eur Urol. 2014;66:1054–64.
18. Key TJ. Nutrition, hormones and prostate cancer risk: results from the European prospective investigation into cancer and nutrition. Recent Results Cancer Res. 2014;202:39–46.
19. Lippi G, et al. Fried food and prostate cancer risk: systematic review and meta-analysis. Int J Food Sci Nutr. 2015;66:587–9.
20. Ju-Kun S, et al. Association between Cd exposure and risk of prostate cancer: a PRISMA compliant systematic review and meta-analysis. Medicine (Baltimore). 2016;95:e2708.
21. Abrams DI. An integrative approach to prostate cancer. J Altern Complement Med (New York, NY). 2018;24(9–10):872–80.
22. Lippman SM, et al. Effect of selenium and vitamin E on risk of prostate cancer and other cancers: the selenium and vitamin E cancer prevention trial (SELECT). JAMA. 2009;301:39–51.
23. Chen P, et al. Lycopene and risk of prostate cancer: a systematic review and meta-analysis. Medicine (Baltimore). 2015;94:e1260.
24. Zhang M, et al. Is phytoestrogen intake associated with decreased risk of prostate cancer? A systematic review of epidemiological studies based on 17,546 cases. Andrology. 2016;4:745–56.
25. Schröder FH, Roobol MJ. ERSPC and PLCO prostate cancer screening studies: what are the differences? Eur Urol. 2010;58(1):46–52.
26. Schroder FH, et al. Screening and prostate cancer mortality: results of the European Randomised Study of Screening for Prostate Cancer (ERSPC) at 13 years of follow-up. Lancet. 2014;384:2027–35.
27. Punnen S, et al. Finding the wolf in sheep's clothing: the 4Kscore is a novel blood test that can accurately identify the risk of aggressive prostate cancer. Rev Urol. 2015;17(1):3–13.
28. Au D, et al. Prehabilitation and acute postoperative physical activity in patients undergoing radical prostatectomy: a secondary analysis from an Rct. Sports Med Open. 2019;5(1):1–7.
29. Santa Mina D, et al. Prehabilitation for radical prostatectomy: a multicentre randomized controlled trial. Surg Oncol. 2018;27(2):289–98.
30. West MA, Wischmeyer PE, Grocott MPW. Prehabilitation and nutritional support to improve perioperative outcomes. Curr Anesthesiol Rep. 2017;7(4):340–9.
31. Katz AE. Integrative urology and prevention of prostate cancer. Altern Complement Ther. 2013;19(2):67–70.
32. Moyad MA. Preventing lethal prostate cancer with diet, supplements, and rx: heart healthy continues to be prostate healthy and "first do no harm" part I. Curr Urol Rep. 2018;19(12):1–9.
33. Fujita K, Hayashi T, Matsushita M, Uemura M, Nonomura N. Obesity, inflammation, and prostate cancer. J Clin Med. 2019;8(2). pii: E201.
34. World Cancer Research Fund/American Institute for Cancer Research. Food, nutrition, physical activity and the prevention of cancer: a global perspective. Washington, DC: AICR; 2007.
35. Chan JM, Gann PH, Giovannucci EL. Role of diet in prostate cancer development and progression. J Clin Oncol. 2005;23:8152–60.
36. Gann PH, Deaton RJ, Rueter EE, et al. A phase II randomized trial of lycopene-rich tomato extract among men with high-grade prostatic intraepithelial neoplasia. Nutr Cancer. 2015;67:1104–12.
37. Kristal AR, Lampe JW. Brassica vegetables and prostate cancer risk: a review of the epidemiological evidence. Nutr Cancer. 2002;42:1–9.

38. Capodice JL, Gorroochurn P, Cammack AS, et al. Zyflamend in men with high-grade prostatic intraepithelial neoplasia: results of a phase I clinical trial. J Soc Integr Oncol. 2009;7:43–51.

39. Thomas R, Williams M, Sharma H, et al. A double-blind, placebo-controlled randomised trial evaluating the effect of a polyphenol-rich whole food supplement on PSA progression in men with prostate cancer—the UK NCRN Pomi-T study. Prostate Cancer Prostatic Dis. 2014;17:180–6.

40. Alumkal JJ, Slottke R, Schwartzman J, et al. A phase II study of sulforaphane-rich broccoli sprout extracts in men with recurrent prostate cancer. Invest New Drugs. 2015;33:480–9.

41. Keizman D, et al. Effect of pectasol-C modified citrus pectin (p-Mcp) treatment (Tx) on psa dynamics in non-metastatic biochemically relapsed prostate cancer (Brpc) patients (Pts): results of a prospective phase II study. J Clin Oncol. 2018;36(6_suppl):14.

42. Xu Y, Shao X, Yao Y, et al. Positive association between circulating 25-hydroxyvitamin D levels and prostate cancer risk: new findings from an updated meta-analysis. J Cancer Res Clin Oncol. 2014;140:1465–77.

43. Tretli S, Hernes E, Berg JP, et al. Association between serum 25 (OH) D and death from prostate cancer. Br J Cancer. 2009;100:450–4.

44. Carlson LE, Speca M, Faris P, Patel KD. One year pre– post intervention follow-up of psychological, immune, endocrine and blood pressure outcomes of mindfulness based stress reduction (MBSR) in breast and prostate cancer outpatients. Brain Behav Immun. 2007;21:1038–49.

45. Victorson D, Hankin V, Burns J, et al. Feasibility, acceptability and preliminary psychological benefits of mindfulness meditation training in a sample of men diagnosed with prostate cancer on active surveillance: results from a randomized controlled pilot trial. Psychooncology. 2017;26:1155–63.

46. Klotz L. Active surveillance for low-risk prostate cancer. Curr Urol Rep. 2015;16(4):1–10.

47. Ornish D, Weidner G, Fair WR, et al. Intensive lifestyle changes may affect the progression of prostate cancer. J Urol. 2005;174:1065–70.

48. Ornish D, Magbanua MJ, Weidner G, et al. Changes in prostate gene expression in men undergoing an intensive nutrition and lifestyle intervention. Proc Natl Acad Sci U S A. 2008;105:8369–74.

49. Ornish D, Lin J, Chan JM, et al. Effect of comprehensive lifestyle changes on telomerase activity and telomere length in men with biopsy-proven low-risk prostate cancer: 5-year follow-up of a descriptive pilot study. Lancet Oncol. 2013;14:1112–20.

University of Arizona Andrew Weil Center for Integrative Medicine: Lifestyle Medicine Approaches in an Integrative Primary Care Model

29

Robert L. Crocker

Abbreviations

AWCIM   Andrew Weil Center for Integrative Medicine
EHR   Electronic health record
HCP   Healthcare professional
IMPACT   Integrative Medicine Primary Care Trial
MBSR   Mindfulness-based stress reduction
UAIHC   University of Arizona Integrative Health Center

Introduction

Integrative medicine, as defined by the Andrew Weil Center for Integrative Medicine (AWCIM) at the University of Arizona, is "healing-oriented medicine that takes account of the whole person, including all aspects of lifestyle. It emphasizes the therapeutic relationship between practitioner and patient, is informed by evidence, and makes use of all appropriate therapies" [1]. This definition is further explained by the eight defining principles of integrative medicine set forth by AWCIM (Fig. 29.1). At the heart of an integrative approach to health is a focus on evidence-based, patient-centered care that heavily emphasizes the importance of lifestyle on optimal health. Although AWCIM teaches this in educational programs, many AWCIM graduates struggle with how to apply these principles in clinical practices that are primarily supported by the current US healthcare reimbursement system. The mainstream US healthcare system predominantly addresses illness, not wellness, and incentivizes healthcare professionals (HCPs) to spend less, not more,

R. L. Crocker (✉)
Director, Strategic Clinical Planning and Implementation, Andrew Weil Center for Integrative Medicine, Clinical Assistant Professor of Medicine, College of Medicine, University of Arizona, Tucson, AZ, USA
e-mail: crocker@email.arizona.edu

time with their patients. This system still does not seem to fully grasp the importance of lifestyle choices on the prevalence of chronic illness in the United States and the subsequent burden this places on individuals and the economy.

Development of the University of Arizona Integrative Health Center

In 2011, AWCIM embarked on a course to conceptualize a model for integrative primary care that would incorporate all of the principles of integrative medicine and primary care while being financially viable, sustainable, and replicable. AWCIM envisioned a model that would make integrative primary care accessible to a broad segment of the population. Over a 6-month period, with the help of an outside consultant and a team comprised of AWCIM staff, consumers, and complementary HCPs, a new model for integrative primary care was developed and then conceptually presented to seven focus groups, some of which were comprised of consumers and others of integrative HCPs. Upon finalization of the conceptual model, development of the business plan, and identification of an operating partner, implementation of this model was undertaken. The University of Arizona Integrative Health Center (UAIHC) opened its doors in Phoenix, Arizona, in September 2012.

The UAIHC was an innovative integrative health facility that provided patient-centered, team-based integrative primary care for adults in a free-standing location. UAIHC was staffed by two fellowship-trained physicians and later a fellowship-trained physician assistant or nurse practitioner, a chiropractor, 1–2 acupuncturists, a behavioral health clinician, a nutritionist, a health coach, a holistic nurse, and a certified nurse assistant, in addition to an office manager and a receptionist. One of the physicians served as the medical director and, in addition to providing direct integrative patient care, also facilitated staff training, program development, and support for collaborating employer groups.

© Springer Nature Switzerland AG 2020
J. I. Mechanick, R. F. Kushner (eds.), *Creating a Lifestyle Medicine Center*, https://doi.org/10.1007/978-3-030-48088-2_29

Fig. 29.1 Andrew Weil Center for Integrative Medicine: The Defining Principles of Integrative Medicine. © 2019 The Arizona Board of Regents on behalf of The University of Arizona Andrew Weil Center for Integrative Medicine

- Patient and practitioner are partners in the healing process.
- All factors that influence health, wellness, and disease are taken into consideration, including mind, spirit, and community, as well as the body.
- Appropriate use of both conventional and alternative methods facilitates the body's innate healing response.
- Effective interventions that are natural and less invasive should be used whenever possible.
- Integrative medicine neither rejects conventional medicine nor accepts alternative therapies uncritically.
- Good medicine is based in good science. It is inquiry-driven and open to new paradigms.
- Alongside the concept of treatment, the broader concepts of health promotion and the prevention of illness are paramount.
- Practitioners of integrative medicine should exemplify its principles and commit themselves to self-exploration and self-development.

The University of Arizona Andrew Weil Center for Integrative Medicine website. Accessed 1 Aug 2019. https://integrativemedicine.arizona.edu/about/definition.html

Prior to opening, all UAIHC staff, both clinical and nonclinical, completed AWCIM's online *Introduction to Integrative Medicine* course and participated in a 2-week orientation and training. During this training, the new model was discussed in detail, training on clinic processes and workflows was provided, and each staff member received introductory training in motivational interviewing and mindfulness-based stress reduction (MBSR). Additionally, an in-depth overview of current multidisciplinary literature on the effectiveness of various conventional and complementary medical interventions in the treatment of certain common conditions was provided, including cardiovascular disease, metabolic syndrome, diabetes, and chronic pain. The importance of respect and delivering a high level of customer service was stressed. This training was invaluable in establishing a shared vision and an understanding of the clinic model along with its purpose, philosophy, and processes, as well as serving as a team-building exercise.

Key Elements of the Integrative Primary Care Practice Model

Integrative Medicine Philosophy and Principles

The UAIHC fully embodied the philosophy and principles of integrative medicine and evidence-based primary care. The care delivered was high touch, patient-centered, relationally oriented, and experienced by patients as a true health partnership. The goal was to assist patients in finding their individual path to optimal health while addressing lifestyle risk factors. This was accomplished by the clinical staff spending adequate, high quality time with patients while providing evidence-based interventions, education, and empowerment, without creating dependency on the practitioners or the healthcare system.

Health Partnership Acknowledgement

The clinic model was designed to be a true health partnership, in which each patient was seen as an indivisible whole of mind-body-spirit. The role of the HCP was to support each patient on their personal journey toward optimal health. One of the unique features of the UAIHC was the use of a *Health Partnership Acknowledgement* (Fig. 29.2). Every patient and their physician signed a *Health Partnership Acknowledgement* at the onset of patient participation in the practice, agreeing to be accountable to one another and to do their best so that the patient could succeed in making and sustaining important changes in eight lifestyle areas. The patient would then choose the area or areas of lifestyle on which they wanted to initially focus their efforts. This document was intended to communicate that ultimately the

Welcome to our Center. We recognize that achieving and maintaining optimum health requires a commitment on both our parts—yours and ours. In our meetings together, we will set the stage to help you promote health in your daily life, since most healing is actually self-healing. In multiple areas, your lifestyle choices can significantly affect your health. We are here to walk the path with you and to support and help guide you, but ultimately, it is your path.

As we develop a healing relationship, we will both gain insight into what you need to be healthy. While it is vital to accurately diagnose and treat specific conditions, we also want to focus on you as a whole person. That means paying attention to emotions, thoughts, beliefs, cultural and physical environments, and relationships – all the things that make you who you are. We believe that this approach will keep you healthy, and frequently enable you to use fewer medications or procedures, while providing for a better quality of life. Please join us in committing to your wellness.

These are some of the components of health that we feel are most important. We hope that you share these beliefs, and will endeavor to make them a part of your life:

1. Movement and/or exercise. We favor some form of vigorous movement or exercise most days of the week. We will tailor a regimen to your individual needs, abilities, goals and lifestyle.

2. A healthy diet. For most of you, we hope that you will try to eat ample amounts of fresh fruits and vegetables daily—organic or locally produced food if possible. You will probably want to limit your consumption of processed or "fast" foods. Again, specific recommendations will vary according to your own needs.

3. Sleep. Healthy sleep is essential to help your body heal and stay healthy.

4. A healthy weight. We will agree upon a healthy body weight, and together decide on how best to achieve or maintain that weight.

5. Avoiding harmful habits. Some people have trouble decreasing (or stopping) the use of a substance that may interfere with a healthy lifestyle (excess food, caffeine, tobacco, alcohol, drugs). If this applies to you, we will work together to find a plan to help eliminate unhealthy habits.

6. Healthy relationships. Healthy connections to others, including family, friends, and your community are essential.

7. Managing stress. We believe that the body and mind are intimately related. Stress affects all of us, and we need to pay attention to where and how stress manifests in our own body and explore paths to reduce the harmful effects of stress.

8. Maintaining balance. Finally, establishing a mindful balance in life is extremely important. We all need to allow quality time for ourselves, for others, and for play.

I will do my best to practice these healthy lifestyle habits. I feel I need to start with number/s_____.

_____
Patient Health Partner

As your health care practitioner, I will help you work toward these goals. I will do my best to provide care that is thoughtful and personalized. I will honor your own capacity to heal.

_____
Physician Health Partner

Fig. 29.2 Health Partnership Acknowledgement. © 2019 The Arizona Board of Regents on behalf of The University of Arizona Andrew Weil Center for Integrative Medicine

patient is in charge of, and accountable for, his/her health and was also intended to empower patients to speak up if they did not feel they were getting what they needed from the HCPs. In this model, it was imperative that each patient receive care in a manner that was based not just on their physiological needs but also on their individual goals, beliefs, and values.

Team Care Model

Much of the care in the conventional Western medical system is provided by HCPs acting in an authoritarian manner with individual patients during very brief encounters. This prevailing model is problem oriented – not patient oriented – and patients are often hesitant to ask questions or share certain aspects of their history, in part because of time limitations and in part due to the nature of the relationship. The team care model implemented at UAIHC supported individual patients by first spending time with them to better get to know them personally, not just as a diagnosis code. In addition to understanding their medical history, an assessment was made of their lifestyle and the social, relational, and spiritual aspect of their lives. As a treatment plan was being developed, the patient's goals, beliefs, and values were considered, and various evidence-based treatment options were presented to them, including lifestyle and complementary options. Using a shared decision-making process, a treatment plan would be agreed upon, and then the complementary HCPs supporting the treatment plan would be chosen, thereby forming the individual patient's care team. For instance, the physician might feel acupuncture would be very helpful, but the patient has such a fear of needles that selecting this treatment would not be consistent with a patient-centered approach. Each patient would choose the evidence-supported complementary modalities they wished to pursue and, accordingly, the composition of their care team. The patient's interprofessional team supported them not only by providing their clinical expertise but also delivered their interventions with the goal of helping each patient actively engage in self-care and lifestyle change.

Case presentation meetings involving all HCPs were regularly scheduled to provide an opportunity for review and discussion of complex cases. This provided an opportunity to obtain insights from all of the healing traditions represented by the clinical staff, ultimately benefiting both patients and HCPs.

Health Coach

Health coaches are becoming more prevalent in healthcare delivery systems. Their purpose is to help individuals succeed in making meaningful and sustainable changes in various areas of lifestyle. The coach is not primarily an educator, but a change agent, trained in goal setting, motivational interviewing, and behavioral change theory and techniques. Health and wellness coaches have been noted to be effective in helping individuals achieve lifestyle change in support of the attainment of better clinical outcomes and personal transformation. The health coach at UAIHC also participated in educational program design and delivery and supported the social media activities for the Center.

Groups and Classes

The UAIHC was designed to be a space where patients came not only for services that were "sickness" related but also for activities that promote wellness. Accordingly, space was planned in the clinic for group activities, such as weekly yoga and Tai Chi groups. Additionally, there were classes provided for patients on topics such as nutrition, healthy meal preparation, and food shopping and MBSR. There was also a 6-month optimal weight and lifestyle program designed to provide intensive support to individuals seeking both a healthy weight and lifestyle transformation. Individuals who chose to participate in this program attended regular group sessions, in which there was instruction and discussion regarding all areas of lifestyle, in addition to receiving peer support from the other participants.

Yoga, Tai Chi, and MBSR classes were taught by contracted instructors. The other groups and classes were developed and taught by UAIHC clinical staff. All of these activities were made available to patients as benefits of being enrolled in the practice.

Hybrid Financial Model

The current US health insurance reimbursement methodology has consistently proven inadequate to support the optimal practice of patient-centered medicine; hence, several alternative reimbursement methodologies have emerged. The UAIHC model applied lessons learned from some of these new models to the financing of an innovative model for the delivery of integrative primary care in the current healthcare environment.

In the UAIHC model, insurance reimbursement was accepted for those primary care services covered under patients' health insurance benefit plans. In addition to these services, patients would pay a health partnership fee annually or monthly for participation in the practice. This provided patients access to Complementary and Alternative Medical HCPs and a health coach, as well as to groups and classes typically not covered by third-party payers. Patients would choose between three intensity levels of bundled services based upon their personally anticipated level of usage providing them access to the complementary HCPs, health coach, groups, and classes as they desired. If a patient wished to exceed the number of visits covered in their initially selected service bundle, they could purchase individual visits with the complementary care HCPs or health coaches at a discounted rate, or they could pay the differential between their chosen bundle of services and a larger bundle should more than a few additional services be needed. All patients receiving ongoing primary care services at UAIHC had a membership, and of approximately 1800 members, 80% purchased the *Basic* bundle, 15% purchased the *Core* bundle, and 5% purchased the *Expanded* bundle.

The membership bundle prices at the UAIHC were developed using a proprietary financial modeling tool that included estimated income from third-party payers as well as salary, space, and other expenses. Prior to setting membership fees, feedback from the seven focus groups was used to inform both the model and pricing of the bundles. Revenue from the membership fees roughly equaled that from third-party reimbursement sources. Although supplements were available for purchase at the UAIHC, this was a very small percentage of the revenue, and primarily limited to products not commercially available, such as some traditional Chinese medicine products.

Many patients who came to the UAIHC were already spending money on an ongoing basis for complementary healthcare services that they now could access at UAIHC as a part of their membership in the practice. Some individuals utilized their employer-based health savings accounts or flexible spending accounts to cover a portion of these expenses, as defined by their employer/health plan and Internal Revenue Service rules. This lessened the out-of-pocket expenses for the patients. Additionally, two large employers paid 40–80% of their employees' memberships fees, thereby further reducing barriers for participation at UAIHC. Longer office visits, shorter wait times for appointments, same-day appointments when clinically warranted, and increased access to HCPs via telephone and secure email were also a standard part of the design.

There were a few patients who sought an integrative medicine consult only and did not initially wish to receive ongoing primary care services at the clinic. For these individuals, integrative physician consults were provided, and the physician's time was billed for third-party reimbursement. These integrative consults also included two visits with complementary HCPs, with nutritionist and health coach visits being the most popular consult choices. Individuals were billed on a fee-for-service basis for these two complementary consult visits; if they decided they wanted to receive ongoing care at the Center, the amount paid for the complementary HCP-portion of the consult was applied toward purchase of a practice membership. Approximately 35% of individuals who came for a consult purchased a membership at the end of their integrative consult visit.

Patient Care and Process Flows

Patients in the Center were typically self-referred. Prior to their initial visit, they were sent a secure link to an in-depth intake form, which included questions addressing not only their medical history but also their lifestyle, relationships, social support, and spirituality. This became part of the medical record and would be reviewed by the integrative physician prior to the patient's first visit. First visits were always with the integrative physician. During the first visit, the patient's comprehensive medical and lifestyle histories were reviewed, an exam performed, labs obtained as appropriate, and discussions regarding various treatment options presented. During this first visit, the *Health Partnership Acknowledgement* form (Fig. 29.2) would be discussed and signed by both the patient and physician. Decisions would be made jointly regarding which complementary HCPs the patient desired to include as a part of their treatment team and also about groups or classes in which they might wish to participate. The patient chose their membership level and payment option at the end of the first visit. Follow-up visits would then be scheduled using a scheduling tool that permitted the office administrative staff to view all of the HCPs' schedules for each day in a single view. This allowed for the scheduling of members for return visits with their various HCPs on the same day, avoiding the inconvenience of having to make multiple trips.

Initial physician visits were scheduled for 60–75 minutes and follow-up physician visits typically for 30 minutes. Visits with the complementary HCPs varied by specialization desired, but these visits were usually 60 minutes for new patients and 30–45 minutes for follow-up. On average, physicians would see 2–3 new patients per day and 8–10 follow-up visits per day, for a total of 10–12 visits per day. All HCPs, regardless of their healing tradition, charted in an electronic health record (EHR), thereby providing all the HCPs access to the latest information regarding each patient. The office-based practice had business hours Monday through Friday, from 8 am to 5 pm. One of the physicians was available by phone after hours, but no hospital care was provided.

Physical Setting

The UAIHC was located on the 7th floor of a professional office building in downtown Phoenix, Arizona. This location was chosen because of its proximity to a large employer who promoted the Center to their employees, but also because of its proximity to light rail transportation and dedicated parking. The space was approximately 7000 square feet in size and was created specifically to be a *healing space*. As such, architectural design was undertaken to create a calming space that placed an emphasis on natural light and views of the nearby mountains (Fig. 29.3). Natural materials and colors inspired by the Sonoran Desert were used, and additional amenities included a meditation room and a health information resource center in the lobby (Fig. 29.4). Low-energy lighting was used, and interior finishes with low volatile organic compounds were chosen to ensure an efficient and healthy environment. The design defined a comfortable and meditative environment

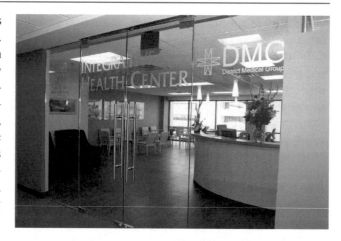

Fig. 29.4 Waiting room for the University of Arizona Integrative Health Center

where nature and good design fostered the well-being of mind, body, and spirit for both members and staff.

The space included a room to host groups and classes. Also provided was a large area where the HCPs could be together between patient visits for charting. This design was chosen to architecturally encourage team building and ready access to the expertise of other HCPs when developing treatment plans for patients with more complex medical conditions.

Health Outcomes Research and Results

One of the challenges in demonstrating health outcomes related to integrative medicine is the lack of coordinated clinical networks designed to collect health outcome data. The integrative primary care clinic provided a unique opportunity to study the model and its outcomes. Subsequently, the Integrative Medicine Primary Care Trial (IMPACT), which was jointly funded by the Adolph Coors Family Foundation and AWCIM, was designed to evaluate the impact of integrative primary care delivered at UAIHC on the health and utilization patterns of patients cared for at this clinic. Research professionals from the Center for Health Outcomes and PharmacoEconomic Research at the University of Arizona College of Pharmacy participated in the study design and analysis.

In this study, integrative primary care was the intervention. Therefore, it was important to establish whether or not the care received by participants was delivered as designed (Fidelity). The development of the *Fidelity* portion of the IMPACT study was described in detail in an article previously published [2]. The *Outcomes* portion of the study was

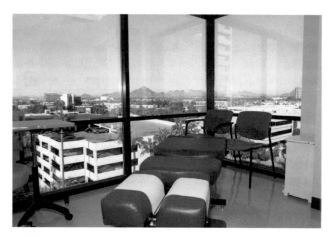

Fig. 29.3 Exam room in the University of Arizona Integrative Health Center

designed to measure specific clinical and cost outcomes of clinic study participants; the full protocol for this portion of the study was described in a separate published article [3].

Among the questions evaluated in the IMPACT study were the following:

1. Did the staff at UAIHC actually deliver patient-centered, integrative primary care as designed? (Fidelity portion of the study)
2. Did patients note meaningful change as a result of care received at UAIHC? (Patient-Reported Outcomes portion of the study)
3. Did employees of participating employer groups who received care at UAIHC have comparable or better cost and/or utilization outcomes when compared to similar employees receiving care as usual? (Cost and Utilization Outcomes – this comparison is underway using a limited employer health claims data set as defined by the Health Insurance Portability and Accountability Act, but analysis is not yet complete.)

After Institutional Review Board approval was obtained, a dedicated study coordinator was hired and worked from a designated space in the clinic designed specifically for this function. Data collection began in 2013, and analysis was begun in 2016. Results from both the Fidelity portion of the study and Patient-Reported Outcomes portion of the study have been very encouraging.

The Fidelity portion of the IMPACT study revealed that study participants felt they received holistic care and established caring relationships with integrative HCPs who promoted self-care and well-being. When asked about their satisfaction with various aspects of their care experience, extremely high percentages (91–99%) of the respondents expressed that they felt their physician explained things clearly, listened carefully, cared as much about the patient's health as the patient did, and spent enough time with them. A summary of the complete findings from the Fidelity portion of the IMPACT study was presented in a poster session at the International Congress on Integrative Medicine and Health (ICIHM) in 2016. Full analysis and discussion of the Fidelity study findings were subsequently published [4].

The Patient-Reported Outcomes revealed statistically significant improvements in the following measures: general, mental, and physical health scores, overall well-being, work productivity with decreased activity impairment, sleep quality, pain, fatigue, and physical activity. A summary of the full Patient-Reported Outcomes findings of the IMPACT study

was also presented in a poster session at the ICIHM in 2016. Full analysis and discussion of the IMPACT Patient-Reported Outcome findings can be found in an article recently published [5].

In summary, based upon responses from UAIHC patients who were study participants, the staff at the UAIHC in Phoenix delivered integrative primary care in the manner described in the model resulting in extremely high levels of satisfaction. The patients also found the care to be impactful on their lifestyle, health, and well-being.

Clinic Closure

The UAIHC and respective clinic experienced many wonderful successes including having a waiting list for new members. More than 1800 patients joined the clinic as members, and IMPACT study data indicates positive results. By state law, the University of Arizona cannot directly operate a clinic but must work with an operating affiliate partner. When the University of Arizona signed a long-term affiliation with a key competitor of the clinic's operating affiliate partner, the affiliate made a strategic decision to cease their involvement with UAIHC, resulting in closure of the clinic. The many successes of the UAIHC were a great source of pride, particularly that it was possible to create a viable model for integrative primary care that could produce meaningful patient outcomes. Plans are underway to open a second clinic under the AWCIM auspices utilizing this same model in Tucson, Arizona, in 2020.

Lessons Learned from the Integrative Medicine Primary Care Model

Much analysis and thought has gone into identifying lessons to be learned from our experience at the UAIHC in Phoenix. The following key lessons learned also identify attributes of the clinic model that contributed to its success:

1. *Start with a clear mission, vision, and plan.*
   The time spent clarifying these elements prior to opening the clinic or even hiring staff proved invaluable. By having a clearly articulated mission and vision for this clinic, AWCIM was able to effectively develop a plan, identify key metrics of success, design a team-based model of care, hire the right staff, and ensure full embodiment of the principles of integrative medicine and primary care.

2. *Choose business partners well.*

In any relationship, it is important to have shared vision, good communication, mutually agreed upon priorities, clearly articulated roles and responsibilities, and a good understanding of accountability and authority. Discussing these areas in depth, early and often, while coming to a shared understanding, strengthens the relationship and promotes success.

3. *Understand the target market.*

It was important to take time to identify the target market for this clinic and ensure that the model being designed would be desired by and meet the needs of individuals in that segment of the market. The AWCIM wanted to offer an integrative primary care model that would be attractive not just to adults of significant financial means but also be accessible to a broader segment of the population. During the design of the integrative primary care model, seven focus groups explored whether or not an integrative, team-based, primary care model would be attractive. The AWCIM also scrutinized various price point options for the memberships to ensure financial accessibility. This was time well spent in identifying a starting point that would appeal to the target audience.

4. *Hire well.*

The UACIM was fortunate to have a large number of qualified applicants for this interdisciplinary team. There were certainly many who had the technical skills to perform their clinical duties, but the final selection of employees was strongly influenced by whether or not applicants had a shared vision, would be able to work interdependently as a part of a team, and would be genuinely patient/member focused. This was a significant factor in being able to deliver integrative, patient-centered, team-based care. Additionally, the AWCIM designed the model to be scalable. This meant that initially some staff positions were part-time, either using employees or contractors. As the practice grew, hours for some staff members were increased, or additional staff members were added to meet the growing demand. This supported the UAIHC in better controlling expenses during growth of the practice while meeting the needs of the members.

5. *Training is important.*

In view of the fact that this was a new integrative primary care model being delivered in a new clinic setting with an interdisciplinary team that had never worked together, the AWCIM prioritized having a detailed and rigorous plan for training and orientation. This started with the requirement that any physicians and advanced practice providers (nurse practitioners or physician assistants) who would work at the clinic be AWCIM Fellowship trained. This provided an assurance that these HCPs would be entering into this new practice with a shared understanding and philosophy of integrative medicine. The 2-week training provided prior to opening the UAIHC was instrumental in creating a shared understanding of the vision, model, philosophy, process flows, and clinical literature while helping to build a cohesive team.

6. *Continue to build and strengthen your team.*

The importance of team building was not only talked about in orientation but embodied in an ongoing manner. In addition to regular staff meetings, staff members were brought together as needed to discuss any challenges and address concerns or celebrate successes, and team building exercises were periodically held. Creating an integrative, patient-centered team culture was key to the clinic's success.

7. *Ensure the technology supports the model.*

UAIHC experienced several technology-related challenges along the way. This began with a temporary EHR solution while awaiting the clinic operating affiliate's conversion to a new EHR. Both the timing of the new EHR implementation and the lack of some needed functionality in the EHR presented challenges for several months. Specifically, the EHR lacked a membership tracking system which proved problematic. Additionally, there were no well-established means to collect recurring payments for membership fees. This created an inconvenience, especially for members who chose the monthly payment option, and in some cases put membership retention at risk. There were also recurring phone system issues that created scheduling difficulties. These technology challenges temporarily slowed clinic processes but did not negatively impact the quality of care being delivered. It is important to have key system functionality to support clinic operations and carefully plan the timing of any system conversion.

8. *Collaborate with employers.*

Many employers are looking for ways to promote wellness, healthy lifestyle, and overall health of their employees. Such efforts have the potential of increasing employee satisfaction while decreasing health claims costs, absenteeism, and lost job productivity, which can result in significant savings for the employer. Data from the IMPACT study demonstrated that the integrative primary care delivered at the UAIHC resulted in improvements in health, well-being, productivity, and satisfaction measures. Collaboration, particularly with one large employer, provided a patient referral source and access to a de-identified limited data set for health service utilization and cost analysis that was part of the IMPACT study. In return, UAIHC clinical staff members regularly presented on various topics of interest to employees at "lunch and learn" sessions, which also generated new patients for UAIHC. This employer collaboration was mutually beneficial and is strongly recommended for consideration as a strategy for growth.

9. *Be patient.*

Building relationships with patients takes time. In a practice model built on longer office visits, there are fewer new and return patients who can be seen in a day. That means it also takes more time to fill the practice and reach financial targets. It is important to plan a long ramp up time to bring and retain new members into the practice. This requires careful management of expense. However, the improved care and patient satisfaction are worth the wait.

10. *Never lose sight that it is always about the patient.*

AWCIM's goal was to establish an effective integrative primary care model that was team-based and truly patient-centered. This was not just about good customer service but also about shared decision-making and considering each individual patient's needs, goals, beliefs, and values. This began at the first visit by establishing shared accountability through use of the *Health Partnership Acknowledgement* (Fig. 29.2) and continued throughout the operation of UAIHC. Time spent initially to establish an integrative patient-centered relationship-based culture was extremely beneficial for patients and staff alike.

Additional Challenges

Certainly, in a system that focuses on disease, not health, and on volume rather than quality, it is not surprising that the prevailing US healthcare system is slow to embrace integrative medicine. This is why it is important to have clearly designed integrative clinical models that are collecting data on meaningful patient metrics in an attempt to make a business case for integrative care and ultimately for the overhaul of the current medical reimbursement system.

As the field of integrative medicine has matured, patient demand for integrative interventions has increased. The body of scientific evidence in support of integrative approaches has also continued to increase. There are now a number of well-recognized robust integrative health and medicine programs providing training to broad array of HCPs, both allopathic and complementary. In 2014, the American Board of Integrative Medicine was established, and a national board certification for integrative physicians was first offered. "Integrative medicine" has become a buzz

word used in marketing various types of practices because of its growing appeal to the general public. However, many of the practices appropriating the term "integrative" in their business are not truly integrative and may be operated by HCPs with no formal training in integrative health and medicine.

The AWCIM frequently receives requests from individuals or organizations that wish to collaborate on clinical initiatives. However, there were struggles internally with how to identify a good clinical partner. Consequently, AWCIM embarked on an effort to establish a set of integrative health and medicine practice standards that could be used to guide decisions regarding clinical alliances, as well as to communicate key elements of integrative practices to various parties. The main goals in creating these integrative medicine practice standards are as follows:

1. To educate interprofessional students in training programs regarding key elements of an integrative practice
2. To aid the AWCIM in determining which sites, institutions, and/or organizations would be suitable for collaboration in comparative health outcomes research
3. To assist the AWCIM in evaluating collaborative opportunities regarding the development of integrative clinics or clinical networks
4. To inform the field and marketplace regarding what to look for in an integrative practice

Ultimately, these standards could be the basis for the development of a set of national standards for integrative health and medicine practices.

To date, the AWCIM has worked with staff and external integrative HCPs in the development of a set of standards that will be tested at various integrative clinic sites. These standards were created and grouped in six domains: embracing defined integrative principles, delivery of patient-centered and relationship-based care, quality and safety, demonstration of integrative medical competencies, education and certification, and ethical business practices. Initial testing and review of these standards is in progress. AWCIM then hopes to promote discussions that would help integrative medicine practices differentiate themselves while assisting potential patients in knowing whether or not a practice is truly integrative.

Summary

When working in a clinical field, such as integrative medicine, in which there is no prevailing model of care, it is important to share thoughts, models, and experiences in an effort to support one another in the creation of practices of safe and effective whole-person care. Integrative medicine, with its emphasis on lifestyle, and the AWCIM, with its mission to educate, heal, and transform, seek to create a new paradigm of whole-person healing that is accessible worldwide.

References

1. AWCIM: The University of Arizona Andrew Weil Center for Integrative Medicine website. What is integrative medicine? https://integrativemedicine.arizona.edu/about/definition.html. Accessed on 20 July 2019.

2. Dodds SE, Herman PM, Sechrest L, et al. When a whole practice model is the intervention: developing fidelity evaluation components using program theory-driven science for an integrative medicine primary care clinic. Evid Based Complement Alternat Med. 2013;2013:652047.

3. Herman PM, Dodds SE, Logue MD, et al. IMPACT— integrative medicine primary care trial: protocol for a comparative effectiveness study of the clinical and cost outcomes of an integrative primary care clinic model. BMC Complement Altern Med. 2014;14:132.

4. Crocker RL, Grizzle AJ, Hurwitz JT, et al. Integrative medicine primary care: assessing the practice model through patients' experiences. BMC Complement Altern Med. 2017;17:490.

5. Crocker RL, Hurwitz JT, Grizzle AJ, et al. Real-world evidence from the Integrative Medicine Primary Care Trial (IMPACT): assessing patient-reported outcomes at baseline and 12-month follow-up. Evid Based Complement Alternat Med. 2019;2019:8595409.

Ramfis Nieto-Martínez, Juan P. González-Rivas, and Jeffrey I. Mechanick

Abbreviations

ACLM	American College of Lifestyle Medicine
CHIP	Complete Health Improvement Program
HCP	Healthcare Professional
IRR	Incident Rate Ratio
LMGA	Lifestyle Medicine Global Alliance
SDOH	Social Determinants of Health

Introduction

Lifestyle medicine has seen enormous growth in recent years, and most clinical practice guidelines now incorporate lifestyle recommendations for the prevention or treatment of chronic diseases [1]. In response to this emerging field of medicine, the

The original version of this chapter was revised and updated. The correction to this chapter can be found at https://doi.org/10.1007/978-3-030-48088-2_32

R. Nieto-Martínez (✉)
LifeDoc Health, Memphis, TN, USA

Harvard TH Chan School of Public Health, Harvard University, Boston, MA, USA

Foundation for Clinical, Public Health, and Epidemiological Research of Venezuela (FISPEVEN), Caracas, Venezuela
e-mail: nietoramfis@hsph.harvard.edu

J. P. González-Rivas
International Clinical Research Center,
St Anne's University Hospital, Brno, Czech Republic

Harvard TH Chan School of Public Health, Harvard University, Boston, MA, USA

Foundation for Clinical, Public Health, and Epidemiological Research of Venezuela (FISPEVEN), Caracas, Venezuela

J. I. Mechanick
The Marie-Josée and Henry R. Kravis Center for Cardiovascular Health at Mount Sinai Heart, and the Division of Endocrinology, Diabetes and Bone Disease, Icahn School of Medicine at Mount Sinai, New York, NY, USA
e-mail: jeffrey.mechanick@mountsinai.org

American College of Lifestyle Medicine (ACLM) [2] and the Institute of Lifestyle Medicine were created in 2004 and 2007, respectively. These organizations and others have promoted medical education, public advocacy, and the formation of Lifestyle Medicine Centers to protocolize evidence-based lifestyle interventions in research and clinical settings, including primary care. In 2015, the Lifestyle Medicine Global Alliance (LMGA) [3] started as an initiative of the ACLM to increase the communication among lifestyle medicine professional organizations in the world, representing different regions (Asia, Europe, Latin America, Africa, South Pacific, and Australasia) and countries (USA, Canada, United Kingdom, Philippines, Korea, Poland, Lithuania, Italy [Mediterranean], Albania, Brazil, Israel, China, India, Iran, Japan, Portugal, and Romanian). A listing of these lifestyle medicine associations and their respective websites is given in Table 30.1.

Experts from ACLM, European, and Australian organizations defined lifestyle medicine as a branch of evidence-based medicine in which comprehensive lifestyle changes (including nutrition, physical activity, stress management, social support, and environmental exposures) are used to prevent, treat, and reverse the progression of chronic diseases by addressing their underlying causes [4]. More simply put, lifestyle medicine is the non-pharmacological and non-procedural management of chronic disease. Different cultural attributes impact chronic diseases globally, primarily through a host of social determinants of health (SDOH). In contrast to biological determinants of health (genetic, epigenetic, physiological, biochemical, and anatomical factors), which also vary among different ethnicities, examples of SDOH include disparities in access to good health care, food preferences and culinary practices, religion, socioeconomic status, food security, education, language, health policies, politics, environmental exposures, pollution, crime and discrimination, demographic transitions, displaced populations, alcohol use, and tobacco use. Additional factors include availability of qualified lifestyle medicine health-care professionals (HCPs), local health-care practices, and traditional/alternative medical practices, all of which require a

Table 30.1 Scientific organizations of lifestyle medicine[a]

Region/country	Name	Activities	Link
Asia	Asian Society of Lifestyle Medicine (ASLM)	1. Certification 2. Conferences 3. Courses	https://aslm.asia/
Australasia	The Australasian Society of Lifestyle Medicine (ASLM)	1. Certification 2. Congresses 3. Webinars 4. Workshops 5. Fellowships	https://www.lifestylemedicine.org.au/
Europe	The European Lifestyle Medicine Organization (ELMO)	1. Congresses 2. Courses	https://eulm.org/
Japan	Japanese Society of Lifestyle Medicine	1. Congress	http://www.lifestylemedicinejapan.org/
Korea	Korean College of Lifestyle Medicine (KCLM)	1. Certification 2. Conferences 3. Workshops	http://lifestylemedicinekorea.org/
Latin America	Latin American Lifestyle Medicine Association (LALMA)	1. Certification 2. Workshops 3. Webinars 4. Congresses	https://www.lalma.co/home
Nigeria	Society of Lifestyle Medicine of Nigeria (SLMN)	1. Conferences 2. Training 3. Certification	https://www.lifestylemedicineng.com/
Mediterranean	Mediterranean Society of Lifestyle Medicine (MSLM)	1. Conferences 2. Training	https://www.mslm.it/
Philippine	Philippine College of Lifestyle Medicine	1. Certification 2. Congresses 3. Training	https://lifestylemedicinephilippines.org/
United Kingdom	British Society of Lifestyle Medicine (BSLM)	1. Certification 2. Conferences 3. Training	https://bslm.org.uk/
United States	American Board of Lifestyle Medicine (ABLM)	1. Certification 2. Training	https://ablm.co/
United States	American College of Lifestyle Medicine (ACLM)	1. Certification 2. Programs 3. Congresses 4. Webinars	https://lifestylemedicine.org/
United States	Lifestyle Medicine Education Collaborative (LMEd)	1. Implementation of lifestyle curriculum in US medical schools	http://lifestylemedicineeducation.org/
Worldwide	Lifestyle Medicine Global Alliance	1. Congresses 2. Courses	https://lifestylemedicineglobal.org/

[a]All websites accessed on March 27, 2020

protocolized approach lifestyle medicine interventions. Accordingly, the process of "transculturalization" can facilitate and expedite the flow of scientific information from a source culture to a target culture; this occurs through organized meetings of credentialed experts from different cultures to adapt information so lifestyle medicine implementation can be optimized [5, 6].

Lifestyle Medicine Centers are a valuable tool, in fact "force multipliers" (entities that increase effects from the same amount of effort), to disseminate scientific information, implement strategies, and produce high-impact clinical results for individuals and populations. These centers are physical areas with structured operations that implement specific lifestyle components in different ethno-cultural settings and have proliferated throughout the world, though with great heterogeneity. Obtaining information from these centers can highlight the transcultural components that must be included for the successful implementation of lifestyle interventions in the chronic disease model.

Search Strategy

The initial computerized search (i.e., PubMed) was designed to detect Lifestyle Medicine Centers worldwide that implemented successful and scientific lifestyle medicine protocols with results published in peer-reviewed journals. However, most centers do not have academic programs with reported clinical outcomes, and therefore, evading detection using this approach. Consequently, the search was revised and expanded to better identify Lifestyle Medicine Centers incorporating evidence-based routine protocols and interventions, with the added consideration of transcultural and implementation aspects.

This more ambitious, revised search approach targeted information published in English up to August 2019. Four sequential methods to detect the Lifestyle Medicine Center with the characteristics mentioned were conducted. First, MEDLINE database included the terms "center," "medical center," "lifestyle medical center," "lifestyle center," "lifestyle," "lifestyle medicine," "institute," "research," "research institute," "lifestyle research," "lifestyle intervention," "outcomes," "transcultural," "implementation," "transculturalization," "culture," "ethnic," "evidence based," "institution," "recommendations," "program," "chronic disease," "chronic diseases," and "protocol." Second, the "[country name]" AND "lifestyle medicine" AND "publications" were searched using Google. When a Lifestyle Medicine Center was detected, its name was then searched in the MEDLINE database, and, additionally, a search in the webpage of the center was performed; both of these searches focused on identifying posted scientific publications. Third, the website of all lifestyle medicine professional organizations registered in the LMGA was reviewed to capture additional leads to pursue using the methods above. Finally, all centers were vetted in terms of peer-reviewed journal publications; these references were reviewed with respect to scientific interventions or protocols for the prevention and treatment of any chronic disease to determine whether the Center should be included in the final listing.

Results

The main challenge in evaluating centers was to delineate process (planning, building, operating, and other aspects of implementing lifestyle intervention programs, including transcultural adaptation) and performance (clinical results, published or unpublished). Moreover, many Lifestyle Medicine Centers offered descriptive information about culturally tailored lifestyle interventions but without any formal publication in peer-reviewed journals of the implementation process or intervention effectiveness. Informative examples are described below.

The Center for Cultural Competence in Health Care in Doha, Qatar

In 2012, Elnashar et al. [7] described the creation of the Center for Cultural Competence in Health Care, at the Weill Cornell Medical College, in Doha, the capital city of Qatar. This country, located in the Arabian Gulf, is considered an "extremely high-density multicultural setting" with people speaking more than 190 languages in Doha. This creates a major challenge for medical students to communicate with patients, usually needing unofficial, untrained, and incidental interpreters (e.g., family members), imposing risks of miscommunications [8]. The medical interpretation program for medical students, consisting of training community members to be fluent in English plus a local common language (e.g., Hindi), was created to tackle this problem. Associated with this training, educational campaigns targeting medical students to increase awareness to use professional medical interpretation were implemented, including sessions and DVDs. Despite implementation of the initiative, the use of these interpreters was very low. Logistic issues (e.g., limited working hours of interpreters), bias in the selection of English patients, unfamiliarity with the interpreters' function, lost time, etc., were some of the comments by students that explained the low adoption rate [7].

The Center for Cultural Competence in Health Care was created to solve these significant cross-cultural challenges. Additionally, the main scope of the center includes training students, residents, and staff to be culturally competent [7]. After a pilot intervention, a content curriculum was developed using the tool for assessing cultural competence training [9] including five domains: (1) cultural competence rationale, context, and definition, (2) key aspects of cultural competence, (3) understanding the impact of stereotyping on medical decision-making, (4) health disparities and factors influencing health, and (5) cross-cultural clinical skills.

From 2012 to 2019, the Center for Cultural Competence in Health Care has trained more than 300 professionals in the Bridging the Gap Medical Interpreters Training, to support the effective communication in the Qatar health-care system. Other programs are also currently implemented [10]. This experience can serve as a model for other international medical centers to develop and implement culturally tailored programs using local resources.

The Complete Health Improvement Program (CHIP) in Australia

The Lifestyle Research Center in Australasia is a multidisciplinary institution relating to lifestyle, health, and well-being [11] and includes diverse health-care programs, among them, the Complete Health Improvement Program (CHIP) [12]. The CHIP is a lifestyle intervention program implemented in several centers in Canada, the United States, and Australasia, aiming to improve lifestyle habits of participants by promoting healthy eating, increasing physical activity and sleep, achieving weight loss, avoiding substance use, reducing stress, and addressing mental and emotional health. This program includes 18 group sessions for 6–12 weeks. During each session of about 1.5 hours in duration, attendees view a prerecorded educational video and then participate in group activities, such as cooking demonstrations, physical exercises, and a discussion [12]. The intervention is centered on self-monitoring, goal setting, and problem-solving strategies. The program has demonstrated effectiveness in different settings, such as improvement in cardiometabolic risk factors and mental health [12].

A feasibility study including 836 participants of the CHIP program in Australasia (731 from 14 centers in New Zealand; 105 from 4 centers in Australia) was evaluated in a single-arm, non-randomized intervention. After 30 days, a significant improvement of cardiometabolic risk factors was observed compared with baseline, body mass index −3.8%, systolic blood pressure −5.6%, diastolic blood pressure −4.6%, total cholesterol −14.7%, low-density lipoprotein cholesterol −17.9%, triglycerides −12.5%, and fasting plasma glucose −5.6% [13]. The transcultural adaptation process of the CHIP from the United States to Australasian population was not described. In the future, further research is required to determine the long-term benefit of this intervention, and more information it is necessary about the implementation process to serve as a model for the creation of future Lifestyle Medicine Centers.

Healthy Lifestyle Centers in Sri Lanka

Sri Lanka is an island country in South Asia, located in the Indian Ocean, with a public health system organized in preventive and curative services, ranking from primary medical care units to divisional hospitals, in addition to secondary and tertiary care institutions. Since 2011, the Ministry of Health established the Healthy Lifestyle Centers in the primary medical care units. The main objective was to reduce the risk of noncommunicable disease by early detection of individuals with risk factors, ages 40–65 years old, and improving access to specialized care [14].

Using a local guideline for management of noncommunicable diseases in primary health care [15], the screening process included determination of unhealthy behaviors and risks, such as smoking, alcohol consumption, unhealthy diet, low physical activity levels, high fasting capillary blood glucose, high blood pressure, and elevated body mass index. Those individuals with a 10-year cardiovascular disease risk ≥30% were referred to specialized medical attention, and those at <30% were recommended to visit the Healthy Lifestyle Center according to their risk [15]. Lifestyle intervention included group health-education sessions using brochures, flip charts, and videos designed and developed specifically for these centers. Staff was also encouraged to counsel high-risk individuals on physical activity [14].

The number of Healthy Lifestyle Centers has grown from 126 in 2011 to 826 in 2016, and coverage of the targeted population has increased from 2.5% in 2011 to 25% during the same period. Challenges included increasing the attendance rate of the target population, especially men, improving the follow-up of the individuals, reducing the drop out, and increasing the capacity of the health-care system, and human resources dedicated to reducing cardiovascular diseases [14]. More details about the effectiveness of these centers to improve the risk profile of the participants and details of the implementation process should be published to understand the effect of this policy. Nonetheless, it is a good example of policy-makers commitment to create, implement, and sustain lifestyle medical centers, especially in low-resource and underserved populations.

The National Diabetes Center in Sri Lanka

The Diabetes Association of Sri Lanka was created in 1984, and the headquarters were established at the National

Diabetes Center in Rajagiriya, the capital city, in 1995 [16]. This center provides education and awareness programs, clinical screening for diabetes complications, laboratory services, care for patients with type 1 diabetes, and research programs [16]. A pragmatic clinical trial was initiated aiming to assess the effectiveness of a trimonthly lifestyle modification program (intensive) versus a less-intensive 12-monthly (control) arm in young individuals with high-risk for cardiometabolic diseases, ranging from 5 to 40 years [17]. Inclusion criteria included a family history of diabetes, elevated body mass index, low physical activity level, and abdominal obesity. Subjects with ≥2 of these elements were invited to participate. In total, 4672 individuals with a mean age of 22.5 years (48% males) were randomly assigned to each group. The intensive group intervention was delivered face-to-face by a locally trained peer educator who provided guidance every 3 months on the importance of a healthy diet, increased physical activity, and managing psychological stress [17]. In those with increased weight, a target of >5% weight loss over 12 months was recommended. Control group participants received lifestyle recommendations annually. The primary composite cardiometabolic endpoint was incident diabetes, prediabetes, hypertension, cardiovascular disease, or renal disease. After a median follow-up of 3 years, the cumulative incidence of the primary composite endpoint was 479 in the intensive group (74/1000 person-years) versus 561 in the control group (96/1000 person-years) and an incident rate ratio (IRR) of 0.89 (95% CI 0.83–0.96, $p = 0.02$) [18]. Noteworthy, the effect on the composite outcome was only significant in the group <18 years old (IRR of 0.83; 95% CI 0.73–0.94, $p = 0.004$), but not in those ≥18 years old (IRR of 0.93; 95% CI 0.86–1.03, $p = 0.11$). This program, implemented at the National Diabetes Center in Sri Lanka, demonstrated significant reduction in the incidence of cardiometabolic risk factors in young individuals with high risk for cardiovascular disease [18]. This program is also an example of successful integration among a scientific medical society, a medical center, and a high-quality research endeavor.

Conclusions and Recommendations

Lifestyle recommendations remain elusive for daily clinical practice, and cultural differences increase the challenge related to prescription and implementation. A broad survey of Lifestyle Medicine Centers around the world has emphasized how evidence-based recommendations can be translated to affect locally adapted interventions. Some of these centers are freestanding or associated with sponsoring institutions, while others are embedded in public health systems Table 30.2 [7, 8, 11, 12, 14, 17–23]. However, the process, tools, and frameworks used to

Table 30.2 International Lifestyle Medicine Centers[a]

Center	Scope	General practice (dimension and resources)					Impact of Interventions
Country/name/website	Target	Chronic disease focus[b]	Structure	Lifestyle component[c]	Resources	Transcultural factors and implementation	Results
Panel A. Lifestyle Medicine Centers (freestanding or associated with sponsoring institutions)							
Qatar/Center for Cultural Competence in Health Care. Weill Cornell Medicine Qatar/https://qatar-weill.cornell.edu/institute-for-population-health/center-for-cultural-competence-in-health-care	Educational center to promote culturally and linguistically appropriate health-care services in Qatar, to achieve equity and eliminate healthcare disparities	Nonspecific	Institute for population health lectures, group discussions, exercises, and videos Education	Nonspecific	Weill Cornell Medicine – Qatar professors and researchers	Bedouins, Hadar, and African origin. Cultural competence curriculum	A culturally competent training program Students and physicians trained [7, 8]
Australia/Lifestyle Research Center at Avondale College of Higher Education/http://www.avondale.edu.au/Departments/Research/LRC-Report-2018.pdf	Multidisciplinary research center to promote healthy lifestyle, well-being, and research Three targets: 1. complete health Improvement Program (CHIP) 2. Health care -associated infections 3. holistic health and well-being	CM (CVD, OWOB, DM, HTN, CHOL)	N/A	N, PA, WB, SLP, SR, T, A	Researchers, physicians, nurses, and volunteers	The theory of planned behavior The health belief model The social cognitive theory The transtheoretical model educative sessions focused on the improvement of lifestyle habits	Significative improvement of cardiometabolic risk factors [11, 12]
Australia/Lifestyle Medicine Centre/https://www.lifestylemedcentre.com.au/	Interdisciplinary approach with medical doctors and coaches focused on weight loss and healthy lifestyle habits The I Can Change Me Program	CM (CVD, OWOB, DM, HTN, CHOL) DP (ANX, DEPR)	Medical assistance	B, N, PA, SR	General practitioners, registered nurse, psychologists, physiotherapists, exercise physiologist, coaches, mentors, and occupational therapists	The program is implemented in 10 modules for 12 months	N/A
Sri Lanka/National Diabetes Centre Sri Lanka/ http://www.diabetessrilanka.org/index.php	The center provides screening, medical attention, and laboratory services to the population, and to implement high-quality research for the urban population	CM (CVD, OWOB, DM, HTN, CHOL)	Medical assistance	N, PA	Laboratory services, screening packages, a wellness program, and insulin bank. General and specialist physicians, nurses, researchers, and laboratory personnel	South Asians peer educator provided lifestyle recommendations	A pragmatic lifestyle modification program reduced cardiometabolic disease and dysglycemia risk factors in a young healthy population [14, 17, 18]

(continued)

Table 30.2 (continued)

Center	Scope		General practice (dimension and resources)					Impact of Interventions
Country/name/website	Target	Chronic disease focus[b]	Structure	Lifestyle component[c]	Resources	Transcultural factors and implementation		Results
Canada/Alberta Center for Active Living/https://www.centre4activeliving.ca/	Obesity and mobility issues Facilitators that help to overcome barriers that prevent or limit people of being physically active supporting and/or encouraging an active lifestyle	CM (OWOB)	Creation of networks with community, government, practitioners, and researchers Implementation of strategies on diffusion of information	PA	Human: front-line HCPs, social workers, and recreation staff	Ecological validity model Groups: people from rural areas, aboriginal, newcomers to Canada, and older adults		The most common reason for limited physical activity was a "lack of time." Reasons varied among and within each group [19]
United Kingdom/Lifestyle Medicine Center/https://www.lifestylemedicinecentre.co.uk/index.php	Interdisciplinary approach on lifestyle counseling	CM (CVD, OWOB, DM, HTN, CHOL)	Face-to-face group interventions	B, N, PA, SLP, SR, T	Physical activity specialist, physiotherapist, nutritionist, and therapist	N/A		N/A
United Kingdom/One Wellness Mowbray Square Medical Center/http://www.onewellnessharrogate.co.uk/	General practitioner services and lifestyle programs	CM (CVD, OWOB, DM, HTN, CHOL) DP (ANX, DEPR)	Face-t- face individual interventions	B, N, PA, SLP, SR	General practitioners, and coaches	N/A		N/A
Singapore/PALM Preventive and Lifestyle Medicine/https://www.palmcentre.sg/	Specialized center on implementation of lifestyle programs to prevent and treat chronic conditions	CM (CVD, OWOB, DM, HTN, CHOL)	Face-to-face individual interventions	N, PA	Specialist, nutritionist, and coaches	Programs related to screening, prevention, and/or treatment of chronic diseases		N/A
Nigeria/Brookfield Centre for Lifestyle Medicine/https://www.brookfieldhealth.org	Multidisciplinary health-care center	CM (CVD, OWOB, DM, HTN, CHOL) DP (ARTH, OSTEO, ALZ, DEM, DEPR) C	Education Medical assistance	A, B, N, PA, SLP, SR, T, WB	Specialist, general practitioners, and researchers	Health promotion at schools. Certification of lifestyle medicine specialist		N/A

Country/Center	Description	Category	Intervention	Disciplines	Staff	Population	Outcomes
Ghana/Sweden Ghana Cancer Centre/https://www.sgmcancercentre.com/	Multidisciplinary center on cancer diagnosis, prevention, and treatment	C	Face-to-face individual intervention with nutritionists	N	Specialist, general practitioners, researchers, and nutritionist	N/A	N/A

Panel B. Lifestyle Medicine Centers (embedded in the public health system)

Country/Center	Description	Category	Intervention	Disciplines	Staff	Population	Outcomes
Sri Lanka/Healthy Life Centers/http://healthdept.wp.gov.lk/web/?page_id=420	Primary health care centers provide culturally adapted standardized lifestyle recommendations	CM (CVD, OWOB, DM, HTN, CHOL)	826 centers were working in 2016	A, B, N, PA, SLP, SR, T	Each center is staffed with one medical officer and one health assistant and/or a dispenser	Proactive identification of risk factors. Stratification by their 10 years cardiovascular risk score. Lifestyle intervention includes group health-education sessions	Ongoing [14, 17, 18]
Rwanda/Tertiary center in Kigali/	Suboptimal diabetes care. Education in standard care	CM (DM)	Process not described	B, N, PA, T	University hospital facilitators (5 physicians, 4 nurses, 3 nutritionists, and 3 psychologists). Receives three sessions of training	Africans	RCT: 251 adults with diabetes. Standard care vs. standard care plus monthly lifestyle group counseling and education sessions. Goal: improve A1C levels. After 12 months, A1C level was 1.18% lower in the intervention group than control group [20]
Canada/Primary care centers/Rural area	Lifestyle intervention in clinical practice is difficult to implement	Nonspecific	Caloric and dietary fat restriction, weight goal, and increased physical activity. Provided by local physicians	N, PA	Process not described. Retrospective analysis of electronical medical records	Whites	372 adults with metabolic syndrome and type 2 diabetes. Metabolic syndrome components improved in participants of two rural centers [21]

(continued)

Table 30.2 (continued)

Center	Scope		General practice (dimension and resources)					Impact of Interventions
Country/name/website	Target	Chronic disease focus[b]	Structure	Lifestyle component[c]	Resources	Transcultural factors and implementation		Results
Iran/Primary care centers/	A structured lifestyle intervention program to reduce blood pressure and cardiometabolic risk factors	Nonspecific	Four sessions weekly Theme +20 minute-guided relaxation DASH diet for Iranians Physical activity according to AHA Stress management Breathing awareness Meditation and progressive muscle relaxation Standard care: no defined program	N, PA, SR	Provided by nurses	Iranian women		RCT: women with hypertension $N = 161$ women aged 35–65 years After 6 months, compared with standard care, a significant reduction in blood pressure, weight, physical activity, and salt intake was observed [22]
Iran/Urban government public health centers	N/A	CM (HTN)	Iranian women	N, PA	Six public health-care centers in Isfahan Provided by a psychologist, nutritionist, and sports coach	Six sessions weekly: group sessions of 2 to 2.5 hours Content: SMART goal setting and self-care Dietary recommendation using DASH diet, physical activity Standard care: no defined program		RCT: women with overweight and hypertension $N = 146$ women aged 30–65 years After 6 months, compared with standard care, self-efficacy, physical activity, and blood pressure improved Education and self-efficacy programs improve quality of control in hypertensive women in Iran [23]

[a]All websites accessed on March 27, 2020. Abbreviations not defined below: A1C, Hemoglobin A1c; AHA, American Heart Association; DASH, Dietary Approaches to Stop Hypertension; HCP, Healthcare Professional; N/A, Not Available; RCT, Randomized Controlled Trial; SMART, Specific, Measurable, Achievable, Relevant, Time-bound

[b]Chronic diseases codes

CM (Group 1; Cardiometabolic diseases) - Cardiovascular disease [CVD], Overweight/obesity [OWOB], Diabetes Mellitus [DM], Hypertension [HTN], Hypercholesterolemia [CHOL];
DP (Group 2; Degenerative/Psychiatric) - Alzheimer [AD]; Anxiety [ANX]; Arthritis [ARTH]; Dementia [DEM]; Depression [DEPR]; Osteoporosis [OSTEO];
CA (Group 3; Cancer);
KP (Group 4; Kidney/Pulmonary) - Chronic Kidney disease [CKD], Asthma [ASTH], Chronic Obstructive Pulmonary Disease [COPD];
ID (Group 5; Infectious Disease)

[c]Lifestyle components: Alcohol Moderation (A); Behavior (B); Nutrition (N); Physical Activity (PA); Sleep Hygiene (SLP); Stress Reduction (SR); Tobacco Use (T); Well-Being (WB)

implement these lifestyle interventions in different cultures and settings have been very rarely described in centers outside the United States. Current centers need to publish their protocols, experiences, and clinical trial results to promulgate this information. The current underrepresentation of this information in the medical literature is a major knowledge gap that needs to be closed in short order to optimize the implementation of Lifestyle Medicine Centers and nurture a culture of preventive medicine with a global footprint.

Disclosures Received honoraria from Abbott Nutrition for lectures and program development.

References

1. Rippe JM. Lifestyle medicine: the health promoting power of daily habits and practices. Am J Lifestyle Med. 2018;12:499–512.
2. American College of Lifestyle Medicine (ACLM). https://www.lifestylemedicine.org/. Accessed on 29 Aug 2019.
3. Lifestyle Medicine Global Alliance (LMGA). https://lifestylemedicineglobal.org/. Accessed on 28 Aug 2019.
4. Sagner M, Katz D, Egger G, et al. Lifestyle medicine potential for reversing a world of chronic disease epidemics: from cell to community. Int J Clin Pract. 2014;68:1289–92.
5. Hamdy O, Mechanick JI. Transcultural applications to lifestyle medicine. In: Mechanick JI, Kushner RF, editors. Lifestyle medicine. A manual for clinical practice. New York, NY: Springer; 2016. p. 183–90.
6. Nieto-Martinez R, Gonzalez-Rivas JP, Florez H, et al. Transcultural endocrinology: adapting Type-2 diabetes guidelines on a global scale. Endocrinol Metab Clin N Am. 2016;45:967–1009.
7. Elnashar M, Abdelrahim H, Fetters MD. Cultural competence springs up in the desert: the story of the center for cultural competence in health care at Weill Cornell Medical College in Qatar. Academic Med. 2012;87:759–66.
8. Abdelrahim H, Elnashar M, Khidir A, et al. Patient perspectives on language discordance during healthcare visits: findings from the extremely high-density multicultural State of Qatar. J Health Communic. 2017;22:355–63.
9. Association of American Medical Colleges (AAMC). Tool for Assessing Cultural Competence Training (TACCT). https://www.aamc.org/initiatives/tacct. Accessed on 10 Aug 2019.
10. Center for Cultural Competence in Health Care. Weil-Cornell Medicine Qatar. https://qatar-weill.cornell.edu/institute-for-population-health/center-for-cultural-competence-in-health-care. Accessed on 10 Aug 2019.
11. Mitchell BG. Lifestyle Research Centre Annual Report 2017. Avondale Cooranbong: College of Higher Education, 2018. http://www.avondale.edu.au/Departments/Research/LRC-Report-2018.pdf. Accessed on 25 Aug 2019.
12. Morton D, Rankin P, Kent L, et al. The Complete Health Improvement Program (CHIP): history, evaluation, and outcomes. Am J Lifestyle Med. 2014;10:64–73.
13. Morton DP, Rankin P, Morey P, et al. The effectiveness of the Complete Health Improvement Program (CHIP) in Australasia for reducing selected chronic disease risk factors: a feasibility study. N Z Med J. 2013;126:43–54.
14. Mallawaarachchi DSV, Wickremasinghe SC, Somatunga LC, et al. Healthy Lifestyle Centres: a service for screening noncommunicable diseases through primary health-care institutions in Sri Lanka. WHO South-East Asia J Public Health. 2016;5:89–95.
15. Guideline for management of NCDs in primary health care (total risk assessment approach). Colombo: Ministry of Health; 2012. https://extranet.who.int/ncdccs/Data/LKA_D1_NCD%20Management%20Protocol.pdf. Accessed on 27 July 2019.
16. Diabetes Association of Sri Lanka, National Diabetes Center, Rajagiriya, Sri Lanka. http://www.diabetessrilanka.org/index.php. Accessed on 10 Aug 2019.
17. Wijesuriya M, Gulliford M, Vasantharajah L, et al. DIABRISK-SL prevention of cardio-metabolic disease with life style modification in young urban Sri Lankan's–study protocol for a randomized controlled trial. Trials. 2011;12:209.
18. Wijesuriya M, Fountoulakis N, Guess N, et al. A pragmatic lifestyle modification programme reduces the incidence of predictors of cardio-metabolic disease and dysglycaemia in a young healthy urban South Asian population: a randomised controlled trial. BMC Med. 2017;15:146.
19. Loitz C, Khalema E, Spencer-Cavaliere N. Using an ecological approach to understanding the barriers and facilitators to physical activity promotion among seniors in rural and urban contexts. Poster presentation at The 15th International Interdisciplinary Conference Qualitative Health Research. October 4-6, 2009, Vancouver, Canada. Int J Qual Methods. 2009;8:36.
20. Amendezo E, Walker Timothy D, Karamuka V, et al. Effects of a lifestyle education program on glycemic control among patients with diabetes at Kigali University Hospital, Rwanda: a randomized controlled trial. Diabetes Res Clin Pract. 2017;126:129–37.
21. Mark S, Du Toit S, Noakes TD, et al. A successful lifestyle intervention model replicated in diverse clinical settings. South Afr Med J. 2016;106:763–6.
22. Hasandokht T, Farajzadegan Z, Siadat ZD, et al. Lifestyle interventions for hypertension treatment among Iranian women in primary health-care settings: results of a randomized controlled trial. J Res Med Sci. 2015;20:54–61.
23. Daniali SS, Eslami AA, Maracy MR, et al. The impact of educational intervention on self-care behaviors in overweight hypertensive women: a randomized control trial. ARYA Atheroscler. 2017;13:20–8.

Synthesis: Deriving a Core Set of Recommendations for Planning, Building, and Operating a Lifestyle Medicine Center

Jeffrey I. Mechanick and Robert F. Kushner

Introduction

Our first book on lifestyle medicine, *Lifestyle Medicine: A Manual for Clinical Practice*, focused on the scientific grounding of lifestyle medicine and using evidence to promote wider acceptance of this new branch of medicine. The purpose of this second book on lifestyle medicine, *Creating a Lifestyle Medicine Center: From Concept to Clinical Practice*, is to provide the reader with the necessary information and intellectual tools for effective and sustainable translation into action. This takes the form of a formal Lifestyle Medicine Center, predicated on the growing and validated need to prevent chronic disease risks and progression in order to optimize individual and population health.

Various drivers of chronic disease are listed in Table 31.1 along with corresponding roles for lifestyle medicine. Primary drivers are genetics, environment, and behavior, all interacting to initiate the disease process and determine a specific phenotypic expression. Secondary drivers relate to a more specific, downstream disease process that impels disease progression on a chronic basis. Although pharmacotherapy and procedures (surgical or nonsurgical) can mitigate this progression, it is argued and generally accepted that lifestyle medicine (the nonpharmacological, nonprocedural management of chronic disease) confers sufficient mitigation in many cases but with far less potential for adverse effects or harm.

This current book is oriented to being a "how-to" guide, which now culminates in a systematic chapter review, analysis for recurring themes and emergent con-

cepts, and then synthesis into a set of core recommendations. This exercise has been performed elsewhere for diabetes care among different countries, ethnicities, and cultures [1].

Methods

There are several discrete and reproducible steps to this thought-provoking process, performed by the co-editors (JM, RK) (Fig. 31.1). In the first step, all chapters were reviewed, key messages summarized as bullet points, and an overall implication derived. Many of the chapters were didactic in nature to build a framework for action, particularly with a socioeconomic context for healthcare. Others were more concrete in terms of itemized, defined actions in a more pragmatic context. Additional chapters provided examples to illustrate real-world challenges and obstacles to improve the potential for adaptation and optimization. The resulting set of implications were therefore valuable, but they needed to be understood based on needs.

In the second step, *a priori* classifiers were identified based on needs and actions to create a Lifestyle Medicine Center. Needs are represented as three types of "gaps" and take the form of:

1. *Research gaps*: correspond to research questions without evidentiary answers and where commentary moves ahead of evidence for educational purposes [2]
2. *Knowledge gaps*: correspond to a non-uniform distribution of information (scientific and experiential evidence) in a population, resulting from, e.g., differences in knowledge transmission or accessibility by healthcare professionals or poor health literacy by the general public and resulting in, e.g., poor health policy [3]
3. *Practice gaps*: correspond to differences between knowledge/theory and experience/practice, due to complexity and educational shortfalls in the real world [4]

J. I. Mechanick (✉)
The Marie-Josée and Henry R. Kravis Center for Cardiovascular Health at Mount Sinai Heart, and the Division of Endocrinology, Diabetes and Bone Disease, Icahn School of Medicine at Mount Sinai, New York, NY, USA
e-mail: jeffrey.mechanick@mountsinai.org

R. F. Kushner
Departments of Medicine and Medical Education, Northwestern University, Chicago, IL, USA

© Springer Nature Switzerland AG 2020
J. I. Mechanick, R. F. Kushner (eds.), *Creating a Lifestyle Medicine Center*, https://doi.org/10.1007/978-3-030-48088-2_31

355

Table 31.1 Drivers of chronic disease and role of lifestyle medicine[a]

Classification	Drivers of chronic disease	Role of lifestyle medicine
Primary	1. Molecular	
	• Genetic	Not available
	• Epigenetic	Indirect effect of, e.g., healthy eating (molecular nutrition), physical activity, and avoidance of disruptors
	2. Environmental	
	• Physical	
	– Geography/climate	
	– Pollution	Education and avoidance
	– Other disruptors	Education and avoidance
	• Nonphysical	
	– Cultural	Transcultural adaptations
	– Social determinants	Community engagement, behavioral counseling, education
	3. Behavioral	
	• Physiological	
	– Stress response	Stress reduction and behavioral counseling
	– Other adaptive	Stress reduction and behavioral counseling
	• Pathological	
	– Psychiatric disease	Healthy eating and physical activity as adjuncts to primary psycho- and pharmacotherapy
	– Other maladaptive	Behavioral counseling
Secondary	1. Metabolic	
	• Adiposity-based	Achieve normal ethnicity-adjusted body composition; healthy eating and physical activity to reduce insulin resistance and inflammation
	• Dysglycemia-based	Above + medical nutrition therapy, healthy eating, physical activity
	• Cardiometabolic-based	Above + address MetS traits (e.g., DASH diet)
	2. Inflammatory	Healthy eating (molecular nutrition) and physical activity
	3. Infectious	Healthy behaviors and eating patterns
	4. Neoplastic	Healthy eating patterns and physical activity
	5. Degenerative (aging)	Healthy lifestyles, eating patterns, and physical activity

[a]This is a partial list of drivers and roles. Lifestyle medicine roles or interventions (including healthy eating patterns, physical activity, sleep hygiene, stress reduction, behavioral counseling, tobacco cessation, alcohol moderation, community engagement, etc.) are mapped to chronic disease drivers; entries are those with a particularly strong effect. Abbreviations: *DASH* Dietary Approaches to Stop Hypertension, *MetS* metabolic syndrome

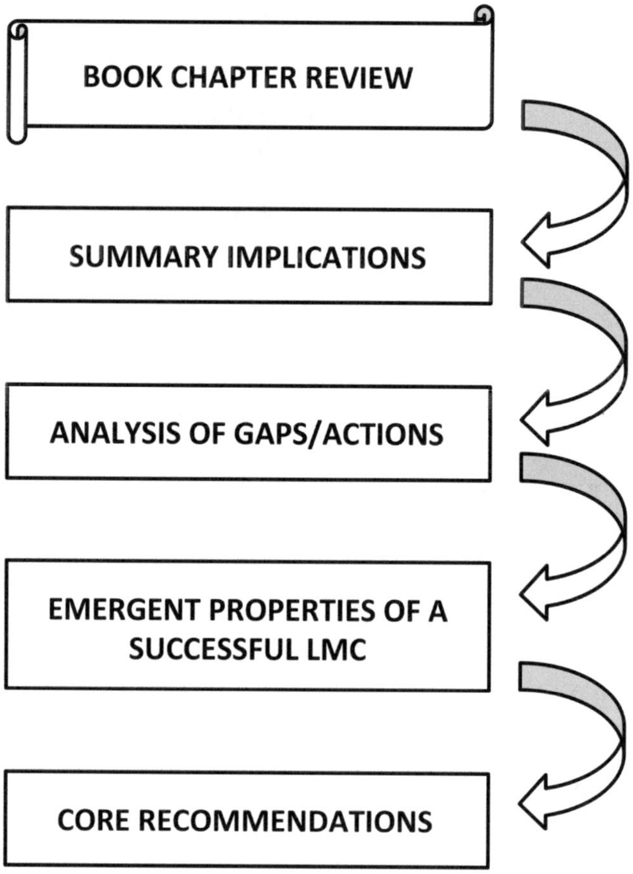

Fig. 31.1 Methodology.* (*Methods used to derive core recommendations in planning, building, and operating a Lifestyle Medicine Center). Abbreviation: *LMC* Lifestyle Medicine Center

Actions to create a Lifestyle Medicine Center are divided into three discrete stages: planning, building, and operating. By organizing ideas gleaned from the individual chapters in step 1 into this 3 × 3 gap-action matrix, analyses can be facilitated. Certain patterns and concepts are revealed, or emerge, in the form of phrases that can be used for specific recommendations.

In the third step, key phrases from the analysis in step 2 are assembled and extended in nine core recommendations for each 3 × 3 gap-action pair. These core recommendations are intended to serve as action steps by those interested in developing a Lifestyle Medicine Center.

Results

Thirty chapters are reviewed with results and implications provided in Table 31.2. In the introductory Chaps. 1, 2 and 3, lifestyle medicine is found to be much more scientifically substantiated in the past few years according to PubMed citations of published clinical trials. Strategically targeting lifestyle factors is decreasing the risk and progression of

Table 31.2 Step 1: Primary results of chapters[a]

Chapter # and description	Primary findings	Implications
1. Purpose of LM	• Increased LM clinical trials • Strategic target = CD • Tactics (research, practice, education) • LMC are force multipliers	• LMC are transformative: translating drivers of chronic disease to LM strategies to LMC actions
2. Burden of CD and Role of LM	• Allostatic stress and SDOH cause CD • Role for LM guidelines • Role for population health	• LMC to provide preventive and precision medical care
3. Translation of LM to LMC	• Multi-morbid CCM useful • Translate LM need and opportunity to idea and then LMC materialization (conceptualization and operationalization) and optimization	• Need formal implementation science for LMC
4. Implementation Science	• Address research-practice gap • Use specific models strategies, tools, training, and stakeholders	• Provides details on how to leverage implementation science for LMC
5. Models for Complex Care	• Bridging inpatient and outpatient LM • Role of community health worker • Defragment healthcare	• Develop comprehensive care program in LM with novel work and reimbursement models
6. Urban Infrastructure	• Effect of local physical environment with health outcomes • Roles of environmental health, SDOH, urban planning, and policy	• LMC need to be integrated with urban environments
7. Preventive Medicine	• Population health scale • Defining the magnitude, determinants, interventional strategies, and outcomes of population-based problems	• Applying preventive medicine informs the behavioral medicine component of LMC
8. Clinical Service Lines	• "Macro" demands for superior value-performance • Emergence of CSL programming • Financial and management models	• Vision to structure LMC as CSLs for success and durability
9. Medical Economics	• Practice and big picture maps guide business plans • Operationalizing business plans	• The unique nature of LM, costs of building and operating a LMC, and relatively low reimbursement rates require novel business plans
10. Immersive Phys. Environment	• Plans based on IPE based on VR· • Optimize cost, volume, impact, and potential failure	• Optimal and immersive LMC physical settings can be guided by IPE and use of VR
11. Immersive Nonphys. Environment	• High-touch behaviors and infras-structure contribute to the immersive environment and better outcomes • Human resources and teamwork	• Selecting and training LMC personnel is critical to an immersive environment; a gym, teaching kitchen, or meditation room can facilitate this immersion
12. Gym	• Details on gym equipment • Need for innovative payment models • Need expertise for gym operations	• Having an onsite, dedicated gym for medical fitness and specialized programs can enhance an immersive experience, facilitation of services, and superior outcomes
13. Wearable Technologies	• Survey of wearable devices that monitor chronic disease metrics • Nutrition, physical activity, and cardiovascular monitoring are most common	• LMC can optimize patient engagement and clinical outcomes with wearables
14. Patient Education Tools	• Use of easy-to-read educational materials can improve outcomes • Details of creating this materials are provided	• The use of LM educational tools is part of LMC planning and operations
15. Behavioral Medicine	• Based on models of change • Intervention strategies, especially motivational interviewing and cognitive-behavioral therapy • Benefits facilitated with wearable technologies • Importance of ethno-cultural sensitivities	• Behavioral medicine is a fundamental part of LM and therefore needs to be included and enhanced in the LMCs, e.g., hiring and training of personnel, writing of policies and protocols, and part of outcome metrics
16. Interprofessional – RDN	• MNT provided by RDNs is critical part of LM • Payment models are discussed • RDNs are part of a LM team	• Formal RDN services are necessary in an LMC
17. Interprofessional – EP	• An EP provides specialized supervision of medical fitness, cardiac rehabilitation, etc. • Payment models are discussed EPs are part of a LM team	• Though costly, the incorporation of a gym with credentialed EPs is desired in an LMC

(continued)

Table 31.2 (continued)

Chapter # and description	Primary findings	Implications
18. Inpatient LM	• Acute episodes occur with chronic disease • Inpatient LM programs are rare • Specific services are described	• Inpatient LM consultative services canenhance CD prevention, LMC engagement, and healthcare defragmentation
19. Transcultural	• Transcultural adaptation is part of precision medicine and can optimize LM • Validated transcultural programs provide supporting clinical evidence	• LMC should be planned, built, and run with ethno-cultural sensitivities and adaptations in mind
20. Spirituality	• Spirituality plays an important role in health, acute illness, and CD • Specific spirituality services are highlighted in community and various healthcare scenarios	• Spiritual dimensions to LM and inclusion of chaplains in LMC teams is important and may be necessary
21. Community Engagement	• Details how LMC can reach underserved populations community health advisors and peer-based health education are discussed	• Community engagement by HCPs in the LMC helps to fulfill the mission
22. Epidemiological Research	• LM applications to population health requires epidemiological evidence • How to build infrastructure to conduct epidemiological research	• LMC should aspire to conduct quality and funded epidemiological research
23. Introduction to Case Studies	• LMC examples provide guidance·about realizing successes, managing challenges, and avoiding setbacks • An environmental scan informs decision-making, the strategic and business plans, operations, scalability, and sustainability	• One should study other LMCs before embarking on plans to build their own LMC
24. Academic Wellness Center	• Patients participate in clinical research • HCPs oriented toward research, writing/publishing, and lecturing	• Revenue generation is a principal challenge to academic LMCs
25. Obesity Center	• Large healthcare system sponsored center • Emphasizes teamwork among HCPs • Educational mission • Fiscal viability as major challenge	• Obesity care well suited for formal LM and delivery by a LMC
26. Neurodegenerative Dis. Ctr.	• Focus on metabolic drivers • Multidisciplinary teamwork and use of a live-in program	• Emerging population for LMC
27. Cardiometabolic Center	• Goals are optimal cardiometabolichealth with (aggregated) revenue neutrality • Onsite, dedicated gym for secondary prevention and cardiac rehabilitation • Based on *Lifestyle Medicine* 2016	• Proof-of-concept LMC
28. Prostate Cancer Center	• Incorporation of mind-body services·with state-of-the-art medical-surgical management in large academic system • Holistic approach	• Research gap identified to determine if mind-body services improves clinical outcomes in cancer therapy
29. Integrative Medicine Center	• Innovative, membership-supported primary care • Whole-person, team-based care model • Importance of business partners	• Persistent problems with healthcare system adopting/accepting integrative medicine, contributes to financial pressures
30. Global LM Centers	• First published survey of international LMCs • Low number of these LMCs • High variability in LMC operations	• Need for transculturalization in international LMC • Opportunity for all international LMC to capture data for their own ethno cultural LM adaptations

[a]Abbreviations: *CD* chronic disease, *CSL* clinical service line, *Ctr* Center, *Dis* Disease, *EP* Exercise Physiologist, *HCP* healthcare professional, *IPE* immersive physical environment, *LM* lifestyle medicine, *LMC* Lifestyle Medicine Center (includes LM clinical service lines), *MNT* medical nutrition therapy, *Phys* physical, *RDN* registered dietician nutritionist, *SDOH* social determinants of health, *VR* virtual reality

chronic disease with greater precision, especially when considering allostatic stress and other social determinants of health, all in the context of a multi-morbid model to improve population health. However, the thrust of these chapters, and this book in general, is how do you actually accomplish this? The tactical solution is through implementation – to translate lifestyle medicine concepts into clinical practice. However,

simply being educated about concepts, or even studying translational approaches, is insufficient. The true answer lies in the follow-up with materialization of a Lifestyle Medicine Center, consisting of conceptualization and operationalization steps, and then optimization of the whole process, which ideally results in scaling up and out with improved population-based metrics. Building multiple Lifestyle

Medicine Centers that produce clear benefits across a population leads to a transformative culture in healthcare, from both economic and clinical outcome standpoints. At this point in the book, after reading the first 3 chapters, the reader's interest is piqued, with subsequent chapters providing details and concrete guideposts to implementing the process of developing Lifestyle Medicine Centers.

In the next 19 chapters, important elements of the implementation process are discussed for the reader that cover the planning, building, and operating processes for a Lifestyle Medicine Center. The concepts in these chapters are critical for the inception of the implementation process and may represent new ideas that challenge the reader. In Chap. 4, the authors explain implementation science, research-practice gaps, and potential methods. Once empowered with knowledge about implementation science and information from subsequent chapters on models for complex patient care, urban infrastructure, and preventive medicine, the reader can better fashion strategic plans and mission and vision statements and more effectively communicate these proposals to others in leadership roles, such as committees, board members, or department chairs. Without question, the most significant potential stumbling block is economic feasibility. The creation of clinical service lines within a larger sponsoring organization (in the case of an academic setting) and other economic models is discussed in detail in Chaps. 8 and 9. Since lifestyle medicine, by its very nature, is poorly reimbursed at best, or non-reimbursable at worse, novel business structures need to be engaged. Fiscal responsibility is necessary not only for the short-term success of a Lifestyle Medicine Center but also for long-term sustainability that is needed to be truly transformative. Depending on the specific goals of the Center, various programs can be developed and built. Physical and nonphysical components of the Center are discussed in detail to provide proper tailoring according to the aspirational blueprint put forth during the planning and funding process. Examples include the extent of patient immersion; high-touch training of personnel; including a *bona fide* gym, teaching kitchen, or meditation room, with exercise physiologists, registered dietitian nutritionists, and behaviorists, respectively; expertise with wearable technologies, patient education tools, and community engagement; transcultural and spiritual sensitivities; clinical research efforts; and collaboration with an inpatient lifestyle medicine program to defragment care. None of these programs are sufficient nor necessary for the success of a Lifestyle Medicine Center, further asserting the need for early, diligent planning and conceptualization for optimal design and functionality.

The last eight chapters instantiate the aforementioned implementation concepts. Case studies of exemplary Lifestyle Medicine Centers address the practice gap issue where almost invariably, pen and paper ideas fail to translate into brick and mortar, real-world conditions. First, unpredictable environmental settings and financial pressures dictate adjustments to architectural and business plans, respectively. Second, the innate complexity of human physiology, not to mention capricious patient behaviors and detrimental mandates by third-party payers and pharmacy benefit managers, contributes to problems of adherence, miscommunications, and unexpected clinical outcomes (positive and negative). For these reasons, a survey across the range of practice settings, models, and disease targets is presented with reverse engineering of these enterprises to appreciate pitfalls, shortcomings, and challenges, as well as potential grounds for success.

Analysis

There are many primary findings and implications captured from a review of each book chapter, but to advance these items to core recommendations, simple and understandable analyses need to be performed. These items are distilled down to a set of common phrases, which are then curated in a 3 × 3 matrix of questions (or gaps) and answers (or implementation stages) (Table 31.3). These phrase entries are organized as nine cells, in three categories (planning, cells 1–3; building, cells 4–6; and operating, cells 7–9) that will subsequently expose some emergent properties and inform core recommendations.

In cell 1, healthcare professionals planning a Lifestyle Medicine Center will need to be aware of the key research publications in chronic disease and lifestyle medicine, familiar with the evidentiary basis for drivers that can identify target patient populations, and able to convey this information as addressing research gaps to usher in a transformative culture of healthcare. Other planners might include clinicians, administrators, finance personnel, and potential investors or donors. In cell 2, planners will need to familiarize themselves with clinical service line programming and the field of implementation science in order to participate in meaningful discussions addressing social issues and knowledge gaps. In cell 3, planners will need to understand the reasons why theoretical constructs for Lifestyle Medicine Centers may not successfully translate into successful operations in the real world. Here, meaningful concepts are comprehensive care models (i.e., which model[s] to use), inpatient lifestyle medicine consultative services, and urban infrastructure. Ultimately, these concepts, which are particular to lifestyle medicine, shape a novel business plan (consisting of a mission statement, vision statement, strategic plan, and marketing strategy).

In cell 4, the implementation plans have been approved, and now the building process begins. The use of virtual reality to create immersive physical environments is advised and should be based on existing evidence, but more research is still needed to validate this process in terms of better clinical outcomes. In cell 5, one of the greatest challenges is construction of a safe and effective gym, teaching kitchen, or meditation room, depending on the target patient population, resources (especially space), and funding levels. Information

Table 31.3 Step 2: Analytic cross-tabulation of gaps and actions[a]

LM gaps to address	LMC planning	LMC building	LMC operating
Research	• Chronic disease states • Drivers • Transformative impact (Cell 1)	• Immersive physical environments • Virtual reality (Cell 4)	• Community engagement • Mind-Body and integrative health services • Transcultural adaptationswearable • Technologies (Cell 7)
Knowledge	• Clinical service line • Implementation science (Cell 2)	• Onsite dedicated gym, teaching kitchen, or meditation room (Cell 5)	• Behavioral medicine • Patient Educational tools (Cell 8)
Practice	• Comprehensive care • Inpatient LM consultative service • Novel business plans • Urban infrastructure (Cell 3)	• Epidemiological research • Infrastructure (Cell 6)	• Exercise Physiology • High-touch training • Population health • Precision Care • Preventive care • Registered dietician nutritionist • Spirituality (Cell 9)

[a]Tabular entries are derived from summarized implications from each chapter. Cell numbers are provided in parentheses under entries. See text for definitions of research, knowledge, and practice gaps. Abbreviations: *LM* lifestyle medicine, *LMC* Lifestyle Medicine Center

about optimizing these specialized activities should be tapped to narrow this knowledge gap. In cell 6, construction will also need to address infrastructural needs, primarily technological (security, electrical, ventilation, etc.), to support a clinical research program, especially one that focuses on high-volume epidemiological studies, and also educational needs (conference room, audiovisual capabilities, etc.).

In cell 7, the Lifestyle Medicine Center construction stage has finished and a go-live date set. Operations will need to include policies, protocols, identification of duties and selection of needed human resources, and a plan for iterative optimization, adaptation, and eventual scalability. Research gaps exist for many programs deemed important for the success of the Center, including community engagement, mind-body and integrative health, transcultural adaptation, and wearable technologies. However, despite these gaps, each of these services/programs should still be considered. In cell 8, social determinants of health and disparities of care should be incorporated in the execution and reimbursement structures for behavioral medicine, one of the most important facets of lifestyle medicine. Patient educational tools should also be produced and take into account knowledge gaps in the target patient population, generally due to socioeconomic class and education levels. In cell 9, the nuances of clinical practice are addressed by on-boarding various lifestyle medicine programs, ranging from preventive and precision care, to population health, and to the commonly overlooked aspect of spirituality.

Table 31.4 Step 3: Synthesis of core recommendations for a successful Lifestyle Medicine Center[a]

Classifier	Recommendation
Planning (cells 1–3)	1. Further research should be conducted to (a) clarify the effect of specific **primary and metabolic drivers** on **chronic disease states** (existing evidence should be used to define the target population; a decision should be made whether new research should be carried out in the new Lifestyle Medicine Center) and (b) determine how specific, structured lifestyle interventions, delivered by Lifestyle Medicine Centers, can have a **transformative impact** on individual and population-based clinical outcomes and healthcare culture
	2. Basic and advanced concepts of **implementation science** and **clinical service line** programming should be disseminated, particularly obtaining institutional leadership and appropriate levels of technology based on the care model; this applies across the full range of social strata to improve healthcare and facilitate construction of Lifestyle Medicine Centers
	3. **Comprehensive care**, involving not only all aspects of lifestyle medicine, but also the coordination of community-based outpatient, as well as **inpatient** care delivery models, should be part of the initial Lifestyle Medicine Center planning phase. This should also include considerations of the neighboring physical **(urban) environment** on Lifestyle Medicine Center operations. Due to the unique nature of lifestyle medicine and the management of patients who may not yet exhibit symptoms or signs of disease, novel business plans will need to be devised (including the mission and vision statements, strategic plans, and marketing strategies)

(continued)

Table 31.4 (continued)

Classifier	Recommendation
Building (cells 4–6)	1. To consider involving consultants with experience designing healthcare centers, preferably in lifestyle medicine, who use **virtual reality** to create **immersive physical environments** 2. To prioritize building a **gym, teaching kitchen, or meditation room** in the facility, suitable for primary (e.g., medical fitness, healthy eating, and stress reduction) and secondary (e.g., cardiac and/or pulmonary rehabilitation) prevention programs, and including aerobic and strength training equipment, cooking stations, and comfortable furniture. Innovative reimbursement structures and delivery models need to be developed so that this type of supervised physical activity is available to patients of limited financial means and/or in underserved areas 3. To explore resources and capabilities to develop **infrastructure** to conduct clinical trials, **epidemiological research**, and educational activities (e.g., conference room and audio-visual technology)
Operating (cells 7–9)	1. To consider the design and execution of research projects in **community engagement, mind-body and integrative health, transcultural adaptation,** and **wearable technologies** 2. To develop **behavioral medicine** resources and **patient education tools** that can be offered to all patients, regardless of insurance plans and financial status 3. In order for a Lifestyle Medicine Center to succeed, a broad range of services and personnel, with innovative **business** models, should be available: **exercise physiologists, registered dietitian nutritionists, high-touch interactions** and training, **precision** and **preventive** care to positively impact **population health**, and **spirituality**

ᵃPhrases from Table 31.3 are in **bold** and serve to anchor recommendations for each classifier

Synthesis

By analyzing the information in the chapters in a tractable way, significant points (represented as phrases) emerge and can then be pulled together to direct a set of core, actionable, recommendations that implement lifestyle medicine as a Lifestyle Medicine Center (Table 31.4). These recommendations are sorted into three categories (planning, building, and operating) with three parts for each category mapping to cells in Table 31.3. These recommendations are intended to be used as guideposts in creating a Lifestyle Medicine Center. Specifically, these recommendations assist with due diligence as initial committees meet to discuss opportunities, feasibility, logistics, and funding. Readers can refer to individual chapters for detailed explanations and rationales for each of the recommendations. Over time, it is expected that these recommendations will not only grow in number but be reshaped based on changing healthcare trends. The role of lifestyle medicine will undoubtedly need to evolve, reconciling technological advances in medicine with one's own responsibility to lead a healthy life.

References

1. Mechanick JI, Leroith D. Synthesis: deriving a core set of recommendations to optimize diabetes care on a global scale. Ann Global Health. 2015;81:874–83.
2. Philibert I. Review article: closing the research gap at the interface of learning and clinical practice. Can J Anesth. 2012;59:203–12.
3. Zielinski C. Causes of the knowledge gap. Lancet Global Health. 2019;7:e842.
4. Zieber M, Wojtowicz B. To dwell within: bridging the theory-practice gap. Nurs Philosophy. 2019;00:e12296. https://doi.org/10.1111/nup.12296.

Correction to: Creating a Lifestyle Medicine Center

Jeffrey I. Mechanick and Robert F. Kushner

Correction to:

J. I. Mechanick, R. F. Kushner (eds.), *Creating a Lifestyle Medicine Center*, https://doi.org/10.1007/978-3-030-48088-2

The book was inadvertently published with incorrect affiliation of **Ramfis Nieto-Martínez** in Chapter 19 & 30. The first affiliation "International Clinical Research Center, St Anne's University Hospital, Brno, Czech Republic" was amended to "LifeDoc Health, Memphis, TN, USA".

The updated version of the chapters can be found at https://doi.org/10.1007/978-3-030-48088-2_19
https://doi.org/10.1007/978-3-030-48088-2_30

© Springer Nature Switzerland AG 2020
J. I. Mechanick, R. F. Kushner (eds.), *Creating a Lifestyle Medicine Center*, https://doi.org/10.1007/978-3-030-48088-2_32

Appendices

The two appendices that follow present a snapshot of action steps and resources to set up a Lifestyle Medicine Center. These quick references direct the reader to ten action steps to jumpstart the early, formative processes that translate a new idea into action. Key websites and publications are culled from the chapters in this book and organized according to action steps to bring readers and their colleagues up to speed as quickly and diligently as possible. Examples of actual Lifestyle Medicine Centers are provided throughout the chapters, with global examples in Chap. 30. These examples illustrate features, variations, and all the different recipes for success to help the reader imagine and then build a Lifestyle Medicine Center. The reader can find in-depth explanations and further details of these two quick references in the relevant book chapters.

Appendix 1. Quick Reference: Ten Action Steps for Building a Lifestyle Medicine Center[a]

Action step #	Name	Description
1	Activation	A champion reaches a threshold of clinical experience and evidentiary knowledge and recognizes the need for a LMC
2	Scan	Environmental factors affecting healthcare practice and outcomes are explored, analyzed, and interpreted for a LMC

Action step #	Name	Description
3	Pitch	Force multipliers and leaders are identified to introduce/manage the concept; the "ask" is to develop a formal plan to build a LMC
4	Plan	Strategic plans (e.g., chronic disease risk and progression mitigation) and business plans (revenue neutral; profit) are formulated
5	Design	Tactical plans (e.g., funds, resources, logistics, and timeline) are devised to implement strategic/business plans in the form of a physical LMC
6	Build	Engage architects, contractors, consultants, legal, etc. and supervise physical space construction, equipment purchasing, and decorations
7	Recruit	Develop clinical endpoints, policies, and protocols and then focus on identifying and hiring appropriate human resources (HCPs and staff)
8	Operate	Go live! See patients, implement high-tech/high-touch, monitor workflow, manage problems, and capture/report performance metrics
9	Adapt	Review reports, registry, and clinical trial data, prioritize problems, conduct regularly scheduled meetings, and optimize operations
10	Scale	Repeat the above action steps and decide on scaling up and scaling out on evolving mission and vision statements

[a]Force multipliers are tools, or in this case people, that can amplify output with the same effort (e.g., leaders (healthcare professionals and staff), potential donors, and others with track records of success). Abbreviations: *HCP* healthcare professionals, *LMC* Lifestyle Medicine Center

J. I. Mechanick, R. F. Kushner (eds.), *Creating a Lifestyle Medicine Center*, https://doi.org/10.1007/978-3-030-48088-2

Appendix 2. Quick Reference: Resources for Lifestyle Medicine Center Planning, Building, and Operating Stages[a]

Stage	Description	Website	Appendix 1 action step	Book Chapter #
Planning	NextGenU.org online lifestyle medicine training	https://nextgenu.org/course/view.php?id=205	1,2	1
	Healthy People 2020	https://www.lifestylemedicine.org/	1,2	2
	Dietary Guidelines for Americans 2015	https://www.healthypeople.gov/	1,2	2
	Physical Activity Guidelines for Americans 2018	https://health.gov/paguidelines/	1,2	2
	Standards of Medicine Care in Diabetes	Diabetes Care 2019; 42 (Supplement 1)	1,2	2
	Cancer Prevention Guidelines	CA Cancer J Clin 2012; 62: 30-67	1,2	2
	Primary Prevention Cardiovascular Disease	JAMA Cardiol 2019; 4: 1043-1044	1,2	2
	Hypertension Guidelines	Circulation 2018; 138: e484-e594.	1,2	2
	Obesity Guidelines	Endocrine Pract 2016; 22 (Suppl 3) : 1-203	1,2	2
	High Cholesterol Guidelines	Circulation 2019; 139: e1082-e1143	1,2	2
	Metabolic Syndrome Lifestyle Recommendations	Nutr Rev 2017; 75: 307-326	1,2	2
	World Cancer Research Fund	https://www.wcrf.org/dietandcancer/about	1,2	2
	2018 Sleep in America Poll	https://www.sleepfoundation.org/press-release/national-sleep-foundations-2018-sleep-americar-poll-shows-americans-failing	1,2	2
	Gallup 2019 Global Emotions Report	https://www.gallup.com/analytics/248909/gallup-2019-global-emotions-report-pdf.aspx	1,2	2
	Primary Care Practice Guidelines 2019	https://www.uspreventiveservicestaskforce.org/Page/Name/recommendations	1,2	4
	NIH Training Institute in Implementation	https://www.scgcorp.com/tidirh2019/index.html	1-3,5,7	4
	Community Preventive Services	https://www.thecommunityguide.org/task-force-Findings	1,2	4
	National Health Expenditure Data	https://www.cms.gov/Research-Statistics-Data-and-Systems/Statistics-Trends-and-Reports/NationalHealthExpendData/NationalHealthAccountsHistorical.html	1,2	5
	Institute for Health Metrics and Evaluation	http://www.healthdata.org/results	1,2	5
	Social Isolation and Loneliness	https://www.nia.nih.gov/news/social-isolation-loneliness-older-people-pose-health-risks	1,2	5
	Food Deserts	https://www.marigallagher.com/2006/07/18/examining-the-impact-of-food-deserts-on-public-health-in-chicago-july-18-2006/	1,2	5
	Foresight Obesity System Map	http://www.visualcomplexity.com/vc/project.cfm?id=622	1,2	7
	About Preventive Medicine	https://www.acpm.org/about-acpm/what-is-preventive-medicine/	1,2	7
	Behavioral Health Trends	http://www.samhsa.gov/data/	1,2	7
	Obesity-Related Data and Trends	https://www.tfah.org/report-details/stateofobesity2019/	1,2	7
	Obesity System Atlas	https://assets.publishing.service.gov.uk/government/uploads/system/uploads/attachment_data/file/296290/obesity-map-full-hi-res.pdf	1,2	7
	Behavioral Risk Factor Surveillance System	https://www.cdc.gov/brfss/index.html	1,2	7
	Behavioral Research Program	https://cancercontrol.cancer.gov/brp/	1,2	15
	Motivational Interviewing Network of Trainers	https://motivationalinterviewing.org/	1,2	15

Stage	Description	Website	Appendix 1 action step	Book Chapter #
	Shared Decision-Making	https://www.healthit.gov/sites/default/files/nlc_shared_decision_making_fact_sheet.pdf	1,2	15
	Life's Simple 7	https://www.heart.org/en/professional/workplace-health/lifes-simple-7	1,2	18
	Top 10 Causes of Death	https://www.who.int/news-room/fact-sheets/detail/the-top-10-causes	1,2	18
	Cancer Incidence and Mortality	https://www.ncbi.nlm.nih.gov/pubmed/25220842	1,2	28
	California Department of Public Health	https://www.cdph.ca.gov/Programs/CCDPHP/DEODC/EHIB/EES/pages/wildfire.aspx	2	6
	California Health in All Policies	http://sgc.ca.gov/programs/hiap/	2	6
	CDC Built Environment Assessment Tool	https://www.cdc.gov/nccdphp/dnpao/state-local-programs/built-environment-assessment/index	2	6
	Environmental Atlas	https://enviroatlas.epa.gov/enviroatlas/interactivemap/	2	6
	National Environment Public Health Tracking Network	https://ephtracking.cdc.gov/DataExplorer/#/	2	6
	Healthy Minnesota Partnership	https://www.health.state.mn.us/communities/practice/healthymnpartnership/index.html	2	6
	Walk Score	https://www.walkscore.com/	2	6
	Policy Map	https://www.policymap.com/maps	2	6
	National Household Travel Survey	https://nhts.ornl.gov/	2	6
	Food Environment Atlas	https://www.ers.usda.gov/foodatlas/	2	6
	Neighborhood Atlas	https://www.neighborhoodatlas.medicine.wisc.edu/	2	6
	Limited Supermarket Access Analysis	https://www.reinvestment.com/wp-content/uploads/2018/08/LSA_2018_Report_web.pdf	2	6
	Healthy Food Access	https://www.healthyfoodaccess.org/access-101-research-your-community	2	6
	ParkServe	https://www.tpl.org/parkserve	2	6
	Social Determinants of Health Atlas	https://sdohatlas.github.io/	2	6
	Housing and Transportation Index	https://htaindex.cnt.org/	2	6
	Atlas of Inequality	https://inequality.media.mit.edu/	2	6
	Pew Health Impact Assessments	https://www.pewtrusts.org/en/research-and-analysis/data-visualizations/2015/hia-map?sortBy=relevance&sortOrder=asc&page=1	2	6
	500 Cities Project	https://www.cdc.gov/500Cities/	2,4	6
	Community Commons	http://www.communitycommons.org/collections/Maps-and-Data	2,4	6
	Medical Professionals as Force Multipliers	Cureus 2019; 11: e6469	3	1
	Care Models	https://innovation.cms.gov/	4	5
	Social Determinants of Health	https://healthleadsusa.org/resource-library/	4	5
	Fully Capitated Payment Model	https://www.iorahealth.com	4	9
	Lifestyle Medicine Economics	Am J Lifestyle Med 2017; 11: 404-407	4	9
	Dietitian Insurance and Reimbursement	https://www.todaysdietitian.com/newarchives/0217p40.shtml	4	16
	Medicare Diagnosis Codes for Nutritionist	https://www.eatrightpro.org/payment/coding-and-billing/diagnosis-and-procedure-codes/diagnosis-codes-for-medicare-mnt	4	16
Building				
	Agency for Healthcare Research and Quality	https://www.ahrq.gov/research/findings/factsheets/translating/index.html	3,5	4
	Quality Enhancement Research Institute	https://www.queri.research.va.gov/	3,5	4
	NIH Grants and Funding	https://grants.nih.gov/grants/guide/pa-files/PAR-19-274.html	3,5	4
	Implementation Science at a Glance	https://cancercontrol.cancer.gov/IS/docs/NCI-ISaaG-Workbook.pdf	3,5	4
	Stanford School of Design: Design for Health	https://dschool.stanford.edu/classes/design-for-health-fall	5	6

Stage	Description	Website	Appendix 1 action step	Book Chapter #
	Jefferson University Design Track	https://www.jefferson.edu/university/skmc/programs/scholarly-inquiry/tracks/design.html	5	6
	University of Virginia Medical Design Program	http://uvamedical.design/	5	6
	University of Texas Austin Design Institute for Health	https://dellmed.utexas.edu/units/design-institute-for-health	5	6
	Integrated Health System and Leaning Organizations	https://www.governanceinstitute.com/	5	8
	Shared Beliefs and Managing Strategic Risk	https://www.governanceinstitute.com/	5	8
	Social Psychology of Clinical Service Lines	https://www.castlingpartners.com/leadership-coaching-corner/2017/4/3/the-social-psychology-of-clinical-service-line-management	5	8
	Culture Alignment – Board's Game Plan	https://www.keystoneculturegroup.com/2018/03/01/culture-alignment-high-performing-healthcare-organizations-and-the-role-of-the-governing-board-part-one/	5	8
	Culture Alignment – High Performance	https://www.keystoneculturegroup.com/2018/05/01/culture-alignment-high-performing-healthcare-organizations-and-the-role-of-the-governing-board-part-two/	5	8
	Patient-Centered Outcomes Research Institute	https://www.pcori.org/	5,7	4
	Management Culture	http://www.biomedcentral.com/1472-6963/11/195	5,7	3
		http://www.implementationscience.com/content/7/1/104	5,7	3
	Whole Building Design Guide	https://www.wbdg.org/building-types/health-care-facilities/hospital	6	10
	Virtual Reality Design	https://www.beckershospitalreview.com/healthcare-information-technology/four-ways-virtual-reality-can-help-us-design-and-create-better-healthcare-facilities.html	6	10
	Immersive Virtual Environment and Behavior Change	http://www.bmedreport.com/archives/25986	6	10
	Choosing Paint Colors for Healthcare	https://www.healthcaredesignmagazine.com/architecture/healing-hues-choosing-paint-colors-healthcare/	6	10
	Fire Protection Requirements for Healthcare Facilities	https://www.sfpe.org/page/FPE_2015_Q1_4/Fire-Protection-Requirements-for-Health-Care-Facilities%2D%2D-An-Overview-.htm	6	10
	Essential Elements of Office Design	https://www.dentaleconomics.com/articles/print/volume-92/issue-5/features/one-dozen-essential-elements-of-a-great-office-design-part-2.html	6	10
	Acoustics in Healthcare Environments	http://www.cisca.org/files/public/Acoustics%20in%20Healthcare%20Environments_CISCA.pdf	6	10
	Health and Safety Executive	http://www.hse.gov.uk/temperature/thermal/factors.htm	6	10
	Gym equipment – Amazon	www.amazon.com	6	12
	Gym equipment – Schwinn Fitness	http://www.schwinnfitness.com	6	12
	Gym equipment – Rogue Fitness	www.roguefitness.com	6	12
	Gym equipment – Nautilus	http://www.nautilus.com	6	12
	Patient Navigator Training Collaborative	http://www.patientnavigatortraining.org/healthcare_system/module3/1_index.htm	7	10
Operating				
	Concierge High-Touch Care	www.chenmed.com	7	11
	Patient Communication	https://kresserinstitute.com/patient-communication-provide-high-touch-care-without-burning/	7	11
	Patient-Centered Team-Based Primary Care	www.pcmh.ahrq.gov/page/creating-patient-centered-team-based-primary-care	7	11

Stage	Description	Website	Appendix 1 action step	Book Chapter #
	Lay Healthcare Workers and High-Touch	www.healthaffairs.org/do/10.1377/hblog20150611.048452/full/	7	11
	Warm Hand-Off	www.ahrq.gov/sites/default/files/wysiwyg/professionals/quality-patient-safety/patient- family-engagement/pfeprimarycare/warmhandoff-quickstartfull.pdf	7	11
	Team-Based Care for Hypertension	www.cdc.gov/dhdsp/pubs/guides/best-practices/team-based-care.htm	7	11
	High-Touch Care for Diabetes	www.brookings.edu/wp-content/uploads/2016/06/Rio-Valley-ACO.pdf	7	11
	Commission on Dietetic Registration	https://www.cdrnet.org/news/rdncredentialfaq	7	16
	Nutrition Source	https://www.hsph.harvard.edu/nutritionsource/healthy-weight/diet-reviews/dash-diet/	7	16
	Qualifications of a Registered Dietitian Nutritionist	www.eatright.org https://www.eatright.org/food/resources/learn-more-about-rdns/qualifications-of-a-registered-dietitian-nutritionist	7	16
	National Board for Health and Wellness Coaching	www.nbhwc.org	7	16
	Group Versus Individual Nutritional Counseling	https://www.andeal.org/topic.cfm?menu=3151&cat=3549	7	16
	Telehealth	https://www.eatrightpro.org/practice/practice-resources/telehealth/practicing-telehealth	7	16
	Lifestyle Data Analytics Platform	www.healthsnap.io	8	13
	Wearables and Weight Loss	JAMA 2016; 316: 1161-1171	8	13
	mHealth in Diabetes, Physical Inactivity, and Smoking	Curr Atheroscl Rep 2017; 19: 16	8	13
	Newest Vital Sign – To Assess Patient Numeracy	www.pfizer.com/health/literacy/public-policy-researchers/nvs-toolkit	8	14
	Screening Tools for Health Literacy	https://www.ncbi.nlm.nih.gov/pmc/articles/PMC5882442/	8	14
	Functional Health Literacy	https://link.springer.com/article/10.1007/BF02640361	8	14
	Senior Friendly Website Content	http://www.lgma.ca/assets/Programs~and~Events/Clerks~Forum/2013~Clerks~Forum/COMMUNICATIONS-Making-Your-Website-Senior-Friendly%2D%2DTip-Sheet.pdf	8	14
	Courses for Writing for Health Literacy	https://www.cdc.gov/healthliteracy/gettraining.html	8	14
	CMS Toolkit for Clear Written Materials	https://www.cms.gov/Outreach-and-Education/Outreach/writtenmaterialstoolkit/	8	14
	Converts Images to Line Drawings	www.rapidresizer.com	8	14
	CDC Public Health Image Library	https://phil.cdc.gov/	8	14
	Conversational Health Literacy Assessment Tool	https://www.ncbi.nlm.nih.gov/pmc/articles/PMC5863801/	8	14
	Dietitian – Physician Partnerships	https://www.eatrightpro.org/payment/nutrition-services/private-payers/items-to-consider-when-establishing-an-rdnmd-partnership	8	16
	Vegetarian Nutrition	https://www.andeal.org/topic.cfm?menu=5271	8	16
	Exercise Prescription	https://www.ajpmonline.org/article/S0749-3797(09)00549-2/abstract	8	17
	Art Therapy in Inpatients with Schizophrenia	http://www.biomedcentral.com/1471-244X/10/65	8	18
	Louis Armstrong Department of Music Therapy	https://www.mountsinai.org/locations/music-Therapy	8	18
	Transculturalization	Endocr Pract 2019; 25: 729-765	8	19
	Religious Landscape Study	https://www.pewforum.org/religious-landscape-study/	8	20
	Church-Health System Partnership	https://innovations.ahrq.gov/profiles/church-health-system-partnership-facilitates-transitions-hospital-home-urban-low-income	8	20
	Community Engagement	BMC Public Health 2017; 17: 944	8	21

Stage	Description	Website	Appendix 1 action step	Book Chapter #
	Patient Portal	EGEMS 2016; 4: 1262	8	27
	Zyflamend Prostate Cancer Supplements	www.newchapter.com/products/zyflamend-whole-body/	8	28
	Pomi-T™	www.pomi-t.com	8	28
	Chronic Disease Registries to Optimize Performance	Curr Vasc Pharmacol 2016; 14: 426-431	9	3,22
	Intervention Scalability Assessment Tool	Health Res Policy Syst 2020; 18: 1	10	3
	Scale-Up and Scale-Out Program for Obesity	Int J Environ Res Public Health 2020; 17: e584	10	3

[a]All websites accessed on February 29, 2020. Abbreviations: *CDC* Centers for Disease Control and Prevention, *CMS* Centers for Medicare & Medicaid Services, *NIH* National Institutes of Health

Index

A

Academy of Nutrition and Dietetics (AND), 296
Accreditation Council for Education in Nutrition and Dietetics (ACEND), 187
Acoustics, immersive physical environments, 105
Active surveillance programs, 328
Adiposity-based chronic disease (ABCD), 119, 241, 310
Advance Practice Provider (APP), 7, 112
Aerobic, 119, 120, 122
After-visit summary (AVS), 294
A-ICU model, 112, 115
Air quality, immersive physical environment, 105
Allergens, 105
Allostasis, 13
Allostatic load, 13
Allostatic state, 13
Alzheimer's disease (AD), 299
American Association of Cardiovascular and Pulmonary Rehabilitation (AACVPR), 202
American Board of Integrative Medicine, 343
American Board of Obesity Medicine (ABOM), 290
American College of Cardiology (ACC), 201
American College of Lifestyle Medicine (ACLM), 345
American Disability Act Guidelines, 157
American Heart Association (AHA), 201–202, 309
Anaerobic, 122
Andrew Weil Center for Integrative Medicine (AWCIM), 335, 336
Anthropogenes, 10
Area deprivation index, 52
Artful Living Program, 40
Atherosclerotic cardiovascular disease (ASCVD), 202
Audiovisuals, 149
Aural literacy, 146

B

Back office, 83
Bariatric Surgery program, 292
Behavioral economics theory, 165, 166
Behavioral medicine
    change talk, 170
    chronic care model, 163
    cultural sensitivity, 174
    definition, 161
    five A's framework, 168, 169
    goal setting, 167
    health belief model, 165
    identifying behavioral change experts, 174
    integrated care approach, 161, 162

    interventions, 166
    mobile health, 172, 173
    motivational interviewing approach, 169–171
    My Own Health Report, 172
    online technology, 174
    prospect theory, 165
    self-monitoring, 167
    sensors, 173
    shared decision making, 167, 168
    short message service text reminders, 173, 174
    social cognitive theory, 164
    social ecology model, 162
    social learning theory, 164
    stages of change, 164, 165
    stimulus-response theory, 163, 164
    techniques, evidence-based behavior change, 167
    two substitute A's, 169
Behavioral models, 50
Behavioral Risk Surveillance System, 284
Better Exercise Adherence after Treatment for Cancer (BEAT-Cancer), 30
Big Picture Map, 83
Board for Certification of Nutrition Specialists (CBNS), 188
Bona fide gym, 359
Brain aging and neurodegenerative disorders
    Alzheimer's disease, Parkinson's disease and stroke, 299
    challenges, 306
    clinical diagnosis and patient care, 299, 300
    eating and exercise patterns, 304–305
    eating behavior modification, 299
    education and outreach, 306
    electronic communication, 306
    exercise programs, 299
    expanded roles and responsibilities, 303
    intellectual challenges, 305–306
    lifestyle modification, 305
    Lifestyle Medicine Center for Brain Aging and Neurodegenerative Diseases, 302
    organization of lifestyle medicine center
        human resources, 302–303
        Lifestyle Medicine Center for Brain Aging and Neurodegenerative Diseases, 301
        participant evaluation equipment, 302
        physical setting and environment, 301–302
    patient care and flow, 303
    prevention and treatment, 301
    risk factor for, 300, 301
    risk-reduction and treatment plans, 299
    take home messages, 307